Food, Cuisine, and Cultural Competency for Culinary, Hospitality, and Nutrition Professionals

Edited by:

Sari Edelstein, PhD, RD

Associate Professor of Nutrition

Simmons College
Boston, Massachusetts

JONES AND BARTLETT PUBLISHERS

Sudbury, Massachusetts

BOSTON   TORONTO   LONDON   SINGAPORE

World Headquarters
Jones and Bartlett Publishers
40 Tall Pine Drive
Sudbury, MA 01776
978-443-5000
info@jbpub.com
www.jbpub.com

Jones and Bartlett Publishers
Canada
6339 Ormindale Way
Mississauga, Ontario L5V 1J2
Canada

Jones and Bartlett Publishers
International
Barb House, Barb Mews
London W6 7PA
United Kingdom

Jones and Bartlett's books and products are available through most bookstores and online booksellers. To contact Jones and Bartlett Publishers directly, call 800-832-0034, fax 978-443-8000, or visit our website, www.jbpub.com.

Substantial discounts on bulk quantities of Jones and Bartlett's publications are available to corporations, professional associations, and other qualified organizations. For details and specific discount information, contact the special sales department at Jones and Bartlett via the above contact information or send an email to specialsales@jbpub.com.

This publication is designed to provide accurate and authoritative information in regard to the Subject Matter covered. It is sold with the understanding that the publisher is not engaged in rendering legal, accounting, or other professional service. If legal advice or other expert assistance is required, the service of a competent professional person should be sought.

Production Credits
Publisher: Cathleen Sether
Acquisitions Editor: Shoshanna Goldberg
Senior Associate Editor: Amy Bloom
Production Manager: Tracey Chapman
Associate Production Editor: Kate Stein
Marketing Manager: Jody Sullivan
Manufacturing and Inventory Control Supervisor: Amy Bacus
Composition and Art: Publishers' Design and Production Services, Inc.
Associate Photo Researcher: Jessica Elias
Cover Design: Kristin E. Parker
Cover Image: © Jupiterimages/age fotostock
Printing and Binding: Malloy, Inc.
Cover Printing: Malloy, Inc.

Library of Congress Cataloging-in-Publication Data
Food, cuisine, and cultural competency : for culinary, hospitality, and nutrition professionals / Sari Edelstein.
    p. cm.
    Includes bibliographical references and index.
    ISBN-13: 978-0-7637-5965-0 (pbk.)
    ISBN-10: 0-7637-5965-1 (pbk.)
    1. Diet.   2. Food habits.   3. Cookery.   I. Edelstein, Sari.

TX357.F637 2010
641.5—dc22

2009044578

6048

Printed in the United States of America
14 13 12 11 10   10 9 8 7 6 5 4 3 2 1

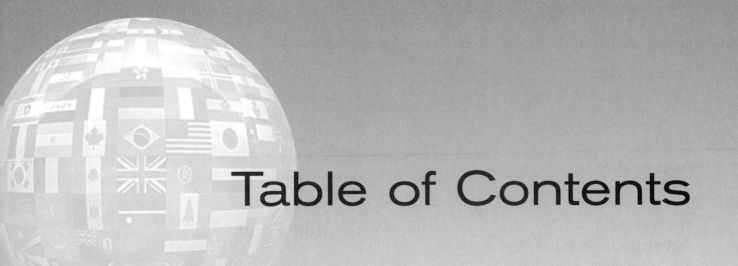

Table of Contents

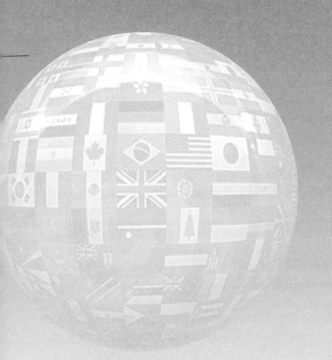

Preface

Sari Edelstein, PhD, RD

Food, Cuisine, and Cultural Competency for Culinary, Hospitality, and Nutrition Professionals provides the food and nutrition expert with insights into many cultures of the world through the history and traditions of the people themselves as well as the foods they grow, gather, and prepare. From these insights, readers will become more culturally aware about the diverse world in which we live today. To become culturally competent in the face of this diversity, one must understand the food traditions that unite people and the significance that food plays as an integral part of culture. Each chapter thus provides a description of the culture's history and explains how food is utilized for religious customs, nutritional health, traditional celebrations, medicinal treatments, and international commerce. To provide this level of detail, each culture is analyzed in terms of its protein, starch, fat, vegetable, fruit, spice, and beverage choices. In addition, typical and holiday meals, with recipes, are provided, as well as food-name translations.

FOODS IN EACH CULTURE

Particular foods often exist in a culture because of the climate, terrain, and robustness of the crop. Cultures have flourished or floundered based on the availability of crops and livestock, which provide vital proteins and nutrients for sustainability. The following chapter excerpts characterize the cultures to which they relate:

"Traditional African cooking methods include steaming food in banana or corn-husk leaves, boiling, frying in oil, or grilling over an open fire." —Ethiopia (Chapter 31)

"The cattle and horses left behind from the first failed Spanish settlement began multiplying and formed the basis for the cattle and horse industry of today." —Argentina (Chapter 42)

"Dates (*tamar*) are a delicacy cherished and demanded all year long. In fact, the palm tree is also highly prized and considered *barakah* (a blessing) in any proximity. It is the only tree indigenous to the region, the one that survived the desert heat." —Arabian Peninsula (Chapter 47)

"'Bush foods,' such as berries, roots, and nectars, were a vital part of the aboriginal diet in many areas." —Australia (Chapter 44)

"It is a common misconception that all Chinese people eat rice as a staple food." —Far East (Chapter 22)

"The perfect meal follows the ancient Chinese model containing five colors (purple, white, red, yellow, and green) using a variety of preparation methods (raw, grilling, steaming, boiling, braising, and deep-fat frying) and is composed of six tastes (sweet, bitter, salty, sour, peppery, and umami)." —Japan (Chapter 25)

"Another significant vegetable is the sweet potato, which is increasing in importance in Kenya and other areas of sub-Saharan Africa due to its ability to be cultivated for both food security and income production." —Kenya (Chapter 32)

"Historically, the national diet was divided regionally: people who grew rice consumed rice almost exclusively and those who produced wheat consumed wheat almost exclusively." —Persia (Chapter 52)

"The poor ate porridge made from coarse millet, barley, and oats. By the 15th century, buckwheat groats were cultivated. Today, they are called kasha and are closely identified with Russian foods." —Russia (Chapter 27)

FOODS WITH CULTURAL SIGNIFICANCE

Food means more than just sustenance; it defines many of the traditions and customs found in each culture. The following chapter excerpts are examples of how food is culturally significant:

"Wat is Ethiopia's national dish. It is placed on top of injera bread and served in a large basket. Typically, the food is eaten with the fingers by tearing off pieces of injera and dipping it into the wat." —Ethiopia (Chapter 31)

"In the early afternoon in Argentina, long lines form at empanada shops. Empanadas came to Argentina with the first Spanish immigrants and now are a cultural phenomenon." —Argentina (Chapter 42)

"Muslims do not eat any form of pork, or any meat that has been slaughtered without invoking God's name (known as *halal* meat or *thabiha*), although some consider any nonpork meats to be *halal* and substitute *thabiha* for kosher." —Arabian Peninsula (Chapter 47)

"Vegemite is probably the most notable cultural food in Australia today." —Australia (Chapter 44)

"Traditionally, children were expected not to eat certain foods, for example, girls were not supposed to eat meat from birds but boys were expected to eat such meat." —Botswana (Chapter 30)

"Pregnant women are discouraged from eating too much and taking prenatal vitamins, or from taking showers at night, because this is believed to make the baby too large and the labor difficult." —Cambodia (Chapter 21)

"There are numerous Greek desserts that are popular in Greece and internationally. A hallmark of Greek desserts is that they are very sweet. There are sweets that use phyllo dough and are topped with syrup. Two such popular Greek desserts include baklava, which is layers of phyllo dough filled with walnuts, almonds, or a combination of both, and galaktobouriko (custard pie). In addition, kadaifi is a wheat-based (i.e., like shredded wheat) dessert filled with nuts and topped with syrup." —Greece (Chapter 14)

"Eating eel on Christmas Eve symbolizes renewal and new beginning in the coming year, because eels shed their skin and replace it with new skin." —Italy (Chapter 17)

"Most of the traditional vegetables used by the Luo are considered to be medicinal and are used in a variety of ways: treating simple wounds; dealing with *chira* (a curse or an illness caused by breaking social rules and customs related to cultivation, marriage, and sexuality), spirit possession, and the evil eye; and creating love potions and protective charms." —Kenya (Chapter 32)

"The belief that beef has hot qualities for the body is commonly held by most Pakistanis in the Punjab region in particular, which is the reason for its low consumption." —Pakistan (Chapter 22)

"Many Iranians believe in 'hot' and 'cold' properties of food, and making a dish that combines foods with opposing properties is the cornerstone of a balanced diet." —Persia (Chapter 52)

"Kasha is believed to have healing properties and it is given to children and the sick. Honey is considered to have healing powers as well, and it is often mixed with milk, mineral water, or lemon juice to treat colds and coughs." —Russia (Chapter 27)

"The smörgåsbord, literally translated 'sandwich table,' is often an important part of the festivities that mark special events and holidays, from weddings to Christmas." —Sweden (Chapter 19)

COMMUNICATION AND COUNSELING TIPS FOR CULTURAL COMPETENCY

Cultural competency, or the lack therefore, plays an important role in the communication and counseling carried out by food and nutrition professionals. When cultural customs are unwittingly ignored or violated, the result can be rejection of necessary information. The following chapter excerpts are examples of contexts for which cultural competency is desirable:

"When it came to social activities, men and women never socialized together." —Arabian Peninsula (Chapter 47)

"'Mateship' is an Australian cultural idiom that embodies the working-class ethos: equality, loyalty, and friendship." —Australia (Chapter 44)

"Batswana also have totems in the form of animals that signify the tribe to which they belong, and it may not be culturally proper to offer a person a food item that is part of their totem." —Botswana (Chapter 30)

"The Dutch are characteristically direct and straightforward. Although this directness may be misinterpreted as rudeness, when read through the lens of pragmatism the Dutch simply want to get to the heart of the matter immediately." —The Netherlands (Chapter 12)

"The French prefer subtlety and discretion to bluntness and detail. The French are known to talk around an issue. In a counseling setting it is important to listen for nuances and hidden messages in their communications." —France (Chapter 13)

"Keeping warm is considered an important measure to prevent illnesses such as colds or flu." —Greece (Chapter 14)

"Haitians will appear to agree with a person of higher socioeconomic status even if they are not truly in agreement." —Haiti (Chapter 38)

"For both men and women, the standard form of greeting is a handshake; however, a man should pause for a woman to extend her hand first." —Hungary (Chapter 15)

"It is considered taboo to point directly at somebody because it might cause disease." —Kenya (Chapter 32)

"Nepalese are very family/friend oriented. They do not like to do anything alone, so communicating any health information will most likely be better received with family or friend(s) present." —Nepal (Chapter 24)

GENERAL HEALTH AND NUTRITIONAL INDICATORS

This book contains vital information regarding the various health and nutritional indicators that are used to assess the overall health status of a culture. For instance, while some cultures experience an increase in the incidence of obesity, others suffer from malnutrition, undernutrition, anemia, and vitamin A deficiency. The following chapter excerpts provide a sample of the health and nutritional challenges that we face in the world today:

"Arabians prefer fermented forms of dairy products and have a high incidence of lactose intolerance." —Arabian Peninsula (Chapter 47)

"In Australia, low iron stores have been reported in up to one third of children aged 1–3 years." —Australia (Chapter 44)

"While undernourishment is not a significant threat, increasing rates of overweight and obesity have become a major public health concern. Data from the World Health Organization indicate that the per capita daily food consumption in Great Britain totals over 3400 calories." —Great Britain (Chapter 11)

"Overall, the results showed a reduced presence of undernutrition and, importantly, increased overweight and obesity." —Costa Rica (Chapter 37)

"Common health problems among Haitians include diabetes and hypertension. In children, malnutrition and anemia are frequently seen. HIV is also a big problem in Haiti." —Haiti (Chapter 38)

"Hungary has one of the highest smoking rates in Europe. In the year 2000, 38.3% of males and 23% of females reported being 'regular smokers.' Standardized mortality rates for cardiovascular disorders in Hungarians less than 65 years are three times higher than the European average." —Hungary (Chapter 15)

"Overall, Italians are one of the healthiest and longest-lived people; men live to an average age of 78.6 years and women live to an average age of 84.1 years. This is the highest life expectancy among Europeans, and many people believe it to be related to the Mediterranean diet, which includes red wine and olive oil." —Italy (Chapter 17)

"Lactose intolerance was very common in Japan, because after weaning, children rarely had access to milk." —Japan (Chapter 25)

"Diarrhea is a leading cause of mortality among Nepali infants and children. Food and water are withheld in the belief that such action will cure the illness, but it often compounds the dehydration problem." —Nepal (Chapter 24)

"Nigerian children have suffered the most due to poor prevalence of breastfeeding, inadequate calories per person, crop failure, and lack of iron, vitamin A, and iodine-containing foods. Compared with the rest of the world, Nigeria ranks high in infant mortality, iron-deficiency anemia, stunting, and wasting. With lack of safe water in some areas and poor immunity due to nutritional inadequacy, children are at high risk of infectious disease." —Nigeria (Chapter 33)

"Sweden has a long history of public health care policy which includes national responsibility to provide health care to all and preventative health measures that underscore the country's commitment to equality and security." —Sweden (Chapter 19)

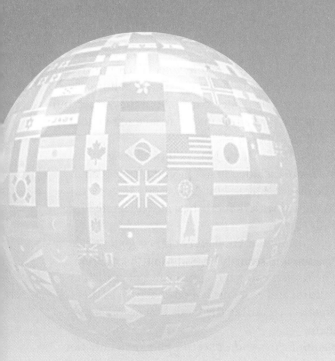

Introduction

Sari Edelstein, PhD, RD

Food, Cuisine, and Cultural Competency for Culinary, Hospitality, and Nutrition Professionals was created to provide useful information about various cuisines and cultures, including the traditions and sensibilities that characterize them. The book is coauthored primarily by nutrition experts and food lovers whose origins are rooted in the cultures about which they report. The text covers many more cultures, such as Botswana, Nigeria, Rwanda, Sudan, Ghana, Sierra Leone, Liberia, Afghanistan, and Bangladesh, than explored previously in other books. This is because the present era is more conducive to immigration, and people from diverse regions are now found all over the world. As food professionals, it behooves us to become familiar with as many cultures of the world as possible, because we will be serving clients from around the globe. Being properly informed when interacting with a person from another culture will empower the professional in terms of understanding cultural differences and developing the cross-cultural skills necessary to be effective in any counseling environment. Awareness of this fact, combined with actions taken to address it, leads to "cultural competency," which, in this book, refers to an individual's ability to interact consciously and effectively with persons of diverse cultures.

The book was created such that the instructor may hand-pick cultures from a larger selection for students to learn and become competent about. Thus, each chapter provides a stand-alone culture description. This allows the text to be customized for each classroom. Each chapter also provides cultural and history-related information as to how cuisines have evolved over the centuries to their present state, with regard to menus and recipes, as well as exploration of the cultural and religious traditions that have shaped them. Each chapter includes information on the following:

- *Culture and World Region.* In this section, the reader is given the geography of the region along with information about the climate, indigenous food supply, and the ethnic groups that reside there.
- *Language.* The number of languages spoken globally is staggering. Languages generally indicate the diversity and origin of the peoples in a given region; thus, each culture has its unique composition of languages and/or dialects.
- *Culture History.* Many cultures derive their identities from a combination of age-old traditions and the influence of recent immigration, which

adds to the diversity and richness of their cultural practices today. This section weighs the significance of such factors.

- *Food History Within the Culture.* In this section the reader encounters the culture's history in the context of its relevance to the cuisine. Determining factors, such as famines, floods, or degree of soil richness, are described to inform the reader as to why specific foods are plentiful in some civilizations and scarce in others.
- *Major Foods.* Each culture enjoys foods that represent religious, geographic, social, and economic choices. The reader learns pertinent details about each major food and what those foods represent to the culture.
  - *Protein Sources.* Each culture depends on a prominent protein source. Whether the country is located by the sea, which implies a diet plentiful in fish, or is a land-locked country dependent on animals for protein, the reader learns about the vital connection between geography and food resources of each culture.
  - *Starch Sources.* Soil cultivation often defines the starch sources of each culture, whether they be tubers or grains.
  - *Fat Sources.* The main fat sources of each culture are of particular interest in relation to health and potential longevity of its people. The reader is introduced to the Mediterranean diet in cultures that use olive oil prominently as compared with the trans- and saturated fats used more in the westernized world. The spread of fast food around the world has led to health problems that mirror those of the United States.
  - *Prominent Vegetables.* Similar to starches, the choice and quality of vegetables depends on soil quality along with climate and access to water.
  - *Prominent Fruits.* Fruit variability is vast, depending on distance from the equator, and prominent fruits change significantly from region to region.
  - *Spices and Seasonings.* Each culture has given the world an array of unique spice blends that define their culture's recipes and dishes.
  - *Beverages.* A diverse variety of beverages, from ancient mystical teas to malt beer, define many cultures.
  - *Desserts.* The joy of each culture is celebrated in its desserts!

- *Foods with Cultural Significance.* Each culture has recipes and foods that carry special cultural significance. The reader learns about the recipes and foods that play a role in the social and religious traditions of each society.
- *Typical Day's Menu.* Many culturally significant foods are included in a typical day's meal plan. The reader learns about how foods are served, combined with other dishes, and integrated into daily life.
- *Holiday Menus.* Food and holidays go together and often represent the traditions of a culture. The reader learns the significance of particular cultural and religious holidays, as well as the practices regarding the foods that accompany them.
- *Health Beliefs and Concerns.* Food and nutrition professionals will be interested in the health beliefs of each culture as well as some of the major dietary concerns facing their population.
- *General Health and Nutritional Indicators Summary.* This section discusses statistics that reflect the nutritional status of the country. Table I-1 provides the comprehensive table from UNICEF which lists the nutritional summary from many cultures and countries around the world.
- *Communication and Counseling Tips.* When serving clients from various cultures, professionals need to be culturally competent in communicating within the social norms of each culture. This section provides the necessary information in a practical manner, using the standard counseling model in most instances.
- *Primary Language of Food Names with English Translation.* Because language can be a barrier to providing cultural competence, the reader is given the names of foods in the culture's native tongue, and in most instances the phonetic pronunciation as well.
- *Observations from the Author.* Snippets of personal experience from authors enhance many chapters and give the reader an inside view of what it is like to be among people of another culture in their native country. Many authors offer whimsical lessons learned and amusing scenarios for readers to enjoy.
- *Featured Recipe.* Enjoy trying representative recipes from each culture.

TABLE I-1 Nutrition

Countries and Territories	Percent of infants with low birthweight 1998-2005*	exclusively breastfed (<6 months)	breastfed with complementary food (6-9 months)	still breastfeeding (20-23 months)	underweight moderate & severe	underweight severe	wasting moderate & severe	stunting moderate & severe	Vitamin A supplementation coverage rate (6-59 months) 2004	Percent of households consuming iodized salt 1998-2005*
Afghanistan	–	–	29	54	39	12	7	54	96t	28
Albania	5	6	24	6	14	1	11	34	–	62
Algeria	7	13	38	22	10	3	8	19	–	69
Andorra	–	–	–	–	–	–	–	–	–	–
Angola	12	11	77	37	31	8	6	45	77	35
Antigua and Barbuda	8	–	–	–	–	–	–	–	–	–
Argentina	8	–	–	–	4	–	1	4	–	90x
Armenia	7	33	57	15	4	0	5	13	–	97
Australia	7	–	–	–	–	–	–	–	–	–
Austria	7	–	–	–	–	–	–	–	–	–
Azerbaijan	12	7	39	16	7	1	2	13	14	26
Bahamas	7	–	–	–	–	–	–	–	–	–
Bahrain	8	34x,k	65x	41x	9x	2x	5x	10x	–	–
Bangladesh	36	36	69	90	48	13	13	43	83t	70
Barbados	11	–	–	–	–	–	–	–	–	–
Belarus	5	–	–	–	–	–	–	–	–	55
Belgium	8x	–	–	–	–	–	–	–	–	–
Belize	6	24k	54	23	–	–	–	–	–	90x
Benin	16	38	66	62	23	5	8	31	94t	72
Bhutan	15	–	–	–	19	3	3	40	–	95
Bolivia	7	54	74	46	8	1	1	27	42	90
Bosnia and Herzegovina	4	6	–	–	4	1	6	10	–	62
Botswana	10	34	57	11	13	2	5	23	62w	66
Brazil	8	–	30	17	6	1	2	11	–	88
Brunei Darussalam	10	–	–	–	–	–	–	–	–	–
Bulgaria	10	–	–	–	–	–	–	–	–	98
Burkina Faso	19	19	38	81	38	14	19	39	95t	45
Burundi	16	62	46	85	45	13	8	57	94	96
Cambodia	11	12	72	59	45	13	15	45	72t	14
Cameroon	13	24	79	29	18	4	5	32	81	88
Canada	6	–	–	–	–	–	–	–	–	–
Cape Verde	13	57k	64	13	–	–	–	–	–	0x
Central African Republic	14	17	77	53	24	6	9	39	79	86
Chad	22	2	77	65	37	14	14	41	84t	56
Chile	6	63	47	–	1	–	0	1	–	100
China	4	51	32	15	8	–	–	14	–	93
Colombia	9	47	65	32	7	1	1	12	–	92x
Comoros	25	21	34	45	25	–	8	44	7	82
Congo	–	19	78	21	15	3	7	26	94	–
Congo, Democratic Republic of the	12	24	79	52	31	9	13	38	81t	72
Cook Islands	3	19k	–	–	–	–	–	–	–	–
Costa Rica	7	35x,k	47x	12x	5	0	2	6	–	97x
Côte d'Ivoire	17	5	73	38	17	5	7	21	60	84
Croatia	6	23	–	–	1	–	1	1	–	90
Cuba	5	41	42	9	4	0	2	5	–	88
Cyprus	–	–	–	–	–	–	–	–	–	–
Czech Republic	7	–	–	–	–	–	–	–	–	–
Denmark	5	–	–	–	–	–	–	–	–	–
Djibouti	16	–	–	–	27	8	18	23	–	–
Dominica	11	–	–	–	–	–	–	–	–	–
Dominican Republic	11	10	41	16	5	1	2	9	–	18
Ecuador	16	35	70	25	12	–	–	26	–	99

(continues)

TABLE I-1 Nutrition (Continued)

Countries and Territories	Percent of infants with low birthweight 1998–2005*	Percent of children (1996–2005*) who are:			Percent of under-fives (1996–2005*) suffering from:						Vitamin A supplementation coverage rate (6–59 months) 2004	Percent of households consuming iodized salt 1998–2005*
		exclusively breastfed (<6 months)	breastfed with complementary food (6–9 months)	still breastfeeding (20–23 months)	underweight		wasting	stunting				
					moderate & severe	severe	moderate & severe	moderate & severe				
Egypt	12	38	67	37	6	1	4	18	–	78
El Salvador	7	24	76	43	10	1	1	19	–	62
Equatorial Guinea	13	24	–	–	19	4	7	39	–	33
Eritrea	14	52	43	62	40	12	13	38	50	68
Estonia	4	–	–	–	–	–	–	–	–	–
Ethiopia	15	49	54	86	38	11	11	47	52	28
Fiji	10	47x,k	–	–	–	–	–	–	–	31x
Finland	4	–	–	–	–	–	–	–	–	–
France	7	–	–	–	–	–	–	–	–	–
Gabon	14	6	62	9	12	2	3	21	–	36
Gambia	17	26	37	54	17	4	8	19	27	8
Georgia	7	18k	12	12	3	0	2	12	–	68
Germany	7	–	–	–	–	–	–	–	–	–
Ghana	16	53	62	67	22	5	7	30	95	28
Greece	8	–	–	–	–	–	–	–	–	–
Grenada	8	39k	–	–	–	–	–	–	–	–
Guatemala	12	51	67	47	23	4	2	49	18w	67
Guinea	16	27	41	71	26	7	9	35	95t	68
Guinea-Bissau	22	37	36	67	25	7	10	30	64	2
Guyana	13	11	42	31	14	3	11	11	–	–
Haiti	21	24	73	30	17	4	5	23	–	11
Holy See	–	–	–	–	–	–	–	–	–	–
Honduras	14	35	61	34	17	2	1	29	40	80
Hungary	9	–	–	–	–	–	–	–	–	–
Iceland	4	–	–	–	–	–	–	–	–	–
India	30	37k	44	66	47	18	16	46	51w	57
Indonesia	9	40	75	59	28	9	–	–	73t	73
Iran (Islamic Republic of)	7x	44	–	0	11	2	5	15	–	94
Iraq	15	12	51	27	12	3	8	23	–	40
Ireland	6	–	–	–	–	–	–	–	–	–
Israel	8	–	–	–	–	–	–	–	–	–
Italy	6	–	–	–	–	–	–	–	–	–
Jamaica	10	–	–	–	4	–	4	3	–	100
Japan	8	–	–	–	–	–	–	–	–	–
Jordan	12	27	70	12	4	1	2	9	–	88
Kazakhstan	8	36	73	17	4	0	2	10	–	83
Kenya	10	13	84	57	20	4	6	30	63	91
Kiribati	5	80x,k	–	–	–	–	–	–	58	–
Korea, Democratic People's Republic of	7	65	31	37	23	8	7	37	95t	40
Korea, Republic of	4	–	–	–	–	–	–	–	–	–
Kuwait	7	12k	26	9	10	3	11	24	–	–
Kyrgyzstan	7x	24	77	21	11	2	3	25	95	42
Lao People's Democratic Republic	14	23	10	47	40	13	15	42	48	75
Latvia	5	–	–	–	–	–	–	–	–	–
Lebanon	6	27k	35	11	4	–	5	11	–	92
Lesotho	13	36	79	60	20	4	4	38	71	91
Liberia	–	35	70	45	26	8	6	39	95	–
Libyan Arab Jamahiriya	7x	–	–	23x	5x	1x	3x	15x	–	90x
Liechtenstein	–	–	–	–	–	–	–	–	–	–
Lithuania	4	–	–	–	–	–	–	–	–	–
Luxembourg	8	–	–	–	–	–	–	–	–	–
Madagascar	17	67	78	64	42	11	13	48	89t	75

TABLE I-1   Nutrition (Continued)

| Countries and Territories | Percent of infants with low birthweight 1998–2005* | Percent of children (1996–2005*) who are: | | | Percent of under-fives (1996–2005*) suffering from: | | | | Vitamin A supplementation coverage rate (6–59 months) 2004 | Percent of households consuming iodized salt 1998–2005* |
		exclusively breastfed (<6 months)	breastfed with complementary food (6–9 months)	still breastfeeding (20–23 months)	underweight moderate & severe	underweight severe	wasting moderate & severe	stunting moderate & severe		
Malawi	16	53	78	80	22	5	5	48	57	49
Malaysia	9	29k	–	12	11	1	–	–	–	–
Maldives	22	10	85	–	30	7	13	25	–	44
Mali	23	25	32	69	33	11	11	38	97	74
Malta	6	–	–	–	–	–	–	–	–	–
Marshall Islands	12	63x,k	–	–	–	–	–	–	24	–
Mauritania	–	20	78	57	32	10	13	35	95t	2
Mauritius	14	21k	–	–	15x	2x	14x	10x	–	0x
Mexico	8	–	–	–	8	1	2	18	–	91
Micronesia (Federated States of)	18	60k	–	–	–	–	–	–	74	–
Moldova, Republic of	5	46	66	2	4	1	4	8	–	59
Monaco	–	–	–	–	–	–	–	–	–	–
Mongolia	7	51	55	57	7	1	3	20	93t	75
Montenegro‡	–	–	–	–	–	–	–	–	–	–
Morocco	15	31	66	15	10	2	9	18	–	59
Mozambique	15	30	80	65	24	6	4	41	26	54
Myanmar	15	15k	66	67	32	7	9	32	96t	60
Namibia	14	19	57	37	24	5	9	24	–	63
Nauru	–	–	–	–	–	–	–	–	–	–
Nepal	21	68	66	92	48	13	10	51	97t	63
Netherlands	–	–	–	–	–	–	–	–	–	–
New Zealand	6	–	–	–	–	–	–	–	–	83
Nicaragua	12	31	68	39	10	2	2	20	98	97
Niger	13	1	56	61	40	14	14	40	–	15
Nigeria	14	17	64	34	29	9	9	38	85t	97
Niue	0	–	–	–	–	–	–	–	–	–
Norway	5	–	–	–	–	–	–	–	–	–
Occupied Palestinian Territory	9	29k	78	11	5	1	3	10	–	64
Oman	8	–	92	73	18	1	7	10	95w	61
Pakistan	19x	16x,k	31x	56x	38	13	13	37	95t	17
Palau	9	59x,k	–	–	–	–	–	–	–	–
Panama	10	25x	38x	21x	8	1	1	18	–	95
Papua New Guinea	11x	59	74	66	–	–	–	–	32	–
Paraguay	9	22	60	–	5	–	1	14	–	88
Peru	11	64	81	41	8	0	1	24	–	91
Philippines	20	34	58	32	28	–	6	30	85t	56
Poland	6	–	–	–	–	–	–	–	–	–
Portugal	8	–	–	–	–	–	–	–	–	–
Qatar	10	12k	48	21	6x	–	2x	8x	–	–
Romania	8	16	41	–	3	0	2	10	–	53
Russian Federation	6	–	–	–	3x	1x	4x	13x	–	35
Rwanda	9	90	69	77	23	4	4	45	95t	90
Saint Kitts and Nevis	9	56k	–	–	–	–	–	–	–	100
Saint Lucia	10	–	–	–	–	–	–	–	–	–
Saint Vincent and the Grenadines	10	–	–	–	–	–	–	–	–	–
Samoa	4x	–	–	–	–	–	–	–	–	–
San Marino	–	–	–	–	–	–	–	–	–	–
Sao Tome and Principe	20	56	53	42	13	2	4	29	76t	74
Saudi Arabia	11x	31k	60	30	14	3	11	20	–	–
Senegal	18	34	61	42	17	3	8	16	95	41
Serbia‡	–	–	–	–	–	–	–	–	–	–
Seychelles	–	–	–	–	–	–	–	–	–	–

(*continues*)

TABLE I-1 Nutrition (Continued)

Countries and Territories	Percent of infants with low birthweight 1998–2005*	Percent of children (1996–2005*) who are: exclusively breastfed (<6 months)	breastfed with complementary food (6–9 months)	still breastfeeding (20–23 months)	Percent of under-fives (1996–2005*) suffering from: underweight moderate & severe	underweight severe	wasting moderate & severe	stunting moderate & severe	Vitamin A supplementation coverage rate (6–59 months) 2004	Percent of households consuming iodized salt 1998–2005*
Sierra Leone	23	4	51	53	27	9	10	34	95t	23
Singapore	8	–	–	–	3	0	2	2	–	–
Slovakia	7	–	–	–	–	–	–	–	–	–
Slovenia	6	–	–	–	–	–	–	–	–	–
Solomon Islands	13x	65k	–	–	–	–	–	–	–	–
Somalia	–	9	13	8	26	7	17	23	6	–
South Africa	15	7	46	–	12	2	3	25	37	62
Spain	6x	–	–	–	–	–	–	–	–	–
Sri Lanka	22	53	–	73	29	–	14	14	57w	94
Sudan	31	16	47	40	41	15	16	43	70	1
Suriname	13	9	25	11	13	2	7	10	–	–
Swaziland	9	24	60	25	10	2	1	30	86	59
Sweden	4	–	–	–	–	–	–	–	–	–
Switzerland	6	–	–	–	–	–	–	–	–	–
Syrian Arab Republic	6	81k	50	6	7	1	4	18	–	79
Tajikistan	15	41	91	55	–	–	5	36	98t	28
Tanzania, United Republic of	10	41	91	55	22	4	3	38	94t	43
Thailand	9	4x,k	71x	27x	18x	2x	5x	13x	–	63
The former Yugoslav Republic of Macedonia	6	37	8	10	6	1	4	7	–	94
Timor-Leste	12	31	82	35	46	15	12	49	43	72
Togo	18	18	65	65	25	7	12	22	95t	67
Tonga	0	62k	–	–	–	–	–	–	–	–
Trinidad and Tobago	23	2	19	10	6	1	4	4	–	1
Tunisia	7	47	–	22	4	1	2	12	–	97
Turkey	16	21	38	24	4	1	1	12	–	64
Turkmenistan	6	13	71	27	12	2	6	22	–	100
Tuvalu	5	–	–	–	–	–	–	–	–	–
Uganda	12	63	75	50	23	5	4	39	68	95
Ukraine	5	22	–	–	1	0	0	3	–	32
United Arab Emirates	15x	34x,k	52x	29x	14x	3x	15x	17x	–	–
United Kingdom	8	–	–	–	–	–	–	–	–	–
United States	8	–	–	–	2	0	6	1	–	–
Uruguay	8	–	–	–	5x	1x	1x	8x	–	–
Uzbekistan	7	19	49	45	8	2	7	21	86t	57
Vanuatu	6	50k	–	–	–	–	–	–	–	–
Venezuela (Bolivarian Republic of)	9	7k	50	31	5	1	4	13	–	90
Viet Nam	9	15	–	26	27	4	8	31	95t,w	83
Yemen	32x	12	76	–	46	15	12	53	20	30
Zambia	12	40	87	58	20	–	6	50	50	77
Zimbabwe	11	33	90	35	17	3	5	26	20	93
MEMORANDUM										
Serbia and Montenegro (pre-cession)	4	11k	33	11	2	0	4	5	–	73
SUMMARY INDICATORS										
Sub-Saharan Africa	14	30	67	55	28	8	9	37	73	67
Eastern and Southern Africa	13	40	69	63	27	7	7	40	60	60
West and Central Africa	15	20	65	48	28	9	10	35	85	73
Middle East and North Africa	15	30	59	24	16	4	8	24	–	65
South Asia	29	38	47	69	45	16	14	44	62	54
East Asia and Pacific	7	43	43	27	15	–	–	19	81**	85
Latin America and Caribbean	9	–	49	26	7	1	2	15	–	86

TABLE I-1   Nutrition (Continued)

Countries and Territories	Percent of infants with low birthweight 1998–2005*	Percent of children (1996–2005*) who are:			Percent of under-fives (1996–2005*) suffering from:					Vitamin A supplementation coverage rate (6–59 months) 2004	Percent of households consuming iodized salt 1998–2005*
		exclusively breastfed (<6 months)	breastfed with complementary food (6–9 months)	still breastfeeding (20–23 months)	underweight		wasting	stunting			
					moderate & severe	severe	moderate & severe	moderate & severe			
CEE/CIS	9	22	47	28	5	1	3	14	–	50	
Industrialized countries§	7	–	–	–	–	–	–	–	–	–	
Developing countries§	16	36	52	46	27	10	10	31	68**	71	
Least developed countries§	19	34	64	65	35	10	10	42	75	53	
World	15	36	52	46	25	9	9	30	68**	70	

‡ Due to the cession in June 2006 of Montenegro from the State Union of Serbia and Montenegro, and its subsequent admission to the UN on 28 June 2006, disaggregated data for Montenegro and Serbia as separate States are not yet available. Aggregated data presented are for Serbia and Montenegro pre-cession (see Memorandum item).

§ Also includes territories within each country category or regional group. Countries and territories in each country category or regional group are listed on page XX.

NOTES

–   Data not available.

x   Data refer to years or periods other than those specified in the column heading, differ from the standard definition, or refer to only part of a country.

k   Refers to exclusive breastfeeding for less than four months.

*   Data refer to the most recent year available during the period specifies in the column heading.

t   Identifies countries that have achieved a second round of vitamin A coverage great than or equal to 70%.

** Excludes China.

w   Indentifies countries with vitamin A supplementation programs that do not target children all the way up to 59 months of age.

DEFINITIONS OF THE INDICATORS

Low birthweight: Infants who weigh less than 2500 grams (or 5 lbs. 8 oz.).

Underweight (moderate and severe): Below minus two standard deviations from median weight for age of reference population.

Underweight (severe): Below minus three standard deviations from median weight for age of reference population.

Wasting (moderate and severe): Below minus two standard deviations from median weight for height of reference population.

Stunting (moderate and severe): Below minus two standard deviations from median height for age of reference population.

Vitamin A: Percentage of children aged 6–59 months who have received at least one high dose of vitamin A capsules in 2004.

Iodized salt consumption: Percentage of households consuming adequately iodized salt (15 ppm or more).

Reproduced with permission from UNICEF, *The State of the World's Children 2007: Women and Children, the Double Dividend of Gender Equality.* http://www.unicef.org/sow

Jones and Bartlett Publishers also provides text adopters with the following materials that can enhance the learning environment:

- Student study guides
- Student activity sheets
- Multiple-choice and short-answer chapter quizzes
- Instructor TestBank
- Sample course syllabus
- PowerPoint presentations with color photos from each culture
- Additional recipes from many of the cultures discussed in the text

See http://nutrition.jbpub.com/foodculture/ for more information.

About the Editor

Dr. Sari Edelstein's present position is as Associate Professor in the Nutrition and Dietetics Department at Simmons College in Boston, Massachusetts. She presently teaches both food-science and food-service classes. Before coming to Simmons College, Dr. Edelstein was in private practice and served as a hospital food service director and chief dietitian. She is the author of many research articles and author/editor of several books with Jones and Bartlett Publishers, which include:

Nutrition Pocket Guide for Nurses, 2007

Managing Food and Nutrition Services: For the Culinary, Hospitality, and Nutrition Professions, 2008

Lifecycle Nutrition: An Evidence-Based Approach, 2008

Food and Nutrition at Risk in America, 2009

Nutrition Pocket Guide for Dietitians, 2010

Essentials of Lifecycle Nutrition, 2010

Nutrition in Public Health, Third Edition, 2011

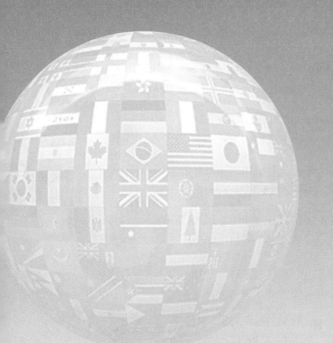

Contributing Authors

Dalal U.Z. Alkazemi, MSc, PhD Candidate
McGill University

Denise Bailey, MEd
Public Health Consultant

Roula Barake, MSc, PhD Candidate
McGill University

Sara Brass, MPH

Constance Brown-Riggs, MSEd, RD, CDE, CDN
Consultant

Emily J. Burritt, MS, RD, CNSD
Long Beach Memorial Medical Center

Simone Camel, MS, RD
Nicholls State University

Joseph M. Carlin, MS, MA, RD, LDN, FADA
U.S. Administration on Aging

Chandra Carty, MMSc, RD
Nutrition in the Now

Katherine L. Cason, PhD, RD
Clemson University

Cynthia Chandler, MS, RD, LD, CDM, CFFP
Sullivan University

Karen Chapman-Novakofski, RD, PhD
University of Illinois at Urbana-Champaign

Gary S. Chong, PhD
Jackson State University

Felicia Cohen-Egger, BS
Yeshiva University

Sara Dietrich, MS
Simmons College

Goulda A. Downer, PhD, RD, LN, CNS
Howard University College of Medicine

Sari Edelstein, PhD, RD
Simmons College

Eve V. Essery, PhD
Texas Women's University

Laurie M. Eynon, MPH, RD, CD-N
Bloomington Hospital

Katherine L. Fernald, MS, RD, LDN
The Nutrition Education and Wellness Service

Rachel Fisher, MS, MPH, RD
NIH Division of Nutrition Research Coordination

Marta Eugenia Gamboa-Acuna, BS
Clemson University

Jessica Garay, RD
George Washington University and Washington
Hospital Center

Samia Hamdan, MPH, RD
ADA Public Health and Community Nutrition
Practice Group

Jeffrey I. Harris, DrPH, MPH, RD, LDN
West Chester University

Rachel Hayes, MPH, RD
Nutritionist

Yenory Hernandez Garbanzo, BS
Clemson University

Melissa Ip, BS
Montgomery County Community Action
Development Commission

Colette Janson-Sand, PhD, RD, LD
University of New Hampshire
Dartmouth College

Carolyn King, RD
St. Joseph's Medical Center

Zaheer Ali Kirmani, PhD, RD (Retired)
Sam Houston State University

Beth Klos, BS
Brigham and Women's Hospital

Susan Levine Krantz, MA, RD
AtlantiCare

Mary Louise Kranyak, PhD, MBA, RD
New York Institute of Technology

Marcy J. Leeds, PhD, RD
Slippery Rock University

Colette G. Leistner, PhD, RD
Nicholls State University

Anna M. Love, PhD, RD, CHES
Texas Women's University

Segametsi Ditshebo Maruapula, PhD
University of Botswana

Susan J. Massad, HSD, RD
Framingham State College

Marilyn Massey-Stokes, EdD, CHES, FASHA
Texas Woman's University

Colleen E. McLean, RD, CNSD
Miller Children's Hospital

Hugo Melgar-Quinonez, MD, PhD
Ohio State University

Elizabeth Metallinos-Katsaras, PhD, RD
Simmons College

Jennifer Miller, RD, CNSD
Miller Children's Hospital/Long Beach Memorial
Medical Center

Titilayo O. Ologhobo, BS, MPH Candidate
West Chester University

Carol E. O'Neil, PhD, MPH, LDN, RD
Louisiana State University

Sharon Palmer, RD
Freelance Food/Nutrition Writer

Sudha Raj, PhD, RD
Syracuse University

Bharati Koli Rastogi, PhD, RD
Lowell Community Health Center

Arezoo Rojhani, PhD, RD
Western Michigan University

Miho Sato, MA
Management Sciences for Health

Martine I. Scannavino, DHSc, RD, LDN
Cedar Crest College

Rebecca J. Scritchfield, MA, RD
Consultant

Ahlam Badreldin Ibrahim Al Shikieri, PhD
The National Ribat University

JoAnna Siciliano, RD, LDN
University of Illinois Medical Center

Marta Sovyanhadi, DrPH, RD, LDN
Oakwood College

Lynn Thomas, DrPH, RD, CNSD
University of South Carolina School of Medicine

Margaret Udahogora, MS, RD, PhD Candidate
University of Maryland

Jeannette van der Velde, MPH, MSc
Boston Children's Hospital

Lisa Weber, BS, MS Candidate
Simmons College

Hülya Yüksel, PhD
Dumlupinar University

Some contributing authors are members of The American Overseas Dietetic Association (AODA; Website: http://www.eatrightoverseas.org/), which is the international affiliate of the American Dietetic Association (ADA). We thank them for their help with this project.

REVIEWERS AND STUDY GUIDE CONTRIBUTORS

Tiffany Alongi

Rachel Brady

Melissa Bryant

Katie Burchman

Samantha Cheung

Ryann Collins

Kristen Connolly

Kristen DeLisio

Yoldy Eugene

Kristen Eugley

Riley Fadden

Danielle Gulizia

Crystal Herbosa

Alicia Jamous

Kari Jorgensen

Kimberly Korenewsky

Tiffany Koshis

Brie LeDuc

Elizabeth Marble

Kara Masse

Jenna Merrill

Kelly Muirhead

Kyla Peters

Shawnna Prendergast

Tori Reynolds

Deanna Santanello

Marissa Schmid

Laura Sherburne

Kayla Tirrell

Lisa Weber

Samantha Yagle

Overview of Religions

Although there are literally thousands of religions in the world today, *Food, Cuisine, and Cultural Competency for Culinary, Hospitality, and Nutrition Professionals* draws the reader's attention to four prominent religions. These chapters provide an overview of the religions that, along with other major faiths central to certain cultures, are discussed further in the subsequent country-specific chapters. The religions covered briefly in this section are:

CHAPTER 1 Christianity

CHAPTER 2 Islam

CHAPTER 3 Judaism

CHAPTER 4 Seventh-Day Adventist

RELIGIONS

Christianity, Islam, Judaism, and Seventh-Day Adventist are major religions that are practiced throughout the world.

Christianity

Christianity was rooted in the Abrahamic religious tradition and originated in the eastern Mediterranean. During the Middle Ages, Christianity became a religious minority in the Middle East, North Africa, and India.

Islam

Islam is an Abrahamic religion and is the predominant religion in much of Africa and the Middle East, as well as in major parts of Asia.

Judaism

The world Jewish population lives mostly in Israel and the United States. It too is a religion descended from Abraham.

Seventh-Day Adventist

The Seventh-Day Adventist religion was founded in the United States during the middle of the 19th century and was formally established in 1863. It currently has a worldwide membership and is culturally diverse.

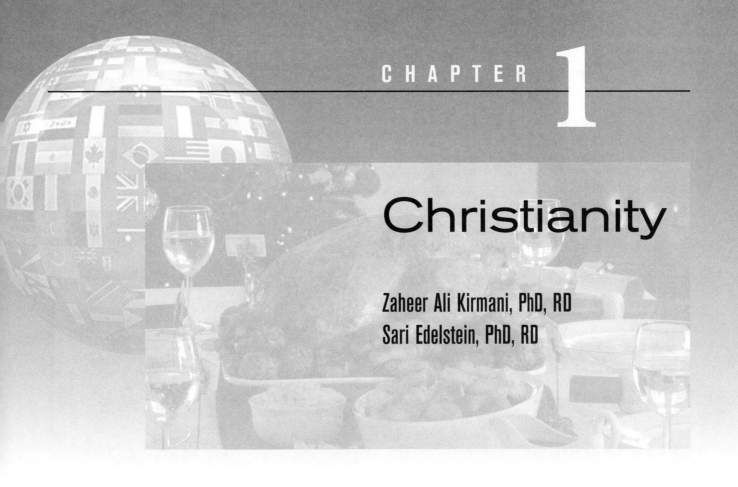

CHAPTER 1

Christianity

Zaheer Ali Kirmani, PhD, RD
Sari Edelstein, PhD, RD

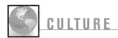 **CULTURE**

Christians celebrate the life of Jesus Christ, whom they believe to have been the son of God and who preached God's message of love and forgiveness in Jerusalem more than 2000 years ago. Having suffered crucifixion because of his teachings, according to Christian belief, Jesus Christ rose from the dead after 3 days and ascended to heaven. Christians believe in only one God, but the concept of the Trinity is an essential part of the faith. The Trinity includes: (1) the Father (God, the Creator of heaven and earth); (2) Jesus, His son, who came to earth to teach love and forgiveness; and (3) the Holy Ghost, the unseen power of God that is working everywhere in the world. It is believed that Christ's crucifixion and rising from the dead signifies forgiveness for wrongdoers so that they can have a fresh start in life.

The Old Testament of the Christian holy book, the Bible, is also recognized by Muslims and Jews, whereas the New Testament, which chronicles Christ's life through to his death and resurrection, is relevant solely to Christianity. With Jesus Christ's teachings as the common thread, Christians are subdivided into various denominations such as Catholic, Protestant, Greek Orthodox, Pentecostal, Baptist, Southern Baptist, Mormon, Anglican, Latter-Day Saint, Jehovah's Witness, Quaker, and Seventh-Day Adventist (SDA), among others. The style of worship and customs differs among the various denominations and sects. For example, although the crucifix is universally recognized in Christianity as the symbol of Christ's suffering and death, some Christians believe that a cross without his figure is a more appropriate symbol because he ascended to heaven after death. Most followers of Christ perform acts of kindness toward people in need. Such endeavors include supporting orphanages, schools for disadvantaged children, hospitals, and schools in developing countries. In most Christian churches, babies are welcomed into the Church in a baptism ceremony in which the baby is either submerged in blessed water or blessed water is sprinkled on the baby. Young Christians may also celebrate First Communion, which commemorates the last meal Christ ate with his disciples the night before his crucifixion.

In many Christian households, although Sunday is the day of formal worship and church attendance, prayers are offered before every meal and before going to bed. In addition, Christians who adhere more fervently to symbolic rituals often engage in special practices. For example, many Christians in South America lead processions on certain days with palm branches in their hands and in the hand of a statue of Christ.

Christians have several holy days. Epiphany marks the visit of the Three Wise Men to the Baby Jesus. Ash Wednesday signifies the beginning of Lent (a period of prayer and self-denial before Easter) in February/March. Holy Week is celebrated in March/April with Palm Sunday, Good Friday, and Easter to commemorate the life, death, and resurrection of Jesus Christ. In June, Pentecost celebrates the coming of the Holy Spirit. The Advent period, in November/December, is observed until Christmas, and Christmas is celebrated as the birthday of Jesus Christ.

Christians number 2 billion worldwide, comprising the world's most popular religion. Because Christians exist across various sects in many different cultures, dietary adherence, traditions, and food availability varies extensively, which makes generalizing or describing a universally standard daily meal plan impossible; thus, this chapter highlights only the dietary preferences and traditions of a few Christian denominations.

 MAJOR FOODS

The major foods utilized in Christianity, inclusive of protein, starch, vegetable, fruit, fat, beverages, and spices, are best illustrated by the food traditions found at holiday meals. This section focuses on those aspects of two holiday meals: Christmas and Easter dinners.

 Christmas Dinner

Just as Christianity has many denominations and sects, Christmas dinner is also celebrated with different cuisines in various regions of the world. In the United States, Christmas dinner may include roast turkey, beef, ham, or pork as the major protein source.

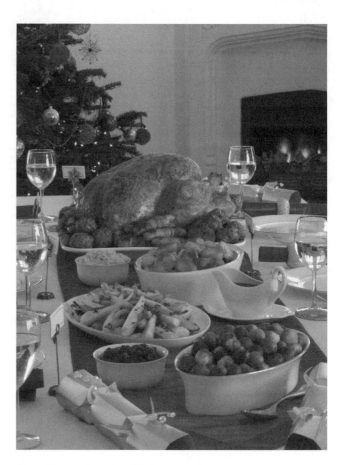

One Example of a Christmas Dinner

This will be accompanied by stuffing and mashed potatoes as the starch source, and corn, squash, or green beans as a vegetable. Desserts may include fruit pies. Variations within the United States may include black-eyed peas as a starch source in the southern part of the country and the use of pineapple as an Asian influence. Mincemeat pie at Christmas dinner is linked to Spanish/Hispanic traditions.

Other regional Christmas dinner preferences may include the use of Luke fish in Norway, an Edam cheese ball in the Philippines, a turkey stuffed with ground beef and peanuts in Peru, cold potato salad in Brazil, and goose, oysters, and cream cake in France. People in The Netherlands do not always practice the family-meal style in which everyone eats from one large platter of each food; instead, people gather to each cook their own Christmas meal in individual frying pans in smaller portions. Finely chopped vegetables and shrimp are commonly consumed in Dutch cuisine. Mexico makes use of tamales (with chocolate or fruit sauces) as a traditional Christmas dinner dessert dish

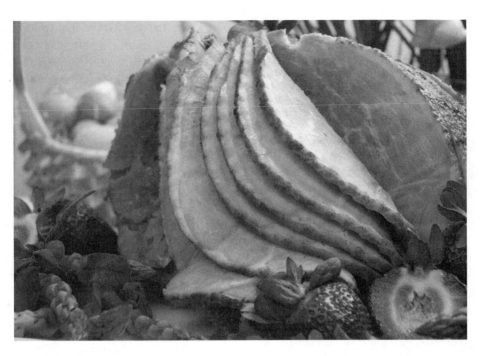

One Example of an Easter Dinner

and stuff their turkeys with sugarcane water solutions and fruit for sweetness.

 Easter Dinner

Easter dinner is celebrated by most Christians as the end of the period of Lent to signify rebirth; thus, the symbol of the Easter egg represents this rebirth or time of renewal. In the United States, ham is the traditional Easter dinner protein source; however, in Europe roasted lamb may be the protein of choice for Easter. A traditional starch consumed during Easter time is the hot cross bun. Hot cross buns link back to the ancient Greeks and relates to Christ's cross. Russians are known for making kulich, a bread shaped in an Easter symbol (sometimes a tall and narrow shape with a bulging top, signifying that Christ has risen) with beautiful decorations made of candied citrus peels.

 FOODS WITH CULTURAL SIGNIFICANCE

The Sabbath for the Mormons is Sunday while SDAs observe Sabbath from sunset on Friday to sundown on Saturday. This is the time to take respite from the daily chores and reflect on God's many blessings in the company of family and friends during Bible studies. Sabbath afternoon meal is the largest meal of the day and includes the family's favorite foods.

Many foods with cultural significance are those that are prohibited in some Christian sects. For example, SDA and Mormon churches recommend that their followers consume food that is considered clean in order to stay healthy. True followers of both of these religions do not consume alcohol or caffeinated beverages. They also avoid smoking and blood in meats. Human health is the main consideration for the imposition of food restriction in both SDA and Mormon churches, and bears a relationship with the Old Testament. The Old Testament provides clear instruction for the consumption of clean animals, which include those with cloven hooves that chew their cud, and fish with fins and scales. Birds of prey, pig, rabbit, bear, raccoon, cat fish, shrimp, lobster, octopus, frog, snake, and lizard are deemed to be unfit for consumption. Tradition, which was established before proper refrigeration was available, insisted that chicken, other poultry, and beef be consumed, and that persons abstain from eating pork, because pig is not deemed a clean animal according to the teachings of these churches. Vegetarian meals have been adopted by many Christians of these denominations. Specifically, vegetarianism is common in SDA faith and health and dietary regimentation seems to be a hallmark of this religion (See Chapter 4).

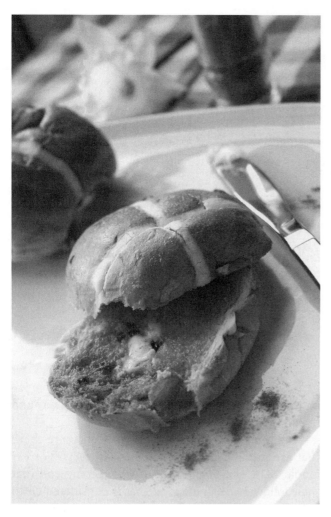

Hot Cross Buns

Many Eastern Orthodox and Oriental Orthodox groups also discourage pork consumption, with the exception of Eritrean Orthodox Tewahdo Church and the Ethiopian Orthodox Church, where the proscription is rarely enforced.

REFERENCES

Ariel, Y.S. (1954). Christianity through reform eyes: Kaufmann Kohler's scholarship on Christianity. *American Jewish History, 89*(2), 181.

Arnett, R.A. (2008). Short world history of Christianity. *Library Journal, 133*(7), 90.

Bainton, R.H. (2000). *Christianity.* Boston: Houghton Mifflin.

Buller, L. (2005). *A faith like mine.* New York: DK Books.

Christian, G. (2008). The attentive life: Discerning God's presence in all things. *Library Journal, 133*(4), 71.

Deveny, K. (2008). Talking to kids about God. *Newsweek, 151*(6), 60.

Ferrero, M. (2008). The triumph of Christianity in the Roman empire: An economic interpretation. *European Journal of Political Economy, 24,* 167.

Gonzalez, T.A. (2008). Simple twist of faith. *Newsweek, 151*(5), 17.

Hart, W.D. (1957). Slavoj Zizek and the imperial/colonial model of religion. *Nepantla: Views from South, 3,* 136.

Hommerding, L. (2008). The faith: What Christians believe, why they believe it, and why it matters. *Library Journal, 133*(4), 85.

Wieseltier, L. (2008). Ring the bells. *New Republic, 238*(7), 56.

Wills, G. (2008). Head and heart: American Christianities. *Publishers Weekly, 255*(8), 75.

CHAPTER 2

Islam

Zaheer Ali Kirmani, PhD, RD

 CULTURE

The followers of Islam, Muslims, number more than a billion throughout the world. Muslim means "submission to the will of the Creator." Muslims believe that this Creator is Allah, which is an Arabic word for God. Muslims must follow the will of Allah as revealed in their holy book, the Qur'an, which was handed down to their prophet, Muhammad. Islam is a simple religion that teaches each Muslim to be a humble servant of Allah while fulfilling all obligations of living. The five pillars of Islam describe what a Muslim must adhere to in order to remain a true believer. These pillars of Islam teach respect and humility toward Allah, and love and caring for all mankind.

The first pillar is faith in Allah, acknowledging that He is the Creator of heaven and earth, and that Muhammad is his prophet. Another pillar of Islam is the offering of prayers (Salah) five times a day. Five prayers, from dawn to the late evening, regulate Muslim everyday life. Prayers involve ablution, standing, bowing, prostrating, and sitting postures facing Kabah, which is situated in Mecca, Saudi Arabia. Every practicing Muslim reads prayers in Arabic as taught by the prophet. Additional prayers are optional. Zakah (charity) is yet another pillar of Islam. The required amount is 2.5% of the yearly earnings. A Muslim must be charitable, and if he or she cannot afford to give money, then he or she must take part in some kind of community-benevolence program. For Muslims, even greeting somebody with a smile is charity. The remaining two pillars, fasting during Ramadan and making a pilgrimage to Mecca, are discussed later in this chapter.

Muslims believe that the Qur'an is the holy word of Allah, brought by the angel Gabriel to Muhammad, the last prophet of Allah. They believe that Muhammad was from a lineage of prophets that ended with him, and claim that he encompasses all other prophets and their scriptures. Muhammad was born in 570 BCE in Mecca to a tribe with lineage to Ishmael, the first son

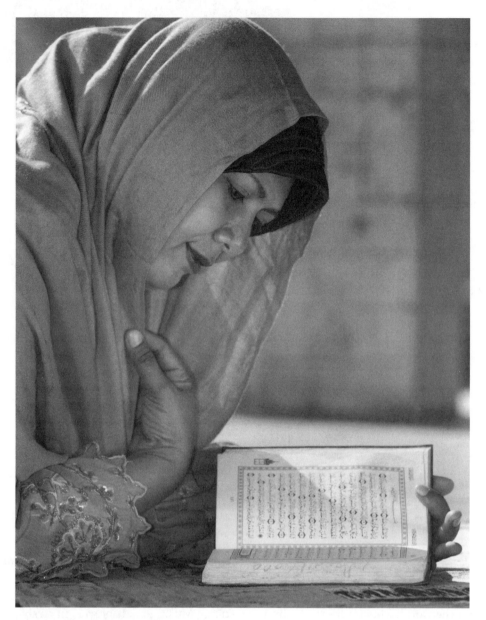

The Qur'an, the Holy Book of Islam

of Abraham. His father, Abdullah, was son of Abdul-Muttalib, leader of the Qureish tribe in Mecca, and his mother, Amina, was the daughter of Wahb, leader of the Bene Zuhra tribe of Medina. His parents died when he was young and he was raised by his uncle, Abu Taalib. Muhammad never received formal education and could not read or write. He received his first message from Allah when he was 40 years old and continued to preach Islam for the next 23 years. According to Muslim belief, it is a miracle of Allah that, after receiving the first revelation from Him, Muhammad could read and recite verses of the Qur'an better than anyone else. The first revelation of the Qur'an occurred during the

month of Ramadan; therefore, recitation of the holy book is a Muslim tradition particularly during that month.

The Qur'an is the only book that believers claim to be nothing but the actual words of Allah, and it is still preserved in its original language, Arabic, in its original form. Muslims all over the world recite the Qur'an in Arabic as well as read and write commentary in their native languages based on the Arabic text, history, and Sunnah (sayings/teachings of Muhammad). Sunnah and Hadith are compilations of approvals and disapprovals of the prophet written in separate books after his death.

Fasting throughout the month of Ramadan is mandatory for Muslims and is one of the pillars of Islam. The Qur'an states, "O ye who believe! Fasting is prescribed to you as it was prescribed to those before you, that ye may (learn) self restraint." Ramadan is the ninth month of the Islamic lunar calendar. Daily dawn to sunset fast is prescribed for 29–30 days and includes prohibition of food, drink, and any sexual activity. The fast is broken by a meal called Iftar, which is usually more substantial than an ordinary dinner. Eid al-Fitr is the holiday celebrated at the end of Ramadan.

Pilgrimage to Mecca, called hajj, at least once in their lifetime is one of the pillars of Islam and is obligatory to all able-bodied Muslims who can afford it. About two to three million Muslims from all over the world perform the hajj every year. Every Muslim who performs the hajj wears a simple white robe that consists of two pieces of cloth that can be used for burial at the time of the person's death.

Eid al-Adha is the celebration the next day after pilgrimage is over. Sheep, goat, lamb, and camels are sacrificed to revive the memory of the prophet Abraham's unwavering obedience to God: when asked, he was willing to sacrifice his own son. God accepted his virtuous deed in spirit and asked him to sacrifice a lamb instead. Meat of the sacrificed animals is distributed among the poor. People wear fine clothes, special prayers are held, children receive gifts, and families get together for a special meal that includes the meat from the sacrificed animals to mark this joyous occasion.

Islamic prescription for food prohibits meat from animals that are found dead, blood, the flesh and other products from swine, scavengers, birds of prey, alcohol in any form (including any food that contains alcohol as an ingredient) and any other substance that can intoxicate (except for legitimate medical prescriptions), meat from animals (those that are permitted) on which the name of Allah is not invoked at the time of slaughter, and meat from an animal on which the name of someone else is invoked at the time of slaughter.

The meats that pass the Muslim criteria for helping to maintain a body and soul healthy and clean are branded as "halal." Muslims in the United States look for the seal of halal on meats and other products, such as gelatin, which come from animals. Food products that contain tallow (beef fat) and lard (pig fat) are not consumed by Muslims. Sausages, hot dogs, and any cold cut will not be acceptable to Muslims unless they

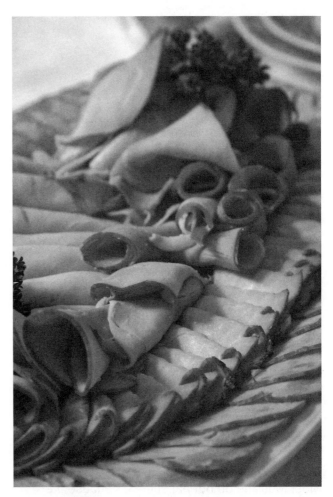

Kosher meats and cold cuts are acceptable to Muslims.

are halal or kosher. Cheese is another product that Muslims must approach cautiously because the rennet (an animal byproduct) used in the manufacturing process for certain types of cheese does not come from halal or kosher animals.

 MAJOR FOODS

 Protein Sources

Beef, goat, lamb, sheep, chicken, quail, duck, turkey, and fish are the main sources of protein in a Muslim diet. Eggs as well as milk, cheese, and other dairy products are additional sources of animal protein, and lentils/beans are a source of vegetable protein. Peanuts, cashews, almonds, walnuts, pecans, and hazelnuts are used in various recipes and complement other sources of protein. Processed meats, such as sausage, bologna,

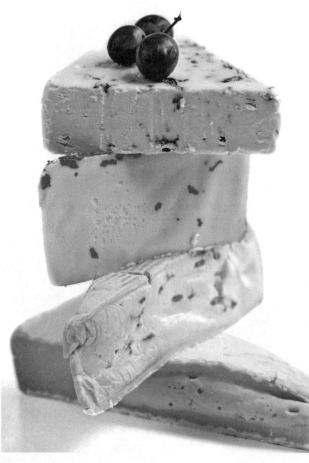

Most Muslims do not eat cheese because the rennet in the manufacturing of the cheese does not come from halal or kosher animals.

and beef or turkey bacon, are used but must be labeled as halal. Tofu, tempeh, textured vegetable, roasted soy, various grains, and wheat gluten are used frequently with meats or separately.

 Starch Sources

Various lentils and beans, wheat, corn, rice, barley, oats, buckwheat, rye, millet, triticale, and all types of potatoes are major sources of starch. Other sources of starch include pilaf, cold and hot cereals, tacos, tortillas, and all types of baked products such as cakes, pastries, bagels, muffins, and biscuits.

 Fat Sources

Whole milk, sour cream, vegetable oils, butter, margarine, mayonnaise, peanuts and peanut butter, salad dressings, coconut, cream cheese, goat cheese, and olives are sources of fat.

 Vegetables and Fruits

All types of fruits and vegetables are consumed by Muslims, depending on the region in which they live.

 Spices, Seasonings, and Other Ingredients

Spices and herbs used in recipes vary by region. Salt, pepper, cayenne, cumin, cloves, celery, cinnamon, curry powder, and cardamom are most commonly used in the United States. However, died herbs, such as oregano, rosemary, thyme, sage, and savory, also often find their way into Muslim recipes. Baking soda, baking powder, and baker's yeast are used to make homemade bread and other baked products such as muffins and rolls.

 Beverages

Coffee, tea, colas, and various types of punches are most commonly consumed.

 Desserts

A variety of desserts, such as cakes, pastries, and pies, are consumed. Muslims look for halal ingredients for desserts, especially with regard to the fat sources that must be vegetable oil, margarine, or butter. Halal or kosher gelatin is frequently consumed as a dessert.

 TYPICAL DAY'S MENU

Islam does not dictate diets for Muslims, but it does forbid certain food items in the interest of health for its followers. Muslims, wherever they happen to live, can formulate recipes according to their own personal traditions and cultures, as long as they avoid foods that have been proscribed. The meals given below are an example of Muslim dietary practices in the United States.

Breakfast

- Fried eggs
- Wheat toast with jam or jelly
- Coffee or tea

Lunch

- Hamburger (made from halal ground beef)
- Cola

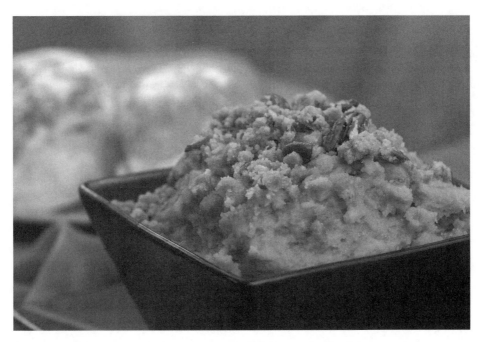

Sweet potato casserole is a common dish served at holiday meals.

Dinner

- Baked halal lamb
- Brown rice
- Mixed vegetable salad with Italian dressing
- Water with ice
- Tea or coffee

 ## HOLIDAY MEALS

Eid al-Fitr and Eid al-Adha are two major religious holidays on the Islamic lunar calendar. American Muslims also celebrate Thanksgiving, a time when family and friends gather, with great fervor. Halal meat can be a baked turkey, lamb, or goat prepared with salt, pepper, butter, carrots, celery, and giblet gravy with turkey. Baked green beans with olive oil, onions, garlic, salt, peppers, bread crumbs, Parmesan cheese (fermented without animal byproducts), and butter is another favorite dish. Sweet potato casserole is often prepared with eggs, sugar, butter, milk, vanilla, and mashed sweet potatoes. Topping for the sweet potatoes is prepared with brown sugar, flour, butter, and chopped pecans; several variations to this recipe are prevalent. Dinner rolls and croissants usually accompany the dinner. Apple pie or other fruit pies are often served as dessert. Colas, water, fruit juices, tea, and coffee are the beverages of choice.

The halal method of slaughtering and preparing animal meat is certified by the U.S. Department of Agriculture. Halal meats, such as beef, lamb, goat, and poultry, can be purchased from Middle Eastern or Pakistani food stores in cities throughout the United States or can be ordered from certain vendors on the Internet.

REFERENCES

Aandahl, K. (2003). *Islam i Sudan. Hasan al-Turabis ideologi: En teoretisk modell av en islamsk stat.* Unpublished master's thesis, University of Oslo, Oslo, Norway.

Abdo, G. (1951). *No God but God: Egypt and the triumph of Islam.* London: Oxford University Press.

Buller, L. (2005). *A faith like mine.* New York: DK Books.

Columbia University Press. (2006). Islam. In P. Lagasse, L. Goldman, A. Hobson, & S.R. Norton, (Eds.) *Columbia Encyclopedia* (6th ed.) Retrieved February 16, 2008, from http://www.education.yahoo.com/reference/encyclopedia/entry/Islam.html/

Grube, E. (1967). *The world of Islam.* New York: McGraw-Hill.

Ibrahim, A.A.A. (1999). A theology of modernity: Hasan al-Turabi and Islamic renewal in Sudan. *Africa Today, 46*(3/4), 195–222.

Ismael, T.Y. (1985). *Government and politics in Islam.* New York: St. Martin's Press.

Khalidi, T. (1985). *Classical Arab Islam: The culture and heritage of the golden age.* Princeton, NJ: Darwin Press.

Malik, M.F. (1998). *English translation of the meaning of Al-Qur'an: The guidance for mankind.* Houston, TX: The Institute of Islamic Knowledge.

Nasr, S.H. (1976). *Islam and the Arab world: faith, people, culture.* New York: Knopf (in association with American Heritage).

Nasr, S.H. (1987). *Traditional Islam in the modern world.* London: KPI.

O'Brien, S. (1999). Pilgrimage, power, and identity: The role of the Hajj in the lives of Nigerian Hausa Bori Adepts. *Africa Today, 46*(3/4), 11–40.

Qutb, S. (2007). *The Sayyid Qutb reader: Selected writings on politics, religion, and society 1906–1966.* London: Routledge.

Unknown. (2008). *Religious and dietary practices: Religious belief expressed as food customs.* Retrieved February 16, 2008, from http://www.faqs.org/nutrition/Pre-Sma/Religion-and-Dietary-Practices.html/

Watt, W.M. (1968). *What is Islam?* New York: Praeger.

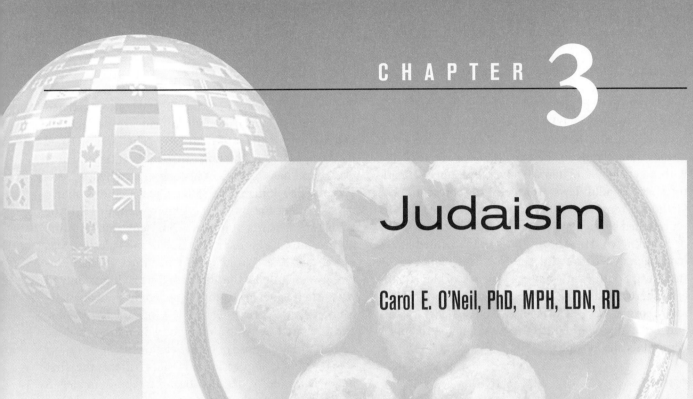

CHAPTER 3

Judaism

Carol E. O'Neil, PhD, MPH, LDN, RD

 CULTURE AND WORLD REGION

Judaism is the oldest monotheistic religion. Over 4000 years ago at Mount Sinai, God (sometimes written as G_d) entered into a covenant (*B'rit*) with the people of Israel, which contains 613 commandments that cover all aspects of Jewish life. Included among these commandments are the Jewish dietary laws (*Kashrut*). Prior to the end of the 19th century all Jews followed *Kashrut*. At that time the Conservative and Reform movements in Judaism arose in Germany and spread to other parts of the world. Early leaders in the Reform movement argued that, because of the destruction of the second Temple (70 CE), there was no longer a reason to observe *Kashrut*—the laws were no longer relevant because they were instituted in connection with the Temple sacrificial system. Recently, however, attitudes have changed and there are Reform Jews who observe *Kashrut*, but it is a personal preference, not a law. Observance may be full or modified; for example,

eschewing pork and shellfish only or eating *matzah* at Passover; however, the intricacies of *Kashrut*, coupled with their long history and the fact that Jews could not eat in the home of a non-Jew, have tended to preserve Jewish food practices. Today, Orthodox Jews, including Chassidic Jews, who are sometimes called ultra-Orthodox Jews, follow the dietary laws, as do many Conservative and some Reform Jews.

Jews are found throughout the world. In 2006, Israel had the largest population of Jews, surpassing the United States for the first time; if this trend continues, it is projected that half the world's Jewry will be living in Israel by 2015 (The Jewish People Policy Planning Institute, 2006). Determining an accurate number of Jews in the United States is difficult because the U.S. Census Bureau is prohibited (Public Law 94-521) from asking a question on religious affiliation on a mandatory basis. Available surveys in the United States are dated, with the most recent in 2001, when The American Jewish Identity Survey determined that the number of individuals who regard themselves as Jewish by religion or say they are of Jewish parentage or upbringing but have no religion declined from about 5.5 million in 1990 to about 5.3 million in 2001 (Mayer, Kosmin, & Kaysov, 2003). Approximately 1 million households in the United States are affiliated with a synagogue or temple. Overall, Reform constitutes 38% of adult Jews, Conservative represents 32%, Orthodox represents 10%, and the remaining 20% is represented by Secular Humanists, Reconstructionists, or is unknown. Historically, Jews in the United States have been concentrated in the Northeast, followed by the West, South, and Midwest. Outside of the Northeast, there are significant populations of Jews in Florida, Georgia, Texas, Chicago, St. Louis, New Orleans, and Los Angeles (see http://www.simpletoremember.com/vitals/ajisbook.pdf).

 LANGUAGES

The languages usually associated with the Jews are Hebrew and Yiddish; however, they speak a polyglot of languages that reflect the country in which they live, and possibly the country of their origin. Hebrew is a Semitic language of the Afro-Asiatic language family spoken by more than 7 million people in Israel and by an unknown number of people in Jewish communities around the world. It is one of the two official languages (with Arabic) of Israel, and is spoken by the majority of the population there. Hebrew is the language of the *Tanakh* as well, the idiom in which Jews wrote literature and verse.

To Jews, it is the "language of sanctity, the holy tongue" (Sáenz-Badillos, 1996). The *Talmud*, the record of the rabbinic discussions about Jewish law, is in Hebrew and Aramaic.

Yiddish (literally the Yiddish word for "Jewish") arose between 900 and 1100 CE from Middle High German and Hebrew in the Ashkenazi culture; it is written using the Hebrew alphabet and is spoken by approximately 3 million people, principally Orthodox Jews, around the world. It is the official language of Jewish Autonomous Oblast, and is officially recognized as a minority language in Sweden, the Netherlands, and Moldova.

Yiddish was never a part of Sephardic culture. Their international language is known as Judesmo, and is a hybrid of medieval Spanish and Hebrew. Ladino, a language derived principally from Old Castilian, Hebrew, and Turkish, is also spoken by some Sephardic Jews.

 CULTURE HISTORY

Throughout history, the two principal concepts related to the Jewish political environment are persecution coupled with exile and migration. The land of Israel has been sacred to the Jews since Biblical times. However, Israel has a turbulent history—ruled by Jews, Assyrians, Babylonians, Persians, Greeks, and Romans; it was part of the Byzantine Empire and, in 1561, the Ottomans began a rule that would continue into the 20th century. The British Mandate for Palestine was established after World War I when the Ottoman Empire was split up by the Treaty of Sèvres. It was only in 1948 when Israel declared its independence that a Jewish homeland was established. It is the only Jewish state and is shared by Arabs, many of whom are Muslims, Christians, and those of other religions.

To escape oppression by these rulers, the first major Diaspora of the Jews began in approximately 8 BCE when they moved across Asia, Spain, and Portugal (to become the Sephardic Jews), and northern Europe (to become the Ashkenazi Jews). At times they were welcomed and they lived in peace and prosperity with their neighbors, but at other times they were not. Jews flourished in Muslim Spain; Toledo, Córdoba, Grenada, and Seville became important Jewish centers. Jews were integrated into every aspect of community life and they were artisans, statesmen, and agriculturists. Where Jews were driven out, they were forced to settle in other countries that would take them in: Holland, northern France, Italy, North Africa, and the Ottoman Empire in Turkey. The first Jews in the United States were these Sephardic Jews. Often they were welcomed readily, although as times changed, not all countries were open to them and some countries, such as Italy, confined them to ghettos. The emigration of these Jews continued until the end of the 16th century.

In the strictest sense, Sephardic Jews are those only from the Iberian Peninsula; "Sepharad" means Spain in modern Hebrew. In the broader sense, in which the term is usually used, Sephardic refers to Jews from the Middle East, the Mediterranean, and Asia. Sephardic Jews were more integrated into their community than were the Ashkenazi; for example, when living in Muslim Spain, the Sephardim dressed as Arabs and spoke Arabic and they had many secular pursuits. They ate a wide variety of foods including olive oil, peppers, eggplant, cracked wheat, and saltwater fish. Their eating style was similar to their Muslim neighbors and they were less likely than the Ashkenazis to observe *Kashrut* strictly.

Ashkenazi Jews are of middle European ancestry. *Ashkenaz* means Germany in medieval Hebrew. Between the 10th and 19th centuries, they migrated eastward into Poland and Russia. Their food and culture developed in the cold bitter winters. The overwhelming majority of Jews in the United States are Ashkenazis, descended from Jews who emigrated from Germany and eastern Europe from the mid 1800s to the early 1900s. What is generally thought of in the United States as "Jewish food" is that of the Ashkenazis—the "peasant food of the shetl" (Rhoden, 2001).

Everywhere Jews went they incorporated local foods into their cooking, adapted these to *Kashrut*, and developed their own cuisine. They have also produced a lasting impact on world cuisine, especially that of Spain and Portugal, but also in France and Italy. This stems in part from the length of time spent in those countries, although, ironically, due to the persecution they experienced there. Pork and other forbidden foods were often added to traditional dishes to show the sincerity of conversion and to prove that one was not a Jew. *Cocido*, the Spanish meat stew, is the only dish found in every region in Spain and is thought to have derived from the Sabbath dish *adafina*; pork, and sometimes *morcilla* (blood sausage), was added. *Olla podrida* is another dish similar to *adafina*; the dish has chicken and eggs, chick peas, cabbage, and spices; again, pork was added. Chorizo, a dried pork sausage, or a dried ham, was also hung by the rafters as proof that no Jew lived in the house.

The Jewish tradition of cooking one-pot meals overnight is ancient and has to do with the interdiction of lighting fires on the Sabbath coupled with the mitzvah of providing a hot meal to the family. *Cholent* is the classic Sabbath stew. Because no light can be lit on the Sabbath ("Ye shall kindle no fire throughout your habitations upon the Sabbath day" [Exodus 35:3]), and it is a mitzvah to provide a family with a hot meal, the long-cooking *cholent* arose. The name is believed to come from the medieval French *chaud* (hot) and *lent* (slow). The basic *cholent* is barley, beans, potatoes, and meat, although other foods, including eggs, sausages, onions, and garlic, are added. Although typical of the Ashkenazim, *dafina* and *hamin* are similar and are the "Sabbath pot" for the Sephardim. *Dafina* is often made with chickpeas, potatoes, rice, meat, and spices. *Cholent* may have become *cassoulet* in France. In Italy, deep-fried artichokes and caponata, as well as cold fried fish and other cold dishes, are standard. Jews are largely responsible for introducing New World foods to the Mediterranean areas.

After the early dispersion of Jews from the Middle East, there was an almost complete separation of Sephardic and Ashkenazi Jews; they did not "reunite" until the 20th century. At that time, there was a wide difference in their foods and cooking styles. There were also differences in the foods that are allowable for Passover (described below).

FOOD HISTORY WITHIN THE CULTURE

Historically, the principal influence on Jewish food and Jewish cooking is *Kashrut*. Food in accord with Jewish law (*Halakha*) is termed kosher (in English), from the Hebrew word *kasher*, meaning "fit." The word did not originally apply to food, but it was originally used in the Bible (Esther 8:5 and Ecclesiastes 11:6) to mean "good" or "proper." It was later applied to ritual objects, and finally to food. Food that is not kosher is informally called *treife*, although the word actually means "torn" and refers to improperly slaughtered meat.

Throughout history, Jews have endangered their lives for *Kashrut*. Hannah and her seven sons chose death rather than transgress the dietary laws (Apocrypha II Maccabees 6:12–17) and eat pork. The Jewish Dietary Laws, found in the *Tanakh*, evolved stepwise (see Table 3-1). The commandments are brief; thus, they have been interpreted and amplified on "a generous scale" over a time period of several thousand years, notably in the *Talmud*. The *Talmud* is comprised of two components—the *Mishnah* (c. 200 CE), which is the written form of Jewish oral tradition, and the *Gemara* (c. 500 CE), which contains rabbinical commentaries and the analysis of the *Mishnah*.

Although early Jewish and Arab physicians and historians, including Maimonides, al-Demiry, and al-Maqrizy, describe diet and health in relationship to the dietary laws, it was not until the late 19th century that the codified dietary prohibitions received serious study (Grivetti & Pangborn, 1974). A principal point of interest was the prohibition of pork, which is perhaps the best known of the dietary laws to non-Jews. Several theories have been used to explain the dietary laws; however, the three that have received the most attention are health, ethnic identity, and ecological arguments (Grivetti & Pangborn, 1974). When these theories are examined, it is important to consider the historical time in which they arose.

TABLE 3-1   Biblical Injunctions for *Kashrut:* Stepwise Development of the Jewish Dietary Laws

Stage One

Genesis 1:29–31: All products on earth are clean.

"And God said, Behold, I have given you every herb bearing seed . . . to you it should be meat."

Stage Two

Genesis 1:29–31: Plant food constituted the initial diet of humans.

"And to every beast of the earth, and to every fowl of the air, and to everything that creepth upon the earth, wherein there is life, I have given every green herb for meat: and it was so."

Stage Three

At the time of the flood, in Genesis 7:1–2, clean and unclean animals are distinguished, but not identified.

"Of every clean beast, thou shalt take to thee by sevens, the male and his female: and of beasts that are not clean by two: the male and his female."

Stage Four

In Genesis 7:1–2 both clean and unclean animals are brought onto the ark and saved.

Stage Five

In Genesis 9:3–4, Noah and his descendents are permitted all food, except blood, after the flood. The diet is defined as a combination of plant and animal foods.

"Every moving thing that liveth shall be meat for you; even as the green herb have I given you all things . . . . But flesh with the life thereof, which is blood thereof, shall ye not eat."

"Only ye shall not eat the blood; ye shall pour it upon the earth as water."

Blood was prohibited in Genesis 9:3–4; Deuteronomy 12:16, 23–24, 15:12; I Samuel 12:32–34; and Ezekiel 4:14.

Stage Six

Clean and unclean flesh foods are specified and other forbidden foods and food-related behaviors are codified. Clean meats are identified in Leviticus 11:2–3, 9, 21–22; and Deuteronomy 14:4–6, 9, 11, 20.

"Speak unto the children of Israel, saying, 'These are the beasts which ye shall eat among all beasts that are on the earth . . . . Whatsoever parteth the hoof, and is clovenfooted, and cheweth the cud, among the beasts, that shall ye eat . . . . These shall ye eat of all that are in the waters: whatsoever hath fins and scales in the waters, in the seas, and in the rivers them shall ye eat . . . . And these are they which ye shall have in abomination among the fowls: they shall not be eaten, they are in abomination.'"

It is often assumed that health was the reason; however, there is no basis for this belief (Regenstein, 1994). Although pigs are associated with trichinosis, the cyst causing the infection was not observed until 1822, and the association of improperly cooked pork and trichinosis was not shown until 1860. There is also evidence that trichinosis was unknown in the Middle East in antiquity (Grivetti & Pangborn, 1974). Moreover, cooking pork to an internal temperature of at least 144°F will kill trichinosis (United States Food and Drug Administration Title 9 318.10); because most Jews thoroughly cook meat, it is unlikely that this was a problem. Prohibiting carrion is also assumed to have a health basis, although other societies, even those in the tropics, use carrion as a staple food. Most of the unclean foods do not pose health risks, and several of the clean foods are associated with anthrax, brucellosis, tapeworm, and other parasitic diseases that have mortality rates equivalent to those of trichinosis. Finally, there are no prohibitions against toxic plants, including certain mushroom species, which, when consumed, are almost always fatal. The assumption that ancient Hebrews employed sophisticated epidemiological methods to determine dietary laws lacks evidence.

Explanations based on ethnic identity assume that foods that are unclean were consumed or even worshiped by Egyptians, Canaanites, and Romans. This is true; however, meats on the "clean" list, including beef, goat, and lamb, were consumed by the Egyptians, and cattle, goats, and sheep were worshiped by them (Darby, Ghalioungui, & Grivetti, 1977). There is historic support that the codes directed toward pork and the mixing of meat and milk products are linked to this hypothesis. The ancient Egyptian (c. 1341–1085 BCE) ate large quantities of pork and the prohibition may have stemmed from an attempt to remain apart from their oppressors. Ancient Babylonians (5 BCE) not only consumed pork, but used pigs in sacrificial rights. The prohibition of consuming milk and meat during the same meal is thought to have arisen from the commandment not to seethe the kid in the mother's milk, codified in the *Talmud* (Hullin 8:104a-b). There is evidence to suggest that this results from a Canaanite practice of boiling a kid in the milk of its mother and spreading the resulting mixture over the fields as a ritual offering to Astarte, the goddess of fertility (Grivetti & Pangborn, 1974).

Finally, it has been argued that animals such as pigs could not compete economically with sheep and goats and were not suited to the climate; however, these animals were raised in Egypt, which had a similar climate. Pigs did not produce milk or wool and they would have been in direct competition with animals that did. (Darby et al., 1977). It is unlikely that this argument contributed to the development of the dietary laws.

It is interesting to speculate on the "why" of the dietary laws; however, the reality is that the only reason to follow most dietary laws is that they were given as commandments. Blood is the single exception: It was prohibited three times in the Hebrew Bible (see Table 3-1). Ancients saw blood as a substance that might transmit the qualities of the dead to the living. Some tribes drank the blood of a slain hero so that his courage could fill their own bodies, and some used blood of their totem in the hope of being strengthened. For the Jews, because there was to be no other source of life and strength but God, the other "life" was not to be ingested.

Why do any Jews follow the dietary laws when obeying them clearly means a potentially costly and time-consuming process that requires so much dedication? The three most logical answers would be (1) it is a declaration of the covenant and creates a Jewish lifestyle, (2) it is an expression of faith and discipline, and (3) Jews have been commanded to keep these laws. The term holy (*Kadosh*) means to "set apart," and Jews have set themselves apart from the world to link with God and grow in holiness through discipline in diet (Trepp, 1980).

The dietary laws focus primarily on three issues, all concerning animal products: allowed animals, prohibition of blood, and prohibition of mixing milk and meat. These laws dictate the type of animal products that can be eaten and tradition dictates when they can be eaten. The *Torah* divides all beings into four groups: (1) domesticated animals and beasts, (2) birds, (3) fish, and (4) insects and reptiles. Ruminants with split hooves that chew their cud, traditionally consumed domestic birds, and fish with fins and removable scales are generally permitted; thus, cattle, oxen, bison, goats, sheep, deer, and gazelles can be eaten. Foods that are unclean (*treife*) include pigs, bears, horses, camels, rabbits, birds of prey or scavengers, reptiles, amphibians, shellfish, and some fin fish. Milk and eggs from forbidden animals are also forbidden.

Kosher Slaughter (*Shehitah*) and the *Kashering* of Meat

Allowable mammals and birds must be slaughtered in accordance with Jewish law. *Shehitah* is performed by a trained, religious person (*shochet*) with rabbinical authorization. The *shochet* uses a knife (*chalef*) specifically designed for this process. It must be extremely sharp, have no nicks, and have a very straight blade that is at least twice the diameter of the neck of the animal. Prior to the slaughter, the *shochet* makes a blessing; however, it is the process itself that makes the food kosher. Failure to sever the trachea, esophagus, and vessels with one cut renders an animal *neveila* (animals that die from reasons other than ritual slaughter).

Animals are not stunned prior to slaughter, and if done correctly, the animal will die without signs of stress. In 1958, the U.S. Congress declared kosher slaughter to be humane, and included an exemption for preslaughter handing of the animal (Grandin, 2006).

After slaughter, rabbinically trained inspectors inspect the organs of the animal; if visible defects are found, the animal becomes *treife*. The defects cannot be trimmed as is generally permitted under secular law. The lungs must be inspected; lungs without any adhesions (*sirkas*) meet the stricter standard known as glatt kosher ("glatt" is Yiddish for smooth). Glatt only refers to the lungs and only to the lungs of large herd animals.

Meat (cows, veal, lamb, and buffalo) must be prepared further by removing certain veins, arteries, prohibited fats, blood, and sciatic nerve. This process (*nikkur*) is done by a specially trained person

(*Menacker*). It is difficult and time-consuming to remove the sciatic nerve and attendant vessels, so in the United States and most other Western countries, this is not done and renders the hindquarters of the animal unusable. The meat is sold for consumption by non-Jews.

Shehitah allows for rapid draining of blood and is the first step in removing blood from the animals. Blood drained in this manner cannot be used. The remaining blood must be removed from the meat, either by broiling or soaking and salting (*melicha*) within 72 hours of slaughter and before the meat is cooked, frozen, or ground. To kosher meat, it is soaked in cool water for 30 minutes; after allowing excess water to drain, the meat is salted for 1 hour with all surfaces, including all cut surfaces and inside the cavity of fowl, covered with salt. The salted meat must be able to drain and the blood must be able to flow away freely. Following salting, the meat is rinsed three times. Alternately, meat can be broiled; liver must be *kashered* by broiling because of the number of blood vessels. Once the meat is *kashered*, any remaining "red liquid" is not considered blood and the meat can be used as desired; however, by tradition, most meat is served well done.

Koshering salt is chemically similar to other salts but has no additives such as iodine; however, it may contain yellow prussicate of soda as an anti-caking agent. The salt used must have a crystal size large enough that it will not dissolve within the hour, but small enough to completely cover the meat. Typically in the United States meat is *kashered* commercially and primal cuts weighing 20–40 lbs. are used. Salt penetration is less than 0.5 cm in red meat (Regenstein, Chaudry, & Regenstein, 2003a); however, the amount of sodium actually absorbed by the meat is unknown.

To ensure that kosher meat and poultry remain kosher, they must be supervised from the time of slaughter until they reach the consumer. A metal tag called a plumba, bearing the kosher symbol, is often clamped to the meat or fowl or the product is packed in tamper-proof packaging with the kosher logo displayed.

The *Torah* does not identify clean birds, but does identify 24 unclean birds. Kosher birds have a stomach lining that can be removed with the rest of the gizzard, cannot be a bird of prey, and must have a tradition of being eaten; thus, chicken, turkey, squab (not commercially slaughtered in the United States), duck, and goose are kosher. Birds must be slaughtered and *kashered* as described above for meat. Birds cannot be dipped in hot water to remove feathers prior to *kashering* because it will cause the blood to coagulate.

Most fin fish can be eaten. For fish to be acceptable the scales must be visible to the naked eye and be removable without tearing the skin; the ganoid and placoid scales of sharks and gar are not allowable. Conservative authorities permit sturgeon and sturgeon roe, whereas most Orthodox authorities do not. Fish need not be *kashered* because the Biblical injunction does not include them and they have minimal amounts of blood.

Most insects are not kosher. The exception is a few types of grasshoppers where the tradition of eating them has not been lost. Honey and some other products from bees, including beeswax, are also allowed, as are lac resin and shellac used as coatings on candy and fruit.

Prohibition of Mixing Milk and Meat

"Thou shalt not seeth the kid in its mother's milk" appears three times in the *Torah* (see Table 3-1) and has been interpreted as a complete separation of milk and meat. In the *Talmud*, this injunction was extended to poultry, but not to fish. Milk and meat cannot be cooked together, eaten together, and a benefit cannot be derived from mixing them (Regenstein et al., 2003a). Regenstein et al. (2003a) used the example of not owning a cheeseburger business, but more subtle examples can be found: A pet food cannot contain milk and meat because feeding a pet is considered a benefit.

Meat (*fleishig* in Yiddish; *basar* in Hebrew) includes allowable animals and cuts of meat (see Table 3-2), but not fish; and milk includes all milk products (*milchig* in Yiddish; *chalav* in Hebrew) including fluid milk, cheese, and yogurt. To ensure a complete separation, milk and meat cannot touch each other, be cooked together, be served together, or be consumed together. *Pareve*, or neutral foods, such as grains, vegetables, fruit, and eggs, can be served with either a milk or meat meal (human breast milk is *pareve* and breast feeding is encouraged); however, if these foods are mixed with meat or milk, they take on the identity of the product with which they were mixed. For example, if vegetables are buttered, they become a dairy food. Milk or other dairy foods may not be consumed after a meat meal for an interval of several hours (the time varies according to custom). For example, in Holland, the wait is 72 minutes, German Jews wait 3 hours, and those from eastern Europe wait 6 hours. Some authorities base this on the time required for the breakdown of meat particles trapped in the teeth and residue that clings to the palate, whereas others base the waiting time on how long it takes the food to be digested. The length of time between consuming a milk product and a meat product also varies according to custom but is much shorter because it is believed that dairy products do not leave a residue in the mouth. In some cultures there is no formal waiting period, but a person must rinse his or her mouth after eating a dairy food prior to eating meat. Hard cheese is an exception, and because it clings to the palate, many authorities require the full waiting period to be observed. This waiting period is in place so that milk and meat do not mix within the body.

Kosher status is transmitted in the presence of heat. Utensils acquire the kosher status of the foods that are cooked in or eaten from them and they transmit this status to the next food they contact; thus, observant households must have at least two sets of utensils, cutlery, and dishes. In practice, most households have two sets for everyday use, two sets for special meals such as the Sabbath, and two sets for Passover. It is likely that the porous nature of pottery, from which dishes were made originally, led to this injunction. Pottery or ceramic cannot be *kashered*. Because glass dishes are not absorbent, it is widely believed that they can be used interchangeably with milk and meat dishes. Although technically correct, it is the intent of the law to have separate sets of dishes, regardless of the material, and the deliberate use of glass dishes for milk and meat meals weakens the spirit of *Kashrut*. Jewish law permits drinking glasses to be used interchangeably with milk and meat dishes; however, if they are washed in a dishwasher, they should be washed with the respective milk or meat dishes.

Sinks, stoves, and dishwashers are easily made nonkosher. Ideally, homes have a double stainless steel sink with one half used for meat and one half used for dairy. If this is not possible, then the sink should be treated as treif and separate kosher basins must be used to soak or wash the dishes. It is not necessary to have separate ovens and stoves for meat and milk; however, if the same oven is used for both, care should be taken to avoid spills, and meat and dairy cannot be cooked in the same oven at the same time. Many people avoid this problem by having separate ovens. When cooking on a stove, care needs to be taken to avoid splatters. It is best to specify the meat and milk burners, covering the unused side with foil. The same dishwasher can be used for meat and dairy cutlery and dishes; however, separate dish racks must be used or the dishwasher must be run between meat and dairy loads. Explicit instructions are available from kosher certification agencies on koshering kitchen equipment. Separate

TABLE 3-2   Permitted and Prohibited Cuts of Meat Commonly Eaten in the United States

	Permitted[a]	Prohibited
Beef	Brisket, chuck, flanken, rib eye, rib steak, rib top, short rib, standing rib roast, shoulder roast, and skirt steak. Offal from these animals (liver, brain, lungs, feet, and intestines) is also permitted.	Flank, round, rump, porterhouse steaks, shank, T-bone steaks, sirloin, and top loin (strip and shell steaks)
Veal	Breast, brisket, cutlets, shoulder, rib chops, and rib roast. Offal is also permitted.	Flank, hind shank, leg, and loin
Lamb	Breast (roast, brisket), neck, rib (chops, roast), shank, and shoulder (chops, roast). Offal is also permitted.	Leg[b] and loin
Poultry[c]	Capon, chicken, Cornish hen, duck, goose, pigeon, turkey, and the livers, gizzards, necks, and feet of these birds.	All other birds

[a]Other clean meats, such as deer, can be eaten if farm raised or trapped and appropriately slaughtered. Deer that is hunted is not permitted. As with other meats, the hind quarters are not eaten.

[b]The leg may be eaten if the sciatic nerve (the Sinew of Jacob) and attendant vessels are removed. This is difficult and requires special training; thus, it is generally not done in the Diaspora. There are butchers in Israel that do this, and meat from the hindquarters is sold to non-Jews. When done appropriately, this renders the cut kosher.

[c]The Biblical law related to removal of the sciatic nerve does not apply to birds since they do not have a spoon-shaped hip.

towels and potholders should be used. Many Jews have separate condiments because these products often touch food during service. Nonkosher items, including soaps, may not be used in kosher kitchens.

Hospitals, catering operations, and even children's camps (Feitelson & Fiedler, 1982) that prepare kosher meals have two separate kitchens to avoid any possibility of error. If your facility does not have a kosher kitchen or cannot cater a kosher meal, a kosher meal or diet cannot be provided for a patient or client. There is no "kosher-style" food. Most airlines can provide kosher meals with advance notice, although individuals should check with their rabbis about the specifics of certification. Restaurants are generally certified as serving either dairy or meat meals.

A wide range of explanations for not mixing milk and meat have been proposed. These explanations include:

1. The practice was contrary to nature and an abomination.
2. It was not a compassionate act to boil meat in the fluid intended for its own nourishment.
3. The combination gave pleasure and should be denied to demonstrate self-restraint.

Some people have suggested that the reason for prohibiting the mixing of meat and milk might have to do with sympathetic magic, specifically that animals could control their milk after humans had obtained it and the boiling of milk was tantamount to applying fire to the animals' udders. As with all of *Kashrut*, ultimately the reason for doing this is that it is a Biblical injunction that has been interpreted in such a way that meat and milk cannot be consumed together (Grivetti, 2000).

Kosher Certification

It is critical to have a means to identify which foods are kosher. A hechsher (Hebrew for "kosher approval" identifies which foods are kosher. Hechshers are registered trademarks and cannot be used indiscriminately. Care should be taken when a food is marked with the single letter "K" alone because this product may or may not be kosher. To ensure that *Kashrut* is not violated, food service operations should check with a rabbi prior to using these foods. Approximately 75,000 products in the United States, including those from major food companies such as Kraft and Nabisco, have kosher certification (Regenstein, Chaudry, and Regenstein, 2003b). It is not clear how many Jews in the United

States follow the dietary laws, but it has been estimated that fewer than one third, and possibly as few as 20% of kosher consumers, are Jewish, with only 900,000 year-round consumers (Regenstein et al., 2003b). Other consumers who use kosher certification marks are Muslims, Seventh-Day Adventists, vegetarians, people with food allergies, and those who value the quality of kosher products.

Kosher Certification Companies

Orthodox Union	http://www.ou.org
Organized Kashrut	http://www.ok.org
Star-K	http://www.star-k.org
Kof-K	http://www.kof-k.org

In the United States, four large companies dominate the supervision of kosher foods and manufacturing processes: the Orthodox Union (OU; http://www.ou.org/), the Organized Kashrut (OK; http://www.ok.org/), the Star-K (http://www.star-k.org/), and the Kof-K (http://www.kof-k.org/). These companies usually accept each other's kosher products (Regenstein et al., 2003b). The OU and the Star-K are part of a larger community of religious organizations, whereas the Kof-K and the OK are private companies and their only function is to provide kosher certification. There are many smaller companies that also provide supervision and certification. *KASHRUS* magazine (http://www.kashrusmagazine.com) reviews symbols yearly; in 2008, there were 921 kosher symbols and agencies worldwide. It also provides consumer online alerts. (Another resource is found at www.kashrut.com/.) Some companies include whether a food is a dairy (D), meat (M), or *pareve* (P) food, or a food manufactured with dairy equipment (DE). A "P" does not indicate that a food is kosher for Passover; those foods are certified with the word "Passover." Not all companies provide these more detailed markings, and without them, confusion and recalls can occur.

Kashrut and kosher certification of foods is not static. With new food products, including bioengineered food (Chaudry & Regenstein, 1994; Regenstein et al., 2003b) available, and changing manufacturing processes, it is important that modern religious authorities continue to interpret and apply traditional laws.

The other significant influence on Jewish food and cooking is the Sabbath and the Jewish holidays (see Table 3-3). The Sabbath sets the rhythm of the Jewish

TABLE 3-3 The Sabbath and Jewish Holidays Associated with Fasting or Special Food Customs

Holiday	Date(s)	Significance	Food Customs
The Sabbath	Friday from 18 minutes before sunset until Saturday night, when three stars are visible, about 40 minutes after sunset	The Hebrew word "Shabbat" comes from the root *Shin-Bet-Tav*, meaning to cease, to end, or to rest. The Sabbath is a day of rest and spiritual activity. No work can be done on the Sabbath. It is considered the most important day in the Jewish calendar. Keeping the Sabbath means keeping the commandment to "Remember the Sabbath day and keep it holy" (Exodus 20:8) and "Observe the Sabbath day and keep it holy" (Deuteronomy 5:12).	The Sabbath meal (Table 3-4) should be the finest that the family can afford. *Challah* and wine are served, and it is customary for Jews to eat fish on Friday night. Roast chicken is also typically served by Ashkenazi Jews. Since no work can be done, no fires can be lit; thus, stoves and ovens cannot be turned on, and cooking must be finished before the Sabbath starts on Friday night. It is a mitzvah to provide a hot meal on Saturday, and long-cooking foods, such as *cholent*, were developed. The dual nature of the commandment means two loaves of *challah* and two candles.
Rosh Hashanah	First of Tishri; usually falls in late September or early October	The New Year, which begins at sundown and is celebrated for 2 days.	Sweet foods are eaten to ensure a sweet year. Apples dipped in honey are traditionally eaten; figs are another sweet fruit that is eaten. Round foods, such as *challah*, meatballs, peas, and chickpeas, are eaten since this carries the connotation that the year is full and rounded. Green vegetables are eaten to symbolize a new beginning. Fish, a symbol of fertility, is served with the head on to express the hope of being at the head. Carrot slices are associated with gold coins in Jewish folklore, and carrot tzimmes is served. Pomegranates are also eaten since it is said to have 613 seeds—the same number as the commandments.
Tzom Gedaliah[a]	The day after Rosh Hashanah	This day commemorates the assignation of Gedaliah, the last governor of Judea. It is one of the four fast days commemorating the destruction of the Temple.	This is a minor fast day; fasting is required only from sunrise to sunset.
Yom Kippur[a]	The 10th of Tishri, 10 days after Rosh Hashanah	Yom Kippur is the day of atonement.	This is a full fast: no food and water, from sundown until sundown of the next day. The meal before the fast is filling but bland so as not to cause thirst. Ashkenazis typically eat chicken soup with stuffed matzoh balls so that "kindness will cover any strict judgment of misdeeds" at this meal. For breaking the fast, chicken is traditionally served. Sometimes a dairy meal was actually used to break the fast; this was followed by a short wait, and then the chicken meal was consumed.

(continues)

TABLE 3-3 (Continued)

Holiday	Date(s)	Significance	Food Customs
Sukkot	Beginning on the 15th of Tishri and lasting 8 days (7 in Israel); usually falls in early October	Sukkot is the Feast of the Tabernacles and Jews spend time in a sukkah, a booth built with plants and branches to represent both the huts in which the Jews lived during their time in the wilderness and God's protection. Sukkot is also a harvest festival.	Fruit and vegetables are frequently eaten and meals are taken in the sukkah. An Ashkenazi tradition is to consume chicken soup with kreplach on the last day of the festival; the soup symbolizes the covering of God's stringency with his loving kindness.
Shemini Atzeret/ Simhat *Torah*— Reveling with the *Torah*	Immediately following the last day of Sukkot, 8th day of Assembly (Tishri 22, 23)	The conclusion to Sukkot is a full festival day with kiddush and candle lighting and prohibition on working. There is a circling of the scrolls the night of Shemini Atzeret. For Simhat *Torah* water is the theme; the last passage of the *Torah* is read.	Fruit and cookies are often served, but unlike most holidays, symbolic foods are not served.
Chanukah	An 8-day celebration beginning the 25th of Kislev	Chanukah commemorates the victory of the Maccabees against the Greeks and the miracle of the cruise of oil that burned for 8 days instead of 1 day. Although popularized in the United States, this is a minor Jewish holiday.	Fried foods are consumed to commemorate the miracle of the burning oil. In the United States, potato latkes are usually served. Jews from other parts of the world eat fried jelly donuts or other fried foods.
Asarah B'Tevet[a]	The 10th of Tevet	Kaddish is said for those whose date and place of death is unknown; some rabbis have designated this as a day of remembrance for the Holocaust.	This is a minor fast day; fasting is required only from sunrise to sunset.
Tu Bishvat: Tasting of the Tree	The 15th day of Shevat	A minor festival that is one of the four "new years" of the Jewish calendar.	Eating the fruit of Israel is associated with this day.
Ta'anit Esther[a]	The eve of Purim (Adar 14)	The fast of Esther commemorates the 3-day fast of the Jews of Persia at Esther's request.	This is a minor fast with fasting from sunrise to sunset.
Purim	Adar 14 usually falls in March	A holiday of self-mockery and masquerade, Purim celebrates the victory of Mordechai and Esther over Haman. The story is told in the Book of Esther.	Purim is a time of feasting. Ashkenazi Jews serve Hamantaschen, a triangular cake traditionally filled with poppy seeds or prunes and representing Haman's hat. Poppy seeds are in memory of Esther's fast during which she ate only seeds. Sephardic Jews serve orejas de Aman

TABLE 3-3   (Continued)

Holiday	Date(s)	Significance	Food Customs
			(Haman's ears)—fried pastries dipped in syrup. Food is traditionally exchanged with friends. Purim ends with the Purim *seudah*, which traditionally ranks second to the Passover Seder as a special meal. This is the only holiday meal where heavy drinking is encouraged. The meal is usually vegetarian and dairy since Esther consumed a vegetarian diet within the palace so as not to break the dietary laws.
Ta'anit Bechorim[a]	Eve of Passover	Represents the gratitude to God for sparing the first born of Israel.	A minor fast from sunrise to sundown; usually only the first-born son fasts.
Passover (Pesach)	Beginning on the 14th of Nisan and lasting 8 days (7 days in Israel); usually falls in April	Pesach is a major festival ordained in the Bible. The Bible commands that Passover be celebrated for 7 days, and it is in Israel; however, for the Diaspora, it is celebrated for 8 days due to uncertainty about the calendar.	The Seder is celebrated the first night of Passover (outside of Israel, it is celebrated the first 2 nights) and includes reading the Haggaddah, which recounts the story of the exodus, the Seder plate, and a festive meal. The Seder is discussed separately in the text.
Shavuot	The 6th day of Sivan (7th day for those in the Diaspora); usually falls in late May or June	Celebrates the giving of the *Torah* to the Jews at Mount Sinai and their becoming a nation by accepting the commandments.	A dairy meal is eaten; this is attributed to the Biblical citation "And He gave us this land flowing with milk and honey" (Deuteronomy 26:9), and because the Jews did not have time to slaughter and kosher meat after leaving Sinai. Shavuot is also a harvest festival of fruit; fruit puddings and cakes are consumed.
Shiva Asar B'Tammuz[a]	The 17th of Tammuz	A number of catastrophes have been associated with this day, most notably breaching of the walls of Jerusalem by the Romans (70 CE) and the incident of the golden calf at Sinai.	This is a minor fast day; fasting is required only from sunrise to sunset.
Tisha B'Av[a]	Ninth of Av	This day marks the day of the destruction of both Temples, the first by the Babylonians in 586 BCE and the second by the Romans in 70 CE. This is a day of catastrophe because of the incident of the spies.	This is a full fast: no food and water, from sundown until sundown of the next day. It is preceded by a meal called the *seudah ha-mafseket*—literally the meal that "interrupts" or differentiates between a regular day and the fast day. Some eat food customarily provided for mourners: hard-boiled eggs and lentils. Ashes were once put in the food.

[a]Holiday associated with fasting. Note that, in addition, individuals may elect to fast at other times, the most common of which are the anniversary of death of a parent or teacher, by the bride and groom on their wedding day (unless it occurs on a Rosh Chodesh), or when a *Torah* scroll is dropped.

household and is central to Jewish life. Keeping the Sabbath is a sign of the covenant between God and Israel. The Sabbath is observed from 18 minutes before sundown on Friday until three stars can be seen in the sky on Saturday. Work, including lighting a fire, is prohibited on the Sabbath. But to ensure a sense of celebration, three feasts, and in some cultures four, are prescribed for the Sabbath; it is also a mitzvah (commandment) to provide a hot meal on Saturday. The core rituals for the Sabbath are lighting the candles, blessing the wine and bread, and eating the meal. The meal should be the best the family can afford (see Table 3-4).

TABLE 3-4 Sample Menus

Typical Day	Sabbath[a]	Holiday/Pesach
French toast with fruit	Wine	Seder plate
1% milk	Salmon cakes	Hamine eggs, matzoth, haroset, wine
Calcium-fortified orange juice	Cold spinach soup	Chicken soup with poached chicken balls
Tomato soup	Roast chicken	
Toasted cheese sandwiches	Roast potatoes	Cold salmon and parsley sauce
Tabouli	Beet salad	Stuffed lamb shoulder
Pears	Meringues with stewed fruit	Marinated red pepper strips and potato salad
Cookies	Cholent[b]	
Milk	Marinated vegetables	Sautéed spinach with garlic
Brisket cooked with carrots, onions, celery, and red wine	Apple salad	Orange flan[d] and almond macaroons
	Challah[c]	Grapefruit halves
Rice and chickpeas	Herring salad	Leek omelet
Sautéed green beans	Cakes	Matzoth
Fennel salad	Sparkling water	Milk
Applesauce		Pumpkin soup
		Moroccan salad plate
		Carrot salad
		Mixed vegetable salad
		Orange and olive salad
		Plain yogurt
		Lemon granita

Note: The typical day menu and Sabbath menu are consistent with Ashkenazi foods, whereas the Pesach menu is more consistent with foods of the Sephardim.

[a]By tradition, three meals are prescribed to be eaten on the Sabbath. The first meal is Friday night, the second is around noon (after the morning service), and the third is a light meal (*seudah shlishit*) eaten late in the afternoon, usually after the *Mincha* service. The tradition of three meals is from the Biblical verse Exodus 16:25, which describes the miracle of the manna in the desert three times. Many people also eat a fourth meal (*Melaveh Malka*) on Saturday night, which is another way of "bidding farewell to the Sabbath queen." (Kolatch, 2000).

[b]Although no fire can be lit on the Sabbath, it is a mitzvah to provide one's family with a hot meal. *Cholent, dafina, adafina,* or *hamin,* types of stew cooked overnight, are traditionally served; ingredients vary widely, and may include meat, eggs, wheat, rice, potatoes, and beans.

[c]Some groups refrain from eating bread at this meal. *Challah* is given as an example; mideastern Jews might eat pita or another type of bread.

[d]Made with almonds, eggs, and orange juice rather than milk or cream.

There are a total of 39 restrictions for the Sabbath that include limiting growing and preparing food, making clothing, writing, and creating fire.

Jewish holidays can be dichotomized into feast days and fast days (see Table 3-3). Feast days include Purim, Passover (*Pesach*), Shavuot, Rosh Hashanah, Sukkot, and Chanukah. All of them are associated with special foods and food symbolism, but none more so than Passover and the Passover Seder (see Table 3-5), the 8-day festival of freedom that commemorates the Exodus. During this time, no leavening (*chametz*) can be owned or consumed, and benefit cannot occur; this necessitates a thorough cleaning of the house to remove all traces of leavening and leavened agents and a complete change of dishes, cutlery, and other utensils. *Chametz* can be burned or sold prior to Passover. During this time the only grain product that can be consumed is *matzah*, the unleavened bread of Passover. It is also important that during this time observant Jews consume only foods certified "Kosher for Passover."

The word Seder means "order" and the foods are eaten in the order prescribed in the Passover prayer book (*Haggada*). There are five obligations (mitzvahs) performed by each Jew in the course of the Seder, three of which include specific foods or drink: (1) eating matzahs, (2) drinking four cups of wine (*Arbah Kosos*), (3) eating bitter herbs (*Maror*), (4) relating the story of the Exodus (*Haggadah*), and (5) reciting Psalms of Praise (*Hallel*).

Tisha b'Av and Yom Kippur are full 25-hour fasts with no food or water from sunset to sunset for all Jews

TABLE 3-5 The Symbolic Foods of Passover. The Seder Plate (*k'arah*) for Passover (*Pessah*)

Karpas: a green vegetable, such as parsley or Bibb lettuce, which symbolizes spring and rebirth. It is dipped in salt water as a reminder of the tears shed by the Israelites during their years of slavery. *Karpas* is dipped twice to invoke children to ask about this practice. The salt water is placed on the Seder table, but not the Seder plate.

Charoset: a fruit and nut paste that symbolizes the color of mortar that the slaves made for bricks in Egypt. The *maror* is dipped into the *charoset* to lessen the bitter herbs' taste. Ashkenazi Jews often use a mixture of chopped apples, nuts, sweet wine, and spices, whereas Sephardic versions tend to include exotic fruits such as dates or bananas.

Maror: means "bitter herbs" and is used as the symbol of the bitterness of slavery. Romaine, freshly ground horseradish, endive, or escarole can be used.

Beitzah: a roasted egg, which is the symbol of the festival sacrifice (*korban hagigah*) offered by each Jew going to the Temple. The egg should be hard-boiled, then scorched on a stove.

Zeroa is a roasted bone, commonly a lamb shank that is symbolic of the Passover sacrifice (*korban pesah*). The bone should be roasted and then scorched like the egg to simulate the sacrifice that was roasted. For vegetarians, a broiled beet has been suggested as an alternative.

Hazeret: some Seder plates have *hazeret* as a sixth symbol, which is to be used for the *koriekh* sandwich of *matzah* and *maror*. This is done since Hillel believed that they were eaten together.

Matzah: plain flour and water matzah; the plain bread of affliction must be used. Three matzah, not placed on the Seder plate but next to it, are used to represent the three categories of Jews: priests (*kohanim*); Levites; and Israelites. Some people prefer to use *matzah shemurah* (watched matzah) for the Seder; these *matzah* are made from grain that has been watched from the time of harvest to prevent contact with water that could lead to fermentation and possible leavening. This *matzah* will be certified as kosher for Passover.

Wine: one that is kosher for Passover is needed; each person is required to drink four cups. Kosher-for-Passover grape juice can be used instead, and if neither can be drunk for reasons of health, any drink that you would serve guests can be used.

Elijah's Cup: an ornate goblet is set aside for Elijah, since according to legend, Elijah visits every home on Passover and drinks from his cup.

who are bar mitzvah or bat mitzvah. Even toothbrushing is forbidden on these days. Children under the age of 9 and women in childbirth (from the time labor begins until 3 days after birth) are not permitted to fast. Older children and women from the third to the seventh day after childbirth are permitted to fast, but they can break the fast if they feel the need. People with illnesses should consult a physician and a rabbi for advice on whether they should fast and what medications can be taken. Other fasts are minor fasts in which fasting is done from sunrise to sunset only.

MAJOR FOODS

Protein Sources

The forequarters of clean meat (beef, veal, goat, sheep, and bison) can be consumed (see Table 3-2). Because meat must be *kashered* within 72 hours of slaughter and the forequarters do not include the tenderest cuts, this has led to the tradition of braising and other methods of slow cooking. In the Ashkenazi tradition, brisket, corned beef, short ribs, stews, and pot roasts are commonly consumed, as are braised lamb shoulders or lamb shanks. Offal is often consumed; tongue is popular and chopped liver, generally made with chicken livers, is a staple food in Ashkenazi homes.

Chicken is very popular; it is usually associated with Ashkenazim, but it is also consumed by Sephardic Jews. Because it was expensive in eastern Europe, it became associated with special meals, such as the Sabbath. Today, roast chicken is traditionally served on Friday nights.

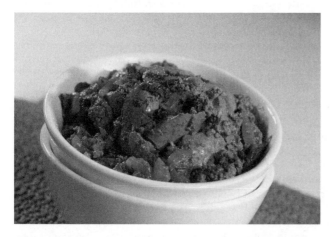

Chopped liver, generally made with chicken livers, is very popular in Ashkenazi homes.

Fish plays an important role in the diet of many Jews. Fish is a symbol of fertility, because Jacob gave his children the blessing that they should be fruitful and multiply like fish in the sea. Fish are also associated with the coming of the Messiah. Fish are often consumed at holidays, especially Rosh Hashanah and Shavuot. The *Talmud* states that fish should be eaten on the Sabbath, and it is customary to eat fish on Friday night (see Table 3-4). Eating fish is also tied to the Creation story, and the *Midrash* (compilation of the homiletic teachings on the *Tanakh*) suggests that because fish were created on the fifth day, man on the sixth, and the Sabbath on the seventh, this combination should be kept with fish eaten to celebrate the Sabbath. The *Mishnah* writings on the Book of Genesis also states that all creatures were annihilated during the time of Noah except fish, because they did not sin. Because fires cannot be lit on the Sabbath, there is a tradition of cold fish dishes.

Fish can be consumed with either a milk or meat meal. If eaten with a meat meal, the fish cannot be served on the same plate, and should be consumed first. In Talmudic times, it was believed that this combination predisposed an individual to leprosy; however, there is no modern support for this theory. Although there is no waiting period between eating fish and meat, many rinse their mouth or eat bread to help dislodge any food remaining in the mouth. At Sabbath meals, soup may be served between the fish and meat dish to clear the palate.

The best known "Jewish" fish dish is gefilte fish, a dish going back to the early Middle Ages. Literally meaning "filled" or "stuffed" fish, this method of preparation reduced the cost of fish because different types of fish could be ground and mixed with matzomeal and eggs. This dish has changed over time; originally fish forcemeat was used to stuff pike or carp skin, whereas today, gefilte fish generally means the forcemeat alone poached in stock. The dish varies in different regions: In Poland it is sweet, whereas others prefer it unsweetened. In the United States, gefilte fish is generally served cold in fish aspic. Very traditional Chassidic Orthodox groups; for example, the Lubavitch, do not mix milk and fish.

Herring has always been another commonly consumed fish among the Ashkenazi Jews, being inexpensive and also widely available because it can be preserved in salt or brine. After soaking, herring can be eaten raw with a wedge of lemon or with sour cream. Salt herring is usually eaten with onion rings, although a variety of "trimmings," such as boiled eggs, apples, and brown bread, can also be served with the fish. Salmon is also a significant fish. The tradition of eating salt-cured fish has long been a custom.

Eggs are another commonly consumed protein food because they are *pareve*. Traditionally, eggs were examined in a glass cup prior to consumption to determine whether they contained blood. In the Sephardic tradition, eggs containing blood in the white may be used if the blood can be removed, but the egg must be discarded if blood is found on the yolk. Ashkenazis do not distinguish between blood in the white or on the yolk; thus, any egg with blood must be discarded. Partially formed eggs found inside slaughtered birds may be eaten, but they are considered meat and therefore must be *kashered*.

 ## Starch Sources

Unprocessed grains and cereals are kosher. Processed foods (e.g., ready-to-eat cereals), however, may contain nonkosher ingredients that cannot be eaten, or dairy ingredients, which would prohibit consumption of the food with a meat meal; thus, the kosher certification of processed foods should be examined prior to consumption of those foods.

For observant Jews, bread defines a meal and is the reminder of the priest's nourishment in the Temple. Jews must ritually wash their hands before consuming a meal with bread, but need not do so if the meal does not include bread. Bread also has its own *bracha* (blessing). If a loaf bread was served with a meat meal, and some is left over, it cannot be served with a dairy meal because there is fear that there may be a greasy meat residue on the bread.

Several breads are associated with Jews. *Challah*, a braided egg bread, is the Jewish Sabbath and holiday bread of the Ashkenazi, and is perhaps the best known. The name is derived from the Hebrew word for "portion" in the Biblical commandment of the first "of your dough shall be given to the Lord a portion of a gift throughout your generations." Jews were commanded to separate one twenty-fourth of their dough and give it to the *kohanim* (priests) every Sabbath. A portion was burned and a portion was eaten by the priest. In post-Temple times, rabbis have ordained that a portion at least the size of an olive had to be separated and burned. Jewish housewives and bakers tear a tiny lump of risen dough and burn it in the oven while making a blessing as a symbolic act. Traditionally, *challah* is dipped in salt before it is eaten, in remembrance of the sacrifices brought to the altar in Temple times.

Because the first two meals eaten on the Sabbath are usually meat meals, *challah* is made without milk and is *pareve*.

Challah became the Jewish ritual bread in Germany, Austria, and Bohemia before being taken to the East. On festive occasions, a blessing is said over two loaves, which represent the double portion of manna God provided on Friday to the children of Israel during their Exodus. When the manna fell to the ground it remained fresh—protected from the dew; this is symbolized by placing a board beneath the bread and a cloth above it. Sesame or poppy seeds are sprinkled to represent the dew. Since the Middle Ages, *challah* has been made in different sizes and shapes that have symbolic meanings. Braided ones are the most common, and with their intertwined arms they represent love. Three braids symbolize truth, peace, and justice. Twelve humps from two small or one large braided bread recall the miracle of the 12 loaves for the 12 tribes of Israel. Round loaves, with no beginning and no end, are baked for Rosh Hashanah to symbolize continuity. At the meal before the Yom Kippur fast, ladder and hand shapes are served so that the great heights can be ascended to, or the loaf may be bird shaped so that "sins be carried away by the bird."

Bagels were the everyday bread of the Jews in eastern Europe. Because they have no beginning and no end, they symbolize eternal life. At one time they were thought to protect against demons and evil spirits by warding off the evil eye and bringing luck. Bagels were served at circumcisions, during labor prior to childbirth, and at funerals. When Jews migrated to the United States, they brought the bagel with them and this commonly consumed bread is now the most

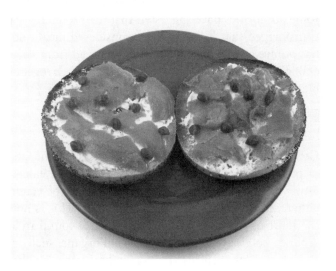

Lox and Bagel

recognized "Jewish" bread. Rye and pumpernickel bread, which are commonly consumed in eastern Europe, are other breads associated with Jews. Common sweet breads include *babka* (a yeasted coffee cake with chocolate or cinnamon) and *lekach* (honey cake).

The Sepahardim do not have such commonly recognized breads. Their traditional breads include pita, saloud (a Yemenite flatbread), and noon Rogani (an Azerbaijani spiral bread).

Matzah was a flat bread eaten by slaves, but it is also the bread of liberation. It is a *Torah* commandment to eat *matzah* the first night of Passover, and it is the only bread allowed during Passover when leavened breads are forbidden. *Matzah* reminds Jews of the Exodus since the Hebrews left Egypt with such haste that there was no time to allow baked bread to rise. Although available all year, *matzah* is the only grain product that can be eaten during Passover—and it must be marked kosher for Passover. For Passover, *matzah* can be made only from one of five grains—wheat, barley, spelt, oats, or rye—and the grains may not be used in any other way during the holiday. What these grains have in common is that they ferment when they are wet. *Matzah* is kneaded quickly, stamped out in a round or square and pricked with holes to prevent it from rising, and baked in a very hot oven. The time it takes for the water to be mixed with the flour and for the bread to be put into the oven cannot exceed 18 minutes. Unlike most commercially prepared breads, *matzah* is not vitamin fortified. During Passover, starch products, including noodles or baked goods, can be prepared with *matzah* or potato flour.

Gelatin is a controversial food. Most gelatin is prepared from the processed hides or bones of animals. Although most gelatins are considered nonkosher, some authorities have suggested that the product is so transformed that it is no longer considered meat and has *pareve* status. Kosher gelatins prepared from vegetable products, such as carrageenan and other vegetable gums, or fish, are also available.

Fat Sources

Certain fats are prohibited by the dietary laws. The fats of prohibited animals, such as lard, cannot be eaten. Other fat (*chelev*) from clean animals cannot be eaten either, and is removed by kosher butchers. This is not the marbled fat in meat, but that which is found in a separate solid layer, surrounding vital organs, such as the kidneys, or is enclosed in a membrane that can be easily peeled off. Because of the real likelihood that these fats can be mixed in a commercial product, it is important to examine products containing fat for kosher certification. Margarines are also of concern since some contain dairy products; thus, to avoid mixing milk and meat, it is important to look for a kosher dairy or kosher *pareve* symbol on margarine. Fats, such as chicken fat (*schmaltz*) or olive and vegetable oils, are often used when preparing meat meals. *Pareve* margarines can also be used with meat meals. When preparing dairy meals, butter, dairy or *pareve* margarines, or oils can be used.

Prominent Vegetables

Vegetables are *pareve* and as such can be eaten with milk or meat meals. Vegetables consumed traditionally are influenced by a Jew's country of origin and tradition, or where they live. For Jews with eastern European roots, vegetables, other than cabbage, potatoes, carrots, beets, onion, and garlic, have not been an especially important part of their cuisine. Potatoes, a New World import, were especially important to these Jews and were eaten daily, alone, or added to soup, stews, breads, or dumplings. Kugels and latkes are special-occasion foods, generally eaten for the Sabbath and Chanukah, respectively. Cabbage was also an important vegetable, and prior to the introduction of the potato, was the only vegetable, apart from carrots, that was commonly available. Caraway or a sweet-and-sour flavoring was often added. Carrot tzimmes is a vegetable dish commonly associated with Ashkenazi Jews. This sweet dish is often served with apples or prunes. Because of their color and shape, sliced carrots are associated with gold coins and this dish is often eaten at Rosh Hashanah as a symbol of prosperity and good fortune; the honey symbolizes the hope of a sweet New Year.

Jews from Hungary, the Balkans, Romania, and Bulgaria were influenced by the Ottomans or by Sephardic settlers and enjoyed a wider variety of vegetables than many Ashkenazi Jews. Eggplant was brought by Arabs to Spain and Italy; however, Jews are credited with introducing it to other cultures during the Diaspora. It is a Jewish tradition in many countries to serve cold fried eggplant on the Sabbath and Italian Jews often serve eggplant in caponata. Artichokes, tomatoes, peppers, pumpkins, beans, onions, and garlic are all associated with the Sephardim. One of the differences in Sephardic compared with Ashkenazi cooking is in food choices. For example, Roman fried artichokes are a classic dish, whereas artichokes are seldom consumed in Ashkenazi cooking. Spanish sofrito with fried onion and tomatoes is a signature of Sephardic cooking.

The prohibition against insects is especially important when considering vegetables, since it is easy for contamination to occur. One insect renders the food unfit for consumption; thus, it is important to inspect many vegetables prior to consumption. Guidebooks and videos are available describing which vegetables and fruit need to be examined, how to do it, and what insects are commonly found on the products. Examples of fruits and vegetables that need to be examined carefully are artichokes (only bottoms are used in the United States), asparagus, broccoli, cabbage, cauliflower, celery, endive, fennel, kale, lettuce, mushrooms, dried fruit, strawberries, and spinach. Bagged salad mixes should also be examined thoroughly. Produce that is very difficult to inspect, for example, Brussels sprouts, watercress, blackberries, and curly parsley, are generally not used. The injunction against insects is for the whole animal; if a food is to be made into a dish where food is to be chopped, such as tabouli, or pureed, such as a vegetable soup, the inspection of fruit and vegetables is not needed.

 ### Prominent Fruits

As with vegetables, fruit is *pareve* and can be eaten with milk or meat meals, although it, too, must be checked for insects. The major restriction of fruit involves grape juice-based products, which must be handled only by observant Jews from grape pressing to final processing. Harvesting cannot occur on the Sabbath, and only Jewish workers can press the grapes. If grape juice is pasteurized (heated), it can be handled by any worker. This practice derives from the laws against using products of idolatry. For the most part, this rule only affects wine and grape juice, but it has become a concern with the many fruit drinks and fruit-flavored drinks, which are often sweetened with grape juice. Some baking powders are not kosher, because baking powder is sometimes made with cream of tartar, a by-product of wine making.

Fruits consumed reflect personal taste, tradition, and availability. Fruits were generally more available to Jews living in warmer climates, rather than those in eastern Europe. The Sephardim have a strong tradition of eating fruit; however, if a single fruit had to be identified with them, it would be the pomegranate. Jewish

tradition teaches that the pomegranate is a symbol for righteousness, because it was believed that the fruit had 613 seeds (it does not), which corresponds to the number of commandments outlined in the *Torah*. Many Jews eat pomegranates on Rosh Hashanah. One fruit that was available to Jews in eastern Europe was the apple. Apples are noted for their sweetness and their healing powers, and were often sent as gifts to people in ill health.

 ### Spices and Seasonings

Since there are so many influences on "Jewish" cooking, the spices used reflect those traditionally used within a community. Sephardic communities are better known for use of a wide range of spices. Cumin and coriander are used by Egyptian Jews, allspice and cinnamon by Turks, and cardamom by Iraqis and Indians. Spice blends are also used, and Jews usually make their own to reduce the chance of insect contamination, although with modern processing this is less common than it once was. Zahtar, a mixture of wild thyme, roasted sesame seeds, and ground sumac berries is very popular in Israel, whereas Moroccans make a blend of black pepper, turmeric, ginger, cumin, and nutmeg.

Some spices are considered *chametz* and cannot be used at Passover. These spices include anise, caraway seeds, coriander, cumin, fennel, fenugreek, pepper, and poppy and sesame seeds (http://www.star-k.org/). Additives to spices or spice blends are a particular concern, and any spice consumed, especially at Passover, should have certification that the food is kosher for Passover.

In Jewish tradition, spices have nonculinary uses. Fragrant spices usher out the Sabbath in the *Havdalah* or "separation." The spices represent a compensation for the loss of the special Sabbath spirit, and are a form of comfort as the new week begins. The spices commonly used are cloves, cinnamon, or bay leaves, and they are typically kept in a special decorated holder called a *b'samim* box. The spice box is passed around for everyone to smell.

 ### Beverages

There are no beverages specifically associated with Judaism; however, there are certain beverages that merit discussion.

Most American Jews drink milk without kosher certification since most farms only produce milk from kosher animals, especially cows, and the U.S.

Department of Agriculture prohibits commercial sale of other types of milk.[1] Most Jews accept this government regulation as adequate supervision; however, there is still concern among some groups. Some Orthodox Jews will drink milk only if a Jew was present at milking and bottling. This milk, called *chalav Yisrael* (milk of Jews), ensures that milk of nonkosher animals, such as mare's or camel's milk, has not been added. This also applies to dairy products, such as cheese.

Tea is a beverage associated with both Ashkenazi and Sephardic Jews. In Russia, tea was drunk from a samovar and sipped from a glass with a lump of sugar held between the teeth. Mint tea has always been drunk in the Middle East. Coffee is also a common beverage. In the United States, carbonated water or seltzer is associated with Jews of Russian descent. The classic "egg cream" (which contains neither eggs nor cream) is a mix of milk, chocolate syrup, and seltzer.

Wine, defined as the "fermented juice of grapes," plays an important role in the Sabbath, Passover, Purim, the Redemption of the First Born, and other holidays. The blessing recited on the wine (*Borei Pri HaGafen*) can also be recited on nonfermented grape beverages. The vast majority of wines available cannot be consumed by observant Jews. It is against Jewish law for Jews to drink wine prepared by non-Jews since historically wine was used for idolatrous worship (*Ya'yin nesach*), thus prohibiting its use by Jews. There is also a rabbinical injunction against drinking unsupervised grape wine (*Stam Yaynom*). Fortunately, many fine kosher wines are available. Israel produces over 13 million gallons of wine per year; kosher wines are also produced in Spain, Italy, New York, California, and Italy. But what makes a wine kosher? Grapes of new vines cannot be used for making wine until the fourth year after planting (true of any fruit crop). From that time, fields must lie fallow every seventh year. Fruit or vegetables cannot be grown between the vines. Once the harvest begins, only kosher tools and storage facilities can be used in the wine-making process, and all of the wine-making equipment must be cleaned so that there are no foreign objects remaining in the equipment or vats. Observant male Jews must initiate, activate, and/or operate every essential step of the crush, including fermentation, standardization, and the taking of samples for quality control. In addition, there is a ritual in which just over 1% of the wine produced is

poured away to symbolize the tithe once paid to the Temple in Jerusalem.

As with other comestibles, the alcoholic beverages consumed reflect traditional choices based on culture. Vodka is consumed by Jews from Poland and Russia, schnapps and slivovitz are consumed by Jews from the Balkans. Jews in the Middle East drink Arak, and those from Morocco drink Mahia.

 Desserts

Sweets for Jews represent joy and happiness and must be present at Sabbath and holiday meals. Cakes and pastries are common and generally adapted from a Jew's country of origin; for example, honey cakes from Germany, butter cookies from Holland, strudel and blintzes from Hungary, and sponge cake from Iberia. Chiffon cakes are popular and because they are made with oil they can be served with either a milk or meat meal. When making these cakes, care should be taken to use cream of tartar with a kosher certification. Sweet kugels are commonly served by Ashkenazi Jews. These traditional Sabbath puddings have been made since the Middle Ages. The principal ingredients are eggs, butter or oil, cinnamon, and sugar; walnuts, apples, and poppy seeds are other common ingredients.

Because of the prohibition of mixing milk and meat, nondairy fruit desserts are common. These desserts range from simple fruit salads and compotes to more elaborate fruit cobblers or fruit served with meringue shells. Fruit sorbets are also good choices. Any dessert to be served with a meat meal can be made with a *pareve* margarine in place of butter.

Honey is traditionally used in cooking and is one of the few insect products allowed by Jewish law. The original ruling was that bees did not make honey, they only carried it. Pure (100%) honey from bees is kosher and does not require kosher certification (http://www.star-k.org/kashrus/kk-palate-honey.htm); however, many companies seek it. Ironically, the "land of milk and honey" and every mention of honey in the *Torah* is thought to refer to date honey.

 FOODS WITH CULTURAL SIGNIFICANCE

Although many foods have cultural significance, it is important to note that the table does, too. Since the destruction of the Second Temple in 70 CE, the table has represented the altar. "When the temple stood, sacri-

---

[1]Recently the water buffalo (whose milk has been approved for cheese manufacture by the USDA) was declared kosher. http://www.israelnationalnews.com/News/News.aspx/103331/

fices would secure atonement for an individual; now the table does" (Hagigah 27a; quoted by Donin, 2001). This has led to many meal-related behaviors including saying grace before and after meals, removing knives (a symbol of war) from the table prior to saying grace, dipping bread into salt, ritual hand washing, and not serving forbidden animals. Bread served with meals took on the symbolism of, and replacement for, the sacrifice that was brought in Temple times, a sacrifice that consisted of a mixture of fine flour, oil, and frankincense, often baked into loaves. The priest burned some of these loaves of bread on the altar to serve as a memorial to God; the burning of the bread continues with the burning of the *challah* as described above.

Salt symbolizes the making of the covenant with Israel ("It is a covenant of salt forever, before the Lord" [Numbers 18:19]) and the offering of sacrifice. It was used with all sacrifices brought on the altar in Temple times since it acted as a preservative, and the custom of dipping bread in salt evolved as a memorial to the sacrificial system. God told Moses, "You shall season all your cereal offerings with salt; you shall not let the salt of the covenant with your God be lacking" (Leviticus 2:10). The Bible commands "On all your meal-offerings shall you sprinkle salt" (Leviticus 2:13), and the *Talmud* (Menachot 20a, b) extended this requirement to all sacrifices.

Many foods have religious or cultural significance to Jews. These foods are discussed elsewhere within the text.

TYPICAL DAY'S MENU AND HOLIDAY MEALS

There is no "kosher-style" food and any meal can be kosher, as long as it is prepared in accordance with Jewish Law. Menu planning can be a challenge for observant Jews; however, the dietary laws have not stifled creativity, they have expanded it. Because of the prohibition against milk and meat, there are many dishes that incorporate dairy products only. Furthermore, there are many dishes that can be enjoyed cold, because fires cannot be lit on the Sabbath.

During Passover (Pesach), it is especially difficult to meet the recommendations for whole grains, although whole-grain matzoth that is kosher for Passover is now available. For most American Jews, beans cannot be eaten during this time. The injunction in the *Torah*, "Seven days shall there be no leaven found in your home," has been interpreted to mean that foods considered leaven (*chametz*) are forbidden; thus, no

wheat, barley, rye, oats, and spelt are eaten—the exception is matzah, which, for Passover, is made from flour milled with new millstones and was guarded from the time of growing through storage to ensure that it did not become wet and have a chance to ferment. During this time, the Ashkenazim are also forbidden to eat *kitniyot* (small things), including rice, corn, dried peas and lentils, soy beans, string beans, peanuts, mustard, sesame, and poppy seeds, and most products derived from these foods. Although these foods are clearly not *chametz*, it was believed that they could be confused with grains and other foods. The Sephardim continue to eat these foods during Passover.

Sample menus are presented in Table 3-4. In the Jewish calendar, all days begin at sundown and extend for 24 hours; thus, the Sabbath meal and Pesach meal are presented in that format. For simplicity, the everyday menu is presented in a more standard form.

HEALTH BELIEFS AND CONCERNS

Jewish Law places life above all other considerations; thus, the expertise of the healthcare provider is very important. Any questions about health that observant Jews have should be referred to their doctor and their rabbi.

Eating in moderation is considered a wholesome and pleasurable activity; overeating is not condoned. The *Talmud* advises to "Eat moderately! Eat simply! Eat slowly! Eat regularly!" (Lepicard, 1994a) Eliahu said "Eat a third, and drink a third, and leave a third" (Lepicard, 1994b); thus, the concept of not overeating is emphasized. The diet should be healthful. "One should not live in a city that does not have a vegetable garden" (Yerushalmi Kiddushin 4:12). Cabbage is considered a nourishing food, and beets are healthful. Lentils, if eaten once in 30 days, are said to protect against respiratory problems.

The tradition of offering chicken to the sick can be traced to Maimonides (1135–1204) and his teacher *Abu Merwan ibn Zohar*. Recent studies have confirmed that chicken soup may have biological effects, including improving hydration and nutritional status (Kunstadter, Kunstadter, Podhisita, & Leepreecha, 1993), accelerating mucosal clearance (Saketkhoo, Januszkiewics & Sackner, 1978), and inhibiting neutrophil chemotaxis (Rennard, Ertl, Gossman, Robbins, & Rennard, 2000).

Studies are lacking that actually link diet intake data from those that follow *Kashrut* with health outcomes, and we were unable to find a recent article that described the dietary intake of Jews in the United States or documenting diet-related health problems. A Canadian study (Shatenstein, Ghadirian, & Lambert, 1993) of ultra-Orthodox Jews in Montreal showed eating habits that closely paralleled those of other North Americans and approximated the recommendations that were in place at that time. Differences in different Hassidic groups were shown and were attributed to differences in Sabbath, fasting days, and holidays, as well as differences in food philosophies.

There are, however, several potential problems related to *Kashrut* and health. The laws against mixing milk and meat, coupled with the 6-hour waiting period that many Jews observe between a meat and dairy meal, may make it difficult to obtain the three servings of dairy recommended for most individuals in the 2005 U.S. Dietary Guidelines. In ultra-Orthodox groups, there have been anecdotal reports of higher than average bone fractures, and decreased bone mineralization in adolescents (Taha et al., 2001). Although the study assessed calcium intake and found it comparable to others of the same age, the sample was small and mean intake was lower than recommended. It is not clear if this is related to low dairy consumption; other behaviors associated with Orthodox Jewry, including lack of physical activity and modest dress, that may decrease vitamin D production; or genetic reasons.

Salt intake is potentially of concern. The salt content of kosher meats has not been well studied (Burns & Neubort, 1984; Gluck, 1985; Kisch, 1953), but it is likely to be higher than that of nonkosher meat. Individuals on salt-restricted diets should be advised of this and advised to buy commercially *kashered* meat, which may absorb less salt than home-*kashered* meats (Regenstein et al., 2003a). Other ways to reduce sodium in the diet should also be discussed with Jews who need a salt restriction. Reduction of meat intake is one option, but reducing consumption of processed foods and increased use of herbs or lemon should also be explored.

Observant Jews wash their hands prior to and after meals at which bread is served. Although no studies were identified that linked this practice in Jews with disease reduction, it is clear that hand hygiene reduces the spread of infection (Jefferson et al., 2008).

Finally, there are health issues associated with fasting. Consequences of short-term intermittent fasts are unknown (Shatenstein & Ghadirian, 1998) and have not been well studied in Judaism. The "Yom Kippur" headache (Mosek & Korczyn, 1995) has been associated with fasting, although this is generally relieved

with over-the-counter medications (Drescher & Elstein, 2006).

Fasting is contraindicated in people with diabetes, hypoglycemia, or renal disease, in surgical/trauma patients, and in other high-risk groups. People with insulin-dependent diabetes are of particular concern. There are several websites available to help with general information (e.g., the Jewish Diabetes Association [http://www.tudiabetes.org/] and Friends with Diabetes [http://www.friendswithdiabetes.org/]); however, these are not a substitute for specific medical information and all observant Jews with health concerns should discuss them with their physician and rabbi to determine if fasting is an appropriate option for them. The majority of recommendations for religious fasting and diabetes have focused on Muslims fasting during Ramadam (Al-Arouj et al., 2005; Elhadd & Al-Amoudi, 2006; Kassem, Zantout, & Azar, 2005; Zargar, Basit, & Mahtab, 2005) rather than the short-term, full fasts of Jews.

 ## COMMUNICATION AND COUNSELING TIPS

It is important to know whether the client is an Orthodox, Conservative, or Reform Jew, and whether he or she observes the dietary laws and what his or her specific beliefs are. It is critical that a health counselor have a working knowledge of the dietary laws so that they can advise clients. If a Jew is hospitalized, it is important to understand his or her practices and to determine whether a kosher meal can be provided if needed. If a kosher kitchen is not available and a kosher meal cannot be catered, a kosher meal obviously cannot be served.

It is also important to be able to refer Jewish clients to kosher meal services within the community; for example, Meals on Wheels, if they are available (Rosenzweig, 2005). Unfortunately, if a large Jewish population is not present in an area, it is probable that access to these services will be limited.

PRIMARY LANGUAGE OF FOOD NAMES WITH ENGLISH AND PHONETIC TRANSLATION

Many foods associated with Jews have become staple menu items in the homes of many Americans; others that may not be as well-known are shown in Table 3-6.

TABLE 3-6   Glossary of Food Terms

Term	Pronunciation	Definition
Babka	băb´ka	A spongy yeast cake
Bagel	bā´gel	A doughnut-shaped yeast roll that is cooked in boiling water and then baked
Blintzes	blĭnts	Thinly rolled pancakes often served with sweetened cottage cheese or fruit
Borscht	bôrsht	A beet soup that can be made with or without meat and served hot or cold
Challah	khä´ lə, hä´	The yeast bread prepared for the Sabbath and holidays
Cholent	khö´ lənt	A long-cooking Sabbath dish made with grains, meats, and eggs
Falafel	fə-lä´ fəl	Ground spiced chickpeas shaped in a ball and fried; a sandwich with the fried chickpeas
Farfel	fär´ fəl	Also called egg barley; a type of pasta
Fleischig	flā-shik	Refers to meat or beef
Gefilte fish	gə-fĭl´ tə	A ground poached-fish mixture often served cold with fish aspic
Hammentashen	hä-mən-tä-shən	A three-cornered pastry filled with poppy seeds or prunes served at Purim
Kasha	kä´ shə	Buckwheat groats
Knish	kə-nĭsh´	A pastry filled with meat or cheese
Kreplach	krĕp´ ləkh	Pasta stuffed with a sweet or savory filling
Kugel	kōō´ gəl	A pudding that can be sweet or savory; often made with noodles but potatoes can be used
Latkes	lät´ kə	A fried vegetable (usually potato) cake served at Chanukah
Lox	lŏks	Smoked salmon
Matzah	mät-sä´	Unleavened bread
Milchig	mil-ḱik	Refers to milk or dairy
Pareve (parve)	pär-(ə)və	Neutral (i.e., assigned to neither dairy nor meat)
Tzimmes	tsĭm´ ĭs	A sweet vegetable or meat and vegetable stew with carrots, prunes, and sweet potatoes

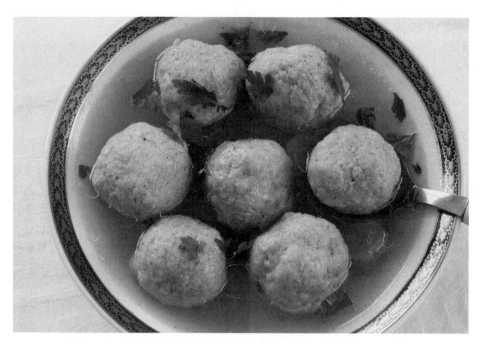

Matzo Ball Soup

FEATURED RECIPE

There is an exciting variety of foods and cookbooks (see list in Additional References section) that are associated with Jewish culture. Familiar recipes include chicken soup, roast chicken, braised brisket, noodle kugel, and carrot tzimmes. Additional recipes can be found at http://nutrition.jbpub.com/foodculture/

Matzo Balls

6 eggs

1½ tsp. baking powder

1½ cups matzo meal

1. Combine all ingredients.
2. Form into walnut-size balls.
3. Place in boiling water.
4. Boil for 30–40 minutes.

Yields 20 balls

REFERENCES

Al-Arouj M., Bouguerra R., Buse J., Hafez S., Hassanein M., Ibrahim M.A., et al. (2005). Recommendations for management of diabetes during Ramadan. *Diabetes Care, 28,* 2305–2311.

Burns, E.R., & Neubort, S. (1984). Sodium content of koshered meat. *Journal of the American Medical Association, 252,* 2960.

Chaudry, M.M., & Regenstein, J.M. (1994). Implications of biotechnology and genetic engineering for kosher and halal foods. *Trends Food Science Technology, 5,* 165–168.

Darby, W.J., Ghalioungui, P., & Grivetti L.E. (1977). *Food: The gift of Osiris* (Vol. 2). London: Academic Press.

Donin, H.H. (2001). *To be a Jew: A guide to Jewish observance in contemporary life.* New York: Basic Books.

Drescher, M.J., & Elstein, Y. (2006). Prophylactic COX 2 inhibitor: An end to the Yom Kippur headache. *Headache, 46,* 1487–1491.

Elhadd, T.A., & Al-Amoudi, A.A. (2006). Recommendations for management of diabetes during Ramadan. *Diabetes Care, 29,* 744–745.

Feitelson, M., & Fiedler, K. (1982). Kosher dietary laws and children's food preferences: Guide to a camp menu plan. *Journal of the American Dietetic Association, 81,* 453–456.

Gluck, S. (1985). Salt content of kosher meat. *Journal of the American Medical Association, 254,* 504.

Grandin, T. (2006). Improving religious slaughter practices in the U.S. *Anthropology of Food, 5,* 2–10.

Grivetti, L.E. (2000). Food prejudices and taboos. In K.F. Kiple & K.C. Ornelas (Eds.), *The Cambridge World History of Food.* (Vol. 2, pp. 1495–1513). New York: Cambridge University Press.

Grivetti, L.E., & Pangborn, R.M. (1974). Origin of selected Old Testament dietary prohibitions. *Journal of the American Dietetic Association, 65,* 634–638.

Jefferson, T., Foxlee, R., Del Mar, C., Dooley, L., Ferroni, E., Hewak, B., et al. (2008). Physical interventions to interrupt or reduce the spread of respiratory viruses: Systematic review. *British Medical Journal, 336,* 77–80.

Kassem, H.S., Zantout, M.S., & Azar, S.T. (2005). Insulin therapy during Ramadan fast for type 1 diabetes patients. *Journal of Endocrinological Investigation, 28,* 802–805.

Kisch, B. (1953). Salt poor diets and Jewish dietary laws. *Journal of the American Medical Association, 153,* 1472.

Kolatch, A.J. (2000). *The Jewish book of why.* Middle Village, NY: Jonathan David.

Kunstadter, P., Kunstadter, S.L., Podhisita, C., & Leepreecha, P. (1993). Demographic variables in fetal and child mortality: Hmong in Thailand. *Social Science Medicine 36,* 1109–1120.

Lepicard, E. (1994a). Medica Judaica. Talmudic aphorisms on diet. *Israel Journal of Medical Sciences, 30,* 314–315.

Lepicard, E. (1994b). Medica Judaica. Talmudic aphorisms on diet: II. *Israel Journal of Medical Sciences, 30,* 554–555.

Mayer E., Kosmin B., & Kaysov S. (2003). AJIS Report American Jewish Identity Survey Center for Jewish Studies. The Graduate Center of the City University of New York. Original issuance date 2001. Retrieved April 27, 2008, from http://www.simpletoremember.com/vitals/ajisbook.pdf/

Mosek, A., & Korczyn, A.D. (1995). Yom Kippur headache. *Neurology, 45,* 1953–1955.

Regenstein, J.M. (1994). Health aspects of kosher foods. Activities report and minutes of working groups and sub-work groups of R&D Associates, *46,* 77–83. San Antonio, TX: Research and Development Associates for Military Food and Packaging Systems.

Regenstein, J.M., Chaudry, M.M., & Regenstein, C.E. (2003a). Kosher and halal in the biotechnology era. *Applied Biotechnology, Food Science, and Policy, 1,* 95–107.

Regenstein, J.M., Chaudry, M.M., & Regenstein, C.E. (2003b). The kosher and halal food laws. *Comprehensive Reviews in Food Science and Food Safety, 2,* 111–127.

Rennard, B.O., Ertl, R.F., Gossman, G.L., Robbins, R.A., & Rennard, S.I. (2000). Chicken soup inhibits neutrophil chemotaxis in vitro. *Chest, 118,* 1150–1157.

Rhoden, C. (2001). *The book of Jewish food: An odyssey from Samarkand to New York.* New York: Alfred A. Knopf.

Rosenzweig, L. (2005). Kosher meal services in the community: need, availability, and limitations. *Journal of Nutrition for the Elderly, 24,* 73–82.

Sáenz-Badillos, A. (1996). *A history of the Hebrew language.* Cambridge, MA: Cambridge University Press.

Saketkhoo, K., Januszkiewics, B.S., & Sackner, M.A. (1978). Effects of drinking hot water, cold water and chicken soup on nasal mucus velocity and nasal airflow resistance. *Chest, 74,* 408–410.

Shatenstein, B., & Ghadirian, P. (1998). Influences on diet, health behaviours and their outcome in select ethnocultural and religious groups. *Nutrition, 14,* 223–230.

Shatenstein, B., Ghadirian, P., & Lambert, J. (1993). Influence of the Jewish religion and Jewish dietary laws (kashrut) on family food habits of an ultra-orthodox population in Montreal. *Ecology of Food and Nutrition, 31,* 27–44.

Taha, W., Chin, D., Silverberg, A., II, Lashiker, L., Khateeb, N., & Anhalt, H. (2001). Reduced spinal bone mineral density in adolescents of an ultra-orthodox Jewish community in Brooklyn. *Pediatrics, 107.* Retrieved April 28, 2008, from http://pediatrics.aappublications.org/cgi/reprint/107/5/e79

The 2005 U.S. Dietary Guidelines. (2005). Retrieved April 28, 2008 from http://www.health.gov/DietaryGuidelines/

Trepp, L. (1980). *The complete book of Jewish observance.* New York: Behrman House; Simon & Schuster.

Yehezkel, D. (2006). *Executive report annual assessment number 3.* Jerusalem, Israel: The Jewish People Policy Planning Institute.

Zargar, A., Basit, A., & Mahtab, H. (2005). Sulphonylureas in the management of type 2 diabetes during the fasting month of Ramadan. *Journal of the Indian Medical Association, 103,* 444–446.

ADDITIONAL REFERENCES: WEBSITES

Cultural and ethnic food and nutrition education materials: A resource list for educators. Retrieved May 11, 2008, from http://www.nal.usda.gov/fnic/pubs/bibs/gen/ethnic.pdf/

Definition of milk. Retrieved April 12, 2008, from http://www.ams.usda.gov/AMSv1.0/getfile?dDocName=STELDEV3004788/

Definition of milk for manufacturing purposes. Retrieved April 12, 2008, from http://www.ams.usda.gov/AMSv1.0/getfile?dDocName=STELDEV3004791/

Friends with Diabetes. Retrieved May 11, 2008, from http://www.friendswithdiabetes.org/guides.html

Information on Kitniot for Passover. Retrieved May 11, 2008 from http://www.kashrut.com/Passover/kitniot_list/

Jewish Diabetes Association. Retrieved May 11, 2008, from http://www.jewishdiabetes.org

Kashrus Magazine, with updates on kosher products. Retrieved April 13, 2008, from http://www.kashrusmagazine.com

K-Star insect checking list. (2008). Retrieved May 11, 2008, from http://star-k.org/cons-appr-vegetables-videos-list.htm/

OK vegetable checking guide. Retrieved May 11, 2008, from http://www.ok.org/PDF/OK_Veggie_Checking_Guide.pdf/

United States Food and Drug Administration Title 9 318.10. Retrieved April 12, 2008, from http://www.cfsan.fda.gov/~lrd/9CF318.html/

Updates on kosher products. Retrieved May 11, 2008, from http://kosherquest.org

ADDITIONAL REFERENCES: COOKBOOKS

Angel, G. (1986). *Sephardic holiday cooking.* New York: Decalogue Books.

Friedland, S.R. (1994). *The Passover table. New and traditional recipes for your seders and the entire Passover week.* New York: William Morrow Cookbooks.

Friedland, S.R. (1999). *Shabbat shalom. Recipes and menus for the sabbath.* Boston: Little, Brown, and Company.

Goldstein, J. (2000). *Sephardic flavors: Jewish cooking of the Mediterranean.* San Francisco: Chronicle Books.

Goldstein, J. (2002). *Saffron shores: Jewish cooking of the southern Mediterranean.* San Francisco: Chronicle Books.

Goldstein, J. (2005). *Cucina Ebraica: Flavors of the Italian Jewish kitchen.* San Francisco: Chronicle Books.

Marks, G. (1996). *The world of Jewish cooking.* New York: Simon & Schuster.

Nathan, J. (1994). *Jewish cooking in America.* New York: Alfred Knopf.

Nathan, J. (1999). *The Jewish holiday baker.* New York: Knopf Publishing Group.

Nathan, J. (2004). *Jewish holiday cookbook.* New York: Schocken Books.

Plotch, B. & Cobe, P. (1992). *The kosher gourmet.* New York: Fawcett Columbine.

Roden, C. (1996). *The book of Jewish food.* New York: Alfred A. Knopf.

Sokolov, R. (1989). *The Jewish–American kitchen.* New York: Stewart, Tabori, and Chang.

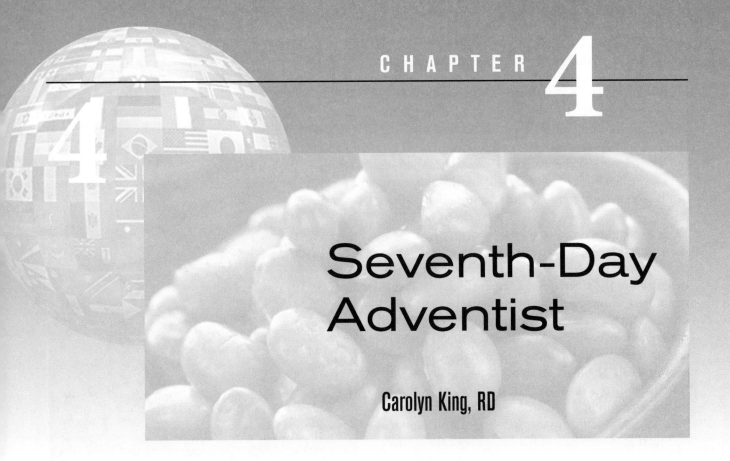

CHAPTER 4

Seventh-Day Adventist

Carolyn King, RD

FOOD HISTORY WITHIN THE CULTURE

The Seventh-Day Adventist (SDA) Church has more than 15 million members worldwide with more than 1 million living in the United States. It is one of the fastest-growing Christian Protestant religions. They are in 204 of the 229 countries recognized by the United Nations.

The SDA Church was officially organized in 1863 in the New England region of the United States, with 3500 members worshiping in 125 churches. The Church was formed of people from various Christian faiths who wanted the Bible as their sole source of guidance. The name Seventh-Day Adventist comes from their belief in the Seventh-Day Sabbath referred to in the 10 commandments of the Old Testament, and the impending second coming, or advent, of Jesus Christ mentioned in the New Testament.

According to SDA beliefs, the Sabbath is a time for rest from the daily work routine, to spend in thoughtful reflection on God's many blessings. The Sabbath is a spiritual illustration of the peace and rest found in salvation. It is also a time for Bible study, church worship services, family and friend togetherness, and Christian witnessing. The Sabbath is observed from Friday sundown to Saturday sundown. Food preparation and other unnecessary work is done the day before or left for later. Sabbath afternoon lunch is usually the largest meal of the day, made special with the family's and guests' favorite foods.

Seventh-Day Adventists also believe that their body is the temple or dwelling place of the Holy Spirit, the method by which God communicates and abides within the individual. It is not only out of respect for His creation that sustaining a healthy body and mind is encouraged; it is also necessary for providing the best service for God in reaching and caring for one's fellow man. Furthermore, SDAs see in the example of Jesus and his apostles the responsibility, as followers of Jesus Christ, to minister to the physical health needs of others. Today, there are 168 SDA hospitals, 138 skilled nursing and retirement centers, and 442 clinics and dispensaries worldwide.

The relationship between religion and health practices stems from the ancient Israelite Levitical laws on health and hygiene found in the Old Testament. These laws give detailed and specific instructions on which foods are appropriate for human consumption. Animals determined as "clean" chew their cud and have a cloven hoof, and fish should have fins and scales. Also included are the clean birds, such as chicken and turkey. Often animals without these characteristics carry disease and are natural scavengers. The SDAs follow the guidelines of eating only "clean" animals and not eating "unclean" animals such as pig, rabbit, bear, raccoon, catfish, shellfish, shrimp, lobster, octopus, vulture, hawk, frog, snake, and lizard, to name a few of the most common. They further refrain from alcohol, tobacco, and illicit drug use due to recommendations and warnings throughout the Bible about their effect on the mind, decision making, and overall health.

 MAJOR FOODS

 Protein Sources

Protein sources are as follows:

- Legumes: dried beans and peas, lentils, peanuts/peanut butter
- Nuts and seeds: walnuts, almonds, cashews, pecans, sunflower seeds
- Soy: edamame (whole green soybeans), tofu, tempeh (baked and seasoned tofu), TVP (dehydrated textured vegetable protein), roasted soy nuts, soy cheese, soy milk, soy yogurt
- Processed meat analogs derived from a mixture of soy, wheat gluten, legumes, grains, and vegetables. Common brand names of canned and frozen meat analogs are: Worthington Foods, Loma Linda Foods, Morningstar Farms, Garden Burger, and Natural Touch
- Eggs
- Dairy foods: milk, cheese, yogurt, cottage cheese
- Meat: beef, chicken, turkey, fish (tuna, salmon, halibut, perch, flounder)

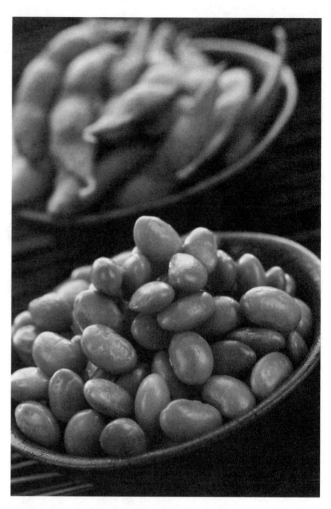

Edamame (whole soybeans) are a popular protein source for Seventh-Day Adventists.

 Starch Sources

Starch sources are as follows:

- Vegetables: potatoes of all kinds, winter squash, green sweet peas, corn
- Grains and cereals: wheat, rice, oat, buckwheat, rye, spelt, millet, quinoa, barley, cornmeal, popcorn
- Various grains and cereals are used in bread, crackers, tortillas, chips, waffles/pancakes, bagels, muffins, biscuits, pilaf, and hot/cold cereal
- Grains are also a basis for numerous homemade vegetarian meat loafs/balls, burger patties, casseroles, pasta dishes, soups, and desserts

 Fat Sources

Fat sources are as follows:

- Olives
- Nuts: almonds, raw cashews, coconut, pecans, walnuts
- Seeds: flax, sunflower, poppy, sesame, tahini (sesame seed paste)
- Avocado
- Oil: olive, canola, soybean, corn, sunflower, lecithin
- Cream cheese
- Sour cream
- Mayonnaise
- Salad dressing
- Margarine

 ## Prominent Vegetables

A wide variety of leafy and non-leafy vegetables are available throughout the United States, typical in the general population, prepared from fresh, frozen, or canned sources. These vegetables include lettuce, greens (spinach, kale, collard, chard), cabbage, broccoli, cauliflower, brussel sprouts, carrots, green beans, beets, eggplant, mushrooms, tomatoes, celery, cucumbers, bell peppers, summer squash, onions, and garlic.

 ## Prominent Fruits

Fruit intake, as with the general U.S. population, varies greatly with the seasons. Common fruits include apples/applesauce, citrus (oranges, grapefruit, lemons), bananas, grapes, melon (cantaloupe, honeydew, watermelon), pineapple, kiwi, strawberries, blueberries, raspberries, cherries, peaches, and pears, as well as dried apricots, dates, cranberries, raisins, and prunes.

 ## Spices, Seasonings, and Other Ingredients

Spices and other comestibles are as follows:

- Salt: season salt, garlic/onion/celery salt, vegetable salt, Bakon seasoning, Spike seasoning, vegetarian soup-base mix such as Vegex paste, McKay's or George Washington chicken/beef-style seasoning, vegetable/chicken/beef bouillon, soy sauce, or Bragg's liquid amino acids
- Spices: celery seed, cumin, curry powder, cayenne pepper, chili powder, cinnamon, onion powder, garlic powder, ginger, paprika, turmeric
- Fresh/dried herbs: basil, cilantro (coriander), dill, oregano, parsley, rosemary, sage, savory, thyme
- Nutritional yeast flakes

- Carob powder
- Kosher gelatin: Emes, Agar-Agar flakes (seaweed)
- Commercial egg replacement: *Ener-G* Egg Replacer (used in baking)

 ## Beverages

Common beverages include the following:

- Juice: orange, grape, apple, lemonade
- Milk: dairy milk, soy milk, rice milk, almond milk
- Carbonated soda: root beer, lemon–lime, ginger ale, orange
- Herbal tea
- Coffee substitute (all brand names): Postum, Roma, Cafix, Teeccino
- Fruit smoothies

 ## Desserts

Desserts include the following:

- Fruit pies/crisp/cobbler
- Fruit and nut cookies/candy bars
- Cake
- Brownies (made with chocolate or carob)
- Pudding (dairy, soy, cashew, or grain based)
- Fruit salad
- Quick breads: banana, apple, date–nut, zucchini, pumpkin
- Sweet rolls/pastries

 ## FOODS WITH CULTURAL SIGNIFICANCE

Because the SDA religion is multicultural, encompassing people with a variety of ethnic backgrounds, it is difficult to capture or summarize the extent of their variable food intake. The following is a list of foods that most SDAs would be familiar with and eat on a regular basis:

- Haystacks. A layered taco salad with tortilla chips on the bottom, then rice, chili/refried beans, lettuce, cucumber, onion, bell pepper, black olives, tomatoes, avocado, salsa, shredded cheese, and sour cream. This is often served at church social gatherings.
- Special K loaf. Homemade cereal-based substitute for meat loaf.

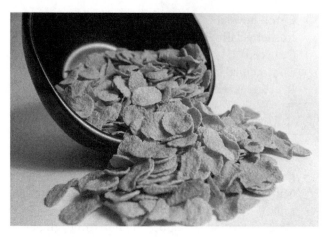

A popular dish for Seventh-Day Adventists, Special K Roast is a homemade cereal-based substitute for meat loaf.

- Grape juice (100% juice). Used for church communion service and a favorite beverage for many people due to its flavor and health benefits. Grape juice is often served with dinner and at church luncheons.
- Popcorn. Often eaten on Saturday nights, after Sabbath, and at church socials. Popcorn is often eaten as a light dinner with fresh fruit, juice, and nuts, or with raw vegetables, dip, and soup.
- Ready-to-Eat cereal. Particularly granola with a variety of nuts, seeds, and dried fruit. The first dry cereals and meat analogs have their history in the SDA culture, starting with Dr. John Harvey Kellogg who worked closely with the SDAs and their health sanitariums in the late 1800s.

 TYPICAL VEGETARIAN DAILY MENUS

Breakfast

The following are typical breakfast choices:

- Hot or cold cereal with milk (dairy or non-dairy) topped with dried/fresh fruit and nuts, whole-grain toast with peanut butter, and half a grapefruit
- Tofu–vegetable scramble or eggs, whole-grain toast with peanut butter, hash browns, and juice

Lunch

The following are typical lunch choices:

- Bean and cheese burrito with lettuce, salsa, and guacamole

- Vegetable- and hummus-filled pita pocket with olives and lentil soup
- Vegetarian deli meat sandwich or veggie burger with salad and chips

Dinner

The following are typical dinner choices:

- Spaghetti topped with sautéed vegetables in marinara sauce (with or without parmesan cheese and vegetarian burger crumbles), tossed salad, corn, green peas, and garlic bread
- Tofu–vegetable stir fry or curry over brown rice
- Baked beans, sautéed kale or collard greens, and corn bread

Snacks

- Fresh/dried fruit, nuts, cookies, yogurt, cheese, or peanut butter with crackers

 TYPICAL NONVEGETARIAN DAILY MENUS

Breakfast

The following are typical nonvegetarian breakfast choices:

- Yogurt and fresh fruit topped with granola
- Pancakes/waffles, turkey ham, fried/poached eggs, fresh fruit, and milk

Lunch

The following is a typical nonvegetarian lunch choice:

- Turkey or egg/tuna salad sandwich, carrot sticks, chips, and fresh fruit or cookies

Dinner

The following are typical nonvegetarian dinner choices:

- Baked mushroom chicken and rice casserole, steamed broccoli, salad, and roll
- Meat loaf, mashed potatoes, gravy, corn, green beans, and bread
- Chili (beef or vegetarian), corn bread, and salad

Snacks

- Fresh/dried fruit, nuts, cookies, yogurt, cheese and crackers, and chips

HOLIDAY MENUS

Thanksgiving and Christmas are the most widely observed holidays among SDAs and the menu is similar for both occasions. There are typically two main meals: breakfast and a late-afternoon dinner meal.

Breakfast Food Items

Breakfast typically includes cinnamon rolls/sticky buns or other sweet bread, blueberry muffins, fresh fruit, pancakes/waffles/French toast with maple syrup or fresh fruit sauce and whipped topping, vegetarian sausage/bacon, tofu or egg scramble/omelet, and hash browns.

Main-Meal Food Items

The main meal typically includes some or much of the following:

- Roasted turkey, homemade vegetarian roast (made from any mixture of the following: meat analog, cottage cheese, eggs, wheat gluten, nuts, seeds, tofu, lentils, bread crumbs, cereal, oats, rice), stuffing, gravy, mashed/scalloped/cottage potatoes, green bean casserole, cranberry relish/sauce, salad, yams, roasted mixed vegetables, vegetable quiche (tofu or egg based), potato–carrot soup, roasted autumn stew, pecan-, lentil-, wild rice-stuffed peppers or acorn squash, bread/rolls/biscuits, vegetable platter with olives, nuts, dip, cheese ball, crackers, sparkling cider, or grape juice.
- Dessert: apple/pumpkin/pecan pie, variety of cookies, cheesecake (dairy or nondairy) with berry sauce.

HEALTH BELIEFS AND CONCERNS

Today, many SDAs are vegetarian because it is thought to be the original diet given by God. It is often described as the most healthful and preferred source of food by God throughout the Bible. The "original diet" includes fruits, vegetables, nuts, seeds, and grains as detailed in the first book of the Bible. It was later modified after "the flood" to include "clean" animals due to the temporary lack of vegetation. In a current study among SDAs in the United States and Canada, 43.7% are non-vegetarian, 8.3% consider themselves semi-vegetarian (eat meat less than once per week), 9.7% are pesco-vegetarian (eat fish), 34% are lacto-ovo vegetarian (eat milk and eggs), and 4.3% are vegan-vegetarians (do not eat any foods of animal origin). Many SDAs continue to adapt their health practices to an ever-increasing awareness of the link between diet and health, currently supported by advanced research and ongoing health discoveries. SDAs may further restrict other food items with particular emphasis on self-control and meal planning. Some members may eat only two meals per day (breakfast and lunch), especially those who lead a more sedentary lifestyle. SDAs often refrain from caffeine-containing foods and beverages due to the caffeine's mind- and body-altering effects. Fermented foods, such as vinegar, pickles, various spices (black pepper, cloves, nutmeg, cinnamon, horseradish, mustard), and condiments using these ingredients, are often also excluded due to their irritating effect on the gastrointestinal tract.

NUTRIENTS OF CONCERN FOR THE VEGETARIAN

A balanced and varied vegetarian diet is healthful and contains all the necessary and essential nutrients needed for growth, maintenance, and healing; however, vegetarians, and vegan-vegetarians in particular, need to take special care in getting sufficient amounts of certain nutrients. Studies show that some vegan-vegetarians have lower intakes of nutrients that are high in meats and dairy foods including vitamin B_{12}, iron, calcium, and vitamin D. On the other hand, vegetarians as a whole typically consume less saturated fat and cholesterol and higher amounts of fiber, potassium, magnesium, folic acid, numerous antioxidants including vitamins C, E, and A (the latter in the form of beta-carotene), as well as countless phytochemicals and flavonoids. The health and nutrient strength of a vegetarian diet comes from a daily variety of whole-plant foods.

There is no reliable and adequate source of vitamin B_{12} in plant foods. Vegan-vegetarians who consume neither dairy products nor eggs need to find alternative sources. Some nondairy beverages are fortified with vitamin B_{12} as well as ready-to-eat cereals, meat analogs, and nutritional yeast flakes. It is recommended that vegan-vegetarians take a daily supplement of the active form of cyanocobalamin or hydroxocobalamin to prevent a deficiency. Iron is of particular importance for both vegan and lacto-ovo-vegetarians. Plant sources include dark green leafy vegetables, legumes, tofu, and whole grains. Consuming a food rich in vitamin C (citrus fruits, tomatoes, strawberries, bell peppers) along with a meal will improve the body's absorption of iron. Calcium is not only found in dairy products but also in dark green leafy vegetables (kale, collard greens, broccoli). Spinach and chard are not recommended sources of calcium due to their high phytate and oxalate content, which decrease calcium absorption. Calcium-precipitated tofu is an excellent source and smaller amounts of calcium can be found in dried beans, tahini, almonds, dried figs, and sweet potatoes. Many common foods are now fortified with calcium, such as nondairy milk, juice, ready-to-eat cereal, and bread. Vegetarians' and nonvegetarians' main source of vitamin D is provided through adequate sun exposure and fortified foods (dairy and nondairy milk, yogurt, cheese, and some ready-to-eat cereals). Good food sources are especially important during winter months. A vitamin D supplement may be needed. With appropriate planning, sufficient amounts of these nutrients can be obtained by incorporating a daily supply of various whole grains, fruits, vegetables, legumes, nuts, and seeds in a vegetarian diet. In some cases, fortified foods and supplements can be helpful in meeting the recommended amounts of these specific nutrients.

 COMMUNICATION AND COUNSELING TIPS

It is difficult to generalize the meal pattern of SDAs due to their varied individual application of health practices. All SDAs abide by the "clean" and "unclean" meat rule and abstain from alcohol and tobacco as part of their doctrine. Further health practices or diet restrictions are a matter of personal conviction; therefore, health behaviors may vary among SDAs and each individual has his or her own specific dietary habits. Respect for his or her health and diet beliefs is essential, and a common interest in the person's overall well-being should be the goal instead of asking him or her to abandon practices that seem overly restrictive or unbeneficial. Naturally, just like anyone (vegetarian or not), his or her diet may not be well-balanced. It may be high in saturated fat, sugar, and sodium. An SDA may be vegetarian because it is widely accepted or expected, and he or she might lack knowledge of general health principles and may rely largely on processed foods. Being familiar with the large variety of meat analogs and dairy substitutes, from burgers, hot dogs, and chicken nuggets to barbequed ribs, bacon, and soy cheese, will be valuable in assessing nutrition adequacy.

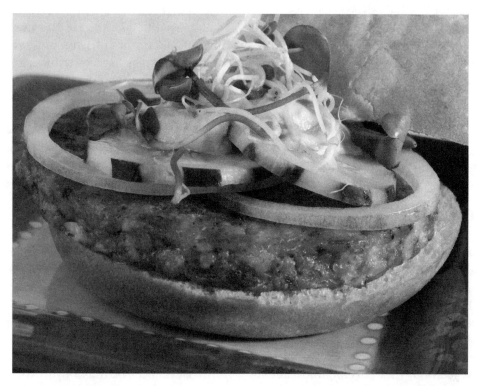

Veggie burgers and other processed meat analogs derived from a mixture of soy, wheat gluten, legumes, grains, and vegetables are a part of the Seventh-Day Adventist diet.

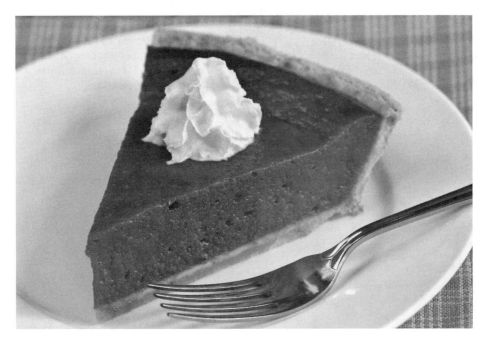

Pumpkin Pie

Lastly, many SDA churches are a health resource within the community, providing numerous seminars on, for example, stopping smoking, nutrition, and vegetarian cooking. Such churches are a source for further information on SDA beliefs and practices.

FEATURED RECIPE

Pumpkin Pie

15 oz. pumpkin puree

½ tsp. salt

1 tsp. pumpkin pie spice

1 pie shell

¾ cup brown sugar or pure maple syrup

½ tsp. vanilla

8 oz. silken extra-firm tofu

1. Blend all ingredients together in a blender until smooth and pour into pie shell.
2. Bake at 425°F for 15 minutes, then lower the temperature to 375°F and bake another 45 minutes.

Praline variation: Top the pie with the following mixture during the last 10–15 minutes of baking: ⅔ cup chopped pecans, ½ cup brown sugar, 1 tsp. pure maple syrup, and 1 tsp. vanilla extract.

More recipes are available at http://nutrition.jbpub.com/foodculture/

REFERENCES

Buettner, D. (2005, November). Secrets of long life. *National Geographic.*

Caviness, C.T. (1994). *Choices: Quick & healthy cooking.* Hagerstown, MD: Review and Herald Publishing Association.

Cooper, A. (Journalist). (2005). Secrets to living longer and stronger. *CNN 360 Degrees* [Television Broadcast]. Atlanta: CNN. Retrieved March 28, 2008, from http://transcripts.cnn.com/TRANSCRIPTS/0511/16/acd.01.html/

General Conference of Seventh-Day Adventists. (2008). *Seventh-Day Adventist world church statistics, health, and history.* Retrieved March 28, 2008, from http://www.adventist.org/

Griffin, V.B., & Griffin, G.M. (1999). *The guilt-free gourmet: A vegan cookbook and lifestyle resource manual.* Coldwater, MI: Remnant Publications.

Loma Linda University. Website for Adventist health study II. Available from http://www.adventisthealthstudy.org. Loma Linda, CA.

McFarland, K. (2004). *Your friends the Seventh-Day Adventists.* Nampa, ID: Pacific Press Publishing Association.

Peters, C.D., Thomas, R.D., & Peters, J.A. (1997). *More choices: for a healthy low-fat you.* Hagerstown, MD: Review and Herald Publishing Association.

Position of the American Dietetic Association and Dietitians of Canada. (2003). Vegetarian diets. *Journal of the American Dietetic Association, 103,* 748–765.

Seventh-Day Adventist Dietetic Association. (2008). *Position statement on the vegetarian diet, the SDA health message, and biblical references to diet.* Retrieved March 28, 2008, from http://www.sdada.org/

United States Department of Agriculture. (2009). *Tips and resources: Vegetarian diets.* Retrieved May 3, 2009, from http://www.mypyramid.gov/

White, E.G. (1938, 1946, 1976). *Counsels on diet and foods.* Hagerstown, MD: Review and Herald Publishing Association.

Willett, W. (2003). Lessons from dietary studies in Adventists and questions for the future. *American Journal of Clinical Nutrition, 78,* 539S–543S.

North America

Food, Cuisine, and Cultural Competency for Culinary, Hospitality, and Nutrition Professionals informs the reader about six regions across North America. Specifically, the Alaskan, Cajun and Creole, Chinese American, and Southeastern cultures of the United States; the French Canadian region of Canada; and Central Mexico are discussed.

Here the reader is introduced to each major country referred to in this section, setting the stage for the chapter presentations on food, cuisine, and cultural competency.

THE UNITED STATES

The United States is located in North America, bordered by both the North Atlantic Ocean and the North Pacific Ocean, between Canada and Mexico. The United States has the largest and most technologically powerful economy in the world. In this market-oriented economy, private individuals and business firms make most of the decisions, and the federal and state governments buy needed goods and services predominantly in the private marketplace. The U.S. firms are at, or near, the forefront in technological advances, especially in computers and in medical, aerospace, and military equipment, although their advantage has narrowed since the end of World War II. Soaring oil prices between 2005 and the first half of 2008 threatened to cause inflation and unemployment, as higher gasoline prices ate into consumers' budgets.

CANADA

Canada is located in northern North America, bordered by the North Atlantic Ocean to the east, North Pacific Ocean to the west, and the Arctic Ocean to the north, north of the conterminous United States. It is a land of vast distances and rich natural resources. As an affluent, high-tech industrial society in the trillion-dollar class, Canada resembles the United States in its market-oriented economic system, pattern of production, and affluent living standards. Canada enjoys a substantial trade surplus with the United States, which absorbs nearly 80% of Canadian exports each year. Canada is the United States' largest foreign supplier of energy, including oil, gas, uranium, and electric power. Canada's major banks are among the most stable in the world.

MEXICO

Mexico is located in the middle of the Americas, bordering the Caribbean Sea and the Gulf of Mexico between Belize and the United States, and bordering the North Pacific Ocean between Guatemala and the United States. A devaluation of the peso in late 1994 threw Mexico into economic turmoil, triggering the worst recession in more than 50 years. The nation had been making an impressive recovery until the global financial crisis hit in late 2008. Per capita income is one fourth that of the United States.

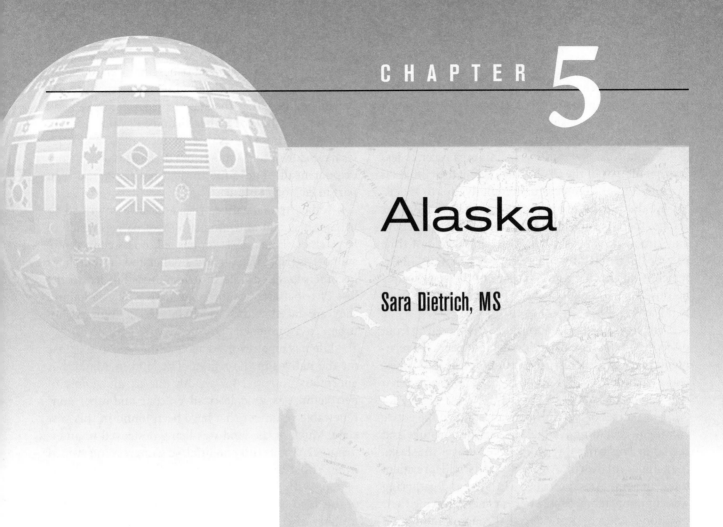

CHAPTER 5

Alaska

Sara Dietrich, MS

 ## CULTURE AND WORLD REGION

Alaska has long been known as the "last frontier," or the last area of America not fully tamed and conquered by civilization. Now, it is more commonly referred to as the "last wilderness" as efforts have been made to preserve much of its wild, untouched land and keep it undeveloped and protected.

Alaska is more than double the size of Texas and stretches across four time zones, making it a varied region of the world. If the state of Alaska were to be superimposed on a map of the United States, the borders of the state would reach from Georgia to California and from Canada to Mexico. There are over 3 million lakes, 33,000 miles of shoreline, 119 million acres of forest, 12 major rivers, and 14 of the highest peaks in North America. Despite this vast size and many wonders, Alaska remains 99% uninhabited. This vast state has a harsh climate making it difficult to inhabit. There is a varied animal population, some of which are not found anywhere else in the United States, including grizzly bears, black and brown bears, wolves, Dall sheep, walruses, polar bears, caribou, fur seals, musk ox, and more.

Alaska, being so vast and separated by three mountain systems, has several climates within the state. The mountain ranges are the Coast Range, the Brooks Range, and the Alaska Range, which includes Mount McKinley, the tallest mountain in North America. These three ranges are each very wide, making them difficult to pass and cutting off parts of the state from each other.

The area known as the panhandle, a narrow strip bordering the Pacific and curving north toward Anchorage, gets warm, humid air from the sea mixing with the cooler air of the mountainous peaks that causes very high levels of precipitation each year. This high level of precipitation promotes plant growth and there are thick forests in this area.

North of the Alaska Range is the interior of Alaska that includes hills, plateaus, and ridges around the Yukon and Kuskokwim Rivers. This area receives less precipitation than the panhandle region; the climate is dry and cold; the temperature regularly dips to –50°F.

At the northern edge of the state is the Brooks Range; there is very little precipitation in this region and almost no plant growth. During the coldest time of year the temperature there can get as low as –24°F, which is not as cold as the interior of the state simply because the Arctic Ocean to the north keeps it from being as frigid.

The revenue in the state of Alaska is primarily from oil found in the region. Both state and federal governments have an interest in developing the resources, using them for revenue while trying to preserve what they can of the land.

The natives of North America wandered the entire continent, including Alaska, subsisting on nature and the land. This early way of life lasted longer in Alaska than much of North America and is still prevalent today in some Alaskan tribes. Hunting and gathering was common, many people were farmers growing their own food, and physical exercise through hunting and gathering was a way of life for people in this region.

Alaska has four major indigenous groups in the region. First, the Aleut, who occupy small villages scattered throughout the Aleutian Islands. Second, the Eskimo reside in the mountainous regions, the tundra, and the flatlands of the Arctic province. The Tlingit and Haida are coastal natives who occupy southeastern Alaska. Finally, the Athabascan are northerners who occupy the interior of Alaska bordered by the Arctic Ocean to the north and the forests to the south. Most Alaskan natives consider themselves hunters and fishermen and many economies in Alaska remained subsistent well into the 20th century. Villages in Alaska continue to use tribal sovereignty and maintain a right to self-rule allowing each village to form their own government. Alaskan natives believe in using their local authority to provide for self-sufficient village economies. Also, all native tribes in Alaska are known for being very rank conscious and elders are treated with the utmost respect in all communities.

According to the United States census less than 1% of the population in the United States is made up of native Alaskans, making it one of the smallest racial minorities in the United States. Currently, there are 561 federally recognized tribes and over 100 state-recognized tribes as well as some tribes that are not recognized by either the state or federal government. Additional assistance for health and education services are given to those tribes that are recognized and studies have shown that some tribes do have a long history of poor health and quite limited health care, due in part to lack of assistance.

Today, many native Alaskans have migrated to urban areas and now almost 50% of natives reside in large cities. This migration has led to less community support as tribes have grown smaller and families have become separated. Life in urban areas has led to the loss of tribal identity for some natives of Alaska and they are faced with new challenges of living in an urban environment.

Life has long revolved around the land and its use for the natives in the region. The land in Alaska has enormous potential for wealth due to the supply of petroleum, gas, zinc, lead, silver, coal, and other non-renewable resources that have been found in this vast state. Much of the land was being destroyed in an effort to exploit its full potential, so Congress intervened in an effort to preserve some of the wildness of this region. With the help of two Acts from Congress some of this land is now considered federal and state parks, military reserves, and wildlife refuges, and is no longer available for development. While it is important to the American economy to use the resources there, such as petroleum, there is always concern over the effect of drilling and a possible spill on the land and its animals. For example, if there were an oil spill in the coastal waters, the migration route of the whales could change and many animals might be killed, lessening the food supply for some natives. There is an ongoing struggle between state, local, and federal governments, whose goals differ; some are attempting to always protect the land and its natural resources, while others are looking out for the good of the country and its energy needs and trade products.

 LANGUAGE

There are 20 known native languages of Alaska: Aleut, Alutiiq, Central Yup'ik Eskimo, St. Lawrence Island Eskimo, Inupiaq Eskimo, Tsimshian, Haida, Tlingit, Eyak, and 11 Athabascan languages. As tribes become less self-sufficient and natives migrate away, the languages are becoming increasingly less prevalent with time. Just two native languages, Siberian Yupik on St.

Lawrence Island and Central Yup'ik in southwestern Alaska, are still taught to children as their first language. English is becoming more common as the first language spoken in the homes of natives. The Alaska Native Language Center was established in 1972 to help document and preserve these native languages.

 ## FOOD HISTORY WITHIN THE CULTURE

On average, one third of the meat and fish eaten by rural Alaskan natives is locally caught. The harvesting, sharing, processing, and consumption of native foods is an important part of the culture and is used to help practice and teach humility and spirituality to children and young adults.

Native sources of meat and fish are higher in many important nutrients as well as more economical than imported sources. Native meats and fish have more protein, thiamin, riboflavin, niacin, and vitamin B_{12}. Many native foods are valuable sources of nutrients that are vitally important in keeping the Alaskan natives healthy and without nutrition or protein deficiencies.

Moose, one of the most common large animals, number over 150,000 throughout the state. Surprisingly, moose have benefited from the destruction of the spruce forest by humans because the first plants to begin growing after the destruction serves as good food for a moose: willow, birch, and aspen thrive first, leaving moose with no shortage of food. Moose can be as tall as 7 feet and weigh as much as 1800 pounds; it is a very mobile animal with great speed and sense of smell, allowing it to get away from enemies early and quickly.

 ## MAJOR FOODS

 ### Protein and Starch Sources

The main protein sources are fish (salmon, cod, halibut), marine mammals (seal, whale), and game animals (moose, caribou, rabbit, reindeer, black bear, muskrat). The main starch sources are potatoes and fried bread.

 ### Prominent Vegetables and Fruits

The prominent vegetables are wild roots, seaweed, and mushrooms, and the prominent fruit is the berry.

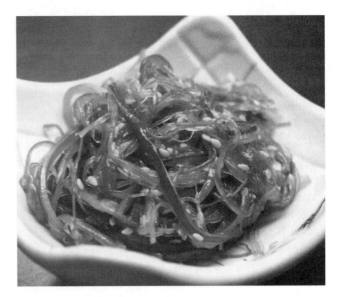

Seaweed is a common vegetable in Alaskan culture.

 ### Desserts and Beverages

Berry pies, fruit cocktail, gelatin, and fruit salad are consumed as desserts, and alcohol is the favored beverage.

 ## FOODS WITH CULTURAL SIGNIFICANCE

Foods that can be obtained through living off the land in a traditional way, such as hunting for game animals, fishing, and gathering berries, are significant in this region. People living in rural areas who adopt the native way of living are legally able to fish and hunt, and living this way is culturally significant.

 ## TYPICAL DAY'S MENU

Breakfast

- Fruit salad
- Sourdough pancakes with salmonberry syrup

Lunch

- Fish soup (cabbage, fish, potato, and carrots)

Dinner

- Salmon pie
- Fried bread

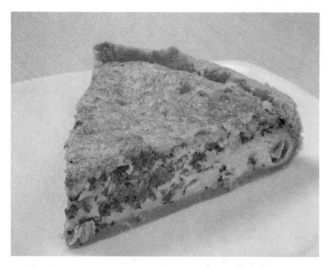

Salmon Pie

 ## HEALTH BELIEFS AND CONCERNS

There are many unique beliefs and practices among native Alaskan tribes. Many of them have ceremonies that they believe help them to maintain their own health and well-being. Medicine men, traditional healers, and herbs are routinely used in the region. One of the beliefs in this culture is that they are all closely connected with nature, and to stay healthy they need to treat the land and the spirits around them with respect.

Diabetes is a major health problem in this region, and getting professionals to help educate Alaskan communities about this serious disease, as well as help them treat it (and prevent it whenever possible), will be an important step in the health of Alaskan natives. Between 1990 and 1998 the total number of young native Americans (both American Indians and native Alaskans) who had been diagnosed with diabetes increased by 71%, and the prevalence of the disease increased by 46%. There is evidence that the per capita expenditures for all native Americans (American Indians and native Alaskans) is lower compared with that of the majority of Americans. This lack of funding may be having a negative effect on the health of the natives in this region.

 ## GENERAL HEALTH AND NUTRITIONAL INDICATORS SUMMARY

According to the Centers for Disease Control and Prevention, there are disparities in the health communication rate among the American Indian/Alaskan native people. Health communication includes Internet access, health literacy, time spent with clients, and whether the health provider spends adequate time with the client and respects the client (both reported by the client). American Indian/Alaska native people were found to have a 50–99% lower rate of Internet access as compared with the group with the highest rate. Basic health literacy was also found to have a large discrepancy; the American Indians/native Alaskans were more likely to have below basic health literacy as compared with the highest group. Being aware of these disparities is helpful, but it is only the first step. It is important to take action to reduce these discrepancies and work to improve the health communications among this group.

American Indians and Alaskan natives live a solitary life due to their isolated location as well as their unique culture and history. The remote location of many of these tribes leads them to form their own healthcare systems, and depending on the tribe, there may be a lack of education and a high rate of poverty contributing to their poor health care.

Specifically, cancer rates have recently received further attention and researchers have worked to determine the cancer incidence among American Indians and Alaskan natives. It was found that cancer incidence rates among this population varied widely by region. Among males and females in the northern and southern plains, American Indian and Alaskan native cancer rates were higher than the rates among non-Hispanic whites; however, in the Southwest, Pacific Coast, and the East regions the opposite was true: the cancer rates among the American Indians and Alaskan natives were lower than among non-Hispanic whites.

Looking at individual types of cancer also showed discrepancies between American Indians/Alaskan natives versus non-Hispanic whites. Lung cancer and colorectal cancer rates for American Indians/Alaska natives were higher than among non-Hispanic whites in Alaska and the northern plains.

Stomach, gallbladder, kidney, and liver cancer rates were higher among the American Indians/Alaskan natives in Alaska, the plains regions, and the Southwest.

It is important to look at regional discrepancies among disease states to become aware of where education and prevention methods may be effective. Recognizing that these natives may lack awareness and have less stringent healthcare guidelines is the first step in correcting the discrepancy of cancer rates in these regions.

Demographic and Health Indicators

Demographic and health indicators are as follows:

- State of Alaska (2006) deaths by number: 3344
- Death rate: 499.1 (per 100,000); age-adjusted death rate: 774.4 (per 100,000)

Rates for American Indians/Alaskan natives (2004) are as follows:

- Fetal mortality rate: 5.84
- Fetal deaths (24 weeks or longer): 258

COMMUNICATION AND COUNSELING TIPS

One of the goals of the program Healthy People 2010 is equitable health status for all racial/ethnic groups by the year 2010. In 1997, just 62% of native Alaskans were covered under health insurance, whereas the national average was 82%. Increasing health coverage is an important goal in this region and with this comes the opportunity for more natives to meet with registered dietitians for counseling and education.

As a counselor in this region it is important to be aware of, and understand the use of, traditional medicines and healing techniques. In all tribes, interactions among people contain the fundamental element of respect. Respect to native Alaskans means "how one presents himself or herself to the world and how one acts" (Huff & Kline, 1999, p. 286). Respect in these tribes is tied to being a native, and as an outsider being aware of this is vital to be an effective counselor and communicate successfully. Respect includes not talking or bragging about oneself, not talking back, and treating others in a kind manner. Also, sharing and being fair to all is important among native Alaskans. In this region a high value is placed on cultural sensitivity and a healthcare worker who is respectful, kind, and understanding of the native culture is truly valued.

There are few native professionals, especially in dietetics, so most natives are treated by nonnatives. As mentioned, there is wide variability among natives and among all the different tribes. A major obstacle found by many counselors and professionals who treat Alaskan natives is a lack of understanding and knowledge about the culture and the differences found between natives of different tribes and in different regions. It is vital that professionals be aware of differences, treat all clients with respect, and be understanding of potential anxiety among their clients. Some professionals have reported cultural mistrust among natives who are unsure that their caregivers know what is best for them. Being aware of this anxiety is helpful in being open to conversation and listening to any concerns clients may have.

Also, specifically for dietitians, it is important to consider that the climate varies widely throughout the year. Because of this, dietary consumption does vary by season, so taking one or even several 24-hour recalls may not be enough unless they are spread throughout the year.

FEATURED RECIPE

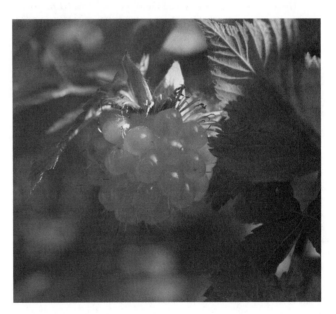

Salmonberries

Salmonberry Syrup

1 pt. salmonberries (found in Alaska)

1 cup sugar

1 tbsp. cornstarch

1. Cook salmonberries over a low heat until the juice leeches out a little.
2. Add the sugar and corn starch.
3. Mix occasionally and continue to cook on a low heat for 30 minutes.

More recipes are available at http://nutrition.jbpub.com/foodculture/

REFERENCES

Acton, K.J., Burrows, N.R., Moore, K., Querec, L., Geiss, L.S., Engelgau, M.M. (2002). Trends in diabetes prevalence among American Indian and Alaska native children, adolescents, and young adults. *American Journal of Public Health, 92*(9), 1485–1490.

Alaska Native Knowledge Network. (2007). *Traditional health, medicine and healing.* Retrieved July 15, 2008 from http://ankn.uaf.edu/iks/health.html/

Alaska Native Language Center. (2001). *Alaska native languages: An overview.* Retrieved July 30, 2008 from http://www.uaf.edu/anlc/languages.html/

Brown, D. (1972). *Wild Alaska. The American Wilderness.* New York: Time-Life Books.

Center for Disease Control and Prevention; National Center for Health Statistics. Retrieved October 29, 2009, from http://www.cdc.gov/nchs/ppt/hpdata2010/focusareas/fa11_2_data_summary_table.xls/

Center for Disease Control and Prevention; National Center for Health Statistics. National Vital Statistics Reports. Retrieved October 29, 2009, from http://www.cdc.gov/nchs/data/nvsr/nvsr56/nvsr56_03.pdf/

Centers for Disease Control and Prevention; United States Cancer Statistics. Retrieved October 29, 2009, from http://apps.nccd.cdc.gov/uscs/Table.aspx?Group=5f&Year=2005&Display=n/

Haycox, S. (2002). *Frigid embrace: Politics, economics, and environment in Alaska.* Corvallis, OR: Oregon State University Press.

Herring, R.D. (1999). *Counseling with native American Indians and Alaska natives: Strategies for helping professionals.* Thousand Oaks, CA: Sage.

Huff, R.M., & Kline, M.V. (1999). *Promoting health in multicultural populations: A handbook for practitioners.* Thousand Oaks, CA: Sage.

Johnston, B.R. (Ed). (1994). *Who pays the price? The sociocultural context of environmental crisis.* Washington, DC: Island Press.

Kunitz, S.J. (2008). Ethics in public health research: Changing patterns of mortality among American Indians. *American Journal of Public Health, 98*(3), 404–411.

CHAPTER 6

Cajun and Creole

Colette G. Leistner, PhD, RD

Simone Camel, MS, RD

 CULTURE AND WORLD REGION

Southern Louisiana is the home of two of America's most unique cultures: Cajun and Creole. The two are often equated by people outside the region; others believe there is a difference but are at a loss to explain it. The two cultures have coexisted in southern Louisiana for over 300 years, yet shared influences of climate, geography, politics, religion, and economics still remained distinct.

Today's Cajuns are descended from the 17th-century French colonists of *Acadie* (present-day Nova Scotia). The result of political conflict between England and France for over 150 years was the end of French control over *Acadie*. In 1755, the English expelled the French colonists in the *Grande Derangement*, or Acadian Diaspora. Most of these Acadians found their way to Louisiana over the next 30 years, some going there directly, some spending time in various eastern seaboard ports, others in English prisons, and still others

in France or French colonies in the Caribbean before making their way to Louisiana (LeBreton, 1980). Over the years in Louisiana the French term "Acadian" was eventually pronounced in a more Anglicized fashion as "Cajun."

A 22-parish (county) area of southern Louisiana is the home of most Cajuns. In 1971, the Louisiana Legislature (Louisiana House of Representatives, 1971) dubbed this area "Acadiana" in recognition of its enduring French Acadian heritage. Cajuns are traditionally a rural people with close ties to extended family. Roman Catholicism remains the predominant religion. English is the major language throughout southern Louisiana, but many Cajuns either speak or understand Louisiana French or have French-speaking family members (Gibson & DelSesto, 1975; Trépanier, 1991).

The term "Creole" can be very confusing depending upon who is using it and who it is describing. It can mean the descendents of early European settlers—French, Spanish, German—who were born in Louisiana before the Louisiana Purchase. Used as an adjective (lowercase "c") creole "refers to the adaptation of a product to a New World environment" (Brasseaux, 1987, p. 322) and was used in this sense to describe slaves born in Louisiana. Black Creoles (uppercase "C") are descendents of *gens de couleur libre*, or blacks who were free prior to the Civil War. "Creole" also refers to a speaker (usually black) of the French Creole dialect in southern Louisiana (Brasseaux, 1987). When "Acadiana" was recognized for its Acadian heritage, black residents residing within the area and not being of Acadian descent began using the "Creole" descriptor to acknowledge their distinct heritage.

Today in New Orleans, Creole "is commonly taken to connote black ancestry or some degree of black ancestry" (Powell, 1992, p. 73). The contributions of this large segment of the population have made New Orleans the distinctive city it is.

FOOD HISTORY WITHIN THE CULTURE

While contributions to the cuisine and culture of southern Louisiana were made by the Africans, Spanish, Germans, Italians, and native Americans, among others, the French influence has remained most evident. Although "[A] French *approach* to cuisine . . . dominates this culinary style, [i.e.,] . . . full utilization of foodstuffs at hand and the expenditure of care, effort, and time in food preparation . . ." (Leistner, 1986) described Cajun cuisine, it is just as applicable to Creole.

A remarkable characteristic of both Cajuns and Creoles is their appreciation of food at every stage of preparation. Conversation among family members and guests gathered for a meal will often center on a detailed review of the dishes being prepared. It should not be forgotten that they have high standards for the foods prepared and consumed.

Traditional Cajun foods featured dishes cooked in one pot; for example, soup, stew, gumbo, and jambalaya. Although other methods of cooking were used, this predispersal method of cooking made the most of the tough meat available—wild game, old hens, salted meat—and suited the limited number of cooking vessels poor families possessed.

New Orleans is renowned for its cuisine, which fits the definition of creole cited earlier: adaptation of a product to a New World environment. Each of the early immigrant groups arriving in this port city,

especially the French, Africans, Spanish, Italians, and Germans, contributed to the mix of ingredients, recipes, and cooking methods that resulted in Creole cuisine. A cosmopolitan approach to dining is evident in New Orleans' neighborhoods. People from one cultural or ethnic group adopt the dishes from others and happily add it to their repertoire.

Men and women in both cultures actively participate in food preparation. Women typically prepare the daily meals, and, as noted by Bienvenu, Brasseaux, and Brasseaux (2005), control the "indoor sphere." Men are associated with preparation of food in the "outdoor sphere." An outdoor cooking event may be for the family (a barbecue or crawfish boil, for example), but it is often for larger groups. Many men are renowned in their communities for particular specialties and are called upon to prepare large quantities of rice dressing, jambalaya, fried fish, or perhaps barbecue for civic or religious organizations, or maybe a pot-roasted duck or doves for a "hunting camp supper" (Bienvenu et al., 2005; Guiterrez, 1983; Leistner, 1993).

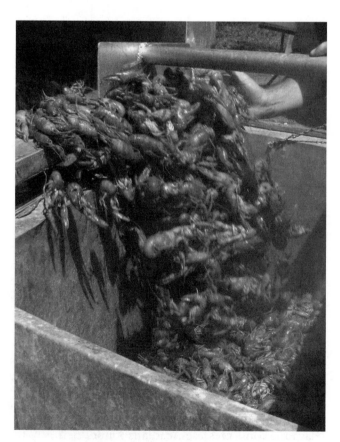

Boiled crawfish donated by local farmers to be served by the pound at a community fundraiser.

Photo by Simone Camel (author)

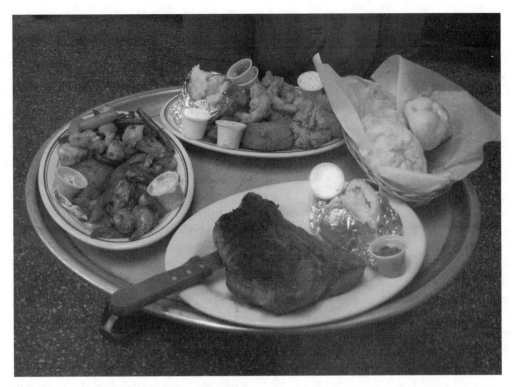

From Left: Grilled Seafood Platter, Fried Seafood Platter, Rolls, Steak, and Potatoes. Seafood platters contain oysters, shrimp, fish, and crab cakes.

Photo by Simone Camel (author)

Not unlike the larger population, changes are seen in food preparation as family members spend more time outside the home and take less time to prepare and serve meals *en famille* (with the family). While ingredients necessary to prepare traditional meals are certainly available in every southern Louisiana grocery store and supermarket, they, along with convenience stores and meat markets, offer convenient forms of traditional food ingredients. One can find packaged mixes for jambalaya, gumbo, bread pudding, and beignets; creole-style canned red and white beans, and canned gumbo; and most recently, frozen dinners produced by regional restaurateurs.

 MAJOR FOODS

There exists in southern Louisiana an informal family/friends food distribution system that supports the retention of traditional food practices in both Cajun and Creole cultures. The beneficiaries of this system are relatives or friends who have moved away, those who may be experiencing difficult financial times, and elderly or ill individuals who are no longer able to hunt,

fish, or garden, all of whom still yearn for familiar traditional foods. Typical of these foods are those that cannot be purchased: wild game, such as venison, rabbit, or squirrel; wild fowl, such as ducks, doves, geese, and quail; those that may be cost-prohibitive, such as seafood; items that benefit from freshness (i.e., homegrown fruits and vegetables); or those that are of superior quality when homemade, such as *boudin*, hog's head cheese, *grattons*, and homemade sausage. Because the genesis of these foods is hunting, fishing, gardening, or animal husbandry, the system may be more prevalent in rural areas; it is not unknown, however, in urban areas where many urban families have generous, thoughtful relatives living in the country.

Another important characteristic of southern Louisiana cuisine is the concept of regional variation, and more specifically, inter- and intraregional variation. This goes beyond the differences that are exhibited by individual or family preferences and illustrates the reality that Cajun and Creole cuisine and culture vary despite common influences. Gumbo is an example of interregional variation: both cuisines feature gumbo, but chicken *filé* gumbo is common in the Cajun region and seafood gumbo in the New Orleans area (Leistner, 1996).

The native Americans of southern Louisiana are the source of a unique ingredient in Cajun cuisine: *filé* or *file* powder. The leaves of the indigenous sassafras tree are dried and then, using a wooden mortar and pestle, crushed or ground into a powder. This powder flavors and thickens poultry-based gumbos. Every household has a source for the small jar in the pantry. Lucky families know someone who continues to make it or know where to purchase it fresh in a roadside stand; everyone else buys it at a grocery store.

Intraregional variation is yet more specific. The chicken *filé* gumbo, or *gombo filé* as it is known in French, starts with a roux. The roux adds flavor and color and is responsible for some of the thickening in a *file* gumbo. Traveling inland from the Gulf Coast, this gumbo will become darker, thicker, and richer due to a preference for using greater quantities of darker roux. In some areas very close to the Gulf, this gumbo is prepared without any roux at all. How dark is a dark roux? Perhaps the best description of this can be found in *Chef Paul Prudhomme's Louisiana Kitchen* (1984) where photos provide guidance. The color of the desired roux is often described in food terms such as caramel, milk chocolate, or dark chocolate in color.

Creole cuisine also exhibits intraregional variation in the use of turtle. Turtle soup is a popular dish on the menus of many New Orleans restaurants. In the black Creole neighborhoods a traditional Easter dish is turtle cooked in a tomato-based or *au jus* gravy (Leistner, 1986).

Cajun cuisine features "one-pot" dishes such as jambalaya, stews, *fricassées*, and gumbos. Creole cuisine falls into two camps: elegant dining in restaurants that reflect a classical French heritage where meals are composed of several courses, and the cooking of the predominately black Creole neighborhoods with the dishes that reflect the diverse cultures of New Orleans as well as the "soul" food of the American south. This is the Creole cuisine that is of primary interest in this chapter.

 Protein Sources

As in other cultures, protein from animal sources is a prestige food in southern Louisiana and is usually served at both the midday ("dinner" in the Cajun region; "lunch" or "dinner" in the Creole region) and evening ("supper" in the Cajun region; "dinner" in the Creole region) meals. Beef, pork, chicken, and turkey, as well as the wild game and wild fowl mentioned previously, are all consumed regularly. The traditional *boucherie* when a hog was slaughtered yielded special dishes that utilized every bit of protein in, and on, the carcass. *Boudin*, a fresh sausage made with pork scraps, cooked rice, and seasoned with cayenne pepper and salt, and perhaps most distinctively, flat-leaf parsley and green onion tops, continues to be popular and virtually iconic. Hog's head cheese utilized the natural gelatin and small bits of meat from the bony parts of the hog. This is seasoned as the *boudin* is. Sausage, fresh and smoked, was produced. The *chaudin* or *ponce* (stomach) was stuffed with a meat and rice mixture and braised. Seafood and egg dishes continue to be served on Fridays year round and not just during the Catholic Lenten season.

Ham, salt pork, pickled pork, and tasso (lean, smoked, seasoned pork) is used to season dried beans. Ground beef and/or pork is a major component of several popular stuffed vegetables, as well as the rice and cornbread dressing that are served as accompaniments in meals that feature meat or poultry.

Fish and other seafood are extremely popular in southern Louisiana due to the proximity to the Gulf, bayous, and lakes, as well as to the strong ties to the traditions of the Catholic Church. The tradition of "fish on Friday" is not limited to those belonging to the Church. Institutions such as hospitals and schools feature seafood and other meatless items on Fridays as a matter of course. Families and restaurants may also prepare shrimp, oysters, crab, crawfish, turtle, or alligator in place of, or in addition to, fish. A noteworthy characteristic of southern Louisiana cuisine that has remained intact since the 1930s is the variety of methods of food preparation that are utilized for meat and seafood. For instance, fish is baked, prepared in a roux-based gravy or stew, fried, cooked in sauce piquant, grilled, and broiled.

Dried beans are traditional across southern Louisiana. Is it Monday in New Orleans? Red beans and rice will appear without fail in homes, in every type of restaurant, hospital cafeterias, and many schools. This dish was, however, uncommon west of New Orleans until the Popeye's restaurant chain introduced it to a wider audience.

White beans are a part of the traditional duck camp supper of southwest Louisiana. That menu features pot-roasted duck (mallards or teals), white beans on rice with *au jus* gravy, and coleslaw (shredded cabbage with apple cider vinegar, salt, and black pepper) served alongside. In the bayou region of southeast Louisiana a typical Friday dinner is fried fish served with white beans over rice.

Starch Sources

Rice is central to dishes in both cultures. For instance, rice is served with every type of gumbo in Cajun and Creole cuisines. It is also one half of the popular "red beans and rice" as well as white beans and rice; however, "rice and gravy," traditionally the focus of almost every noon and evening meal in much of Cajun southern Louisiana, is not common in Creole New Orleans. Another Cajun meal, jambalaya, is predominately rice. Rice and milk was served at breakfast and sometimes for supper before dry cereals were popular.

In southern Louisiana potatoes do not feature prominently on menus as they do in other parts of the United States. They are, however, used in potato salad, a frequent accompaniment for gumbo in both Cajun and Creole cuisines. Traditional recipes for potatoes include potato stew served over rice and in New Orleans, a po-boy featuring fried potatoes.

As one of Louisiana's (major) crops fresh sweet potatoes are available fall through winter and canned year round. They are often served baked whole, in casseroles, candied, or small rounds are pan-fried and sprinkled with sugar. They can be found in tarts, pies, and other baked goods.

French bread remains popular. "Hot" French bread is baked and sold at local supermarkets and in some regional chains. It is sliced and served as is, or as garlic bread. Stale French bread finds its way into bread pudding. When families prepared breakfast "from scratch" stale French bread was often used for *pain perdu*, a type of French toast.

 Fat Sources

Fat in the form of cooking oil and bacon grease are often added to vegetables as they cook. Fatty meats, such as ham hocks and salt pork, season dried beans and some vegetables. The large amount of meat and poultry consumed by residents of southern Louisiana contributes saturated fat to the diet. Fried foods are popular as well.

 Prominent Vegetables

Fresh homegrown vegetables are appreciated in both cultures, but these days fewer families rely on their own skills as gardeners for a steady supply of vegetables. The family/friends food distribution system does provide fresh produce to some people. Oyster mushrooms are gathered from select areas in the wetlands and enjoyed by a limited number of people.

Popular vegetables include tomatoes, okra, corn, onions, peppers of all kinds, eggplant, mirliton (chayote), green beans, and lima beans; cream, purple hull, and crowder peas, beets, turnips, mustard and turnip greens, carrots, and cabbage. While not technically vegetables, flat-leaf parsley and green onions (used primarily for the green "onion tops") are indispensable ingredients for many Cajun dishes and are sometimes the only things planted in a garden. Eggplant and mirliton are often "stuffed" with a mixture of the well-seasoned smothered vegetable combined with rice or bread crumbs and seafood or ground meat. It is worth noting that fat (bacon grease, butter, or margarine) or meat (bacon, ham, sausage, or salt pork) may be added to many of these vegetables in cooking.

 Prominent Fruits

Southern Louisiana produces navel oranges and satsumas (a type of mandarin orange) as a major crop as well as in backyard gardens. This provides a healthy addition to the diet late fall through spring. The wide range of fresh fruit available in supermarkets and grocery stores also contributes to the southern Louisiana diet.

Fig trees are found in many neighborhoods. This is one of the foods shared with family and friends, usually in the form of fig preserves. The receipt of a pint of fig preserves is a treasured gift. In summers past wild blackberries were picked and made into preserves. They can still be found along fence lines in the rural areas and are consumed as ice cream toppings, as well as in cobblers, pies, and tarts. Pear trees provided home-canned pear halves and preserves. They are utilized in fruit breads and salads. Home canning of fruits and vegetables is done less frequently today due to the wide variety of preserves available commercially. Some of the activities associated with the process, such as picking blackberries on a summer day, provide an opportunity for a family outing.

Pecan trees grow across the region. Each fall finds people avidly gathering the fallen nuts. The bounty can be sold for cash at feed stores, hardware stores, and sometimes even convenience stores. These establishments may also offer "cracking," which does just that to the recently picked pecans making it much easier to shell them. Gathering family and friends together to shell the pecans and prepare them for freezing can be another excuse to visit and share a meal. The frozen nutmeat can last until the next crop is available. They are typical ingredients in baked goods, candies such as pralines, fruit salad, or may just be eaten out of hand.

 Spices and Seasonings

Cajun and Creole food has the reputation of being spicy. This is a result of the preference of restaurateurs and does not reflect tradition. Cajun and Creole food is more accurately described as "well seasoned."

Flat-leaf, or Italian, parsley, green onion tops, *file* powder, bay leaves, salt, and thyme are used. The amount of cayenne or black pepper and hot pepper sauce depends upon an individual cook's (or his or her family's) preference. Pork roast, a very popular meat in both cultures, is often "stuffed" with slivers of jalapeno or other hot pepper, bell pepper, garlic, cayenne pepper, salt, and perhaps onion and parsley. Many dishes of southern Louisiana begin with chopped celery, onion, and green or bell pepper (Leistner, 1996).

Cajun seasoning blends (i.e., combinations of salt, peppers, herbs, and spices), have become big sellers in every food market. People are very particular about their favorite brand.

What would be found in a southern Louisiana pantry? It is likely that the shelves would hold a bottle or can of locally or regionally produced dark cane syrup. A baby food jar of *file* powder made by a neighbor or relative and a bottle of cayenne pepper just have to be there. The family's favorite hot sauce may be alongside home-bottled hot vinegar made with hot peppers grown in the backyard garden; however, neither of these items may ever make it to the pantry, remaining instead on the kitchen table always ready for use. Expect a large crock to be holding 20 lbs. of medium- or long-grain rice from a regional rice mill. Dark-roast coffee will be there also, plus a can of "Pet" (evaporated) milk or maybe sweetened condensed milk. A perfectly filled pantry will display several jars of homemade fig preserves, blackberry preserves, and perhaps canned pear halves.

 Beverages

Coffee is the ultimate beverage in the homes of southern Louisiana. Offering a guest (regardless of whether the guest is a relative, friend, or stranger) a cup of coffee is the hallmark of hospitality and to refuse can be interpreted as an insult. At the very least hard feelings may result. In the homes of Cajun Louisiana the *demitasse* (small cup) is the standard-size serving. While coffee makers and percolators have made their way into homes, a "real" cup of coffee is still made using an enameled drip pot. Dark, or French, roast coffee is traditional. Coffee with chicory is used in the famous coffeehouses of New Orleans—*Café du Monde* and Morning Call to prepare the *café au lait*—equal amounts of hot coffee with chicory and hot milk, for which they are known. Many city residents always prepare coffee with chicory in their homes (not necessarily as *café au lait*). Because of its popularity some hospitals and other facilities offer it along with regular dark-roast and decaffeinated coffee. Iced coffee with chicory is a summer tradition in some families in New Orleans (Schwaner-Albright, 2007). While dark-roast coffee is the norm in Cajun southern Louisiana, coffee with chicory is enjoyed by some people.

Sugar and some type of coffee creamer, either powdered milk, half-and-half, evaporated or "Pet" milk, or sweetened condensed milk, are typically added to a cup of coffee.

Iced beverages, such as sweetened iced tea, are very popular in southern Louisiana as they are in much of the South. Root beer, both carbonated and non-carbonated, is popular as well. Barq's, a New Orleans' brand of root beer that is now marketed nationally, is also made by the pitcher with root beer extract and sugar, and is often served in the summer.

Making homemade wine is a hobby of some people. Beer, especially local or regional brands, such as Dixie and Abita, are favorite accompaniments at barbecues, crawfish boils, *boucheries*, and other meals.

 Desserts

While sweets are not necessarily served with coffee or expected after lunch and dinner every day, desserts are often part of a Sunday dinner, a large gathering, or a special occasion. Traditional desserts were made with easily obtainable supplies and include *massepain* or *gateau de sirop*, a gingerbread or spicecake made with the locally produced dark cane syrup. Simple cakes, such as pineapple upside-down cake or a layer cake made with a custard or coconut filling, and rice pudding made use of the eggs and milk produced by the family's hen and dairy cow and supplies available at the local grocery store. Regional cookbooks usually include at least one recipe for fig cake: moist, dense, and rich with the fig preserves and chopped pecans found in the pantry.

Particular favorites of Cajun families are *les tartes douces* (sweet dough pies) and *les petits gâteaux secs* (tea cakes). Made with a basic dough (flour, eggs, sugar, milk, baking powder, and nutmeg), the pies or tarts are filled with fig or blackberry preserves, custard, coconut custard, or sweet potatoes. The custard-filled pie, or *tarte a la bouilli*, is a particular favorite in southeastern Louisiana. Scraps of dough are rolled out and cut into little tea cakes.

Pecan pralines are traditional in Cajun and Creole cultures. There are different styles of this candy—creamy, sugary, those made with dark-brown sugar, others made with light-brown sugar—but all are delicious.

Desserts familiar across the southern United States are also found in Cajun and Creole cuisine. Homemade banana pudding, for instance, makes frequent appearances on the dinner table.

An iconic dessert of New Orleans is bread pudding. It transforms stale French bread, milk, eggs, sugar, and vanilla into a dish that can make (or break) a cook's reputation. Some versions of bread pudding are accompanied by a sauce (e.g., whiskey or rum, custard, or lemon), but a good bread pudding needs no embellishment.

Beignets, the fried, leavened bread dough-like squares sprinkled with powdered sugar and accompanied by a cup of *café au lait*, are a New Orleans specialty associated primarily with the *Café du Monde* and Morning Call. Because these coffeehouses are open 24 hours a day, this confection is sought at any time of day or night.

FOODS WITH CULTURAL SIGNIFICANCE

When someone is asked to name a food associated with south Louisiana it is likely that crawfish will be mentioned. It was not until after 1959 when Breaux Bridge, Louisiana, hosted a Crawfish Festival that crawfish gained much attention (Bienvenu et al., 2005). The popularity of it now has much to do with the success of crawfish farming on the prairies of southern Louisiana.

Across southern Louisiana festivals are held each year to celebrate a variety of foods that are meaningful to the residents. Foods featured at the New Orleans Jazz and Heritage Festival held each spring includes Creole specialties. Other yearly festivals celebrate jambalaya, *cochon de lait* (roast suckling pig), the *boucherie* (slaughter of a hog), gumbo, sauce piquant, frogs' legs, catfish, crawfish, court bouillon, *boudin*, *andouille*, rice, omelets, ducks, and dairy products among other products, dishes, or traditions.

Catholic churches and civic organizations in most communities host bazaars as fund-raising events. A definite highlight of these usually weekend-long events is the food. One dish is highlighted on Friday night, then something else for Saturday lunch and supper. Sunday's finale might be a barbecue at noon.

A much anticipated and much contested feature of most, if not all, of these events is a "cook-off." Whatever the event celebrated is usually the focus of this cooking contest. Teams or individuals will vie for top honors and bragging rights as the winner. Cooking techniques are passed from one generation to the next maintaining the knowledge of preparation of large quantities of culturally significant foods.

TYPICAL DAY'S MENU

The meal pattern in southern Louisiana is based on three meals per day. The midday meal in the Cajun culture is often called "dinner," while in the Creole it may be "lunch" or "dinner." The evening meal is "supper" among Cajuns and more often "dinner" in the Creole culture.

In the Cajun culture breakfast may include dark-roast coffee or coffee milk (milk to which a few tablespoons of hot, sweetened coffee has been added) with biscuits or toast and grits, cold cereal and milk, and perhaps eggs. In recent times, it may also be breakfast picked up at a fast-food restaurant on work days as in other parts of the country. A breakfast in New Orleans' Creole neighborhoods may be lighter and consist of French bread or a biscuit with coffee and chicory or *café au lait*.

The evening meal tends to be heavier in the Cajun culture when the family can share a meal. "Rice and gravy" has been the traditional focus of the meal. Some type of meat or poultry is the source of the gravy. Vegetables, such as smothered green beans, *macque choux*, or some type of field peas, accompany the meat and rice. When gardens are producing, fresh sliced tomatoes and cucumbers or cantaloupe are offered. French bread or sliced white bread may be on the table along with milk and/or iced tea. In winter, gumbo with rice and a bowl of potato salad are typical. Other soups include corn soup and vegetable beef.

The noon meal in the Cajun region varies depending on the employment schedule of the family's adults. In the past, women prepared a heavier meal at noon when husbands returned home for dinner. Supper would have featured leftovers or a simple supper of

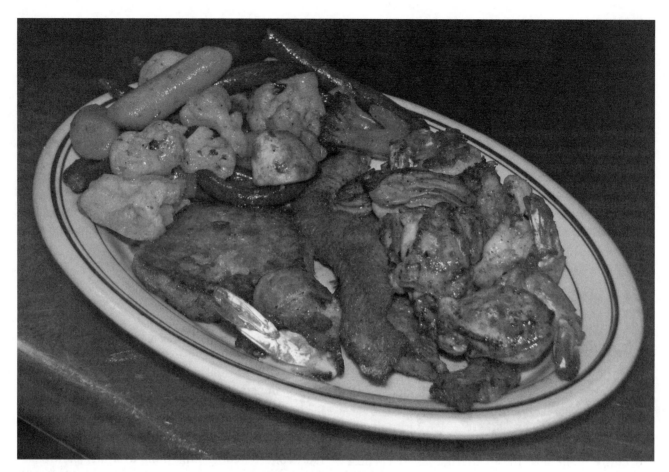

Grilled Seafood Platter: Oysters, Shrimp, Fish, Seafood Cake, and Vegetables

Photo by Simone Camel (author)

scrambled eggs and potatoes or cornbread and milk. Today, dinner may be packed at home and brought to work. At other times fast food will suffice. Another popular alternative is the plate lunch.

Across the region at midday grocery stores, convenience stores, and small local restaurants or lunch counters feature "plate lunches"—southern Louisiana's version of "a meat and three." One of these in Cajun country might feature chicken *fricassée*, rice and gravy, and crowder peas. A slice of white bread would be included. In New Orleans a pork chop or fried chicken may accompany Monday's red beans and rice and French bread. French bread may be included, too.

Po-boys (poor boys), the New Orleans creation that is so much more than a sandwich, may also be on the menu in either region. The best sandwiches are made with crusty French bread, either half a *baguette* or a whole *pistolette*. Fried shrimp-and-oysters po-boys are particularly popular during their respective "seasons." Fried catfish is available year round courtesy of farm-raised catfish. Ham and hot roast beef are also popular. "Do you want it dressed?" is asked when a po-boy is ordered. "Dressed" usually means with mayonnaise, shredded lettuce, and sliced tomatoes.

Many of the establishments in the Cajun region will likely also sell *boudin* (a fresh sausage of ground pork and cooked rice seasoned with fresh flat-leaf parsley and green onion tops, salt, and cayenne pepper) by the pound or by the link. A link of *boudin* stuffed into a *pistolette* (foot-long French bread) makes a filling lunch. It is likely that the *boudin* plus *grattons* (fried pork skin with fat and sometimes meat attached) sold at the neighborhood stores have been purchased for snacks, too.

There is a tradition in New Orleans of having certain meals on set days of the week. For instance, customers expect red beans and rice on Mondays at every restaurant and hospital cafeteria and at home. The same holds for seafood gumbo on Friday. Some families have a tradition of always having meatballs and spaghetti on a certain day regardless of their ethnic background (Leistner, 1996).

HOLIDAY MEALS

A variety of foods traditional in the Cajun and Creole cultures are prepared for holidays. The Thanksgiving menu, for example, will not necessarily be turkey, stuffing, and mashed potatoes. It is very common for the family's favorite gumbo to either begin the meal or be the meal.

Pork roast may well be the most popular meat in both cultures and will usually be included on Thanksgiving, Christmas, and possibly Easter. An additional meat is usually served, such as pot-roasted duck or goose, and in the Cajun area, ham, or deep-fried turkey. More meat or seafood (ground beef and/or pork, crab meat, or shrimp) is present as an ingredient in the rice or cornbread dressing, and stuffed vegetables, such as eggplant, mirliton (chayote), globe artichokes (especially in New Orleans), or cabbage, are also enjoyed.

It is a New Year's Day tradition in the American south and across southern Louisiana as well to find black-eyed peas and some type of greens (e.g., mustard, turnip, or collard) on the table. A few weeks later Carnival season begins (January 6 through Mardi Gras) bringing King Cake (icing-covered sweet yeast bread) to every office and most homes at least once. On Mardi Gras in the Cajun region many families will prepare a chicken *filé* gumbo (Sexton, 1999). In New Orleans, families may enjoy fried chicken and red beans and rice between carnival parades.

Lenten fasting, abstinence from meat on Ash Wednesday and Fridays including Good Friday, and possibly Holy Thursday, continues to be observed throughout much of southern Louisiana. Institutions, including hospitals and schools, and most restaurants, take this into consideration and plan accordingly (Leistner, 1993). In recent years Good Friday has been an occasion for families to gather for a meal, which is often a crawfish boil.

HEALTH BELIEFS AND CONCERNS

It is often the case in southern Louisiana that medical care is sought only after a condition becomes serious. This may be due at least in part to the cultural belief that whatever happens to an individual's health is part of God's plan for his or her life or is "his or her lot in life." This strong faith is apparent when speaking to many people regardless of whether they are Roman Catholic or Protestant.

Assisting individuals in achieving and maintaining a healthy weight can be complicated by the body image that is considered acceptable. In both cultures someone thin (and possibly at a healthy body weight) is sometimes considered "puny" and unhealthy.

Just as in other parts of the United States, the positive impact of regular exercise on good health has yet to be embraced widely in southern Louisiana. Exercise has traditionally been equated with the physical exertion gained through the physical labor of blue collar and agricultural jobs or a "busy day" at work. As a result the transition to urban jobs and modern conveniences common in the home means less physical activity for many people. Other people believe that sports are for children and teenagers; once one is married and has children, participating in sports is no longer appropriate.

Elderly or poorly educated people may still cling to outdated ideas about the causes of diabetes, hypertension, or cardiovascular disease. They may also rely upon home remedies to treat these conditions (Leistner, 1993).

While dietetic practitioners working within the Cajun and Creole cultures of southern Louisiana may find it challenging considering the nutritional content of the typical diet—high calorie, high saturated fat, and high sodium—it must be acknowledged that the appreciation that the people have for food and their ability and willingness to cook are positive aspects of both cultures. It is likely that, with direction, the clients will produce acceptable products incorporating the dietary modifications prescribed.

GENERAL HEALTH AND NUTRITIONAL INDICATORS SUMMARY

Proper diet and adequate physical activity are critical elements in the prevention and treatment of the chronic diseases identified as being leading causes of death in the state of Louisiana where the Cajun and Creole cultures reside. From the statistics cited below, it is clear that Louisiana's dietetics professionals face a challenge in the coming years. The education of the state's future dietetic and culinary professionals should include gaining an understanding of how to incorporate healthier versions of culturally important foods into menus and diet-therapy plans. The role that food plays in these cultures is no less significant than it is in any other culture; it could be argued, in fact, that it is more significant than in some other cultures.

Five of the 10 leading causes of death in Louisiana as reported in the 2003 Louisiana Health Report Card, a publication of the Louisiana Department of Health and Hospital's Office of Public Health, have diet as a modifiable risk factor. The chronic nature of the diseases—heart disease, stroke, cancer, diabetes, and kidney disease—can have a negative effect upon an individual's ability to sustain a productive, satisfying life.

According to the Behavioral Risk Factor Surveillance System Data in 2008, 34.7% of adults in Louisiana were overweight (body mass index 25–29.9) and 28.9% were obese (body mass index ≥30). Only 70.1% of adults reported participating in any physical activity in the previous month. In 2007, 80.4% reported consuming fruits and vegetables less than five times per day. Only with an understanding of the cultures and culinary practices can an impact be made on improving the diets and lifestyles of the Cajun and Creole peoples in order to reduce the rising prevalence of obesity.

COMMUNICATION AND COUNSELING TIPS

The people of southern Louisiana are generally polite and casual in their communication style. To establish rapport, it is customary to inquire about their hometowns and family relations. Initially, they may seem to "protect their privacy" in counseling situations, but they will be more forthcoming as they become more comfortable with the counselor and readily express appreciation for the assistance (S. Camel, personal communication, 2008).

When providing nutrition or health counseling, it is imperative to be culturally sensitive. People tend to be very practical, know how to cook, and are not likely to utilize "specialty" food products. Some have begun to use Louisiana products that are now commercially marketed to reduce food preparation time, such as bottled roux. Many utilize prepared "home-cooked" meal items now found in local groceries to supplement daily

TABLE 6-1 Primary Language of Food Names with Phonetic Pronunciation

Food Name of French Origin	Pronunciation
Etoufeée	Ey-too-fey
Fricassée	Frĭk'ə-sē'
Praline	Prah-leen
Boudin	Boodan
Macque choux	Mok shoo
Filé	Fee-ley
Beignet	Ben-yey
Court bouillon	Ku bē yon
Gratton	Grah tŏn
Andouille	Ahn doo ē

meals (Ten Eyck, 2001). Any diet planning must incorporate those foods important to the culture and the individual. Several cookbooks are available that provide "healthier" versions of common recipes. Many rural people come from farming families or have worked in the oil industry and have not attended college, but they are by no means uneducable. Approaching them with the assumption that no formal education means they will require "simple" instructions can make for an unsuccessful counseling session, and the client is not likely to express dissatisfaction.

Family and their "way of life" is highly valued. Support systems most often consist of extended family members who have very close relationships to each other. For example, cousins may be as close as siblings. Extended families often reside in the same towns or within an hour's drive of each other. It would be unusual to have a client who is "isolated"; even friends take the role of family members when support is needed.

Food resources may not always be purchased. Families still have gardens, fruit and nut trees, hunt and fish, and some foods are foraged. If a family owns livestock, meat products are obtained through private butchering. Roadside stands are a source of fresh, seasonal fruits and vegetables. Diet planning would need to consider the seasonality of these foods.

FEATURED RECIPE

Pot-Roasted Duck

2 mallard ducks or 4 teals

Cayenne pepper

Salt

1–2 onions, cut into quarters

2–4 strips uncooked bacon

2–4 jalapeño peppers, cut into strips

¼–½ cup bacon fat

1. Season the outside and interior cavity of ducks or teals with cayenne pepper and salt. Place ¼ onion and one strip of bacon inside each bird.
2. Make incisions on each side of duck or teal breast about ½ inch deep. Sprinkle cayenne pepper and salt into each incision. Insert several strips of jalapeño pepper into each.
3. Pour bacon fat into cast-iron Dutch oven set over moderate heat. Add ducks or teals and brown evenly on all sides.
4. Reduce heat to low and add 2–3 cups of water. Cover and braise for about 2 hours or until ducks are tender, adding water as necessary. When ducks or teals are tender, remove from Dutch oven and carve. Skim fat from *au jus* gravy and pour it into a gravy boat for serving. Serve over rice.

Variation: Pot-Roasted Duck and Turnips or Jerusalem Artichokes

Prepare 1 lb. of turnips or Jerusalem artichokes, scrubbed and cut into chunks. About 15–20 minutes before serving, scatter the turnips or artichokes around ducks in the Dutch oven. Cover and let cook until tender. Serve over rice.

More recipes are available at http://nutrition.jbpub.com/foodculture/

REFERENCES

Bienvenu, M., Brasseaux, C.A., & Brasseaux, R.A. (2005). *Stir the pot: The history of Cajun cuisine.* New York: Hippocrene Books.

Brasseaux, C.A. (1987). *The Creoles of Louisiana.* In Hamilton & Associates (Ed.), *The Cajuns: Their history and culture* (Vol. 1, pp. 321–337). Opelousas, LA: Hamilton & Associates.

Centers for Disease Control and Prevention. (2007). *Behavioral risk factor surveillance system survey data.* Atlanta, GA: U.S. Department of Health and Human Services, Centers for Disease Control and Prevention.

Centers for Disease Control and Prevention. (2008). *Behavioral risk factor surveillance system survey data.* Atlanta, GA: U.S. Department of Health and Human Services, Centers for Disease Control and Prevention.

Centers for Disease Control and Prevention. (2008). *Louisiana: Burden of chronic diseases.* Retrieved May 12, 2009, from http://www.cdc.gov/nccdphp/states/pdf/louisiana.pdf

Esman, M.R. (1982). Festivals, change, and unity: The celebration of ethnic identity among Louisiana. *Anthropological Quarterly, 55*(4), 199–210.

Gibson, J.L., & DelSesto, S. (1975). The culture of Acadiana: An anthropological perspective. In J.L. Gibson & S. DelSesto (Eds.), *The culture of Acadiana: Tradition and change in South Louisiana* (pp. 1–14). Lafayette, LA: University of Southwestern Louisiana.

Guiterrez, C.P. (1983). *Foodways and Cajun identity.* Unpublished doctoral dissertation, University of North Carolina, Chapel Hill.

LeBreton, A. (1980). *Les pegrots.* Paris, France: LeLiure de Poche.

Leistner, C.G. (1986). *French and Acadian influences upon the Cajun cuisine of southwest Louisiana.* Unpublished master's thesis, Univesity of Southwestern Louisiana, Lafayette.

Leistner, C.G. (1993). *Development of culturally appropriate nutrition education materials for dietetic practitioners working in the Cajun and Creole regions of south Louisiana.* Unpublished doctoral dissertation, Florida State University, Tallahassee.

Leistner, C.G. (1996). *Cajun and Creole food practices, customs, and holidays.* Chicago: American Dietetic Association.

Louisiana House of Representatives. (1971, June 6). House Concurrent Resolution No. 496.

Powell, P. (1992, October 18). Eccentric, authentic New Orleans. *The New York Times Magazine.*

Prudhomme, P. (1984). *Chef Paul Prudhomme's Louisiana kitchen.* New York, NY: William Morrris.

Rowlinson, W., Janes, M., Carpenter, E., & Latiri-Carpenter, D. (1995). *The Oxford paperback: French dictionary and grammar.* New York: Oxford University Press.

Schwaner-Albright, O. (2007). The French are coming. *Gourmet.* Retrieved October 29, 2009, from http://www.gourmet.com/restaurants/2009/06/the-french-are-coming

Sexton, R.L. (1999). Cajun Mardi Gras: Cultural objectification and symbolic appropriation in a French tradition. *Ethnology, 38*(4), 297–313.

Ten Eyck, T.A. (2001). Managing food: Cajun cuisine in economic and cultural terms. *Rural Sociology, 66*(2), 227–243.

Trépanier, C. (1991). The cajunization of French Louisiana: Forging a regional identity. *The Geographical Journal, 157*(2), 161–171.

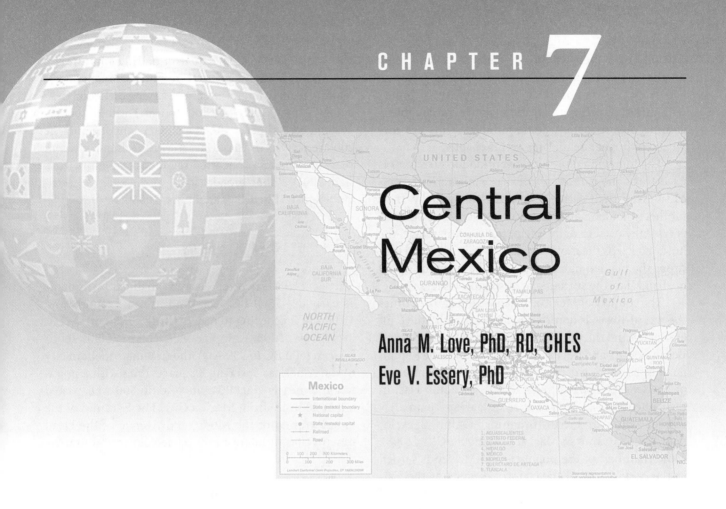

CHAPTER 7

Central Mexico

Anna M. Love, PhD, RD, CHES

Eve V. Essery, PhD

CULTURE AND WORLD REGION

With the first ancient civilizations and the greatest number of volcanoes on the continent, the central region of Mexico (*Estados Unidos Mexicanos*) has the richest history in the country. Today, its beauty can be seen in its Aztec ruins, colonial cities, and museums. In addition, murals on public buildings were commissioned in the 20th century by the postrevolutionary government to reflect the history of the country and the blending of Spanish and European influences with the traditional Amerindian culture (Camp & Mac-Lachlan, 2008).

Mexico's largest ethnic groups are Mestizo (Amerindian–Spanish) and indigenous Amerindian or indigenous Amerindian heritage. Of the total population, estimated at over 108 million in 2007, Mestizo represents 60% (greater in urban areas such as Mexico City) while the indigenous Amerindian comprises 30% (greater in rural regions of Mexico) with most of the

remainder being European (Camp & MacLachlan, 2008; Central Intelligence Agency [CIA], 2008). The predominant religion is Roman Catholicism (population estimates between 76 and 88%), followed by "unspecified" (13.8%), then Protestant (6.3%), and none (3.1%) (Camp & MacLachlan, 2008; CIA, 2008).

As with most of Mexico, this region is largely a patriarchal society that values a man's *machismo* (masculinity; manhood, i.e., sense of pride in fulfilling one's duties to family and community) and a woman's *marianisma* (submissiveness or self-denial in fulfilling duties to family, in reference to the Virgin Mary). Family needs are prioritized over the individual; consequently, often extended family members, sometimes several generations including in-laws and close family friends, share the same roof. Individual family members are honored in death not only by *novenas* (9 days of prayer for the deceased), but by avoiding meat on the day of the death (Kittler & Sucher, 2004). Individuals are honored in life with fiestas. The family hosts fiestas celebrating special days for each member, in particular the *Quincinera or Quinceanera* (analogous to *cumpleanera* meaning "birthday girl"), a girl's 15th birthday party celebrated with music, dancing, and feast to signify the daughter's coming out to society. Some holiday events are discussed in further detail later in this chapter.

The following naming convention for surnames is used throughout most of Mexico. Children are typically given their father's surname followed by their mother's maiden name; however, the father's last name is typically used in daily interactions. At marriage, the husband keeps the mother's maiden name and the wife drops the maiden name to take on the surname of her husband (i.e., the surname of husband's father).

The country of Mexico, which is almost three times the size of Texas, is bordered by Texas (north), the Gulf of Mexico and the Caribbean Sea (east), Guatemala and Belize (south), and the Pacific Ocean (west). The Republic of Mexico is a federal democratic society comprised of one federal district, much like Washington D.C. in the United States, and 31 sovereign states approximately 70% of which are urban (Britannica Online Encyclopedia, 2008; Camp & MacLachlan, 2008; CIA, 2008). More than half of the population of Mexico is settled in the central part of the country. Known as the Valley or Basin of Mexico, the central region consists of an elevated plateau forming a basin surrounded by the Sierra Mountains on all sides but the north. Most of this mountainous region was originally formed by volcanoes; the state of Michoácan alone contains more than 80 volcanoes (Britannica Online Encyclopedia, 2008; Kittler & Sucher, 2008; Long-Solis & Vargas, 2005).

This chapter focuses on Central Mexico including the Federal District (*Distrito Federal*) of Mexico City. With a population of 18.1 million, Mexico City is the second largest city in the world (Tokyo, Japan, is first) (Map of Mexico, 2008). Central Mexico, as defined by the secretary of health, is composed of the following 12 states: Aguascalientes, Colima, Guanajuato, Jalisco, Mexico, Michoácan, Morelos, Nayarit, Queretaro, San Luis Potosi, Sinaloa, and Zacatecas (Rivera & Sepulveda, 2003).

 LANGUAGE

The primary language spoken in Mexico is Spanish, although there are actually 291 living languages in Mexico today including the indigenous languages of Amerindians (Grimes, 2005). Mayan, Náhuatl, Otomi, Tarascan, and other regional indigenous languages are still spoken in the *Mesa Central* or *Highland Mexico* regions. Each language has dozens of regional dialects making translation for precise meaning difficult (CIA, 2008; Grimes, 2005). Although over 1 million people designated Náhuatl as their primary language on the 2000 census, its use has dramatically declined in recent years leading to a concerted revitalization effort (Rolstad, 2001). Public broadcasts in Mexico are in Castilian Spanish (Purnell & Paulanka, 2008).

 CULTURE HISTORY

The Central Mexico region was inhabited by humans as early as ~7500 BC according to some reports and 15,000 BC according to others (Britannica Online Encyclopedia, 2008; Camp & McLachlan, 2008). Teotihuacan (500 BC to 750 AD), the first metropolitan city of the Americas covering 8 square miles with a population of nearly 200,000 at its peak in 600 AD, existed about 30 miles from Mexico City. The Pyramid of the Sun, Pyramid of the Moon, and Avenue of the Dead remain sites of interest for archaeologists and tourists alike. This region was subsequently invaded by the Toltecs (~10 AD), followed by the Uto-Aztec tribe from the north (1428 AD), and the Spaniards (1519 AD) before boundary disputes with Spain, France, Britain, and later the United States began in the 18th century. Independence from Spain was won on September 16, 1821 (Britannica Online Encyclopedia, 2008; Camp & MacLachlan, 2008).

 FOOD HISTORY WITHIN THE CULTURE

The triad of Mexican agriculture in pre-Hispanic times was corn, beans, and squash. The amino acids, tryptophan and lysine, missing from corn were present in beans to provide a balanced diet when meat was unavailable. *Nixtamalización* (the process of grinding corn on *metates* with crushed limestone, wood ashes, and water) is still used in modern Mesoamerica to create *masa harina*. This process prevents pellagra by releasing the niacin bound to protein in the corn (Messer, 2000). Throughout history as invaders and conquerors discovered Mexico, the cuisine became a mix of indigenous ingredients with influences from other cultures including French, English, Chinese, and Japanese; albeit the largest influences are from Spain and America. Examples of nonindigenous foods common in this cuisine include garlic, onions, rice, and spices such as oregano, parsley, coriander, cloves, and livestock from Spain; mainly pigs and cattle. Pigs survived better on the central plains, which increased their popularity as food in this region (Long-Solis & Vargas, 2005).

Mexico City has a flare of all regional cuisines in Mexico, but recently it has had a resurgence of traditional Mexican cuisine due in part to the formation of the Mexican Culinary Circle (*Circulo Mexicano de Arte Culinario*) and another organization called *La Cofradia de la Mayora Mexicana*. The main purpose of the Mexican Culinary Circle is to promote traditional cuisine while *La Cofradia de la Mayora Mexicana* trains and assists *la mayoras* (the "most important" women chefs said to be the "souls of Mexican restaurant kitchens"; Long-Solis & Vargas, 2005, p. 115).

Central Mexico was a part of the cultural history that created one of the world's favorite sweets. In 1519, Hernán Cortés was presented by Montezuma II, the Emperor of the Aztec Empire, with a drink blended with chiles, vanilla, and ground cacao beans called *xocoatl* (chocolatl in Náhuatl). Cortés returned to Spain with cacao beans as part of his precious cargo. Once in Europe, sugar was added to create chocolate as we know it today (Long-Solis & Vargas, 2005). The scientific name for the cacao tree is *Theobroma*, meaning "food of the gods" (Kittler & Sucher, 2004, p. 210).

 ## MAJOR FOODS

Although Mexican cuisine is often considered spicy, many other flavors are found in the dishes of this region. Within Mexico, there are variations in cuisine between northern, central, southern, and coastal regions. In addition, dietary intake varies between urban and rural households. In Central Mexico, corn tortillas and beans form the foundation of the rural dietary pattern with contributions from fruits, vegetables, pasta, and occasional intake of animal products; the urban diet is similar to the rural diet with the inclusion of more animal foods (e.g., meat, eggs, and milk) and refined products (Tovar et al., 2003). In addition, purchasing patterns reveal that urban households buy a higher quantity of food groups than rural households (Rivera et al., 2002). Although traditional food patterns continue, purchase of energy-dense foods, including sugars, refined carbohydrates, and sodas, has increased in recent decades (Rivera et al., 2002). Below is a summary of major foods found within each food group.

 ## Protein Sources

Protein intake in Central Mexico is considered to be adequate (Rivera & Sepulveda, 2003); however, protein sources vary in urban and rural areas. In rural areas, plant products can provide over 90% of dietary energy intake (Black, Allen, Pelto, de Mata, & Chavez, 1994). In contrast, city residents regularly consume animal foods (Tovar et al., 2003).

Legumes such as beans (*frijoles*) are a primary protein source in this cuisine. Examples of legumes consumed in this region include pinto (*pintos*), black (*negros*), fava, chick peas (*garbanzos*), and lentils (*lentejas*), to name a few. In rural areas, beans are the primary protein source, and they are a major staple in urban areas as well. Popular preparations include beans boiled in a seasoned broth (*frijoles de olla*, pot beans), and *frijoles refritos* that are made by mashing and pan-frying *frijoles de olla* in lard. Beans are served as a component of any meal throughout the day. Although legumes are an incomplete protein, when combined

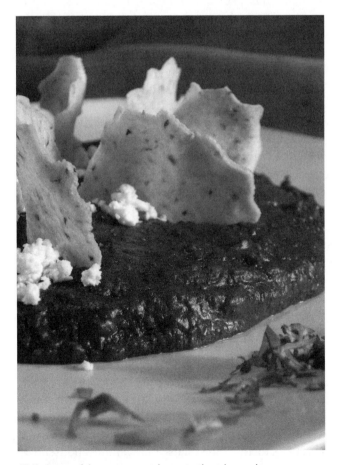

Frijoles refritos are pot beans that have been mashed and pan-fried.

with corn or rice, they provide the necessary protein requirements.

The Spanish provided pork to this region, and it is the most common meat consumed in Central Mexico. Pork is typically prepared using a slow, moist cooking technique. Cooked, shredded pork is added to various stuffed foods including *tacos* (folded soft or fried tortillas filled with beans, vegetables, and/or meat) and *flautas* (deep-fried rolled tacos). Pork is also baked, grilled, and added to stews. One of the most well-known Mexican foods is sausage (*chorizo*). There are many variations of sausage, but they can generally be described as a mixture of pork, lard, *chiles*, and spices that are cased in pig small intestines. As with many traditional cultures, there is little waste in food production. Mexican cuisine aficionado Diana Kennedy explains, "Every part of the pig is used for human consumption except the hair" (Kennedy, 2008, p. 247). Examples include blood sausage, pickled pig's feet, and fried pork rinds.

Chicken is also a common protein source. Chicken is incorporated into soups, shredded, and added to stuffed foods, grilled, or served with sauces. Similar to pork, traditional recipes use most portions of the animal including blood, intestines, and liver.

Milk products, largely cream and cheese, are included in many combination foods in Central Mexico. For example, tortillas or pasta are served in a simple sauce of cream and cheese. Cheese may also be prepared with *chiles* for a dip known as *chile con queso*. The cheeses from this region are made from cow's milk. They are typically mild and include ricotta, *queso fresco*, *queso panela*, and *queso añejo*.

Eggs are a common protein source, particularly during the mid-morning meal. They are often scrambled or fried and prepared with *chiles*, cheese, and/or vegetables including tomatoes and onions.

 Starch Sources

Corn, mainly in the form of tortillas, is the primary starch consumed in this region. Traditional corn tortillas are handmade with dried corn treated with lime (calcium oxide) and moistened with water (Kennedy, 2008). Flour tortillas are more popular in the northern region of the country and are not a substantial starch source in Central Mexico. Although there has been a steady decline in tortilla intake nationwide (Rivera et al., 2002), tortillas are a staple food for most households in Central Mexico (Black et al., 1994). Generally, more

tortillas are purchased in rural than urban households (Rivera et al., 2002). A recent study reported that rural women consumed an average of 11 tortillas per day, while urban women ate fewer than five (Tovar et al., 2003).

Tortillas are often served with meals including soups, stews, and casseroles; however, they have many other functions in Mexican cuisine. For example, tortillas serve as the casing of *enchiladas* (rolled tortillas stuffed with meat, cheese, and/or vegetables and baked in a sauce) and the plate of *tostados* (fried tortillas topped with *frijoles refritos*, chopped fresh vegetables, cheese, and/or meat) (Kennedy, 2008). They can also be added as a component to soups and casseroles or cut into squares or triangles and pan or deep fried as chips.

Beyond tortillas, corn is used in many other recipes in this region. One of the most well-known traditional foods of Mexico is the *tamale*, which is prepared in a time-intensive process from a mixture of ground corn and lard spread onto corn husks and filled with various components including meats, beans, vegetables, or for sweet *tamales*, honey, or raisins. The corn husk is then wrapped and tied, and the *tamale* is steamed. *Tamales* are eaten straight out of the husk or with a sauce or garnish.

Long-grain rice (*arroz*) is also an important component of the Mexican cuisine. Rice is served alone before a meal as a "dry soup" (*sopa seca*), incorporated into soups, or provided with a main dish. It is traditional to pan-fry the rice to a golden brown before cooking. *Arroz a la Mexicana* (Mexican rice) is a popular rice dish prepared with long-grain rice, tomato puree (tomatoes, onion, and garlic), broth, and vegetables (Kennedy, 2008).

Bread is consumed primarily in the form of crusty rolls of various shapes and sizes. The rolls are served with a meal or as a sandwich with fillings such as *frijoles refritos*, cheese, *chiles*, avocado, meat, and/or vegetables. Sweet rolls (*pan dulce*) are also eaten frequently. For example, *conchas* are pastries flavored with cinnamon or cocoa with a sweet topping designed to resemble a seashell (Quintana & Haralson, 1994).

Although many people do not consider pasta when thinking of Mexican cuisine, pasta is used in various forms in Mexican dishes. Fried noodles or pasta soup are often eaten by young children (Romieu, Hernandez-Avila, Rivera, Ruel, & Parra, 1997). In addition, macaroni can be added to casseroles, and various types of pasta are served with a simple tomato sauce.

Fat Sources

Fat intake represents over 30% of energy intake in Central Mexico (Rivera et al., 2002). Pork lard is a major fat source and contributes to the flavors and textures of the traditional Mexican cuisine; however, in recent times, vegetable oils, such as corn and safflower oils, have replaced lard in various recipes.

Nuts are also a fat source in this cuisine. Nuts consumed include almonds, pine nuts, peanuts, pumpkin seeds, sesame seeds, and walnuts. Many nuts, such as almonds and pine nuts, are ground into a paste that is incorporated into savory dishes or desserts. Other nuts, such as peanuts and pumpkin seeds, are toasted, boiled, or fried and eaten as a snack. Several nuts are used in traditional regional sauces (*moles*). Use of nuts varies depending on availability and income. For example, pine nuts are expensive and subsequently not commonly used in all households. Walnuts are grown in this region, and they are used to prepare a walnut sauce known as *nogada* for *chiles en nogada*, a common summer dish (Kennedy, 2008).

Avocados also contribute to the fat intake of individuals in Central Mexico. Avocados are sliced as a topping or blended as a soup base. They are also used to make *guacamole*, a raw dish typically prepared with avocados, onion, *chiles*, tomato, and cilantro.

Prominent Vegetables

Produce consumption in Mexico varies depending on growing conditions and season; however, *chiles* are prolific in Mexican cuisine throughout the year. *Chiles* consumed in Central Mexico vary in heat and include *serranos, poblanos, jalapeños, anchos, pasillas, guajillo, chipotle, chilacas,* and *manzanos. Chiles* have many uses in food preparation. They are included in dishes, sauces, and relishes. They are grilled, charred, fresh, pickled, or dried. They are used whole, sliced, chopped, blended, or ground. Fried *chiles poblanos* stuffed with cheese and/or meat fillings and served with a tomato sauce make up the popular dish *chiles rellenos.*

Similar to *chiles*, red tomatoes (*jitomate*) are common in this cuisine because of their availability. Tomatoes are used in various ways including raw, stewed, blended, or grilled. *Tomate verde*, sometimes referred to as *tomatillo*, is a green tomato that is also commonly included in Central Mexican dishes.

Many other vegetables are consumed in this region. Various squash (and their flowers) including zucchini, pumpkin, *chayote* (vegetable pear), *guicoy,* and summer squash are commonly consumed throughout Mexico. Other key vegetables include onion (primarily white or purple) and cactus leaves (*napoles*). *Napoles* are cleaned and boiled or grilled and then added to salads, eggs, or beans. *Napoles* are particularly common in urban households of lower income (Long-Solis & Vargas, 2005). Other vegetables consumed regularly throughout Central Mexico include indigenous wild greens, cassava or yuca, *maguey* leaves, *jícama*, Swiss chard, potatoes, sweet potatoes, and carrots. Seasonal treats include corn fungus (*cuitlacoche*) and a wide variety of mushrooms.

Vegetables are incorporated into soups and other dishes, served as a relish or other accompaniment, or pickled and eaten as a snack. Combinations of vegetables are served in the many *salsas* of this region. Each salsa contains a unique blend of ingredients, but many contain some form of tomatoes and *chiles,* and onion and cilantro are common. Variations may include garlic, oregano, or other spices. Examples include *salsa de tomate verde* (green tomato sauce) and *salsa Mexicana.*

Prominent Fruits

The most common fruit in this cuisine is the lime (*limón*). A sweet, mild *lima* is grown in Central Mexico and is used in many local dishes. Fruits are eaten raw, dried, or candied, or they are used to prepare beverages, savory dishes, fruit pastes, or desserts. They are also used to decorate serving platters. Raisins and prunes are among the most popular dried fruits. Candied fruits are more variable and include orange peels, lime peels, and papaya. Other fruits consumed in this region include *tuna* (fruit from the prickly pear cactus), *guavas, zapote* (including *chicozapote* and *mamey*), pineapple, mango, bananas, and melons.

Spices and Seasonings

Several spices and herbs are common in central Mexican cuisine. Spices are used extensively, but in moderation; therefore, individual spices do not usually overwhelm a particular dish. The Spanish brought allspice to the region, and it is still a common ingredient in many dishes. Other spices common to this region include cinnamon, cloves, cumin, peppercorns, and salt. Herbs are also important contributors to the flavors of Central Mexican cuisine. Examples include

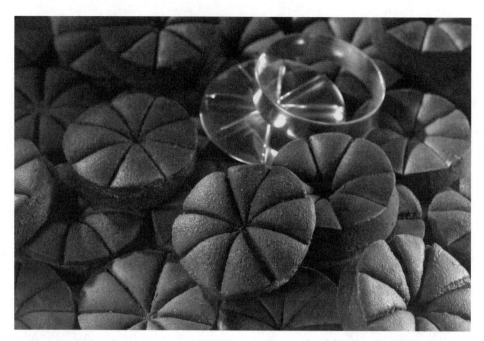

Chocolate tablets are served at funerals, weddings, and New Year's Eve celebrations.

garlic, wild anise, bay leaf, cilantro, marjoram, thyme, *epazote* (Mexican tea), and oregano.

 Beverages

Many beverages are common to the Central Mexican cuisine. Coffee is served in the morning or following a meal with milk and/or cinnamon. Several drinks are flavored with chocolate; for example, hot chocolate remains a favorite drink among children. *Atole*, a traditional corn-based gruel often sweetened with sugar or honey and flavored with fruit, chocolate, or *chiles*, is still regularly consumed. Although water blended with fruit (*aguas naturales*) and teas remain common, the purchase of sodas, such as colas, has increased in recent decades (Long-Solis & Vargas, 2005; Rivera et al., 2002). Immigrants new to the United States often seek Coca-Cola bottled in Mexico, which in place of high-fructose corn syrup uses cane sugar (believed to have a lighter feel in the mouth) (Terhune, 2006).

Several alcoholic beverages are common in Central Mexico. Beer is usually considered the most popular beverage, and whiskey and wine are also consumed. The *maguey* (also known as *agave*) plant is used to produce three alcoholic beverages common in this region: *pulque*, *mescal*, and *tequila*. *Pulque* is considered a distant ancestor of *tequila*, but it is still consumed in Central Mexico (Black et al., 1994). It is made from the fermented juice of the *maguey* plant and has a relatively low alcohol content compared with the other two *maguey*-based beverages. *Mescal* is distilled *pulque,* while *tequila* is distilled twice.

 Desserts

Desserts are an everyday component in the cuisine of Central Mexico. Eggs, nuts, and fruits are chief ingredients to many sweets, and cinnamon and coconut are common additives. Many desserts are custard based and others can be described as intensely sweet and sticky. *Flan*, an egg custard with a crown of caramelized sugar, is probably the most well-known and popular dessert. *Pan dulce* (sweet bread or cake) made with wheat flour, lard, sugar, and eggs is regularly consumed (Romieu et al., 1997). Rice pudding and fruits are also common. Fruits are served fresh, dried, candied, as a paste, or as a frozen treat. For example, candied limes stuffed with coconut are a popular sweet (Quintana & Haralson, 1994).

 FOODS WITH CULTURAL SIGNIFICANCE

The Mexican hot–cold theory of diet and health is still practiced in some households. The hot–cold theory

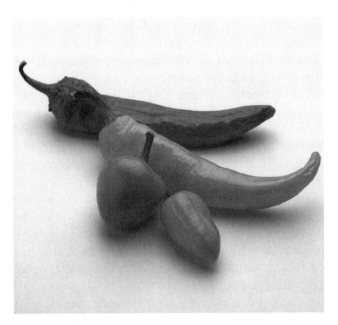

Chiles consumed in Central Mexico vary in heat and include serranos, poblanos, jalapeños, anchos, pasillas, guajillo, chipotle, chilacas, and manzanos.

is based on the premise that the world's resources are limited and must stay in balance. It is said to have been brought to Mexico by the Spaniards and is based on the Arab system of humoral medicine, yet it also mirrors the Asian Yin–Yang Theory (Kittler & Sucher, 2008). The theory suggests that the diet must use hot foods (symbolizing strength) such as alcohol, chiles, onions, beef and pork, radishes, and tamales balanced with cold foods (symbolizing weakness) such as citrus and tropical fruits, dairy foods, goat, and most fresh vegetables. Some foods, such as rice, beans, corn, sugary products, and wheat products, can be prepared to be hot or cold, whereas soups and casseroles serve as a mixture of both. The theory applies to how the food is prepared, proximity to the sun, and how the food affects the body (Kittler & Sucher, 2008). *Empacho* (a digestive ailment with gas and nausea) is thought to result from hot–cold imbalance (Kittler & Sucher, 2004).

Many foods have cultural significance beyond the hot–cold theory. For example, *menudo* is a tripe soup believed to have restorative properties including treatment of hangovers. Tripe is made from the stomach of various animals. Garlic, passion flower, and linden flower are used by some people for hypertension; sage tea, trumpet flower, and bricklebrush are used

by some for diabetes; boiled peanut broth is used for diarrhea (Kittler & Sucher, 2008). Another culturally significant food from this region is the *chile* (spelled *chilli* in traditional Náhuatl), which was used not only as a cooking ingredient but also in medicine and as a weapon. This food was unknown to other continents before being discovered in the Americas in the 15th and 16th centuries (Long-Solis & Vargas, 2005). Chocolate is believed to have at least three medicinal uses consistently found in the literature: (1) to increase appetite in emaciated clients, (2) to stimulate the nervous system and increase energy, and (3) to improve kidney and bowel function; however, Dillinger et al. (2000) compiled a list of over 100 other medicinal uses for chocolate.

 ## TYPICAL DAY'S MENU

A typical day will usually include four to five eating occasions. Breakfast (*desayuno*) is typically light and may include coffee with sweet bread (*pan dulce*). A heavier meal called *almuerzo* is consumed mid-morning. An example of this meal includes eggs scrambled with tomato, onion, and possibly *chiles* or *chorizo* and served with warm corn tortillas, beans, fruit, and coffee. The largest meal of the day, *comida*, is served mid-afternoon. Traditionally, this meal was served as multiple courses, but today, some of these courses are skipped or the foods are simply served with the main course. This meal may begin with an appetizer (*antojito*) such as *tostados*, a soup such as chicken broth (*consumé de pollo*) with vegetables, or a "dry soup" (*sopa seca*) such as Mexican rice (*arroz a la Mexicana*). Chicken tacos (*tacos de pollo*) garnished with chopped vegetables and cheese and served with salsa and beans is a typical main dish that is prepared at home or purchased from a street vendor or restaurant. The meal may be completed with a custard dessert such as *flan*. An early evening snack (*merienda*) may include *atole* (corn-based gruel) and more *pan dulce* or other sweets. Supper (*cena*) is typically light; however, some individuals are adopting a meal pattern that includes a smaller lunch and larger supper. A bowl of *pozole*, pork and hominy stew, might be served with corn tortillas as a traditional evening meal followed by a dessert of fresh fruit or a slice of fruit paste such as *guava* paste (*ate de guayaba*).

Many individuals in Central Mexico prepare foods within their homes as was done traditionally;

however, with the movement of more women into the workforce, there has also been a shift in eating patterns. In 1998, only 11% of households reported food expenditures away from home in the previous week (Rivera et al., 2002). In recent years, various sources for food from street vendors to elegant restaurants have become more popular (Long-Solis & Vargas, 2005). In addition to food service establishments that serve traditional Mexican food, fast-food vendors, including McDonald's, Burger King, and Pizza Hut, are found in many cities. These establishments serve the same basic foods as they do in the United States, but some foods are served with a Mexican twist such as *chiles* on pizza (Long-Solis & Vargas, 2005). It is also noteworthy that restaurants that specialize in other cuisines, such as French, Mediterranean, Caribbean, and Chinese, are also popular in many cities.

 ## HOLIDAY MENUS

Given that over 5000 annual celebrations are listed in Mexico's Calendar of Festivals, this section highlights only the more common holidays. Many of the foods served at *fiestas* are also served for everyday occasions with higher-quality ingredients selected for special occasions. Dishes often served at *fiestas* include turkey with *mole* (*mole de guajolote*), a rich thick sauce typically prepared with ground peanuts, chocolate, chiles, spices, and sesame seeds, vegetable fritters (*tortas de papas*), *torrejas* (an egg-dipped bread that is fried and served with cinnamon syrup and grated lime peel for dessert), and *pozole* (a pork and hominy soup).

A holiday bread pudding (*capirotada*) is prepared for Lent. Tamales are often served at weddings, baptisms (bautismos), and First Communions, as special meals during *Semana Santa* (Holy Week—the week before Easter), and placed on small altars (*ofrendas*) along with chocolate tablets on All Saints Day (November 1) (Britannica Online Encyclopedia, 2008). Chocolate tablets are also served at funerals, weddings, and New Year's Eve celebrations (Long-Solis & Vargas, 2005). *Coachala* is a soup prepared for weddings and baptisms in this region. Other common fare at baptisms include egg-shaped cookies covered in powdered cinnamon sugar (*yemitas*), *tamales*, enchiladas, chicken with *mole*, candied limes, lime crepes, guava filled with coconut crème, and chocolate meringue with mint sauce (Quintana & Haralson, 1994).

All Kings Day (*Dia de los Reyes Magos*), also called Three Kings Day (January 6), commemorates the three wise men bearing gifts for the Baby Jesus, with a ring-shaped sweet bread loaf garnished with dried or candied fruit (*la rosca de reyes*) to represent the crown. A figurine of the Baby Jesus is baked inside. The recipient of the slice of bread containing the figurine customarily throws a party on Candelemas Day (*dia de la Candelaria*, February 2) celebrated with mass, games, and *tamales dulce* and *pink atole* (Kittler & Sucher, 2004; Long-Solis & Vargas, 2005; Quintana & Haralson, 1994).

Garnachos (tortilla-baked snacks), *chiles en nogada* (garnished in white sauce, green cilantro, and red pomegranate seeds to represent the Mexican flag), *gorditas de frijol, picaditas, sopes, green enchiladas, or enchiladas with black mole* are served at Independence Day celebrations (September 15 and 16) commemorating independence from Spain on September 16, 1821 (Long-Solis & Vargas, 2005). The Day of the Dead (*El Dia de los Muertos*, November 1) is the festival welcoming the return of the souls of the dead where bread decorated with extra dough filled on top to form a skull and crossbone (*pan de muerto*) and hollow skulls made of sugar paste are placed at the *ofrenda* with other festive dishes, first for the returning souls, and then for the family members celebrating their return to enjoy (Long-Solis & Vargas, 2005; Quintana & Haralson, 1994).

The *posadas* (inn or refuge) are 9 days, including Christmas Eve (*Noche Buena*), that represent Mary and Joseph wandering in Bethlehem. They are celebrated with costumes, dance, piñata breaking, and refreshments such as *ponche navideno*, *atole*, and hot chocolate. Christmas Eve dinner, usually served after returning from mass, consists of dried cod fish stew (*bacalao*), roast turkey, fricassee of breaded shrimp (*revoltijo de romeritos*), or traditional Mexican Salad (*la ensalada de Noche Buena*), which is prepared with romaine lettuce, beets, *jícama*, apples, oranges, lemons, peanuts, Christmas candy, sugar cane, cloves, and brown sugar (Long-Solis & Vargas, 2005). Turkey with adobo sauce, *quesadillas*, and *chorizo* are served for Christmas Day.

 ## HEALTH BELIEFS AND CONCERNS

A strong belief that all is destined by God influences a perceived locus of control in life events such as illness, birth, and death. These events can be perceived to be due to outside forces, sometimes even as punishment by God for one's sins (Kittler & Sucher, 2004). Prayer is used regardless of the illness. The health experts of the family are the *señoras* and *abuelas* (the mothers, grandmothers, and wives), yet health decisions are not made by the women alone, but rather with the head of the household. Suggested food preparation changes may be perceived that the current method, and thus fulfillment of the woman's role in the family, is inadequate. Building rapport with the food preparers in the house and reinforcing positive behaviors can alleviate this. Home remedies, including various teas (e.g., chamomile, anise, mint, sage), diuretics, laxatives, enemas, or over-the-counter medications used along with traditional remedies found at the herbal pharmacies (*botánicas*) are often sought before going outside the home. *Yerberos* (herbalists), massage/occupational therapists, and midwives will be sought next.

The assistance of a faith healer known as a *curandero* or *curandera* (if the healer is female) is sought to cure conditions not successfully treated by others that are thought to be caused by supernatural powers such as hexes or curses (Kittler & Sucher, 2004, 2008). For example, the evil eye *(mal de ojo)* is thought to be of supernatural origin to which children are particularly susceptible. A person who gazes admiringly at a child without touching the child is thought by some to result in flu-like symptoms for the child (Kittler & Sucher, 2004). Purnell and Paulanka (2008) describe other conditions recognized by many people in this culture (with what is believed to cause them), including *susto* (caused by "magical fright" [p. 321] or excessive emotion); *envidia* (caused by emotion of envy); *caida de la mollera* (displacement of organs in infants); *mal aire* (bad air or wind); *mal puesto* (witchcraft); and *bilis* (imbalance of bile).

GENERAL HEALTH AND NUTRITIONAL INDICATORS SUMMARY

The health of a country is often measured by its infant mortality rate, which for Mexico was 29 infant (defined as <1 year of age) deaths per 1000 live births in 2007 compared with 7 per 1000 in the United States, according to the United Nation's Children's Fund (UNICEF) (2008a). In 2007 the mortality rate for children under 5 years was 35 per 1000 live births compared with 8 per 1000 in the United States. Additional epidemiological data used to measure the health of a population include crude death rate (5 annual deaths per 1000 population compared with 8 per 1000 in the United States), crude birth rate (20 annual births per

1000 population vs 14 per 1000 in the United States), and life expectancy at birth (76 and 78 years for Mexico and the United States, respectively). A particularly striking disparity is found between maternal mortality rates in Mexico (62 per 1000) and the United States (8 per 1000), although the number of low-birth-weight infants (defined as <2500 g) is the same in both countries (approximately 8%).

The prevalence of children under 5 years of age who are dangerously underweight is 5% in Mexico compared with 2% in the United States. As a response to the Millennium Development Goals of the United Nations, UNICEF promotes breastfeeding which specifically addresses the goals focused on reducing child mortality and eradicating extreme poverty and hunger by 2015 (UNICEF, 2008b). Breastfeeding provides a significant protective factor for the future health of the infant. According to UNICEF (2008a), 38% of children in Mexico are breastfed exclusively while the infant is under 6 months of age, 36% are breastfed with complementary food between 6 and 9 months of age, and 21% are still breastfed between the ages of 20 and 23 months.

Dietary intake within Mexico varies by region and by urbanization rate. Mexico's urbanization rate (77%) has reached a level near that of the United States (81%). Dietary changes seen with an urban environment include increases in consumption of animal products and refined products, decreases in the number of food groups or variety in the diet, and decreases in the frequency of tortillas, vegetables, and beans as a primary protein source (Rivera et al., 2002; Tovar et al., 2003). Villalpando et al. (2003) identified levels of micronutrient deficiencies in 966 children and 920 nonpregnant Mexican women by both National Nutrition Survey (1999) and serum levels of vitamins A and C, finding differences between regions of the country (Villalpando et al., 2003). Though clinical vitamin A deficiency was rare in women and children, subclinical deficiency (defined as retinol >10 but <20 ug/dl) was found in 25% of the children, predominantly in rural children under 2 years of age. The highest prevalence (26.5%) was found in Central Mexico.

Furthermore, Villalpando et al. (2003) also found vitamin C deficiency in 30% of children under 2 years of age (33.1% in rural areas) and 40% of women 12–49 years of age, with the lowest prevalence occurring between the ages of 5 and 10 years but reappearing at age 11 years in both urban (32.7%) and rural (27.5%) regions of the country. Higher rates of vitamin C deficiency were also found among nonpregnant women

12–49 years of age living in rural areas. Intakes of energy, fat, fiber, sodium, folate, iron, zinc, and calcium were lower in Central Mexico. Folate deficiency, determined by serum blood concentrations, was most severe in children <4 years of age, with the lowest prevalence of deficiency across age groups found in Central Mexico. Deficiency in this region may have been masked by depleted iron stores given that folic acid intake according to the National Nutrition Survey (1999) was almost half of the recommended level (Villalpando et al., 2003). The prevalence of deficiencies in vitamin A (52%), zinc (58%), folate (77%), vitamin C (67%), and vitamin E (73%) among lactating women in Mexico has been identified previously with nutrient intakes in Central Mexico being significantly lower than in other regions of Mexico (Caire-Juvera, Ortega, Casanueva, Bolaños & Calderón de la Barca, 2007).

According to the World Health Organization Statistical Information System (WHOSIS, 2009), obesity rates among women in Mexico (28.1% in 2000) are similar to those of women in the United States (33.2% in 2004), but men in Mexico have a much lower prevalence of obesity (18.6% in 2000) compared with men in the United States (31.1% in 2004) and women in Mexico. The 1999 National Nutrition Survey ($n = 18,311$ women) allowed for comparison by region of Mexico. The prevalence of overweight or obese women in the northern region (60%) was slightly higher than the prevalence near Mexico City (52%) (Rivera Dommarco et al., 2001).

TABLE 7-1   Communication "Do's and Don'ts"

Verbal Communication Do's	Verbal Communication Don'ts	Nonverbal Communication Do's	Nonverbal Communication Don'ts
Use a direct, action-oriented approach. Use nonconfrontational language. Protect modesty and privacy.	Use the word "stupid"; it's translated very strongly in Spanish. Offer inflexible appointment times. Reject food or drink offered. Reject a dinner offer. Use idiomatic expressions or colloquialisms.	Touch a client with a handshake (men: wait for women to extend their hand first). Leave food on the plate; this is not considered rude (portions are usually large).	Maintain eye contact for long periods of time (could be considered rude). Look admiringly at an infant or child without touching the child.

TABLE 7-2   Primary Language of Food Names with English and Phonetic Translation

Primary Language of Food Names	English Translation	Phonetic Translation
Yemita	Diminutive of egg yolk	yeh-MEE-tah
Xoxocoatl (Náhuatl) or *Chocolatl* (Spanish)	Chocolate and water (bitter water)	shaw-coh-AHT-uhl (cho-ko-LAH-tay)
Manteca de cerdo	Lard	Mahn-TAY-kah deh sair-doh
Chayote	Vegetable pear	chy-OH-teh
Güicoy	Pumpkin-like squash	wee'-koy
Napoles	Cactus leaves	noh-PAHL-es NAPP-oh-les
Huexolotl (Náhuatl) or *guajolote* (Spanish)	Tom turkey	wee-hoh-LOH-teh gwah-hoh-LOH-teh
Cuitlacoche (huitlacoche)	Black mushroom or corn fungus	weet-lah-KOH-cheh

COMMUNICATION AND COUNSELING TIPS

In working with people from this region of Mexico, the main consideration in counseling is that decisions are not often made by one individual, but rather the family as a whole or at least with the head of the household (Purnell & Paulanka, 2008). The belief that the "individual must endure the illness as inevitable," (Kittler & Sucher, 2008, p. 238) also known as *fatalismo*, can be difficult to overcome when working with clients as they feel powerless against their health conditions. Working closely with the family, church leaders, and even *curanderos*, should they be used by clients, can increase the likelihood of behavioral changes being adopted. Although Mexico has a literacy rate of 92.7% (for people over the age of 15 years), the language barrier may lead to misunderstandings with clients from Mexico. Educational materials using clear, simple vocabulary at a second- to fourth-grade reading level and including graphics to assist with word recognition are highly recommended (Institute for Healthcare Advancement, 2008). Approach the client with respect (*respeto*) and *personalismo* (being friend-like), and repeat important points (Purnell & Paulanka, 2008). Realize that to be polite, some clients may not disagree face-to-face with an appointment time known to conflict with their schedule. Not attending a prearranged event or meeting is often not considered rude. Remain flexible when scheduling appointments and offer walk-in services if possible. See Table 7-1 for other "do's and don'ts" of communication with this culture.

FEATURED RECIPE

Tamales

½ tsp. baking powder

½ bag (~4 cups) of masa corn flour (such as Maseca)

½ bag of dried New Mexico red chili peppers

1½ cup of lard or oil (1 cup for corn masa)

Garlic (to taste)

½ tbsp. salt

2 bags of corn husks, soaked in water for 1–2 hours and patted dry

3 lbs. of meat (chicken, pork, beef)

Meat Mixture

1. Cook meat in a little water. Add salt and garlic (to taste). Cook until the meat is tender and shreds easily with a fork, set aside, and let cool. Save the meat broth. Remove the bone of the meat if necessary.
2. Remove seeds from peppers and cover peppers in water to soak for awhile. Pour peppers and water in the blender with salt and garlic to taste.
3. Blend until pureed mixture is smooth. Heat ½ cup of oil/lard, then add peppers (saving some for the corn masa). Add meat and cook while stirring.

Corn Masa

1. In a bowl add corn flour, baking soda, and salt (to taste). Add remaining pepper and the broth from the meat a little at a time while mixing. Add remaining oil while mixing with your hands until a spongy dough forms.
2. When the husks are dry, spread a thin layer of the corn masa on the center of the husk with a spoon leaving ½ inch of the husk empty on the sides, then add 1–2 tbsp. of meat on top of the masa, and fold so that the empty parts of the husk cover the center of the tamale. Cook them in a tamale pot (for about 1 hour) or in a steamer (for about 20 minutes) making sure that you lay them facing the same way.
3. They are ready when you can open up the tamales and the masa does not stick to the husk.

Courtesy of Lila Coronado

More recipes are available at http://nutrition.jbpub.com/foodculture/

ACKNOWLEDGMENTS

We offer our heartfelt thanks to Lila Coronado and Lydia M. Del Rincon for their recipes, sharing with us the delicious taste of Central Mexico.

REFERENCES

Black, A.K., Allen, L.H., Pelto, G.H., de Mata, M.P., & Chavez, A. (1994). Iron, vitamin B-12 and folate status in Mexico: Associated factors in men and women and during pregnancy and lactation. *The Journal of Nutrition, 124*(0022-3166; 8), 1179–1188.

Britannica Online Encyclopedia. (2008). *Mexico.* Retrieved June 24, 2008 from http://www.britannica.com/nations/Mexico/

Caire-Juvera, G., Ortega, M.I., Casanueva, E., Bolaños, E.V., & Calderón de la Barca, A.M. (2007). Food components and dietary patterns of two different groups of Mexican lactating women. *Journal of the American College of Nutrition, 26*(2), 156–162.

Camp, R.A., & MacLachlan, C. (2008). *Mexico: MSN Encarta.* Retrieved June 12, 2008, from http://encarta.msn.com/encyclopedia_761576758/Mexico.html/

Carlos, D. (1951). *Spanish–Mexican cookbook: Continental edition.* Los Angeles: Charles Parnell Leahy.

Central Intelligence Agency. (2008). *The world factbook: Mexico.* Retrieved June 12, 2008, from https://www.cia.gov/library/publications/the-world-factbook/geos/mx.html/

Dillinger, T.L., Barriga, P., Escarcega, S., Jimenez, M., Salazar, L.D., & Grivetti, L.E. (2000). Food of the gods: Cure for humanity? A cultural history of the medicinal and ritual use of chocolate. *The Journal of Nutrition, 130*(0022-3166; 8), 2057S–2072S.

Grimes, B.F. (2005). *Ethnologue: Languages of the world: Maps and indexes.* Dallas, TX: International Academic Bookstore.

Institute for Healthcare Advancement. (2008). *Health literacy.* Retrieved June 24, 2008, from http://www.iha4health.org/index.cfm/MenuItemID/125.htm/

Kennedy, D. (2008). *The art of Mexican cooking.* New York: Clarkson Potter.

Kittler, P.G., & Sucher, K. (2004). *Food and culture.* Belmont, CA: Thomson/Wadsworth.

Kittler, P.G., & Sucher, K. (2008). *Food and culture.* Belmont, CA: Thomson/Wadsworth.

Long-Solis, J., & Vargas, L.A. (2005). *Food culture in Mexico.* Westport, CT: Greenwood Press.

Map of Mexico. (2008). *Mexico map, map of Mexico destinations, Mexico atlas.* Retrieved June 12, 2008, from http://www.worldatlas.com/webimage/countrys/namerica/mx.htm/

Messer, E. (2000). Maize. In K.F. Kiple & C.O. Kriemhold (Eds.), *The Cambridge world history of food* (pp. 103–104). Cambridge, England: Cambridge University Press.

Purnell, L.D., & Paulanka, B.J. (2008). *Transcultural health care: A culturally competent approach* (3rd ed.). Philadelphia: F.A. Davis.

Quintana, P., & Haralson, C. (1994). *Mexico's feasts of life.* Tulsa: Council Oak Books.

Rivera Dommarco J., Shamah-Levy T., Villalpando Hernandez S., Gonzalez de Cossio T., Hernandez Prado B., & Sepulveda J. (2001). *Encuesta Nacional de Nutrición 1999. Estado Nutricio de Niños y Mujeres en México.* Cuernavaca, Morelos, Mexico: Instituto Nacional de Salud Pública.

Rivera, J.A., Barquera, S., Campirano, F., Campos, I., Safdie, M., & Tovar, V. (2002). Epidemiological and nutritional transition in Mexico: Rapid increase of non-communicable chronic diseases and obesity. *Public Health Nutrition, 5*(1368-9800; 1), 113–122.

Rivera, J.A., & Sepulveda, A.J. (2003). Conclusions from the Mexican National Nutrition Survey 1999: Translating results into nutrition policy. *Salud p'Ublica De M'Exico, 45* Suppl 4 (0036-3634), S565–S575.

Rolstad, K. (2001, January–April). Language death in Central Mexico: The decline of Nahuatl and the new bilingual maintenance programs. *The Bilingual Review/La Revista Bilingue, 2001–2002, 26*(1), 3–18.

Romieu, I., Hernandez-Avila, M., Rivera, J.A., Ruel, M.T., & Parra, S. (1997). Dietary studies in countries experiencing a health transition: Mexico and Central America. *The American Journal of Clinical Nutrition, 65*(0002-9165; 4), 1159S–1165S.

Terhune, C. (2006, January 11). Taste test: U.S. thirst for Mexican cola poses sticky problem for Coke; though it's the real thing, soda's route across border breaks company rules; investigating an "irritation." *Wall Street Journal,* pp. A.1.

Tovar, A.R., Torres, N., Barrales-Benitez, O., Lopez, A.M., Diaz, M., & Rosado, J.L. (2003). Plasma total homocysteine in Mexican rural and urban women fed typical model diets. *Nutrition, 19*(0899-9007; 10), 826–831.

United Nation's Children's Fund. (2008a). *The state of the world's children 2009: Maternal and newborn health.* Retrieved April 25, 2009 from http://www.unicef.org/sowc09/docs/SOWC09-FullReport-EN.pdf/

United Nation's Children's Fund. (2008b). *Millennium development goals.* Retrieved April 25, 2009, from http://www.unicef.org/mdg/

Villalpando, S., Montalvo-Velarde, I., Zambrano, N., García-Guerra, A., Ramírez-Silva, C.I., Shamah-Levy, T., et al. (2003). Vitamins A and C and folate status in Mexican children under 12 years and women 12–49 years: A probabilistic national survey. *Salud Pública de México, 45*(Suppl 4), S508–S519.

Wiley-Kleeman, P. (Ed.). (1929). *Ramona's Spanish–Mexican cookery: The first complete and authentic Spanish–Mexican cook book in English.* Los Angeles: West Coast.

World Health Organization Statistical Information System. (2009, February 6). Retrieved April 22, 2009, from http://www.who.int/whosis/en/

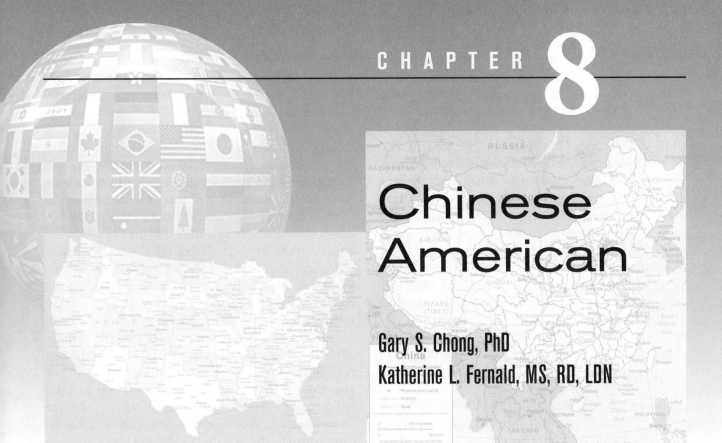

Chinese American

Gary S. Chong, PhD

Katherine L. Fernald, MS, RD, LDN

 CULTURE AND WORLD REGION

During the mid to late 1800s, internecine struggles, war, famine, and dire poverty, particularly in southeastern China, combined to spark and magnify a virtually irresistible desire, predominately in her ambitious young men, to pursue new, more prosperous lives in the faraway lands of South America, the Caribbean Islands, and the "Golden Mountain" (*Gahm Sahn*)—the United States of America. The 1848 discovery of gold at Sutter's Mill, leading to the great Gold Rush, led multitudes of Chinese men to leave wives and family behind to voyage eastward across the great expanse of the Pacific Ocean. Numbering in the tens of thousands, they arrived in America determined to work, sacrifice, provide a better life for their families, and, perhaps, return to China with honor, respect, and wealth. Although the great majority of them settled in the western states, especially California, smaller numbers also immigrated to large cities such as New York, Boston, Philadelphia,

and Chicago (Chang, 1977). From 1852 to 1884, between 18,000 and 25,000 Chinese immigrants ended their eastward journey halfway across the Pacific to work the sugar cane and pineapple plantations in what was then the Kingdom of Hawai'i (Young, 1974).

 LANGUAGE

Descriptions of foods and cuisines vary in the degree to which English- and Chinese-sounding translations are used or mixed with actual Chinese terminology. The degrees of linguistic sophistication and mixture depend on a number of factors. For example, a given menu's author may be from the first, second, third, or subsequent generation of American citizenry. Cultural and educational experiences tend to resemble those of the majority population with each subsequent generation; hence, awkward and, in some cases, embarrassingly humorous Chinese American "translations" of ingredient or food references into English are most often found among new immigrants, compared with first and subsequent generations of Chinese Americans. "One ton" (instead of *won ton*) and "cow yuck" (instead of *kau yuk* or *kau yook*) come to mind. Various Chinese dialects may be used to describe food ingredients and recipes depending on the region (northern, southern, eastern, or western China) from which a given cuisine originates. Since the Han people of China make up about 92% of the population, Chinese American food descriptions are more likely to feature references from the seven major dialects spoken by them: Mandarin (Putonghua), Gan, Hakka (Kejia), Minnan, Wu, Xiang, and Cantonese/Toisanese (Yue). Moreover, each of these language groups contains a large number of subdialects (Anderson, 1988).

CULTURE HISTORY

Along with their dreams and prospects for a better life in the "Golden Mountain," during the 1860s, and for two subsequent decades, Chinese immigrant laborers faced problems with isolation from their families and the rest of society, low pay, indentured work conditions, employment and racial discrimination, and internal struggles familiar to many immigrant minority groups trying to blend into their adopted country while maintaining their cultural identities and traditions. Despite a multitude of hardships and struggles, Chinese immigrants helped settle the American West, in part, by working on the Transcontinental Railroad and other rail or mining projects, and by taking up jobs that held little or no interest for many in the majority population. The proliferation of makeshift, affordable restaurants, laundries, and childcare services provided some of the basis for stereotyped views of these early Chinese immigrants as a service-oriented underclass (Lai, 1991).

As the gold-related economic boom dissipated, and the completion of large rail and mining projects led to more competition for fewer jobs in agricultural work, harder times spread in the western states during the 1870s. Consequently, as Chinese immigrants came to be seen as job-stealing "cheap labor," they faced increased waves of discrimination, threats, and violence. Anti-Chinese governmental and labor practices, which sought to curtail Chinese immigrant rights and economic opportunities, culminated in the 1882 Chinese Exclusion Act passed by Congress, denying them entry into, and citizenship in, the United States. As a psycho-

social and economic adaptation, "Chinatowns" arose to offer welcomed degrees of security and belonging. Eventually, persistent legal actions and a successful constitutional argument before the United States Supreme Court served to reestablish civil rights and protections for legal Chinese immigrants (Strom, 1996).

World War II ushered in more positive changes for Chinese Americans. Positive ripple effects from the Sino–American alliance meant a full welcome for them in the United States war effort and a more rapid progression toward full integration into the mainstream of American society and her labor force. The Civil Rights movement during the 1960s brought further helpful developments including the 1965 Immigration Reform Act, and President Richard Nixon's historic 1972 visit to China sparked a wider interest in Chinese culture among Americans in general. With a strong, traditionally Asian cultural emphasis on education as the best path to success, many Chinese immigrants and first-generation Chinese American parents pushed their children for academic achievement. As a result, the "baby boomers," or second-generation Chinese Americans, began to rise into the middle and upper echelons of society, and to have a growing impact on the wider culture and economy as one of the "model minorities" (Takaki, 1989).

FOOD HISTORY WITHIN THE CULTURE

The origins of Chinese American cuisine can be traced to those men who came to the western United States seeking a better fortune. With the influx of thousands of railroad and other laborers came an equally sizable yearning for familiar tastes of the "old country." Professional Chinese cooks and women were quite rare among their numbers, so the earliest Chinese American cuisines and restaurants were started by relatively unsophisticated, amateurish, labor-class men who had very little knowledge of cooking, and who were forced to improvise with what they could afford from local ingredients (Lau, Ma, & Ng, 1998). The innovative dishes they developed, such as chop suey, may not have been what professional connoisseurs or scholars deem "authentic" or "traditional," but they constituted palatable, affordable, and manageable ways for the pioneering Chinese restaurateurs to feed their compatriots. Soon, they began serving other American workmen. This change led to a restyling of their menus to satisfy broader American tastes, and to take advantage of the local ingredients found in most neighborhood groceries and food markets (Conlin, 1986). From the turn of the century to the rise of the post-World War II "baby boom" generation, Chinese American food adaptations, served right alongside with traditional Chinese cuisine, continued to grow in popularity and accessibility to such a degree that it is now possible for Americans nationwide to experience some form of Chinese American and traditional food without having to go to a "Chinatown." Nonetheless, many Americans, even those of Chinese ancestry, had found the actual prevalence of Chinese American cuisine to be inscrutable until an obscure industry journal, *Chinese Restaurant News* (CRN), was cited in *The New York Times* as estimating between 36,000 and 43,000 Chinese restaurants to be in the United States (Luo, 2004). These figures are more than the total number of McDonald's (13,000+), Burger King (11,000+), and Wendy's (6900+) U.S. franchises combined (Luo, 2004). Moreover, CRN's Web site reports that the Chinese American restaurants are generating about 17.5 billion dollars a year in sales, rivaling the economic heft of the "golden arches" conglomerate (Chinese Restaurant News, 2008).

Chinese–American cooking includes adaptations and traditional versions of foods from all four schools originating in the northern, southern, eastern, and western regions of China. Because most of the immigrant laborers came from the southern Guangdong province, however, the influences of the southern (Cantonese) and western (Sichuan) schools have been more dominant in both restaurant and home menus (Mariani, 1999). Chinese American cuisine adaptations have a very pragmatic history behind them in that many traditional Chinese foods cannot be authentically prepared in the typical American home. Though home cooks may use the venerable wok for simple stir-fry dishes, many traditional recipes call for levels of heat unknown in western cooking. For example, the quick flash-fry, on a high-BTU restaurant stove, seals in flavors in a way that is practically impossible to achieve in typical home kitchens (Lee, 2008). The following are a small sample of popular food dishes that are either purely Chinese American innovations or adaptations from the traditional schools.

Appetizers

Although they were not generally consumed by Chinese immigrants to the United States during the mid to late 1800s, and were unknown to Americans until about 45–50 years ago, Cantonese egg rolls, and the egg-less spring rolls, date back to ancient China and are undeniably a popular appetizer in today's Chinese American cuisine. They were originally made to serve as light, tea snacks for relatives and friends who might visit a family's home in the spring, following Chinese New Year. The finger-length wraps are made with unraised dough surrounding various meat, seafood, and vegetable mixtures, and are usually deep fried (Young, 1999).

Meat Dishes

General Tso's Chicken is a 1970s Chinese American invention that originated in New York, and is absent from traditional Chinese cuisine. If one travels to General Tso's hometown in Hunan Province to make inquiries about the dish, one should be prepared for puzzled or vacant reactions from residents including the general's own descendents. General Tso, whose real name was Tseng Kuo-fan, is better known in China for teaming up with another leader, Li Hung-Chang, to squash the messianic Taiping rebellion (1850–1864) during the Qing (Ching) dynasty at the cost of some 20 million lives (Lee, 2008). To attract American dining tastes, the fried chicken dish included sweet, salty, and spicy flavorings (sugar, soy sauce, onions, peppers, ginger, garlic, wine, and vinegar). The popularity of General Tso's Chicken has led to the witty observation that, in the United States, General Tso, like Colonel Sanders (Kentucky Fried Chicken), is associated with chicken and not warfare; but in China, General Tso is famed for warfare and not chicken.

The beef or chicken with broccoli dishes, so familiar to current American patrons of Chinese American cuisine, represent the successful marketing efforts of the D'Arrigo Brothers Company during the 1920s. The American broccoli (which originated in Italy) used in these dishes is quite different from the kale-like traditional Chinese broccoli. Nonetheless, innovative Chinese American cooks adapted it into an appealing main dish that quickly became a staple of the American diet by the 1930s (Lau et al., 1998). Its popularity as a Chinese–American food dish increased dramatically after World War II with the return of American military personnel from overseas, especially from the European theater of operations. Meanwhile these particular meat and broccoli dishes were all but unknown in China.

Dim-sum (Cantonese: *deem sum*) translates roughly as "so close to the heart." The Mandarin reference, *tien-hsin* translates as "to dot or touch the heart," which some people have taken to mean something like "to hit the spot." As a breakfast and lunch dining tradition that originated among the Cantonese, dim-sum food has always been linked to tea drinking (*yam cha*) giving rise to the phrase: "*dim-sum, yam cha.*" After making its way to the East and West coasts of America with Chinese immigrants, dim-sum grew in popularity, especially in larger American cities where ingredients for the various fillings were more readily available (Barer-Stein, 1999). Dim-sum includes several dozen steamed and deep-fried dishes in the form of nearly bite-sized dough, taro dough, or rice-flour wraps and dumplings. Their centers range across a variety of minced, oiled, and seasoned meat fillings (e.g., shrimp, pork, beef), cooked vegetables, or taro. Popular dips for dim-sum include soy, ginger, oyster, and hot-spiced sauces.

Vegetable Dishes

Chop suey is typically made of leftover vegetables and lesser amounts of meats stir-fried together. Noodles and bean sprouts are very often present, but the rest of the dish can vary according to whatever is around. Of the various folklore accounts surrounding the origins of this quintessential Chinese American dish, the most plausible ones suggest that it was concocted by one or a number of quick-witted Chinese cooks, probably in California, in response to (1) the rude demands of non-Chinese restaurant patrons near closing time, or (2) the needs of poorer miners and railway workers for an inexpensive, palatable, and easily prepared meal that could be made from whatever scraps of food were lying around (Tannahill, 1988). Most historians agree that the dish came into being somewhere between the mid 1800s to 1888, when the term "chop suey" first appeared in the Oxford English Dictionary (Davidson, 1999). In any case, the dish's name is likely to be an anglicized version of either the Toisanese/Cantonese *tsap seui* (mixed bits) or the Mandarin *tsa sui* (chopped up odds and ends).

Noodle Dishes

Chow mein is a dish made of stewed vegetables and meat with fried noodles. The term comes from the Mandarin *chao mien* (fried noodles) and probably was brought to the United States by Chinese cooks serving railroad workers during the mid to late 1850s. Verbal references to chow mein first appeared in English publications in 1900 (Kiple & Ornelas, 2000). Although most chow mein bears very little resemblance to true Mandarin cooking, it has become a staple of Chinese American cuisine. Owing to its inexpensive ingredients, chow mein and adaptations of it have long been a part of American school cafeteria menus.

Rice Dishes

Fried rice is a standard method of cooking leftovers, involving frying cold boiled rice with chopped-up meat and vegetables. In really superior restaurants, rice will be specially boiled and dried for this, but usually old, unused rice is served. The common (and favorite) recipe, however, is not Cantonese, but eastern, deriving from Yon chou in the lower Yangtze region of China. It involves mixing chopped ham, beaten egg, green peas, green onions, and other ingredients to taste, and then sautéing the rice. Ideally, fried rice is neither deep-fried nor stir-fried, but cooked slowly in a little oil to produce a fluffy product with a slight crust (Miller, 1975).

Soups

Won ton, translated from two Chinese words meaning "a small dumpling or roll," consists of a thin, unraised dough wrapper formed around a savory filling of seasoned, minced pork (usually). In addition to appearing in a soup form, won tons may also be steamed, pan-fried, or deep-fried and served along with other dim-sum items. Historical accounts of Chinese stuffed dumplings such as won ton go back for several centuries and have involved a number of cultures. There are accounts of Marco Polo, for example, arriving in China during the 13th century, happily discovering Chinese stuffed noodles including won ton, and returning to Italy with the exotic find (Chang, 1977).

Desserts/Snacks

The ubiquitous "fortune cookie" found in American Chinese restaurants is actually of Japanese origin (Lee, 2008). It was left to Chinese American restaurateurs to popularize the after-dinner snack in their menus during World War II, for the unfortunate reasons that Japanese–American bakeries were shut down, and anything appearing overtly Japanese (including foods) would, understandably, not have been favorably regarded at the time.

Red bean soup is both a popular snack and a sweet dessert soup. The main ingredient, Azuki beans, is a "yang" or warming food. Tangerine peel, used in many recipes, is thought to aid digestion. Brown sugar provides additional sweetening.

If one is ever unsure whether a Chinese-looking dish is purely traditional or a Chinese American adaptation, one way to definitively identify the latter is to look for vegetables and other ingredients that are more typically found in the United States, such as carrots, American onions or sweet onions, American broccoli (Italian in origin), or tomatoes.

Although American tastes still dictate the content of most Chinese menus outside the largest cities, Chinese American food has become more varied since the more recent periods of immigration began from the 1970s onward. The trend for increased variety may also reflect a desire to compete with dozens of cuisines that have also become prevalent as a result of immigration liberalization during the past three decades: Thai, Indian, Vietnamese, Japanese, Korean, and Indonesian, to name just a few of the Asian varieties. "Mongolian Barbecue" restaurants (similar to the Japanese shabu–shabu outlets) allow customers to choose their meats and ingredients to either cook themselves, or to have them cooked on special grills right at their tables (simi-lar to the Japanese *teppanyaki*). The Chinese menu will nearly always feature a "hot" option in deference to the Sichuan and Hunan traditions (Lau et al., 1998). Catering to American health concerns, restaurants will sometimes advertise that they are "MSG free" (monosodium glutamate free) and, more frequently, offer vegetarian options and less greasy dishes that are steamed instead of fried.

MAJOR FOODS

Protein Sources

Chinese American cuisine boasts a wide range of protein sources, including beef, chicken, duck, fish, nuts (almonds, cashews, pine), pork, oxen, oysters (often dried), scallops (often dried), shark's fin, shrimp (cooked or dried), and vegetables (soybeans and soy derivatives like tofu).

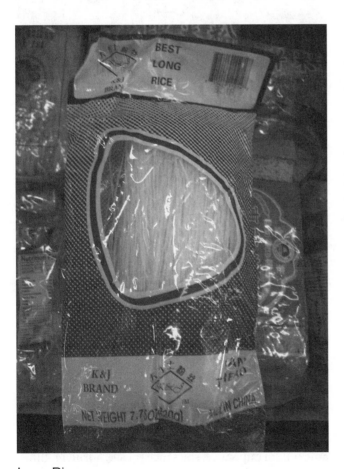

Long Rice
Courtesy of the author

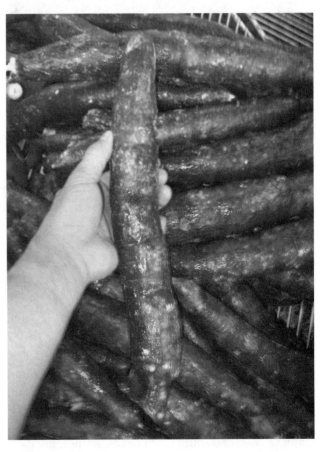

Tapioca
Courtesy of the author

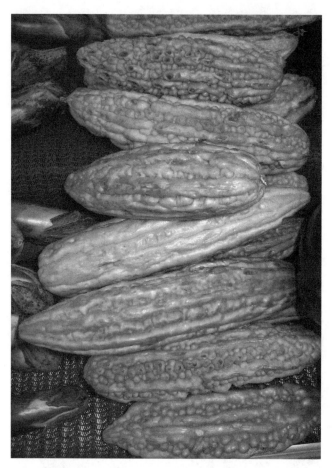

Bitter Melon
Courtesy of the author

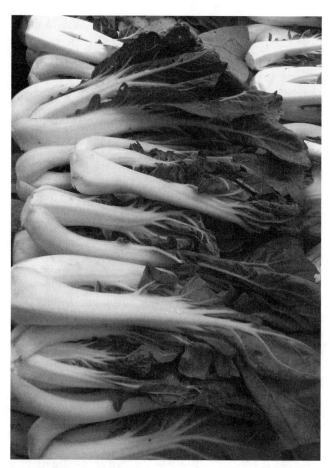

Bok Choy
Courtesy of the author

 Starch Sources

The starch sources are noodles (won ton, chow mein, chow fun), potatoes, rice (short-grain or sweet rice, long rice, rice flour, rice vermicelli), tapioca starch, taro, and wheat starch.

 Fat Sources

Animal fat sources include beef, chicken, duck, and fish; vegetable sources include nuts (almonds, cashews, pine), peanut oil, and vegetable oil.

 Prominent Vegetables

Prominent vegetables are asparagus, bean curd (often dried), bean sprouts, bamboo shoots, bitter melon, black moss, broccoli and Chinese broccoli, carrots, celery, Chinese cabbage (*bok choy*, *pak choi*, or *won bak*), Chinese peas, choi sum, green beans, lettuce, mustard cabbage, mushrooms, *ong choi*, onions (white, green), salted turnip (*teem choy poe* or *chung choy zack*), scal-

lions, snow peas/shoots, spinach, squash, turnips (*chung choi*), water chestnut (dried or flour forms), and watercress.

 Prominent Fruits

Apples, cantaloupe, cherries, honeydew melon, jack fruit, lemon, *lai chi*, oranges, peaches, pears, persimmons, rambutan, tangerine, and watermelon are the prominent fruits.

 Spices and Seasonings

Spices include black bean sauce (liquid, ground, dried), wet bean curd (red, white), black fungus, chili–garlic sauce, chili pepper, Chinese mushrooms (often dried), Chinese parsley, garlic, ginger, hoisin sauce, hot oil, oyster sauce, peppercorns (Sichuan), plum sauce, sesame oil, shrimp sauce, soy sauce (black, *harm ha*, thin), vinegar (red rice, sweetened black), rice cooking wine (*shao hsing*), and XO sauce.

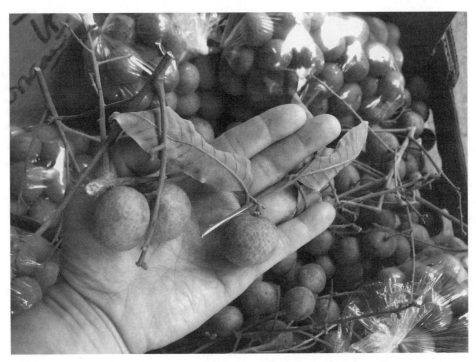

Longan, Fruit Resembling Lai Chi
Courtesy of the author

 Beverages

Teas (black, jasmine, green), fruit juices, and milk (rice, soy, and lactose-free milk for the lactose intolerant) are the preferred beverages.

 Desserts

Almond pudding with fruit cocktail, tapioca pudding, brown candy, rock sugar, and egg custard tarts (*dahn tah*) are favorite desserts.

 FOODS WITH CULTURAL SIGNIFICANCE

Rice (*fan* or *fun*, pronounced "fahn") has always been such a central part of the Chinese diet that its name is considered to be the equivalent in meaning and usage to the English word "food" (Simons, 1991). Other foods symbolize good luck/fortune (tangerines, oranges, pomelo, ginkgo nuts, black moss, dried bean curd, bamboo shoots, vermicelli, scallions), wealth/prosperity (whole fish and chicken, egg or spring rolls, sweet-sticky rice cake, winter bamboo shoots), longevity (uncut noodles, peanuts), fidelity (duck), peace/happiness (apples, prawns), fertility (eggs, seeds: lotus, pumpkin, watermelon), marital goodness (chicken's feet), and love of family (*lai-chee*, lychee nuts, dumplings).

 TYPICAL DAY'S MENU

Chinese American meals may include elements from American, Chinese American, and traditional Chinese cuisines.

Breakfast

Eggs flavored with soy or oyster sauce, toast with orange jelly/jam, a scoop of rice, steamed spinach, and chicken or turkey *jook* (rice porridge) are typical for breakfast. Beverages might include tea, coffee, milk (dairy or nondairy), or a fruit juice.

Lunch

A greater variety of dishes is possible for lunch, probably from Cantonese or Sichuan cuisines. Spring rolls, won ton soup, and *doong* (sticky rice cakes) are popular appetizers, with main dishes including selections such as almond chicken, beef broccoli, some kind of chow fun (noodle dish), chop suey or some other vegetable dish, and dim-sum items. Beverages may be tea, coffee, or a fruit juice. Dessert selections tend to be lighter, such as taro root cake, sponge cake, or New Year's cake.

Dinner

Chinese American culture places great importance on harmony in both family and social gatherings. Dinner selections are meant for savoring, appreciating, and facilitating pleasant exchanges between those present. Appetizers may feature turnip cake, Sichuan cucumber salad, shrimp chips, crispy won ton, and a soup selection (hot-and-sour soup, winter melon soup, or watercress soup). Main dishes are usually more substantial and may be spicier, such as Mongolian beef, spare ribs (sweet/sour or *char siu*), *ma po tofu*, *dan-dan mian* (spicy peanut noodles), Sichuan twice-cooked pork, *kung pao* chicken/shrimp, lemon chicken, steamed whole fish with oyster sauce, fried pork, *bao* (*char siu* or black sugar), chicken with bean sauce, shrimp, pot stickers, *moo goo gai pan*, *moo shoo pork*, long rice, fried tofu, sweet-and-sour spare ribs, eggplant in shrimp sauce, *bok choy*, stir-fried spinach, steamed sponge cake, chicken (ginger, lemon, or almond), pork hash, bitter lemon, and beef.

 HOLIDAY MENUS

Chinese Americans vary in their manner of celebrating any number of both traditional Chinese and traditional Western or American holidays and festivals. East–West–American mixtures often make for a delightful cross-cultural experience, gastronomic and otherwise.

Labor Day/Memorial Day

Traditional hotdogs, hamburgers, potato salad, barbeque ribs, and so on, may be served right alongside with chow fun, crispy pork won ton/*gau gee*, lemon chicken, *char siu bao*, and Mandarin salad.

Thanksgiving and Christmas

Turkey (stuffed Asian style with Sichuan peppercorns, ginger, soy-flavored rice, water chestnuts, dried apricots, and shiitake mushrooms) yams, and corn are as likely to be matched by roast duck, dim-sum selections, and stir-fried garlic lettuce.

"Regular" New Year's Eve and Chinese New Year's Eve

New Year's Eve holidays include champagne, whole fish (symbolizing completeness), persimmons, tangerines, and fruit cocktail (especially with red and orange colors for good fortune), *gin dui* or *zeen doy* (sweet, deep-fried dough balls covered in sesame seeds), taro cake, *nian gao* ("year cake," cooked or fried), noodles (for longevity), dried melon and pumpkin seeds, and candied fruits and nuts (often served with tea by younger family members to their elders as a sign of respect and, in exchange for good luck, *lee-see*—paper money—in small, red envelopes!). On the day after, many Chinese Americans try to avoid meat dishes and eat vegetarian dishes like *Jai* (Buddha's Delight) instead.

Hungry Ghost Festival

The Hungry Ghost Festival (around mid-August) practices, if the holiday is observed at all, may vary from leaving out an untouched, token platter of food for the ghosts (pork, brightly colored cake, and rice for good luck), all the way up to leaving multiple-course meals and a whole, cooked pig.

Mid-Autumn Moon Festival

The Mid-Autumn Moon Festival (around mid-September) includes baked goods, mooncakes with various fillings such as dates, nuts, fruit, and Chinese sausage. More exotic fare would include green-tea mooncakes, and *ping pei* or snow-skin mooncakes.

 HEALTH BELIEFS AND CONCERNS

Mention Traditional Chinese Medicine (TCM) and many Chinese Americans will be able to come up with a smattering of references to yin/yang, acupuncture, Qi (Ch'i), acupressure, herbal medicines, aromatherapy (incense burning), medicinal foods, and meditation techniques. The nature and extent of TCM's influence on their health and nutritional practices is likely to depend on a number of factors such as educational background, American acculturation (often linked to one's generation of American citizenry—first, second, third, etc.), familiarity and experiences with TCM (personal or indirect), and any "renaissance" or reidentification with traditional or modern Chinese culture; hence, Chinese Americans may vary greatly on the degree and manner in which they juxtapose, balance, or blend Eastern and Western health and nutritional beliefs and practices. One Chinese American client or patient may happily use Western medications for headache in the morning and, in the evening, address indigestion with some hot ginger tea. Another person might blend

Observations from the Author (Gary Chong)

As a youngster in Hawai'i, I absorbed the meaning and importance of Chinese American foods through the natural occurrences of family dinners, beachside picnics, and, after my dining etiquette had matured sufficiently, occasional restaurant adventures. During these gatherings, dishes of food were treated almost like honored guests as they arrived at the table. Ooh's, ah's, and other expressions of positive regard were lavishly given, and a few of my uncles or aunts made sure that pictures were taken of each dish until there were nearly as many pictures of the food as there were of family and guests. During New Year and special family celebrations (e.g., birthdays, graduations, or weddings) the pouring of tea for one's elders had both filial and practical aspects, for it not only conveyed respect, but it also significantly improved one's chances of receiving *lee-see* (good-luck money).

No one had to coerce me to learn the Chinese names for all the different foods, or to master using the initially unwieldy chopsticks. One wanted to learn because the older kids and adults knew the Chinese food terms and were adeptly using chopsticks. It provided a developmental rite of passage to clearly demonstrate that I was a more grown-up diner whose skills went beyond the easier use of English terminology and the simpler forks or spoons. (Babies, after all, could neither order food in Chinese nor use chopsticks!) Using chopsticks and Chinese food names also gave me something distinctively Asian to nourish my sense of cultural identity, to share with my friends, and to use in impressing adults. The nine-course dinner also served as a cultural and developmental proving ground. When presented with the challenge of such a gastronomic feat, it was accepted as an unwritten rule that if you did not have the patience, stamina, and courage (or more literally, the stomach) to eat something from each of the nine courses, then you were some kind of gourmet "wimp." Any revulsions to weird or "ugly" looking foods were met by admonishments to "Try it, you'll like it," "If you eat it, then you won't have to look at it," and that perennial parental provocation, "There are starving kids in China who'd love to be eating that." The latter verbal inducement was doubly potent for kids like me, since I was not only a better-off American, but Chinese to boot! Fortunately, I almost always found that the unattractive foods tasted much better than they looked, and eventually took some pride in adopting a few of them (e.g., chicken feet, dried squid, and cuttlefish) as part of my gourmet identity and as badges of consumption courage.

taking a dose of sildenafil citrate (Viagra®) and drinking sea cucumber soup before lovemaking.

The concept of Qi (Ch'i) or biogenic "life force" underlying our existence is a fundamental part of TCM. The world and the human body are seen in terms of invisible energies and vibrations that can be manipulated by various means (e.g., acupuncture, meditation, or diet) to produce healthful changes. Subtle changes in Qi are believed to have effects ranging across medicine, agriculture, all aspects of human life, and even cosmological events. The cultivation of Qi is the "sine qua non" of a healthy, balanced life.

TCM attempts to understand a food's Qi by studying its effects on the body and behavior after it is ingested. Some foods activate or slow metabolism, generate warmth or cold "temperature" in the body, moisten or dry out the body, and nourish the kidneys, liver, or heart.

Eastern nutritional philosophy favors individually tailored interventions rather than standardization or universally "right" diets. The status of factors that affected a patient's Qi (e.g., metabolism rate, "temperature," and moisture levels in the body, gen-

eral circulation, and blood/nutritional supply to the kidneys, liver, or heart) guided the Eastern practitioner's selection of foods to restore proper balance for that individual. He or she may vary from another client in being excessive or deficient, hot or cold, dry or moist, or imbalanced in certain organs or elements, so a diet that is "right" for one person may not work as well for another.

GENERAL HEALTH AND NUTRITIONAL INDICATORS SUMMARY

The current health statistics of Chinese Americans will depend upon year of immigration and adaptation to the American cuisine. UNICEF (2005) gives China a better report card on low-birth-weight infants (4%) as compared with the United States (8%), but a worse grade in the percentage of children (under 5 years of age) underweight in the moderate to severe level (8%) as compared with the United States (2%). The life expectancy in China is 73 years, as compared with 77.8 years in the United States (UNICEF, 2005).

Observations from the Author (Katherine Fernald)

I first became interested in Chinese American foods because I became a vegetarian when I was an undergraduate in college. Within a couple of years, I developed severe lactose intolerance. Unless I suggested a Chinese restaurant to my friends, I had precious little I could eat without appearing to be picky or to have an eating disorder. College, for me, was in the Midwest, where there was a plethora of hearty beef-oriented family-style restaurants, but only the occasional Italian restaurant, for example, that actually served a variety of meatless fare. Many other vegetarians could feel very comfortable in Italian restaurants, but so much Italian food includes cheese on or in it; protein in Italian food comes from cheese, red meat, poultry, or fish. As a vegetarian with lactose intolerance, there simply were not many options.

When I first became a vegetarian, there were not many fast-food restaurants with vegetarian options. My graduate school was located in the panhandle of Texas that, at the time, was even worse for vegetarians, because of the emphasis on meals with meat. When I first arrived there, I went with my internship group to a place that had only one item on the menu that I could eat because it did not have meat or cheese: cole slaw.

As I have drifted back and forth between strict vegetarian and the less-limiting meat-restrictor or lacto-ovo-pesco vegetarian (milk products, eggs, and fish/seafood) eating practices, Chinese restaurants have always been the most accommodating to my taste needs. I later developed reactive hypoglycemia, which meant that I needed a reasonable amount of protein in each major meal; otherwise, I would become dizzy from reacting to high levels of carbohydrates, or I would need food again sooner than expected. I had always relied upon soy, so when I first developed hypoglycemia, I leaned even more on soy foods including tofu. Eating out was simpler if I just went to a Chinese American restaurant and ordered a tofu-containing dish.

To this day, I feel more comfortable eating Asian foods than I do eating other foods, due to the former's wider use of nonanimal (e.g., soy and nut) proteins. Furthermore, because lactose intolerance is very common among Asians (Sahi, 1994), their cuisines usually do not provide or cook with dairy (lactose) products (unless one counts Crab Rangoon and other foods placed on menus for Anglo Americans).

I wanted to learn to cook Chinese food at home. My Chinese American friends made it easier and more fun. While it has become more fashionable to eschew meat, eat lots of soy, and generally try to be heart conscious, there are few places to eat out once you leave the larger cities. In my almost 30 years of meat restricting, I still find comfort and variety in the Chinese style of cooking. Fortunately, there is always a decent Chinese restaurant within easy reach and they usually have chopsticks, which makes the eating more fun and authentic. (I find that some Asian foods are more easily eaten with chopsticks. I have always found cultures different from my own very interesting, and enjoy engaging people from those cultures in conversation about their customs.)

When I received the invitation to contribute to this book, it seemed natural for me, from a personal as well as professional standpoint. Of course, when I talk with people about their cultures, I often meet them in restaurants or think and ask about food anyway. I love food so much that I pursued two degrees in it! Professionally, when I have counseled Chinese Americans, my knowledge of the cuisine and customs certainly has helped me be more effective.

COMMUNICATION AND COUNSELING TIPS

With regard to communication and/or counseling, first determine the degree to which your client subscribes to traditionally Chinese beliefs and thinking about foods and nutrition, independent of what Chinese or Chinese American foods are present in his or her diet. Chinese Americans who subscribe to Western, science-based medical and nutritional health care require little or no special adaptations in counseling. Traditionally minded clients may be more open and compliant regarding dietary modifications if such changes are discussed in terms of restoring a health-

ful "balance" not only nutritionally, but also in terms of their Qi, "temperature," blood, yin, and yang. Given the variety of cuisines and food choices, though, with a little research and care it should be possible to find menu compromises that satisfy both Eastern and Western perspectives of a client's health and nutritional needs. If traditionally minded clients inquire about the use of unfamiliar Chinese medicinal foods or herbal preparations, you may want to consider framing your consultations with Western medical and pharmacology professionals in the context obtaining, again, the best balance of what Eastern and Western health traditions have to offer. Consultations may then proceed to check for possible side effects, allergic reactions, or interactions with other prescription and nonprescription medications or herbs, Eastern or Western.

Nonverbal aspects of counseling may also deserve some attention. Traditionally minded Chinese American clients who are relatively inexperienced (e.g., first generation) with American norms for social interactions may seem more demure, deferential, reserved or passive, disengaged, or polite than more acculturated individuals in your practice. To treat you with the proper amount of traditional respect, they may seem less inclined to make eye contact and gesticulate, for example, or to bring up matters that are either potentially embarrassing or might lead to any disagreements or conflicts with you as a healthcare "authority." The counselor may experience occasions when clients may say "yes" when they mean "no" (or wish to say "no") as a way of being traditionally polite and respectful. Later, however, they may not follow through on therapeutic plans or advice. Such instances are not likely to be cases of either passive aggression or indirect defiance meant to frustrate the counselor. It may be helpful to then gently clarify and normalize the fact that disagreement, questioning, and the discussion of possibly embarrassing material in the context of counseling is actually quite acceptable or even desirable, certainly not disrespectful or impolite, and is indeed very helpful to cultivating a more "balanced" understanding between you and your client, and, subsequently, a more "harmoniously effective" working relationship.

Specific dietary concerns might include the higher salt, saturated fat, and calories found in a number of Chinese American dishes, as noted in a recent 2007 study by the Center for Science in the Public Interest (CSPI). The following recommendations from CSPI may serve as discussion points with your client:

1. Choose dishes that feature vegetables instead of meat or noodles, and include or ask for extra broccoli, snow peas, or other vegetables.
2. Steer clear of deep-fried meat, seafood, or tofu. Substitute it with stir-fried or braised options.
3. Minimize the use of sauce by using forks or chopsticks to leave more sauce behind.
4. Avoid or minimize salt by steering clear of duck sauce, hot mustard, hoisin sauce, and soy sauce.
5. Share your meal, or take half of it home for later.
6. Use or ask for brown rice instead of white rice.

Regarding the estimation of healthy weight ranges, it may not be unusual for the practitioner to see a number of Chinese American clients, both women and some men, who have a significantly lighter skeletal framing relative to individuals from other ethnic groups. Clinical experience and judgment may be needed in considering adjustments to estimations of ideal body-weight range. A careful weight history will likely be helpful in determining healthy weight ranges for such individuals.

PRIMARY LANGUAGE OF FOOD NAMES WITH ENGLISH AND PHONETIC TRANSLATION

Just as many traditional Chinese foods have been adapted and modified to suit both Chinese American and wider American tastes, food names reflect both authentic Chinese and Chinese-sounding references that, it is hoped, have some level of exotic appeal among the English-speaking public. Below is a brief sample of names for some popular Chinese American food items. The pronunciation guide in parentheses is followed by the English description.

- *Bao / Baozi* (bough / bough zhee): steamed bun with a pork and vegetable filling
- *Cai* (kai): Mandarin for dish or vegetable
- *Cha* (chah): any tea
- Cassia bark: a type of bark with a cinnamon-like odor, used in Western Chinese cooking
- *Dou fu / Tofu* (doe-foo / toe-foo): soybean curd
- *Fan* (fahn or fun): rice, or a general reference for food
- *Jiaozi* (chiao-zhee): boiled dumplings with meat and vegetable fillings
- *Jiu* (jee-ew): wine
- *Litchi / lychee / lai chi* (lye-chee): a small, round sweet fruit with a brown peel and white flesh grown in southern China
- *Longan* (lung-gun): fruit resembling *lai chi*
- *Mantou* (mahn-toe): steamed bun
- *Mien* (minn): noodles
- *Rou* (row): meat; *jirou* (jee-row): chicken; *zhurou* (zoo-row): pork
- *Sichuan* (see-chew-on) peppercorn: tiny reddish peppercorn with a flower-like appearance and a "numbing" taste used in Sichuan cooking
- *Taro* root: a starchy, potato-like root used in soups and stews
- *Yue bing* (you-eh-bing): mooncake, small round cakes with various sweet fillings, eaten during the Moon Festival
- *Zhou* (zoh) or *Jook*: rice porridge

Vegetarian *Jai* (Buddha's Delight)

¼ cup cloud ears (*wun yee*)

¼ cup lily buds (*gum tzum*)

¼ cup packed black moss (*fat choy*)

¼ cup unshelled ginko nuts (*bock guo*)

2 sticks (about 1.5 oz.) of dried bean curd (*foo jook*)

1 (3.5-oz.) package of cellophane noodles

4 large Napa cabbage leaves (about 8 oz.)

8 Chinese dried oysters

8 Chinese dried mushrooms

6 fried bean curds (*dul foo gok*) cut into 2 pieces

1 tsp. and 3 tbsp. vegetable oil

Oyster sauce and ginger (to taste)

1. Thoroughly rinse and dry cabbage leaves in colander.
2. Wash and soak oysters in 1½ cups of cold water for 3–4 hours or until softened. Drain and squeeze dry (save soaking water for later).
3. Soak cloud ears, lily buds, and mushrooms in ½ cup of cold water for 30 minutes to soften. Remove all hard spots from cloud ears. Remove hard ends from lily buds and tie each bud into a loose knot. Drain and squeeze dry the mushrooms (save soaking water for later). Discard soaking water of cloud ears and lily buds. Trim off mushroom stems and halve the caps.
4. Cover black moss with water in a bowl. Add the 1 tsp. oil and soak for 15 minutes or until soft. Drain and discard the water.
5. Soak cellophane noodles in cold water for 15 minutes or until soft, then drain.
6. Boil 3 cups of water in a 2-qt. saucepan. Break up bean curd sticks into bite-size pieces and add to boiling water. Cook and stir 1–2 minutes or until sticks turn almost ivory color or soften. Transfer to colander to drain and rinse with cold water.
7. Similarly, boil (until puffy), drain, rinse, and squeeze out the fried bean curd.
8. Shell and blanch the gingko nuts in 1 cup of boiling water for about 1 minute. Rinse the nuts in cold water and remove their skins.
9. Trim off about ½ inch from ends of cabbage leave stems. Chop up cabbage leaves into half pieces. Stir-fry cabbage leaves 2–3 minutes (or until limp) in a wok or skillet using 2 tbsp. vegetable oil with optional ginger flavoring.
10. Add 1 tbsp. of vegetable oil along with the oysters, wet bean curd, and mushrooms, and stir-fry 30 seconds. Add bean curd sticks, blanched fried bean curd, gingko nuts, and black moss, and stir-fry while breaking up the bean curd. Add the soaking water of the mushrooms and oysters and bring mixture to medium boil.
11. Stir, cover, and simmer for 20 minutes. Add more water as needed to keep the wok or skillet from drying out.
12. Add cellophane noodles, cloud ears, lily buds, cabbage, and optional oyster sauce (to taste). Bring mixture to full boil, then cover and let simmer at medium heat until cellophane noodles are translucent and vegetables are tender (about 5 minutes). Serve hot or warm.

Yields 6–8 servings

Courtesy of Jeanette Chong

More recipes are available at http://nutrition.jbpub.com/foodculture/

REFERENCES

Anderson, E.N. (1988). *The food of China*. New Haven, CT: Yale University Press.

Barer-Stein, T. (1999). *You eat what you are: People, culture and food traditions*. Ontario, Canada: Firefly Books.

Chang, K.C. (Ed.). (1977). *Food in Chinese culture: Anthropological and historical perspectives*. New Haven, CT: Yale University Press.

Chinese Restaurant News. (2008). Retrieved January 26, 2010, from www.c-r-n.com

Conlin, J.R. (1986). *Bacon, beans and galantines: Food and foodways on the western mining frontier*. Reno, NV: University of Nevada Press.

Davidson, A. (1999). *Oxford companion to food*. Oxford, UK: Oxford University Press.

Kiple, K.F., & Ornelas, K.C. (2000). *Cambridge world encyclopedia of food*. Cambridge, UK: Cambridge University Press.

Lai, H.M. (1991). *Island: Poetry and history of Chinese immigrants on Angel Island, 1910–1940*. Seattle, WA: University of Washington Press.

Lau, G., Ma, K.M., & Ng, A. (1998). *Chinese American food practices, customs, and holidays*. Chicago, IL: American Dietetic Association, American Diabetes Association.

Lee, J. (2008). *Fortune cookie chronicles: Adventures in the world of Chinese food*. New York: Twelve (Hachette Book Group).

Luo, M. (2004, September 22). As all American as egg foo yong. *The New York Times*. Retrieved October 29, 2009, from: http://travel.nytimes.com/2004/09/22/dining/22CHIN.html?_r=1&fta=y&pagewanted=print&position=

Mariani, J.F. (1999). *Encyclopedia of American food and drink*. New York: Lebhar-Friedman.

Miller, G.B. (1975). *The thousand recipe Chinese cook book*. New York: Grosset & Dunlap.

Sahi, T. (1994). Genetics and epidemiology of adult-type hypolactasia. *Scand. J. Gastroenterol, (Suppl.)*, 202:7–20.

Simons, F.J. (1991). *Food in China: A cultural and historical inquiry*. Boca Raton, FL: CRC Press.

Strom, Y. (1996). *Quilted landscape: Conversations with young immigrants*. New York: Simon & Schuster.

Takaki, R. (1989). *Strangers from a different shore*. New York: Penguin Books.

Tannahill, R. (1988). *Food in history*. New York: Three Rivers Press.

UNICEF. (2005). *The state of the world's children 2007: Women and children, the double dividend of gender equality*. Retrieved April 14, 2009, from http://www.unicef.org/sowc07/statistics/tables.php/

Young, G. (1999). *The wisdom of the Chinese kitchen*. New York: Simon & Schuster.

Young, M. (1974). *Hawaii's people from China*. Honolulu, HI: Hogarth Press.

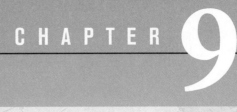

CHAPTER 9

French Canadian

Sara Brass, MPH

Felicia Cohen-Egger, BS

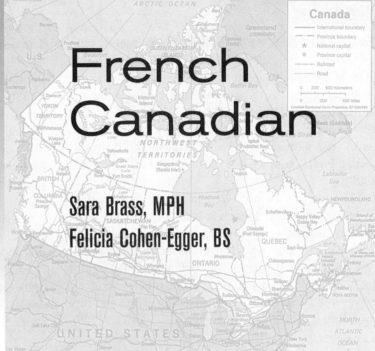

 ## CULTURE AND WORLD REGION

The term "French Canadian" refers to Canadian citizens who are descended from the French settlers of the 17th and 18th centuries, and speak French as their primary language. As of 2006, more than 6.8 million Canadians (roughly 22% of the population) identify French as their mother tongue (Statistics Canada, 2006a). This is the largest French-speaking community in North America (Wartik, 1989).

French Canadians have a vibrant culture that combines contemporary values and a modern lifestyle with long-held traditions from their colonial past. French Canadians are passionate about hockey, and they have been represented on every team in the National Hockey League (Wartik, 1989). Performing arts, winter sports, literature, radio, and television are popular entertainment. In Quebec, international cultural festivals are held throughout the year, including the Winter Carnival, Montreal World Film Festival, Just for Laughs Comedy Festival, and International Jazz Festival. The Canadian Grand Prix, part of the Formula One World Championship, is another popular annual event. Well-known French Canadians include Celine Dion, Jack Kerouac, Mario Lemieux, Former Prime Minister Pierre-Elliot Trudeau, and the performing group Cirque du Soleil (Ferry, 2003).

The majority of French Canadians reside in Quebec, where 80% of the population is French speaking (Statistics Canada, 2006b). The Maritime Provinces, particularly New Brunswick, also have a significant concentration of francophones, known as Acadians. Some French Canadians are also found in Ontario and across the western provinces of Canada (Statistics Canada, 2006b).

More than 2 million French Canadian descendents live in the United States, and many families retain strong roots to their heritage. It is especially common to find these individuals in northern New England, the Great Lakes region, and Louisiana (US Census Bureau, 2005).

LANGUAGE

French Canadians speak a dialect of French, with an accent and vocabulary that differs from Parisian French. Although the particular characteristics differ by geographic region, in general, French Canadians pronounce their consonants sharply while drawing out vowel sounds. Their lexicon combines typical French terms with words derived from English and from Canadian First Nations tribes (Battye, Hintze, & Rowlett, 2000).

Language is a central element of French Canadian identity. In Quebec, French is "the normal and everyday language of work, communication, commerce and business in the civil administration and in enterprises," according to the Charter of the French Language of 1977. French Canadians who live in other provinces, however, have tended to assimilate more into the surrounding English-speaking culture (Wartik, 1989). The country of Canada is officially bilingual, meaning that all national activities are conducted in both French and English.

CULTURE HISTORY

The original French Canadians were settlers from France who came to develop the land and resources of northern North America, which had been discovered by French explorers in the early 1500s. French rule extended from the Atlantic Ocean to the St. Lawrence River Valley (modern-day Maritime Provinces and Quebec), and this territory was called New France, with Quebec City as its capital. The area was valued for its abundance of fishing, farmland, and furs. Roman Catholicism flourished under French rule, and became an essential component of French Canadian life (Moogk, 2000).

Great Britain attempted to win control of New France through several wars in the 18th century. Newfoundland and part of Nova Scotia came under British control in 1713. When French-speaking Acadians in these regions refused to give their allegiance to Great Britain, they were forced from their land in what is known as the "Great Upheaval." France formally ceded control of New France to the British at the end of the Seven Years' War in 1763 (Dickinson & Young, 2001). Britain divided New France into two regions, called Upper and Lower Canada. While Upper Canada was English-speaking and followed the British social system, Lower Canada retained its French ties (Moogk, 2000).

Upper and Lower Canada were reunified in 1841. The Canadian provinces moved toward further unification in 1864 when they formed a coalition. Canada became an independent dominion of Great Britain in 1867, effectively forming its own country. Canada achieved full independence in 1982 (Dickinson & Young, 2001).

The Quiet Revolution of 1960 was a watershed moment in Quebec, when the new political leadership reinvigorated the concept of French Canadian nationalism with the motto, "masters in our own house." The renewed sense of nationalism brought about the establishment of a new political party in 1969, the Parti Quebecois, whose platform centered on achieving sovereignty for the nation of Quebec. Referendums to separate Quebec from the rest of Canada have been held, the first in 1980, but they have not received majority support to date (Dickinson & Young, 2001).

FOOD HISTORY WITHIN THE CULTURE

French Canadian cuisine reflects the adaptation of French cooking techniques and traditions to local Canadian ingredients. Culinary influences from Normandy are particularly evident, as this is a region from which many settlers hailed. Heavily spiced stews, soups, and meat pies were common in the diet of early French Canadians. In coastal communities, shellfish and cod were abundant, and were often served smoked, salted, pickled, or baked. Large loaves of multigrain bread baked in a hearth or wood oven were another staple (Kiple & Ornelas, 2000).

Regional foods, such as maple syrup, salt pork, potatoes, dried peas, and oats, worked their way into many of the recipes over time. Many dishes were made with a high fat content, typically from lard, which provided some warmth in the cold Canadian climate. Fruits and vegetables were incorporated into the diet through local agriculture and from French imports. Alcoholic beverages were distilled from local grains and produce. Ingredients from the United States, such as beans, chili peppers, and cornmeal, were introduced to the cuisine due to the immigration of American loyalists following the Revolutionary War. Trade with the French colonies of the Caribbean also brought new flavors, such as rum and cane sugar. Under British occupation, French Canadians discovered puddings, cakes, pies, and molasses (Kiple & Ornelas, 2000).

MAJOR FOODS

Protein Sources

Quebec is rich in local game and fish, such as duck, venison, cod, herring, and sardines, among others (Armstrong, 2001). Beef and pork are other main sources of protein, and eggs, cheese, and legumes are also featured in the local diet. In particular, Oka cheese, named after the town in which it originated, is a renowned type of local artisanal cheese (Kiple & Ornelas, 2000). Other examples of traditional protein sources include *cretons*, a chilled, spiced pork pate that is redolent of cloves, garlic, and cinnamon, and is commonly eaten at breakfast as a spread on toast; pea soup; and baked beans (Barer-Stein, 1999).

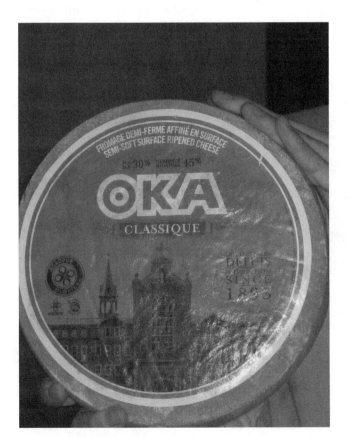

A Wheel of Oka Cheese
Courtesy of the author

It is estimated that protein comprises approximately 16–17% of the diet for French Canadian adults and children (Ghadirian & Shatenstein, 1996; Shatenstein & Ghadirian, 1996).

Starch Sources

The sources of starch in the traditional French Canadian diet have been adapted from, and bear a close resemblance to, the starch-based food types that frequently appear in Europe and elsewhere in North America. While potatoes, breads, and cereals are ubiquitous, starches have been modified and stylized to reflect local tastes, preferences, and food sources. Examples of these local adaptations include buckwheat pancakes with maple syrup; *poutine*, a dish consisting of French fries covered in gravy and topped with cheese curds; and *crêpes* (Armstrong, 2001).

It is estimated that carbohydrates comprise approximately 45–49% of the diet for French Canadian adults and children (Ghadirian & Shatenstein, 1996; Shatenstein & Ghadirian, 1996).

Fat Sources

Lard, butter, cream, and oil are the main sources of dietary fat. It is estimated that fat intake comprises approximately 34–38% of the diet for French Canadian adults and children (Ghadirian & Shatenstein, 1996; Shatenstein & Ghadirian, 1996).

Prominent Vegetables

Maïs sucré refers to a sweet corn that is indigenous to the region and commonly served as part of traditional meals. Onions, mushrooms, potatoes, squash, pumpkins, cabbage, carrots, and turnips are also commonly incorporated in French Canadian food preparation. Fiddleheads are fronds harvested from young fern plants. They are more common in rural areas and can only be picked during certain seasons and in certain regions. White asparagus and artichokes are also commonly used vegetables (Armstrong, 2001).

Prominent Fruits

The fruits that dominate the French Canadian diet trace their roots back to the indigenous plant sources of the Canadian wilderness. Local wild fruits, such as strawberries, raspberries, blueberries, cranberries, gooseberries, and apples, are served fresh or prepared as jams, jellies, and compotes (Armstrong, 2001).

According to Canada's Nutrition and Health Atlas, 65% of Quebecois consume at least five servings of fruits and vegetables daily (Health Canada, 2004).

 Spices and Seasonings

Examples of typical spice additives include juniper berries, shallots, parsley, chives, savory, cloves, garlic, and chervil (Lafrance, 1989).

 Beverages

Several popular Canadian beverages, such as coffee and tea, are derived from imported food sources; however, other beverages owe their popularity to the local availability of key ingredients. Cider is distilled from apples obtained from regional orchards (Armstrong, 2001). Popular regional beers include LaBatt and Molson. There are also many vineyards in Quebec. Popular wines include blueberry wine and ice wine.

 Desserts

Sucre à la crème (sugar cream) and maple syrup tarts are traditional desserts (Benoit, 1970). Sugar, blueberry, and apple pie are also common desserts that are prepared with locally sourced fruits (Armstrong, 2001).

Other Food Sources

Maple syrup is used as both a seasoning and a sweetener. It is used as a glaze on ham, a sweetening agent in the preparation of baked beans, and a key ingredient in candies, fudge, and many local desserts (Armstrong, 2001; Barer-Stein, 1999).

Honey is also popular among French Canadians. In addition to traditional honey, locals enjoy a variety of flavored honey, including apple, blueberry, and buckwheat (Benoit, 1970). Honey is used as an additive in the preparation of both cooked foods and beverages.

 FOODS WITH CULTURAL SIGNIFICANCE

Maple syrup production factors prominently into French Canadian culture, as 80% of the world's maple syrup comes from Quebec (Armstrong, 2001). In the early spring, the sap is tapped from the maple trees and then taken to "sugar cabins" to boil into syrup in a process called "sugaring off." Sugar cabins become gathering spots for the community at this time of year. Children play games and watch as *tire* (maple sugar

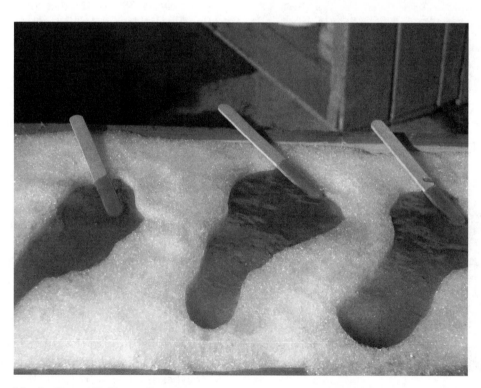

Maple Sugar Taffy on Snow
Courtesy of the author

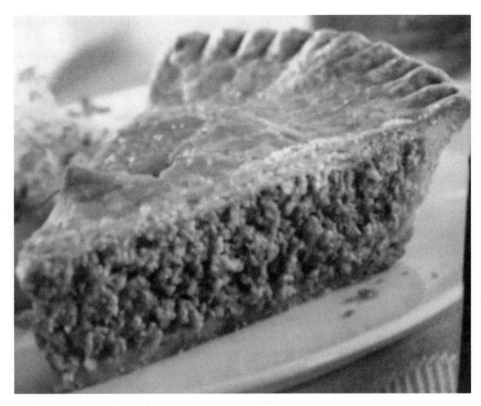

Tourtière
Courtesy of the author

taffy) is made by pouring hot syrup on snow and rolling it onto popsicle sticks, while adults sit down for a multicourse meal of traditional French Canadian foods that can often fill much of the day. Most items are flavored with maple syrup, and meals are typically served either family style or as a buffet (Armstrong, 2001). Music and dancing are also frequently part of the experience.

 ## TYPICAL DAY'S MENU

Contemporary French Canadians eat a fairly typical Western diet. Meats and starches still predominate (Barer-Stein, 1999), although the Canadian health ministry has tried in recent years to encourage lighter diets that include reductions in fat, increases in the consumption of fruits and vegetables, and moderations of sugar intake (Health Canada, 2007). Many French Canadians can also enjoy a wide variety of ethnic cuisines, which now figure prominently in the restaurant scene of most cities.

A visit to local markets and cafés reveals that a typical breakfast may include bacon, eggs, fruit, breads, pastries, or pancakes. A typical lunch may include sandwiches, soup, or fast food. A hot chicken sandwich on white bread with gravy and peas is a distinctly Quebecois dish. A typical dinner may include roast pork, veal, or chicken, potatoes, vegetables, and wine or beer. Pork and beans is a traditional dish. Desserts are sugary, often served with fresh cream.

A recent study of adults in Montréal, Québec, found that men consume approximately 2200 calories and women consume approximately 1700 calories per day. Only 20–30% of adults followed a diet that met recommended nutritional guidelines; many diets were excessively high in saturated fats and simple carbohydrates, and low on calcium intake (Shatenstein, Nadon, Godin, & Ferland, 2005). A separate survey of food habits in Montréal found that 90% of respondents ate breakfast on a regular basis, 96% ate lunch, and 99% ate dinner. Morning and afternoon snacks were common. The vast majority of respondents ate their main meals at home (Ghadirian et al., 1995).

 ## HOLIDAY MENU

A typical Christmas menu includes turkey or goose, a soup or stew, pickled vegetables, fresh breads, and a meat pie called *tourtière*. A chocolate-covered Yule log cake called *bûche de noel* or apple dumplings may be served for dessert, along with coffee or tea. Frequently this meal is served after midnight Mass, in a celebration called *Réveillon* (Barer-Stein, 1999).

 ## HEALTH BELIEFS AND CONCERNS

Canadians benefit from a socialized healthcare system that is funded and administered by the government. As a result, every French Canadian has access to medical care. The Canadian healthcare system emphasizes public health and preventive medicine, as well as cost-effectiveness (Health Canada, 2008).

A series of focus groups found that French Canadians considered their health and nutrition to be important. The emphasis that they placed on their health was reported to increase with age and with the presence of health problems (Health Canada, 1990). Moderation was recognized as an important principle related to nutrition.

Issues related to being overweight and having eating disorders affect French Canadians to a similar degree as much of North America. The Canadian Community Health Survey reports that 21% of adult men and 23% of adult women in Québec are considered obese, and 23% of children ages 2–17 years are considered overweight or obese (Statistics Canada, 2005). A survey also estimated that 2% of Québecers are at risk for an eating disorder (Statistics Canada, 2002). In addition, 8.6% of households in Quebec experience food insecurity (Health Canada, 2004).

COMMUNICATION AND COUNSELING TIPS

The determination of an individual's nutritional needs should address French Canadian taste preferences and food habits, in addition to being adequate and balanced in general (Mahan & Escott-Stump, 1996). Canada's Food Guide lists recommended servings for each food group according to age and gender, and is published in both English and French (Health Canada, 2007).

The creation of a new diet plan requires close cooperation between the counselor and the counseling subject. The first step in providing nutritional counseling is to determine to which population cohort the individual subject belongs. Men and women have different nutritional requirements, as do children, adolescents, senior citizens, pregnant women, and nursing mothers. The next step in providing nutritional advice involves assessing the client's activity level. An individual who runs three miles a day three times per week requires more calories/energy than someone who leads a sedentary lifestyle. One must also collect the client's personal and family medical history, including the incidence of heart disease, high blood pressure, and diabetes. An understanding of the client's medications and dietary supplements is also important, inasmuch as some medications can affect the absorption of certain vitamins and minerals. In addition, the safety and availability of the food supply should be considered (Mahan & Escott-Stump, 1996). For example, individuals who face financial constraints may have difficulties obtaining meat, fish, or fruits and vegetables, especially when they are out of season (Health Canada, 1990).

While it may not be practical to effect immediate changes in a person's diet, it is important to take gradual steps to accomplish some progress. Pursuing too many changes too quickly increases the risk that the client will revert back to preexisting dietary habits without achieving material success. Once dietary adjustments have been achieved during the first several weeks of counseling, additional changes can be introduced incrementally. In this vein, existing recipes can be modified to include healthier ingredients, including leaner meats, lower-fat dairy products, and higher-quality oils.

In terms of effectively communicating with French Canadians, it is important to be aware of both verbal and nonverbal cues. French Canadians often raise their voice when speaking about issues that are particularly important or emotional. Hand gestures and facial expressions are common. Counselors can demonstrate respect for their clients by shaking hands upon meeting and maintaining a respectful distance during the encounter (Coutu-Wakulczyk, Beckingham, & Moreau, 1998). In addition, a focus group found that French Canadians respond best to nutritional messages that are stated in positive, simple, and practical terms (Health Canada, 1990).

PRIMARY LANGUAGE OF FOOD NAMES WITH ENGLISH AND PHONETIC TRANSLATION

French Canadians use French terms for their food. A standard French–English dictionary can be a useful

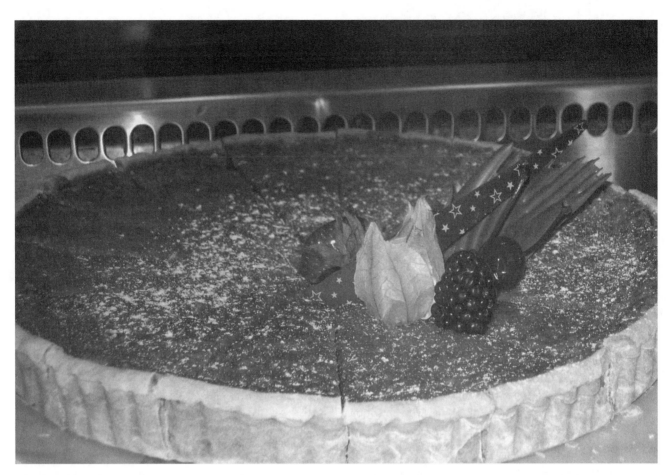

Maple Syrup Tart
Courtesy of the author

tool when communicating with a French Canadian. Among the most important words to know are as follows (compiled by Leete & Wald, 1997):

fruit (frwee)—fruit

fromage (fro-mahzh)—cheese

oeuf (uhf)—egg

legume (lay-gewm)—vegetable

pain (pan)—bread

poisson (pwa-sohn)—fish

poulet (poo-leh)—chicken

salade (sa-lad)—salad

sel (sehl)—salt

viande (vee-ond)—meat

petit déjeuner (ptee day-zheu-nay)—breakfast

dîner (dee-nay)—lunch

souper (soo-pay)—dinner

FEATURED RECIPE

Maple Syrup Tart

10 oz. tart dough

1 cup heavy cream

2 cups maple syrup

2 whole eggs

3½ tbsp. cornstarch

1. Combine the ingredients for the filling.
2. Preheat the oven to 315°F.
3. Roll the tart dough to ¼ inch thickness and place in two tart pans.
4. Pour in the filling. Bake for 40 minutes.

Yields 2 tarts

(Reprinted with permission from http://www. infomag.ca.)

REFERENCES

Armstrong, J. (2001). *A taste of Québec.* New York: Hippocrene Books.

Barer-Stein, T. (1999). *You eat what you are: People, culture and food traditions.* Ontario, Canada: Firefly Books.

Battye, A., Hintze, M.A., & Rowlett, P. (2000). *The French language today: A linguistic introduction* (2nd ed.). London: Routledge.

Benoit, J. (1970). *The Canadiana cookbook.* Toronto, Canada: Pagurian Press.

Coutu-Wakulczyk, G., Beckingham, A.C., & Moreau, D. (1998). French Canadians. In L.D. Purnell & B.J. Paulanka (Eds.), *Transcultural health care: A culturally competent approach* (pp. 273–300). Philadelphia: F.A. Davis.

Dickinson, J.A., & Young, B. (2001). *A short history of Quebec* (2nd ed.). Montreal, Canada: McGill-Queen's University Press.

Energy Information Administration, U.S. Department of Energy. Map of Canada. Retrieved August 18, 2008, from http://www.eia.doe.gov/emeu/cabs/Canada/images/canada_map.gif/

Ferry, S. (2003). *Exploring Canada: Quebec.* San Diego, CA: Lucent Books.

Ghadirian, P., & Shatenstein, B. (1996). Nutrient patterns, nutritional adequacy, and comparisons with nutrition recommendations among French-Canadian adults in Montréal. *Journal of the American College of Nutrition, 15*(3), 255–263.

Ghadirian, P., Shatenstein, B., Lambert, J., Thouez, J.P., Petit-Clerc, C., Parent, M.E., et al. (1995). Food habits of French Canadians in Montréal, Québec. *Journal of the American College of Nutrition, 14*(1), 37–45.

Health Canada. (1990). *Action towards healthy eating: Canada's guidelines for healthy eating and recommended strategies for implementation.* Retrieved March 23, 2008, from http://www.hc-sc.gc.ca/fn-an/nutrition/pol/action_healthy_eating-action_saine_alimentation-07_e.html/

Health Canada. (2004). *Canada's nutrition and health atlas.* Retrieved March 23, 2008, from http://www.hc-sc.gc.ca/fn-an/surveill/atlas/index_e.html/

Health Canada. (2007). *Eating well with Canada's food guide.* Retrieved January 27, 2008, from http://www.hc-sc.gc.ca/fn-an/food-guide-aliment/index_e.html/

Health Canada. (2008). *About Health Canada.* Retrieved February 23, 2008, from http://www.hc-sc.gc.ca/ahc-asc/index_e.html/

Kiple, K.F., & Ornelas, K.C. (Eds.). (2000). *The Cambridge world history of food* (Vol. 2). New York: Cambridge University Press.

Lafrance, M. (1989). *A taste of history: The origins of Québec's gastronomy.* Québec, Canada: Editions de la Cheneliere.

Leete, E.B., & Wald, H. (1997). *Learn French the fast and fun way.* New York: Barrons Educational Series.

Mahan, L., & Escott-Stump, S. (1996). *Krause's food, nutrition & diet therapy.* Philadelphia, PA: W.B Saunders.

Moogk, P.N. (2000). *La Nouvelle France: The making of French Canada: A cultural history.* East Lansing, MI: Michigan State University Press.

Shatenstein, B., & Ghadirian, P. (1996). Nutrient patterns and nutritional adequacy among French-Canadian children in Montréal. *Journal of the American College of Nutrition, 15*(3), 264–272.

Shatenstein, B., Nadon, S., Godin, C., & Ferland, G. (2005). Diet quality of Montréal-area adults needs improvement: Estimates from a self-administered food frequency questionnaire furnishing a dietary indicator score. *Journal of the American Dietetic Association, 105,* 1251–1260.

Statistics Canada. (2002). Risk of eating disorder, by sex, household population aged 15 and over, Canada and provinces, 2002. Retrieved February 23, 2008, from http://www.statcan.ca/english/freepub/82-617-XIE/htm/5110086.htm/

Statistics Canada. (2005). Measured obesity. Retrieved February 23, 2008, from http://www.statcan.ca/english/research/82-620-MIE/82-620-MIE2005001.htm/

Statistics Canada. (2006a). Population by mother tongue and age groups, 2006 counts, for Canada, provinces and territories – 20% sample data. Retrieved January 6, 2008, from http://www12.statcan.ca/english/census06/data/highlights/language/Table401.cfm?Lang=E&T=401&GH=4&SC=1&S=99&O=A/

Statistics Canada. (2006b). Population by mother tongue, by province and territory. Retrieved January 6, 2008, from http://www40.statcan.ca/l01/cst01/demo11b.htm/

US Census Bureau. (2005). American community survey. People reporting ancestry: 2005. Retrieved January 6, 2008, from http://factfinder.census.gov/

Wartik, C. (1989). *The French Canadians.* New York: Chelsea House.

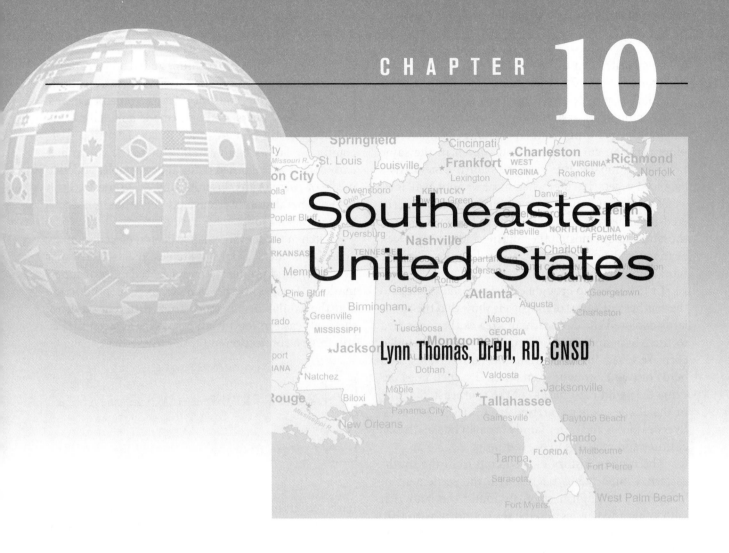

CHAPTER 10

Southeastern United States

Lynn Thomas, DrPH, RD, CNSD

 CULTURE AND WORLD REGION

The states of Virginia, West Virginia, North Carolina, and South Carolina, plus the eastern-most border of Georgia, comprise the southeastern region of the United States. The western to eastern boundaries extend from the Appalachian Mountain range to the Atlantic Ocean. The region has a mild climate, warm winters, and hot, humid summers. The landscape varies from tree-covered mountain terrain to sandy beaches.

This expanse of North America was one of the first destinations for early explorers from the British Isles, France, and Spain. Once the new villages were sustainable, additional settlers arrived from the British Isles. French pioneers migrated south from what is present-day Canada. Spanish explorers came from the Florida coast to the western areas of Virginia looking for territory to claim for the Spanish nobility. The many tribes of Native Americans who called the southeast home were pushed inward from the coast as the number of

settlements increased. Later the Native Americans would either be eliminated or driven into the Appalachian frontier. By the middle of the 18th century, a rush of immigrants was arriving daily from all over Europe. Every group of settlers brought favorite recipes from home to add to the new southeastern Native American menu.

The original settlers were Native Americans. The tribes included the Apalachee, Catawba, Cherokee, Chickasaw, Lumbee, Santee, Shawnee, and Tuscarora, among others. Differing in language and tradition, they managed to coexist albeit with alternating periods of war and peace.

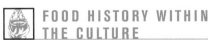 **FOOD HISTORY WITHIN THE CULTURE**

The southeastern Native Americans had an abundant food supply. The constant in their diets was corn. One of the favorite corn dishes was *sofkee*, made by boiling ground corn. Today we know this food as grits. The southeastern Native Americans also grew beans, squash, pumpkins, and sunflowers (for the seeds). They employed a planting technique known as intercropping: planting corns, beans, and squash in the same field. Nutritionally, this gave the Native Americans a balanced vegetarian diet when meat was not available.

The Native American women farmed and gathered nuts, berries, and wild plants. The men cleared the land and did most of the hunting and fishing. Deer, bear, squirrel, possum, rabbit, and wild turkey were the most common game in their diets.

In 1539, DeSoto brought early Spanish explorers to the southeast. Diaries of his travels show that the Spaniards explored the Appalachian area as they marched to the Mississippi River. Their food supply included corn, received in trade from the native tribes, and herds of swine brought from Spain. Escaped hogs became the "wild razorbacks" of the southeast. Starting in the 1600s, pioneers arrived from the British Isles. Every explorer and every family brought bits of diverse cultures and religions to the southeast.

The written history of food culture in the southeastern United States begins with the settlement of Virginia. The English colonists found the land rich with game and berries and the sea bountiful with fish. Unfortunately, the settlers were not able farmers. They depended on the generosity of the Native Americans to feed them in exchange for small amounts of copper. The Native Americans introduced the Jamestown population to hominy (ripe maize, whole or ground as grits), succotash (fresh or dried maize cooked with beans), and cornpone (a pancake preparation), all products from maize that were cultivated in large fields. The Native Americans used two or three sequential plantings each year in order to have fresh corn through late fall. Corn was also dried and stored for use during the winter months. In addition, shad, duck, terrapin, and oysters were plentiful in the Virginia coastal regions.

As the settlements grew, every household had at least a kitchen garden. One famous gardener was Thomas Jefferson, the third President of the United States (1801–1809). He kept garden diaries of the food grown at his Virginia home, Monticello. From these diaries we know that he planted vegetables such as peas, cabbage, lettuce, spinach, and carrots, as well as snap and lima beans in his house garden. He also cultivated fruit and nut trees: plums, apple, peaches, and walnuts. These foods were typical of those found in the Virginias, Maryland, North Carolina, and South Carolina.

Colonists in the 19th century added home canning to their food preservation methods. Almost everything grown in the garden could be canned. Tomatoes, beans, beets, peaches, pears, and homemade jam, jellies, and relishes are still home canned today. Thrifty settlers could now eat reasonably well through the winter and early spring with canned fruits and vegetables added to meals of corn, beans, biscuits, and dried meats. Trips to the general store were usually for milled products, coffee, tea, and sugar.

Kitchen gardens have since been replaced in many areas by farmers' markets. Staples, meats, and other necessary food products are purchased at local supermarkets. Even with the changes in food production and the availability of foods from different cultures, the southeastern food traditions remain strong. They still forge a connection to those early settlers.

 MAJOR FOODS

 Protein Sources

Wild Game

Early settlers hunted large game: buffalo, bear, elk, deer, and hogs. Small game was also a popular dinner item. Bobcat, fox, possum, rabbit, squirrel, turkey, quail, and dove were hunted from the hillsides down to the coast. Nothing was wasted. Lower-quality meat was used to make sausages and stew. The fat was for seasoning and frying. Today, elk, deer, trout, quail, and dove are still hunted "in season." Brunswick stew (named for Brunswick County, Virginia) is prepared with wild game and a selection of vegetables such as tomatoes, potatoes, carrots, squash, lima beans, and corn. The first game to be used in this recipe was squirrel (one squirrel per two persons). The stew is served with corn muffins.

Domesticated Animals

Cows, chickens, and hogs were farm raised by the early settlers. The first cow was thought to be brought from the island of Jersey in England to Jamestown in 1611. Chickens were also thought to be on the first ships that sailed to the New World. Cows provided milk and butter, so they were not often used for meat. Chickens provided both meat and eggs. Fried chicken, chicken and dumplings, and chicken pies/casseroles are well liked today. Feral hogs lived in the hill country. Pork became a very popular meat and was used to replace the mut-

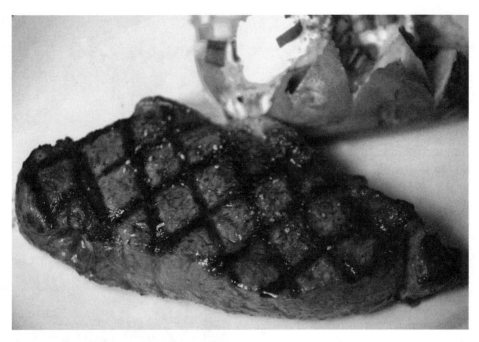

Beef is a popular meat in the United States.

ton from the homeland in many recipes. Salt-cured ham, bacon, and chops are listed on many menus even now. Red-eye gravy is used to make ham and biscuit breakfasts extra special. Good red-eye gravy is made with a generous helping of strong coffee.

Seafood

Shrimp, crab, and trout were among the types of seafood eaten by the colonists that are still enjoyed today. The freshwater areas in the Appalachian hills and the South Carolina midlands are good places to catch trout and bass. Fresh fish is eaten grilled or fried. Shrimp is plentiful throughout the low-country areas of the southeast. A meal of shrimp and grits ranks number one in the minds of many southerners. They would not eat shrimp any other way. Delicious crab cakes can be used as an appetizer or part of the entree. Stews and gumbos, which combine many types of seafood and seasonal vegetables, are frequently steamed in large pots for parties.

Dairy Products

In the early settlement years, farmers raised cows for milk and butter. Cheese was made only on a few farms, mostly in Virginia and North Carolina. Products not needed for the family were taken to neighboring towns for sale or trade. Adults and children alike drank sweet milk for nourishment. Buttermilk was made from the liquid left from churning butter. It was, and still is, a favorite drink in the Appalachian hill country. Often a quick breakfast was crumbled corn bread and buttermilk. Baking soda and buttermilk were used as leavening agents in biscuits, cakes, and other baked goods before yeast was readily available. Buttermilk biscuits are southeastern favorites to this day.

 Starch Sources

Corn

Corn, or maize, introduced to the settlers by Native Americans, is one of the primary starch sources in the southeastern diet. *Suppone* (also known as *appone* or cornpone) was a favorite Indian food. It was a combination of cornmeal, water, grease, and salt. This recipe is the backbone of many contemporary dishes. Cornbread is still a staple throughout the southeast. Variations on the basic cornbread recipe include corn fritters, hush puppies, and Johnny cakes. Some enterprising farmers use dry corn to make mash for moonshine. It is also an ingredient for a popular pudding. Grits and hominy are the breakfast basics in the coastal regions of the southeast.

Today fresh corn (roasting ears) is eaten from the cob, boiled, or grilled. Many salads and vegetable dishes use corn. Popped corn is enjoyed by both young and old. Fresh corn is usually harvested in the summer months but is available all year in canned or frozen products.

Potatoes

White potatoes, often called Irish potatoes, were brought to the southeast by Irish and Scottish immigrants during the 1720s. Cooks combined potatoes and milk to make many of today's very popular recipes such as mashed or scalloped potatoes. Sometimes the potatoes were roasted and eaten plain. Roasted potatoes were popular lunch foods for early school children. There are many stories of children using warm potatoes to keep their hands warm as they walked to school. Potato soup and Irish stew (lamb or beef) with potatoes are still served in southeastern homes. The original Irish stew was only meat and potatoes. Today's stew can be described as a thickened vegetable stew.

German immigrants started settling in the western Carolinas in the 1800s. They made pancakes, soups, salads, and dumplings with white potatoes.

Sweet potatoes are indigenous to North America. Prior to the arrival of the Europeans, they were cultivated by local Native Americans tribes. Sweet potatoes are served as an alternative to the white potato, although during holidays, such as Thanksgiving, both can be found on the dinner table. They are often used in pies, pones, and casseroles. Sweet potatoes are served with butter, cinnamon, and sugar or syrup. Casseroles might include fruits, spices, and heavy cream or yogurt.

Rice

Rice, the long-grain white variety, was introduced to the South Carolina low country region in the 17th century. This crop, along with indigo, made the southern plantation owners and the city merchants very wealthy. The labor-intensive grain flourished in the Charleston area until the end of the Civil War. At that time, when slavery ended, the rice industry all but disappeared in the southeast. Rice is still cultivated in Arkansas and Louisiana, but presently only a small amount of the premium "Carolina Gold" is grown in South Carolina. White, brown, and wild rice remain favorite side dishes in all the southeastern states.

Biscuits

Biscuits deserve a special listing since the country folks throughout the southeast could not survive without them. From the 18th century until early in the 20th century, yeast for bread baking was not readily available. Early settlers brought the recipe for beaten biscuits from England. They are sometimes called Maryland or Virginia biscuits. Unleavened biscuit

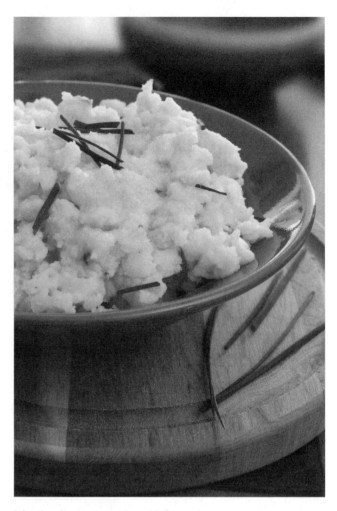

Mashed potatoes is a U.S. mainstay.

dough was beaten until enough air bubbles were created to cause the biscuits to rise when cooked. These biscuits could be made in large batches and then stored for several weeks in tins. South Carolina biscuits made with sweet cream can also be stored for weeks. These biscuits were sent to Civil War soldiers to give them a taste of home. The recipe is similar to the one for beaten biscuits, except sweet cream is substituted for the water and the dough is kneaded instead of beaten. Later biscuits began to be made with baking powder or soda. Baking powder biscuits are served hot from the oven, often with butter, jams and jellies, or gravies. Leftovers are served fried with honey and butter.

 Fat Sources

Traditionally, pan drippings from cooked meats are added to a grease pot that sits by the stove. The drippings are used to make gravies, to season vegetables, or to coat the skillet as it heats. Vegetable shortenings, both solid and liquid, are also used. Butter and lard are also used for baking. Lard is gradually being replaced by other solid shortenings, but many cooks lament the loss of the extra flaky pie crust.

Prominent Vegetables

Beans

Many varieties of beans were being cultivated by Native Americans when the first explorers arrived in the New World. Lima beans, green beans (called snap or string beans in the south), and shell beans; white, navy, and black beans were easily grown in the moderate climates of Virginia and the Carolinas. Early New England colonists learned to bake beans from the Native Americans. As settlers traveled to the south, recipes containing baked beans became popular, but lima and green beans are still the beans of choice with southeastern cooks. Most often beans are used fresh from the garden or market in vegetable soups, salads, and as entrees cooked with ham and new potatoes.

Greens

In the southeastern states, greens are available for picking most of the year. Wild greens are harvested from grassy fields and creek banks. Native Americans taught early settlers how to identify these edible foods. Many cultivated greens are planted starting in early spring and harvested until the first frost. Pokeweed, fiddlehead, dandelion, collards, mustard greens, cresses (upland and water), and ramp (wild leeks) are all popular types of greens. Some greens are mixed uncooked into cold salads; others are served wilted with a hot dressing.

Squash

Cushaw, winter crook-necked squash, pumpkins, zucchini, and summer squash were important foods for the southeastern Native Americans. The Cherokee legend of the "three sisters" gives squash equal importance with corn and beans. Besides food uses, the Native Americans made bowls, dippers, and cups from hollowed-out squashes. Dried strips of pumpkin were used to make sleeping mats. One story says that pumpkin pie was first made when the colonists sliced off the pumpkin top, removed the seeds, and filled the insides with milk, spices, and honey. The pumpkin was then baked in hot ashes. Squashes are important foods today. Squash and pumpkin are used in breads, pies, salads, and casseroles. Other members of the squash family are boiled or fried and served as side dishes.

Tomatoes

Tomatoes were brought to North America by early British colonists. Tomatoes were not eaten but used medicinally since the fruits were valued for pustule-removing properties. In 1781, Thomas Jefferson brought tomatoes to his table, along with French fries. Once they were deemed safe to eat, tomatoes became a fashionable side dish. Tomatoes are easily grown throughout the southeast in many varieties, in gardens and in pots. Heirloom seeds are prized and passed down through families. Tomatoes are eaten fresh from the garden sliced, diced, fried, congealed in aspic, and even made into gravy. Tomato gravy is made from the pan drippings left after making fried green tomatoes.

Prominent Fruits

Apples

Crab apples are the only ones native to North America. In the 17th century, settlers brought apple seeds, cuttings, and the all-important honey bees from the British Isles to the early Virginia settlements. From that time on, most landowners had an apple orchard. Harvest times start in July and run until early November depending on the apple variety. Today, apples are used as healthy snacks and as the basis of butters, chutneys, jellies, cakes, pies, fritters, juices, and ciders (fermented apple juice).

Berries and Nuts

American Indians were already eating blackberries and strawberries when the first colonists arrived in Virginia. Blackberries were gathered and eaten fresh in spring and early summer. The Native Americans crushed strawberries and mixed them with cornbread to make strawberry bread. Colonists "put up" all types of berries as jellies, preserves, and special butters. Figs were introduced to the South Carolina coast by Spanish explorers arriving from Cuba in 1575. Other explorers brought them to Virginia from Bermuda in the 1600s. Besides being used as a sweetener, figs were prized as a diuretic and laxative.

Pecan trees grow naturally in North America. Native Americas were cultivating pecan trees when the first settlers arrived. The name "pecan" is a Native American word of Algonquin origin that was used to describe "all nuts requiring a stone to crack." Pecans were used as a food source during long winters and also as a handy travel food. Today, pecans are frequently used in desserts and candies.

Beechnuts and black walnuts are also native to the southeast. Beechnuts are eaten raw or used as a substitute for pecans. Black walnuts are well liked in cakes, fudge, and cookies for their distinctive flavor.

 ## Spices and Seasonings

Herb gardens planted with rosemary, thyme, chives, sage, garlic, and onions were a common site in the early southeastern settlements. Herbs were dried for winter use. Salt, pepper, and nutmeg were imported. Sage, rosemary, celery, and mustard seeds were used as natural preservatives. Today, spices are grown in kitchen gardens, window boxes, or "store bought." They are still used to add flavor to meats, salads, and vegetables. Spicy sauces and relishes are southern favorites.

 ## Beverages

The southeast is known for beverages with unusual names such as shrubs, syllabubs, and juleps, in addition to punches and the ordinary coffees and teas. Shrubs are generally types of spiced teas. Syllabubs are coffee-based drinks that include a small amount of liquor. Juleps are a cocktail of sugar, mint, and alcohol (mostly bourbon). Punches are special-occasion beverages. Iced and hot teas are pervasive all year long. Coffee is preferred hot and black, but iced coffee and *café au lait* are readily available in the coastal areas. Hot chocolate is a favorite winter drink in all areas.

Ginger ale was the most popular soft drink well into the 20th century. Other flavors have now replaced it including colas and citrus flavors and an imitation ginger-flavored soda. True ginger ale is still available in areas of Virginia and the Carolinas.

 ## Desserts

In the days of the early settlements, many rural households in the southeast ate desserts only as part of a holiday celebration or a birthday. In the cities, where families often held slaves or employed servants, desserts were served more often. The lady of the house frequently held tea parties for her friends and hosted grand balls for the couples in the family's social circle. Desserts were plentiful and lavish. Foods such as crystallized fruits and cakes covered with fresh flowers were among the abundant trifles, tarts, sweetmeats, fresh fruit, puddings, cakes, and peaches preserved in bourbon.

Today, dinner would not be complete without dessert, although it is usually less lavish than in earlier

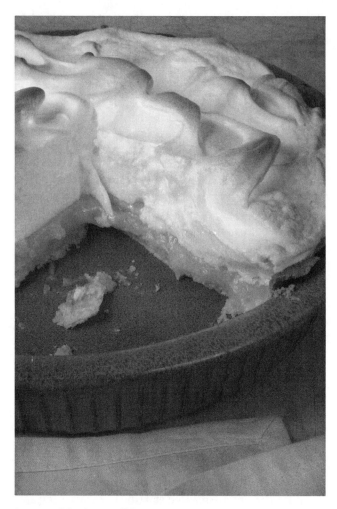

Lemon Meringue Pie

times. The more spectacular desserts are now reserved for parties and weddings. Puddings, pies, and cakes are popular southeastern desserts. In the summer months, fresh fruit with shortcake or homemade ice cream with chocolate sauce over pound cake are frequently served.

 ## TYPICAL DAY'S MENU

Rural Appalachian Breakfast Items

Rural Appalachian breakfast items are as follows:

Fried apples or applesauce

Buttermilk biscuits

Fried potatoes

Bacon, sausage, or ham

Sausage gravy or red-eye gravy

Fried or scrambled eggs

Oatmeal or cream of wheat

Fresh sliced tomatoes or fried green tomatoes

Fresh butter, hot sorghum, honey, jellies, and jam

Coffee (usually black) or tea

Coastal Breakfast Items

Coastal breakfast items are as follows:

Mixed fresh fruit

Hominy or grits

Fried, scrambled, or boiled eggs

Cakes and pastries

Pancakes and waffles

Salmon or fish roe

Coffee with milk or tea

Lunch Menu Items

Lunch menu items are as follows:

Tomato, potato, vegetable, French onion, or pea soup

Coleslaw or homemade potato salad

Cobb salad or fried green tomatoes

Chicken or shrimp salad

Grilled chicken, flounder, or salmon

BLT (bacon, lettuce, and tomato sandwich) or hamburger

Pulled-pork BBQ

Dinner rolls or cornbread muffins

Crème brûlée

Sorbet or ice cream

Tarts or cookies

Iced tea

Dinner or Supper Menu Items

Dinner or supper menu items are as follows:

Ham, fish, and other seafood, geese, mutton, pork, or chicken

Cabbage, asparagus, beets, green beans, lima beans, green peas, corn, tomatoes, side salads, spinach, kale, squash, pumpkin, and onions

Rice, Irish potatoes, or sweet potatoes

Fresh fruit, apple dumplings, sponge cake, short-cake, stack cake, fruit pies, and puddings

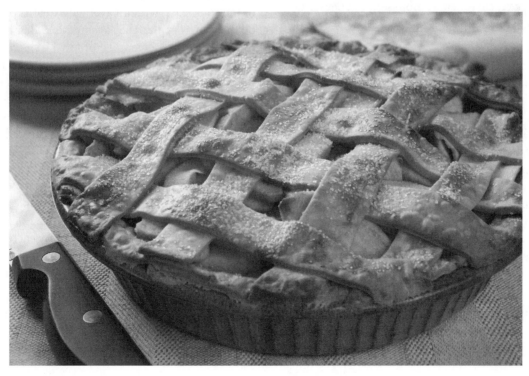

Apple Pie

Biscuits, dinner rolls, or cornbread

Relishes

Homemade wine or iced tea

 HOLIDAY MENUS

Thanksgiving and Other Winter Holidays

Menus for Thanksgiving and other winter holidays are as follows:

Broccoli, pea, and tomato soup

Roasted turkey, peppercorn-crusted ham, rosemary lamb chops, pot roast, and grilled seafood

Pan gravy

Garlic-mashed potatoes, lemon rice, and sour cream and-chives mashed potatoes

Sweet potato casserole

Snap peas with red peppers and corn

Green bean casserole or green beans with bacon and onion bits

Asparagus, corn, squash, and glazed carrots

Tossed salad, fruit salads, and Caesar salad

Cranberry relish

Pumpkin, pecan, and apple pies

Pecan cake, carrot cake, mousse, and cheesecake

Assorted rolls and biscuits

Wines, teas, and coffees

 HEALTH BELIEFS AND CONCERNS

Colonists brought with them a strong belief in the benefits of herbs and barks as medicines. They also acquired knowledge from the Native Americans, who had an extensive formulary of natural remedies. Even though allopathic medicine has replaced most alternative medicine in the southeastern region, there are still pockets of intense use.

The most common uses for alternative medicines are as home remedies for fevers, colds, flu, and female problems. Herbs and barks are generally made into teas or broths. Some practitioners make ointments to use on skin infections; others devise "doses" of herbal brews, which are used to cure a variety of illnesses. As with all medicine, some alternative medications work, such as cranberry juices for urinary tract infections and ginger for morning or motion sickness. Willow tree bark tea contains an aspirin-like ingredient that helps reduce fever.

 GENERAL HEALTH AND NUTRITIONAL INDICATORS SUMMARY

The southeastern states of Georgia, North Carolina, South Carolina, Virginia, and West Virginia house approximately 31.5 million persons. Life expectancy is the same as the rest of the United States (78 years as of 2005). The birth rate (15/1000 vs 14/1000 nationwide) and the crude death rate (900/100,000 vs 812/100,000 nationwide) are slightly higher as reported by the Centers for Disease Control and Prevention (CDC). The increased birth rate can be partially attributed to a tradition of larger families. The death rate is most likely the result of increased prevalence of chronic disease and overweight/obesity. In these five states, over 37% of the population is overweight and 28% are considered obese. Nationally, 36% of the population is overweight and 26% are obese. The southeastern infant mortality rate reflects decreased prenatal care in many rural areas of the southeast, with an average 8 deaths per 1000 live births, whereas the U.S. average is 6 deaths per 1000 live births. The percentage of low-birth-weight babies is approximately 10% compared with the national figure of approximately 9%. Fewer children in the southeast are considered anemic when compared with the national data (14 vs 15%). These figures are available from the 2007 Pediatric Nutrition Surveillance data collected by the CDC.

Nationwide, 24% of Behavioral Risk Factor Surveillance Survey (CDC) participants report consuming at least five servings of fruits and vegetables per day. In the southeast, consumption averages 22%. Physical activity (30 minutes of moderate activity each day) is also less in the southeast (47 vs 49% nationwide). Lower household income and decreased nutrition/physical-activity education opportunities are major influences on the southeastern nutritional indicators.

FEATURED RECIPE

Beaten Biscuits

4 cups all-purpose flour	2 tbsp. unsalted butter, room temperature
1 tsp. salt	1 cup cold milk
¼ cup lard or solid vegetable shortening	

1. In a large bowl, combine flour and salt, tossing with a fork to blend.
2. Add lard or shortening and butter; work fat into flour mixture with your fingertips until mixture resembles coarse meal.
3. Make a well in center of mixture and add milk; stir to combine well. Turn out onto a lightly floured work surface and knead three or four times until dough holds together.
4. Preheat oven to 400°F. Grease baking sheet; set aside.
5. Pat out dough about 1 inch thick and begin to beat it, using a wooden mallet or other implement, with a gentle, rhythmic motion. When entire surface has been well beaten, fold dough in half and repeat the process. Continue to beat and fold until dough is well blistered (20–30 minutes).
6. Roll out dough ½ inch thick and cut into rounds with a floured 2-inch biscuit cutter; reroll and cut scraps. Repeat until all dough has been used.
7. Prick top of each biscuit three times with a fork. Place biscuits on greased baking sheet; bake in preheated oven until golden brown (20–25 minutes). Serve hot.

Yields 24 biscuits

Reprinted from: Chef Rick McDaniel (E-mail: rick@chefrick.com; http://www.chefrick.com).

More recipes are available at http://nutrition.jbpub.com/foodculture/

History of Beaten Biscuits

These were the first biscuits to grace the southern table, dating back to the early days of the Virginia colony. Their exact origin is a mystery; there are English unleavened breads from this period, but none that call for beating the dough. Africa is another possibility, but again, there is no firm proof. A recipe for a similar type of bread is found in Mary Randolph's *The Virginia House-Wife* (1824) with the Indian-sounding name "Apoquiniminc Cakes," but there is nothing to firmly link beaten biscuits to Native Americans, either.

In the 1700s, before the invention of baking soda, baking powder, or commercially available yeast, a substance called pearl ash (calcium carbonate for the chemically curious) started to gain popularity in home baking as a means of rising bread dough without having to wait for yeast to act. Pearl ash did a fine job of leavening, but it had a slight drawback: Pearl ash was made by pouring water over wood ashes and collecting the solid that remained. The problem was that this is the same process used to make lye; add a little animal fat to lye and you have lye soap. When the pearl ash was used to leaven biscuits, there was enough residual lye in it to react with the lard or butter in the dough and give the biscuits a slightly bitter, soapy taste.

Searching for a quicker way to leaven biscuits, cooks found that when unleavened dough was folded over and pounded with a mallet or an axe handle and the process repeated enough times, tiny air pockets formed in the dough. When the dough was baked, the air pockets expanded and caused the biscuits to rise, although the result was somewhere between a cracker and a biscuit rather than the light, fluffy biscuits we know today. Nevertheless, beaten biscuits were a staple in the early South.

Mary Stuart Smith wrote in her *Virginia Cookery-Book* (1885), "In the Virginia of the olden time no breakfast or tea-table was thought to be properly furnished without a plate of these indispensable biscuits." Not everyone shared Mrs. Smith's enthusiasm; Eliza Leslie, writing in her *New Cookery Book* (1857) remarked, "Children would not eat these biscuits—nor grown persons either, if they can get any other sort of bread." After commercial leavening agents came along, beaten biscuits fell out of favor; Mrs. Smith declared them "sadly out of vogue" by the time her book came out.

Beaten biscuits managed to remain popular in Maryland well into the 1930s; old cookbooks sometimes refer to them as Maryland beaten biscuits or simply Maryland biscuits. They are rarely seen today except occasionally at wedding receptions, where they are cut about the size of a quarter and filled with thin, velvety slices of country ham. [Reprinted from: Chef Rick McDaniel (E-mail: rick@chefrick.com; http://www.chefrick.com).]

REFERENCES

Fig Advisory Board. *California Dried Figs.* Retrieved March 10, 2008, from http://www.californiafigs.com/

Garrett, J. (2003). *The Cherokee herbal.* Rochester, VT: Bear and Company.

Glenn, C. (1986). *The heritage of southern cooking.* New York: Black Dog and Leventhal Publishers.

Grivetti, L., Corlett, J., & Lockett, C. (2001a). Food in American history, part 1: Maize. *Nutrition Today, 36,* 20–28.

Grivetti, L., Corlett, J., & Lockett, C. (2001b). Food in American history, part 3: Beans. *Nutrition Today, 36,* 172–181.

Grivetti, L., Corlett, J., & Lockett, C. (2007). Food in American history, part 10(1): Greens. *Nutrition Today, 42,* 88–94.

Library of Congress. *Maps of North America, 1750–1789.* Retrieved March 10, 2008, from http://memory.loc.gov/cgi-bin/map_item.pl/

Metcalfe, G., & Hays, C. (2005). *Being dead is no excuse.* New York: Hyperion.

Mitchell, P. (1991, March 3). Colonial flavors might surprise 20th-century tongue. *Register and Bee.* Danville, VA.

Mitchell, P. (1992). *Delightful dreams of dixie dinners.* Chatham, VA: Mitchell's Publications.

Mitchell, P. (1999). *Specialties from the southern garden.* Chatham, VA: Mitchell's Publications.

Mitchell, P. (2005). *Biscuits and belles.* Chatham, VA: Mitchell's Publications.

Moore, J.H. (1993). *A plantation mistress on the eve of the Civil War.* Columbia, SC: University of South Carolina Press.

North Carolina Extension Service. *Pumpkins.* Retrieved March 21, 2008, from http://mcdowell.ces.ncsu.edu/content/Pumpkin+History/

Pecan Shellers' Organization. *Pecans.* Retrieved February 29, 2008, from http://www.ilovepecans.org/

Randolph, M. (1838). *The Virginia housewife.* Retrieved May 20, 2008, from http://www.gutenberg.org/etext/12519/

Segen, J. (1998). *Dictionary of alternative medicine.* Stamford, CT: Appleton and Lange.

Simmons, A. (1796). *American Cookery.* Retrieved May 20, 2008, from http://www.gutenberg/org/etext/12815

Simpson B.B., & Ogorzaly M.C. (1986). *Economic botany: Plants in our world.* New York: McGraw-Hill.

Sohn, M. (2005). *Appalachian home cooking.* Lexington, KY: University Press of Kentucky.

Southern recipes. Retrieved March 10, 2008, from http://southernfood.about.com/

Swell, B. (1998). *Take two & butter 'em while they're hot!: Heirloom recipes & kitchen wisdom.* Asheville, NC: Native Ground Music.

Tannahill R. (1988). *Food in history.* New York: Crown Publishers.

Taylor, N., & Taylor, R. (2003). In R. Fullinwider, J. Cruchfield, & W. Sparkman-Jeffery (Eds.), *Celebrate Virginia.* Franklin, TN: Cool Springs Press.

UNICEF. (2007). *The state of the world's children 2007: Women and children, the double dividend of gender equality.* Retrieved April 14, 2009, from http://www.unicef.org/sowc07/statistics/tables.php

University of Illinois Extension. *Strawberries.* Retrieved March 7, 2008, from http://www.urbanext.ninc.edu/strawberries/

Villas, J. (2007). *The glory of southern cooking.* Hoboken, NJ: John Wiley and Sons.

Wallace, L. (1908). *The Rumford complete cook book.* Providence, RI: Rumford Chemical Works.

Weaver, W. (2000). *100 vegetables and where they came from.* Chapel Hill, NC: Algonquin Books.

Europe

Food, Cuisine, and Cultural Competency for Culinary, Hospitality, and Nutrition Professionals discusses nine prominent European countries:

GREAT BRITAIN

Britain, also known as the United Kingdom (UK) and/or England, is in western Europe and includes surrounding islands. It is between the North Atlantic Ocean and the North Sea, northwest of France. The UK, a leading trading power and financial center, is one of the quintet of trillion-dollar economies of western Europe. Agriculture is intensive, highly mechanized, and efficient, producing about 60% of food needs with less than 2% of the labor force. The UK has large coal, natural gas, and oil resources, but its oil and natural gas reserves are declining, and the UK became a net importer of energy in 2005. Energy industries now contribute about 4% to the gross domestic product (GDP). Services, particularly banking, insurance, and business services, account for by far the largest proportion of the GDP, while industry continues to decline in importance. Since emerging from recession in 1992, Britain's economy has enjoyed the longest period of expansion on record, during which time the country's growth outpaced most of western Europe. The global economic slowdown, limited credit, and decreasing home prices, however, pushed Britain back into recession in the latter half of 2008.

THE NETHERLANDS

The Netherlands, also known as Holland, is in western Europe, bordering the North Sea, between Belgium and Germany. The country is a leading seafaring and commercial power and is a large exporter of agricultural products. The Netherlands has a prosperous and open economy that depends heavily on foreign trade. The economy is noted for stable industrial relations, moderate unemployment and inflation, and a sizable current account surplus. The country also plays an important role as a European transportation hub. Industrial activity is predominantly in food processing, chemicals, petroleum refining, and electrical machinery. A highly mechanized agricultural sector employs no more than 3% of the labor force but provides large surpluses for the food-processing industry and for exports. The country has been one of the leading European nations for attracting foreign direct investment and is one of the four largest investors in the United States.

FRANCE

France is in western Europe, bordering the Bay of Biscay and the English Channel, between Belgium and Spain, southeast of the UK; it also borders the Mediterranean Sea, between Italy and Spain. France maintains a strong presence in some sectors, particularly the power, public transport, and defense industries. During 2007–2008, the government implemented several significant labor reforms, including a 35-hour work week and the allowance of employees to work longer overtime hours. France's tax burden remains one of the highest in Europe (nearly 50% of the GDP in 2005). With at least 75 million foreign tourists per year, France is the most visited country in the world and maintains the third largest income in the world from tourism.

GREECE

Greece is in southern Europe, bordering the Aegean Sea, Ionian Sea, and Mediterranean Sea, between Albania and Turkey. The Greek economy grew by nearly 4% per year between 2003 and 2007, due partly to infrastructural spending related to the 2004 Athens Olympic Games.

HUNGARY

Hungary is in Central Europe, northwest of Romania. In the past decade, Hungary was listed as the 10th most economically dynamic area and one of the 15 most popular tourist destinations in the world, with its capital, Budapest, regarded as one of the most beautiful urban landscapes in the world. Hungary has made the transition from a centrally planned economy to a market economy, with the private sector accounting for more than 80% of the GDP. Foreign ownership of, and investment in, Hungarian firms is widespread, with cumulative foreign direct investment totaling more than $60 billion since 1989.

IRELAND

Ireland is in western Europe and occupies more than 83% of the Island of Ireland in the North Atlantic

Ocean, west of Great Britain. Ireland has a small, modern, trade-dependent economy. The GDP growth rate averaged 6% during 1995–2007, but economic activity dropped sharply in 2008 and Ireland entered into a recession for the first time in more than a decade, with the onset of the world financial crisis, and subsequent severe slowdown in the property and construction markets ensued. Agriculture, once the most important sector, is now dwarfed by industry and services. Construction most recently fueled economic growth along with strong consumer spending and business investment. Property prices rose more rapidly in Ireland between 1996 and 2006 than in any other developed world economy. Per capita GDP also surged during Ireland's high-growth years, and in 2007 it surpassed that of the United States.

ITALY

Italy, which is in southern Europe, is a peninsula that extends into the central Mediterranean Sea, northeast of Tunisia. Italy has a diversified industrial economy that is divided into the developed industrial north, which is dominated by private companies, and the less-developed, welfare-dependent agricultural south, with high unemployment. The Italian economy is driven in large part by the manufacture of high-quality consumer goods produced by small- and medium-sized enterprises. Italy also has a sizable economy in the agriculture, construction, and service sectors.

SPAIN

Spain is located in southwestern Europe, bordering the Bay of Biscay, Mediterranean Sea, North Atlantic Ocean, and Pyrenees Mountains, southwest of France. The Spanish economy grew every year from 1994 through 2008 before entering a recession that started in the third quarter of 2008. Spain's mixed capitalist economy supports a GDP that, on a per capita basis, is approaching that of the largest western European economies. The Spanish banking system is considered solid, thanks in part to conservative management by the European Central Bank, and government intervention to rescue banks on the scale seen elsewhere in Europe in 2008 was not necessary. After considerable success since the mid-1990s in reducing unemployment to a 2007 low of 8%, Spain suffered a major spike in unemployment in the last months of 2008, finishing the year with an unemployment rate over 13%.

SWEDEN

Sweden is in northern Europe, bordering the Baltic Sea, Gulf of Bothnia, Kattegat, and Skagerrak, between Finland and Norway. A military power during the 17th century, Sweden has not participated in any war in almost 200 years. (Neutrality was preserved in both world wars.) Sweden's long-successful economic formula of a capitalist system interlarded with substantial welfare elements was challenged in the 1990s by high unemployment and in 2000–2002 by the global economic downturn, but fiscal discipline over the past several years has allowed the country to weather economic vagaries. Agriculture accounts for only 1% of the GDP and of employment. Until 2008, Sweden was in the midst of a sustained economic upswing, boosted by increased domestic demand and strong exports.

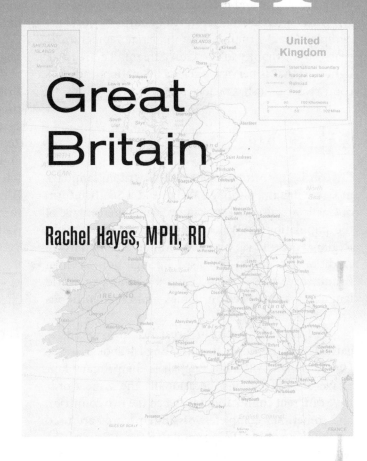

CHAPTER 11

Great Britain

Rachel Hayes, MPH, RD

 CULTURE AND WORLD REGION

With its familiar language, shared pop culture, and ease of travel from the United States, Great Britain is often one of the first countries visited by Americans traveling abroad. Although the Revolutionary War formally cut the ties between the United States and Great Britain, the two nations have grown increasingly similar over time, and have joined forces both politically and culturally over the past century. Looking beyond the modern-day similarities to the United States, though, Great Britain offers a rich history and fascinating cultural study.

The nation is ruled by a bicameral Parliament, including the House of Lords and the House of Commons. The official head of government is the Prime Minister (currently Gordon Brown), who assumes the seat after public election. In addition to the parliamentary democracy, a monarchy still exists, although primarily in a ceremonial role. The current queen, Elizabeth II, has reigned since 1952. Protestant Christianity is the primary religion among the British, although church plays a limited role in the daily life. Catholicism and Judaism are also prevalent, and most other major world religions are practiced by segments of the population. The nation offers both rural and urban landscapes. Picturesque countryside with rolling hills is commonplace in the more rural areas of the country, while bustling city streets are the trademark of the more urban areas. London, the nation's capital, is a vibrant multicultural city, as well as a global economic and political power.

Great Britain lies in the North Atlantic, just 21 miles west of the main European continent, at its closest point. The term Great Britain is used to signify the countries of England, Scotland, and Wales. The nation is part of the sovereign state officially known as The United Kingdom of Great Britain and Northern Ireland (UK), which is a member of the 27-country European Union (EU). The 2006 estimated population of Great Britain was 58,845,700, with the vast majority (86%) dwelling in England. Approximately 90% of the population now lives in urban areas, with London being the largest and most densely populated city.

Although relatively far north in terms of world geography, Great Britain enjoys moderate temperatures year-round, thanks to the Gulf Stream. The regular, light rain that is pervasive across the nation leads to a countryside of lush, spacious pastures.

 ## LANGUAGE

English is the primary spoken and written language in Great Britain, although Welsh and a Scottish form of Gaelic are also still spoken by a small percentage of the population in Wales and Scotland, respectively. Regional accents vary, as do common colloquialisms. Additionally, due to increased immigration to Great Britain over the past 50 years, a plethora of world languages are spoken in homes and neighborhoods around the country.

The English spoken in Great Britain is often regarded as more proper than the English spoken in the United States. Although English is the primary language of both nations, occasionally the same words have different connotations between the two countries, and sometimes completely dissimilar words are used for the same object. For example, in Great Britain, the word "crisps" is used for the American "potato chips," and the word "neeps" is used for "turnips."

 ## CULTURE HISTORY

The roots of modern Great Britain can be traced back to 43 AD, when the Romans invaded, bringing new culture to a previously barbarian land. The Dark Ages/Early Medieval Period began after the withdrawal of the Roman army in 410 AD; society experienced little progress for the next several hundred years. In 1066, the Norman Conquest led to a unified country with a French-influenced ruling class; cultural progress was on the horizon once again.

During the Late Middle Ages/Renaissance, society took a giant leap forward. Queen Elizabeth I, one of the most influential monarchs in history, ruled England from 1558 to 1603. The arts flourished, and world explorers took culture in new directions, both literally and figuratively. New trade routes were established with the Eastern Hemisphere as well as the New

World; the East India Company was founded in 1600 and became a driving force of national culture.

The other most influential monarch in British history came to power three centuries later. The last half of the 19th century was known as the Victorian Era, as Great Britain was ruled by Queen Victoria. During her reign, the nation experienced an industrial revolution and transitioned into a primarily urban society. The British Empire also expanded significantly during this time; at its peak the Empire stretched over 25% of the earth's surface. Just over 100 years later, in the early 20th century, Great Britain was shaken by World War I and then by World War II. The wars took a significant toll on the nation in nearly every way imaginable. The British Empire also significantly diminished over time, forcing the nation to redefine its national identity as well as its role in world politics and culture.

 ## FOOD HISTORY WITHIN THE CULTURE

The Romans ruled the region for nearly 400 years. During this time, they introduced new agricultural and land reclamation techniques, in addition to a host of new foods, including pheasant, figs, walnuts, mulberries, chestnuts, leeks, onions, lettuce, and turnips. They developed a cuisine of complex dishes based on poultry and meats that were stuffed, half-stewed, and finished in sauce. Food culture then took a step backward during the Dark Ages, when people struggled to merely achieve subsistence. Fasting became commonplace; no meat, poultry, animal fats, eggs, or dairy products were consumed on fast days.

After the Norman Invasion, the societal hierarchy was demonstrated through food. The aristocratic diet was highly protein based, with game birds signifying the highest status (due to implications of land ownership). Spices were very scarce and costly, and were thus limited to use by the privileged people. Bread was an important staple in the diets of all people. A variety of crops were commonly grown, including cabbage, leeks, carrots, plums, pears, cherries, and various berries. Butter and honey emerged as the most common fat and sweetener, respectively.

By the 14th century, substantial collections of written recipes were being compiled in English. Pies filled with meat mixtures made their first appearance, although the crusts of these early pies were meant only to protect the contents during cooking and were not meant to be eaten. Fruit was often consumed at the beginning of a meal in hopes of opening the stomach in preparation for digestion. Ale was a very common drink, particularly of the poor, and was brewed by most households. A two-meal-per-day pattern emerged during this time, with the principal meal served midday and a lighter supper served at dusk. Sometimes a small breakfast, consisting of cold meat or fish and ale or wine (!), was also served. The only utensil used regularly up to this point was a knife; most food was eaten by hand and tablecloths were used primarily for wiping messy fingers.

Thanks to the expanding trade routes of the Renaissance period, a variety of new foods, such as turkey, coffee, and tea, were introduced to the region. Tea was first sold in London in 1658; the beverage quickly rose to prominence for use in ceremonies and when entertaining. Potatoes, a food from the New World, grew well in the damp climate and quickly became a staple food for the poor. Spices, aromatic herbs, and sugar became cheaper and more widely available. The word "curry" was introduced during this time to indicate spice mixtures of East Indian origin that were used to flavor meat dishes. Meat pasties and pies became known as English specialties, and puddings (e.g., blood pudding, liver pudding) became a staple. Confectionary flourished, with marmalades, jams, and cakes becoming popular items.

By the late 18th century, the population of London had surpassed 500,000 people; the city became the driving force of cultural trends (including those related to food) nationwide. More efficient agricultural practices allowed for an increased volume of food production, although dependence on imported foods continued to increase as the country became less agrarian and more urban. Vegetables such as asparagus, cauliflower, and kidney beans were newly cultivated during this time. Pubs, or public houses, became popular hangouts for men to converse over alcohol.

The 18th century saw the development of the sandwich and Yorkshire pudding, as well as the proliferation of sweet biscuit (cookie) manufacturing. Tea became the most important British beverage. The idea of a separate dining room was established during this time, and the number of courses in a meal ranged from one to five, depending upon the status of the household and the importance of the occasion. Along with the formal dining room came the widespread use of forks, and the use of gas and electricity for cooking. During this era, food safety advanced by the adoption of pasteurization and the enactment of legislation laying the groundwork for modern food-safety laws.

The early 20th century witnessed an expansion in scientific nutrition knowledge. A 1904 report cited "inadequate diet" as a primary reason that many potential

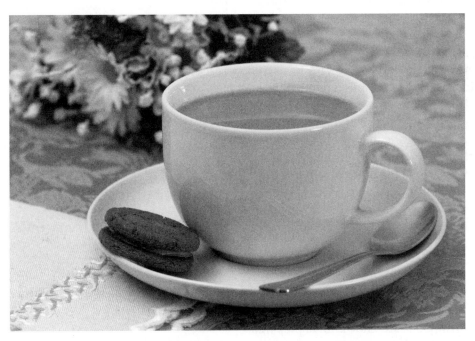

Snacking throughout the day has become a popular alternative to customary high tea in Great Britain.

recruits were rejected from the British armed forces. Poverty and undernutrition were major issues being combated with emerging information on the role of vitamins in health and disease prevention. As a public health measure, vitamin fortification of white flour began during World War II. To ensure that limited food supplies were distributed effectively, a system of food rationing was put into place at the beginning of World War II; the rations continued until 1954, well after the war had ended.

Throughout most of the 20th century, the middle and upper classes followed a daily pattern of breakfast, lunch, afternoon tea, and dinner. The working class and rural population ate an earlier breakfast, a midday dinner (main meal), and a late-afternoon high-tea. The latter half of the 20th century brought a proliferation of convenience foods (e.g., canned fruits, frozen meals) as supermarkets began to dominate food retailing. Agricultural practices evolved into primarily factory farming in order to meet a growing demand with limited natural resources. Some of these practices contributed to a major British health scare in the 1990s: bovine spongiform encephalopathy, or mad cow disease. Food-safety officials responded to this scare by tightening regulations surrounding beef production.

Today, wheat, potatoes, and beef are still important meal staples, but pasta, rice, and poultry are becoming increasingly common. The most obvious change in British food patterns over the past 50 years is the influence of multiculturalism, as witnessed by the almost ubiquitous kebob, curry, and pizza offerings in urban areas. Another major change has been the explosion in popularity and availability of fast food, convenience foods, and preprepared meals. On the opposite end of the spectrum, interest in vegetarianism and media attention on food in terms of both cooking and nutrition is on the rise. Interest in farmers' markets and organic produce has also been growing in tandem. Dining patterns are not followed as rigidly as in the past; afternoon tea/high tea is becoming a less frequent meal and more general snacking is occurring throughout the day. Pubs are increasingly recognized as quality dining establishments rather than simply social drinking venues.

 MAJOR FOODS

Traditionally, British foods are known to be prepared simply and only minimally seasoned; thus, the merits of traditional British dishes have not been highly regarded. Today, there is a growing interest in British cuisine, as some classic dishes have been given a modern makeover.

 Protein Sources

Protein sources include cheese, roast beef, sausages, cod or haddock, chicken, mutton or lamb, herring, and baked beans.

 Starch Sources

Starch sources include cold cereal, oatmeal, white breads, scones, and quick breads.

 Fat Sources

Fat sources include butter, margarine, lard, and suet.

 Prominent Vegetables

Prominent vegetables, which are typically boiled with a little seasoning added, include potatoes, turnips, peas, leeks, onions, brussels sprouts, cabbage, and carrots.

 Prominent Fruits

Prominent fruits, which are mostly consumed in the form of desserts and spreads, include pears, apples, plums, berries, bananas, and dried fruits (raisins, sultanas, currants, prunes, and dates).

 Spices, Seasonings, and Condiments

Spices and condiments include Worcestershire sauce, malt vinegar, ketchup, mustard, jam, marmalade, nutmeg, cinnamon, mint, thyme, garlic, ginger, salt, pepper, and curry powder.

 Beverages

Beverages include tea (primarily black tea of Indian origin), soft drinks, and beer.

 Desserts

Desserts include lemon curd, trifles, crumbles, and chocolate candy.

 FOODS WITH CULTURAL SIGNIFICANCE

Foods with cultural significance include Stilton cheese, haggis, fish and chips, clotted cream, crumpets, Welsh

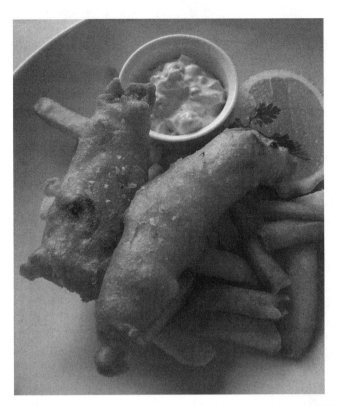

Fish and Chips

rarebit, shepherd's pie, bubble and squeak, chicken tikka masala, cheddar cheese, Doner kebob, and mushy peas.

 TYPICAL DAY'S MENU

As in most Western countries, dining habits have changed dramatically over the past few decades. A typical day's menu is difficult to pinpoint for a number of reasons, including the vast expansion of available food products, a high prevalence of unscheduled snacking, fewer meals eaten together as a family, and significant

differences in intake patterns between age groups. With those caveats, Table 11-1 illustrates a likely menu for an average working adult in Great Britain.

Naturally, eating patterns differ in leisure time versus the work week. For example, a traditional full English/Scottish/Welsh breakfast is commonly served on weekends and holidays, as well as in hotels and inns. This meal always includes bacon, fried eggs, tea, and coffee, as well as any of the following additions: sausage, tomatoes, fried toast, baked beans, fried potatoes, and/or black pudding.

The Sunday roast is another longstanding tradition in Great Britain, although its popularity has waned as fewer families choose to prepare large home-cooked meals. A Sunday roast is a hearty Sunday afternoon meal of oven-roasted beef with gravy, Yorkshire pudding, roasted or boiled potatoes, another boiled vegetable (carrots, peas, or cabbage), and a pudding.

 HOLIDAY MENUS

Some holidays in Great Britain, including Christmas, New Years, Burns Night (Scotland), Shrove Tuesday, Mothering Sunday, and Easter, are celebrated with food traditions. The items served at the most important family celebrations (holidays and otherwise) include fruitcake, large pieces of meat, alcohol, and sweets.

Christmas is celebrated as a two-day public holiday (December 25 and 26). In England and Wales, the main Christmas feast occurs midday and traditionally includes roast turkey, chestnut stuffing, gravy, sausages or bacon rolls, roasted or boiled potatoes, brussels sprouts, and a rich plum pudding (fruitcake) soaked in brandy. Often, a silver coin or other trinket is baked into the pudding; legend claims that the recipient of the silver coin is rewarded with good luck throughout the following year. In Scotland, the Christmas meal is smaller and more low-key, with the largest

TABLE 11-1   Typical Day's Menu

Breakfast	Lunch	Afternoon Tea[a]	Dinner	Other
Cold cereal with semi-skimmed milk	Sandwich	Tea	Pizza, pasta, stir-fry, or meat and vegetable dish	Yogurt
Toast with butter and marmalade	Baked potato or soup	Various breads with butter and marmalade	Pudding	Chocolate candy
Orange juice, tea, or coffee	Soft drink, water, and/or tea	Cake	Water, buttermilk, soft drink, ale, and/or tea	

[a]Tea is always served hot with milk and sugar added.

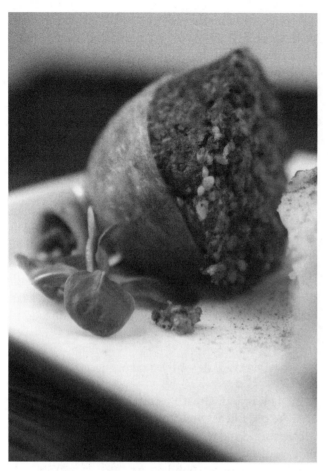

The Scottish national dish is haggis. It is enjoyed with a glass of Scottish whiskey every Burns Night, in honor of the life and work of Scottish poet Robert Burns.

feast occurring over the New Year's holiday. Throughout the Christmas season, mincemeat pie is regularly offered at social gatherings.

In Scotland, typical New Year's treats include shortbread and black bun. Later in the month (January 25), Scotland celebrates Burns Night, in honor of the life and work of Scottish poet Robert Burns. The Scottish national dish, haggis, is the center of the Burns Night meal and is served with Scotch whiskey. Shrove Tuesday is the day before Lent and was traditionally viewed by the British as the day to use up fats and other rich ingredients that one would sacrifice during the Lenten season. The celebratory food on Shrove Tuesday is a large, thin pancake covered with sugar and lemon juice. Some areas around the country celebrate Shrove Tuesday with street races that participants run while flipping pancakes in a skillet.

The fourth Sunday of Lent is known as Mothering Sunday across Great Britain. Simnel cakes are decorated with either 11 or 12 marzipan balls to commemorate the Apostles. In addition to small feasts, Good Friday and Easter are celebrated by the consumption of warm hot cross buns.

 GENERAL HEALTH AND NUTRITIONAL INDICATORS SUMMARY

A high standard of living and access to quality health care help the British maintain an average life expec-

Observations from the Author (Rachel Hayes)

I spent the spring semester of 1996 studying in London, as part of a wonderful university exchange program. The experience was one of the best and most enriching of my life and opened a whole new world to me, both figuratively and literally. That spring was a relatively tumultuous one in Great Britain, both in a political and a public health sense. Politically, ongoing strife with the Irish Republican Army (a private separatist group) led to a series of small bombings around the city. Although the bombs, often placed in mailboxes, barely disrupted daily life in Great Britain, the sensationalized headlines in the United States were enough to cause all of our parents many a sleepless night.

While the bombings were stealing the headlines, a quieter danger was threatening the public health of the nation. In late spring, news broke that ground beef sold and served around the country may have come from cattle suffering from bovine spongiform encephalopathy (BSE), or mad cow disease. The concern was that BSE was directly connected to a rare degenerative brain disease in humans, known as Creutzfeldt–Jakob disease (CJD). The food-safety community, food retailers, and the general public were placed on high alert; all beef was temporarily removed from grocery stores and restaurants. I have a vivid memory of walking past a McDonalds (the quintessential hamburger chain) and seeing its windows lined with giant posters exclaiming that no beef products were available.

Thankfully, the health toll of the BSE scare was minimal; however, the economic costs were steep: British beef exporting was banned for 10 years and beef sales are only recently recovering to the pre-1996 levels.

tancy of 78.7 years. The most recently published data (2005) for the UK as a whole indicate that approximately 8% of infants are born at low birth weight, and infant mortality is 0.5%. Although approximately 3% of the population of the UK was considered underweight (based on body mass index) in 2003–2004, the numbers on undernourishment are so small that they are not statistically significant, according to the United Nations' Food and Agriculture Organization (2004).

While undernourishment is not a significant threat, increasing rates of overweight and obesity have become a major public health concern. Data from the World Health Organization (2007) indicate that the per capita daily food consumption in Great Britain totals over 3400 calories. Given that this level is approximately 1000 calories more than adults typically need to maintain their weight, it is no surprise that nearly two thirds of the adult population is considered overweight, and one fifth is considered obese. Overweight/obesity during childhood is an especially grave concern, as this leads to an increased risk of heart disease, diabetes, and other chronic conditions early in life.

COMMUNICATION AND COUNSELING TIPS

Working with British clients in a nutrition-counseling situation is nearly identical to working with American clients. Of course, the practitioner should have a general knowledge of current and traditional British foods and food patterns for a frame of reference. When offering specific dietary guidance, a practitioner may also want to keep the following in mind:

- Traditionally, consumption of fresh fruit in Great Britain is limited; fruits are primarily used as ingredients.

FEATURED RECIPE

Welsh Rarebit

4 thick slices of
bread, crusts removed

2 tbsp. butter, melted

2 cups grated cheddar cheese

1 tsp. mustard powder

Few drops Worcestershire sauce

4 tbsp. brown ale, beer, or milk

1. Preheat the broiler. Toast the bread until golden-brown, then place in a shallow baking dish (in a single layer). Keep warm.
2. Stir the cheese, mustard powder, and Worcestershire sauce into the melted butter, then slowly pour in the ale (or beer or milk) in a steady stream.
3. Stir the cheese mixture until very well blended.
4. Spoon the cheese mixture onto the toast, then place under the broiler until bubby and golden.
5. Serve immediately.

Yields 4 servings

More recipes are available at http://nutrition.jbpub.com/foodculture/

- Although many common foods are shared between the United States and Great Britain, there are subtle differences (e.g., pizza often includes toppings such as tuna, corn, tandoori chicken, or prawns instead of pepperoni or Italian sausage).
- Oils are not used for cooking to the extent that butter and other fats are used.
- Vegetables are most commonly boiled; fresh salads are not frequently consumed.

TABLE 11-2 Primary Language of Food Names

Biscuits (cookies or crackers)	Almost always offered at tea time
Black bun	Dried fruit, nuts, and spices baked into a flat pastry
Blood pudding	A sausage made by cooking blood (typically from a pig or cow) with a thickener until it congeals
Bubble and squeak	Leftover mashed potatoes, cooked cabbage, and sliced meat mashed together and browned in a skillet; originally named for the sounds made when cooking
Chips	French fries; extremely popular side dish
Cornish pasties	Oblong pastries filled with meat, potatoes, and onions, then oven-baked
Crisps	Potato chips; offered in a wide variety of flavors, including prawn, Worcestershire sauce, and steak/onion
Crumpets	Flat, round, doughy breads cooked on a griddle; served hot with butter at tea time
Doner kebob	Very common takeout food of Turkish origin: lamb meat with salad, yogurt, and tomato sauce, served in pita bread
Fruitcake	Rich dessert cake (often plum) served at most major celebrations, including Christmas, Easter, weddings, birthdays, and christenings
Haggis	Traditional Scottish dish, now served primarily at special banquets: finely ground sheep's heart and liver, beef suet, toasted oatmeal, salt, onions, and pepper stuffed into a clean sheep's stomach and steamed
Jacket potato	Baked potato
Mincemeat	Small, double-crusted pie with currants, raisins, sultanas, candied fruit peel, sugar, spices, apples, and suet
Mushy peas	Dried peas cooked until very soft and then pureed; very popular garnish and side item
Ploughman's lunch	A classic pub lunch. Chunks of bread, wedges of cheese, pickles (or pickled onions), and a pint of ale
Prawns	Shrimp; widely used in salads, sandwiches, sauces, pizzas, and curries
Pudding	Several different groups of dishes, some savory and some sweet; today, assumed to signify a dessert (such as a trifle or crumble) following a meal
Shepherd's pie	Ground meat with onion and seasonings baked under a thick layer of mashed potatoes; also known as cottage pie
Stilton cheese	Blue-veined cheese produced only in the Midlands region of Great Britain
Welsh rarebit	Melted cheese, mixed with beer or milk, then poured over toast and browned; also known as Welsh rabbit

REFERENCES

Barer-Stein, T. (1999). *You eat what you are: People, culture and food traditions.* Buffalo, NY: Firefly Books.

Central Intelligence Agency. (2008). *United Kingdom.* Retrieved March 20, 2008, from The World Factbook. Website: http://www.cia.gov/library/publications/the-world-factbook/geos/uk/html/

Editors of Gourmet Magazine. (Eds.). (1996). *Cuisines of the world: Flavors of England, Ireland, and Scotland. The best of Gourmet* (pp. 241–279). New York: Conde Nast Publications; Random House.

Grigson, J. (1985). *Jane Grigson's British cookery*. New York: Atheneum.

Hoare, J., Henderson, L., Bates, C., Prentice, A., Birch, M., Swan, G., et al. (2004). *The national diet & nutrition survey: Adults aged 19 to 64 years (summary report)*. London: Office for National Statistics; Medical Research Council Human Nutrition Research; Food Standards Agency.

Mason, L. (2004). *Food culture in Great Britain*. Westport, CT: Greenwood.

Menzel, P., & D'Aluisio, F. (2005). *Hungry planet: What the world eats*. Napa, CA: Material World Books; Berkeley, CA: Ten Speed Press.

Office for National Statistics. (2007). *Population estimates*. Retrieved March 30, 2008, from National Statistics Online. Website: http://www.statistics.gov.uk/CCI/nugget.asp?ID=6/

Spencer, C. (2002). *British food: An extraordinary thousand years of history*. New York: Columbia University Press.

UNICEF. (2007). *The state of the world's children 2007: Women and children, the double dividend of gender equality*. Retrieved April 15, 2009, from http://www.unicef.org/sowc07/statistics/tables.php

United Nations Food and Agriculture Organization. Retrieved April 15, 2008, from http://www.fao.org/es/ess/faostat/foodsecurity/index-en.htm

United Nations Food and Agriculture Organization. (2004). *FAO statistical yearbook. Country profiles: United Kingdom*. Retrieved March 20, 2008, from http://www.fao.org/es/ess/yearbook/vol_1_2/pdf/United-Kingdom.pdf/.

Walden, H. (Ed.). (2004). *Traditional British cooking*. London: Southwater.

World Health Organization. (2007). *Core health indicators: United Kingdom*. Retrieved March 20, 2008, from http://www.who.int/whosis/database/core/core_select_process.cfm/

CHAPTER 12

The Netherlands

Jeannette van der Velde, MPH, MSc

 CULTURE AND WORLD REGION

The Kingdom of the Netherlands, as it is officially known, is referred to more commonly as Holland or the Netherlands. The Netherlands is situated in north-western Europe and shares its borders with Germany and Belgium to the east and south, respectively, and with the North Sea to the west and north (CIA World Factbook, 2008). The name Netherlands was bestowed because 27% of the country is below sea level with an average elevation of 37 feet (Hooker, 1999). Except for the southeast part of Holland, where rolling hills make up the landscape, the rest of the country is flat. Holland lays in the deltas of three major rivers—the Rhine, the Meuse, and the Scheldt—as they flow into the North Sea (Hooker, 1999). In the fight to keep water out of Holland's flat topography, the country is interlaced with drainage ditches and dikes. Historically, windmills were used to pump water out of the drainage ditches and into the rivers; today, solar-powered

electric pumps perform the same function (Bol, 2007; Hooker, 1999).

Holland is a small country with a total land surface area of 13,107 square miles (including water surface the total area becomes 16,033 square miles) of which 69% is crop and grassland and 8% is forest (Bol, 2007; OECD, 1973). Over 408,000 acres of land have been reclaimed from the sea (Bol, 2007; Hooker, 1999). Despite its relatively northern location, the climate of Holland is moderate, with mild winters (average temperature 2°C), cool summers (17°C), and annual rainfall between 700 and 800 ml (Hooker, 1999).

The Kingdom of the Netherlands, known then as the Dutch United Provinces, was officially founded in 1579 (CIA World Factbook, 2008; Hooker, 1999; Schama, 1987). Dutch recorded history began when Julius Caesar conquered the Belgian tribes in 57 BC, and again in 15 BC. Augustus called their new territory *Gallica Belgica* (Schama, 1987). Prior to the Roman invasion of 57 BC, no records of Dutch history are found.

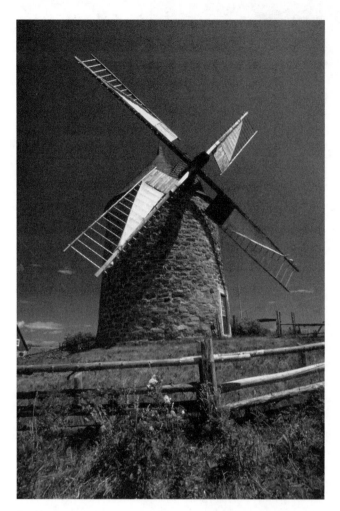

Before the days of electric pumps, windmills were used to pump water out of Holland's drainage ditches and into the rivers.

The territory of *Gallica Belgica* was under Roman dominion for 30 years, when the inhabitants were able to lead a successful revolt against Rome. Another invasion by Rome occurred 20 years later, lasting for 20 years, and again the inhabitants led a revolt (Schama, 1987). The pattern of invasion and revolt continued until the fall of the Roman Empire in 400 AD and, with it, mass migrations of peoples (Schama, 1987). Holland entered the Dark Ages. The Batavians migrated out of Holland to be replaced by Frisians along the coast, Saxons in the west, and Franks in the south (Hooker, 1999; Schama, 1987). For the next 400 years these three peoples vied for power, each ruling at various times until the Viking invasion of 850 AD (Prak, 2002). As with the rest of Europe, which was largely made up of city–states, Holland was divided into four principalities (Hooker, 1999). Because of its proximity to the North Sea and the advantage to use the three major rivers as transpor-

tation routes, these four principalities began to thrive. Over time the dukes and counts lost their power, resulting in 200 years of independence, relative peace, and prosperity (Prak, 2002; Schama, 1987). Holland entered its golden age. In 1464, Philip III, considered the founder of the Netherlands, united its provinces with the Belgian states (Prak, 2002).

The Kingdom of the Netherlands is a constitutional monarchy with an elected parliament (CIA World Factbook, 2008). The current monarch, Queen Beatrix, ascended to the throne on April 30, 1980; her son, Willem Alexander, is the heir apparent. In a constitutional monarchy the monarch is the chief of the executive branch and appoints the cabinet ministers (CIA World Factbook, 2008). The leader of the majority party of the Second Chamber is appointed prime minister by the monarch. The Second Chamber is an elected assembly, with each party holding seats determined by the percentage of the votes received from the public (CIA World Factbook, 2008; Hooker, 1999). More than 12 parties have seats in the Second Chamber; the legislative branch of the government must build consensus in order to pass bills. The Queen's Day (April 30) is Holland's sole national holiday, celebrated to honor the Queen mother Juliana's birthday and Queen Beatrix's ascension to the throne.

LANGUAGE

The latest figures place Holland's population at approximately 16.6 million. With a density of 483 people per square kilometer, it is one of the most densely populated countries in the world (Bol, 2007; CIA World Factbook, 2008; US Census Bureau, 2008). The demographic breakdown is as follows: 17% between 0 and 14 years, 67% between 15 and 64 years, and 14% over 65 years (U.S. Census Data, 2008). For each age cohort the gender ratio is approximately equal; for the first two cohorts males slightly outnumber females, and by the age of 70 years females outnumber males (U.S. Census Bureau, n.d.).

The official language of the Netherlands is Dutch. The other spoken language is Frisian, spoken by approximately 400,000 people in the northern province of Friesland (CIA World Factbook, 2008). In Friesland all official documents must be in both Frisian and Dutch. In addition to these languages, more than 20 distinct dialects exist (Huning, 2008). Most Dutch people converse in formal Dutch in order to understand one another. It is highly probable that people from two different regions will have difficulty understanding one another if they converse in their local dialects. As a result of its merchant past, the Dutch have been in contact with many other countries and therefore value the ability to speak other languages; over 75% of the population speaks English, 67% speak German, and 12% speak French (CIA World Factbook, 2008).

FOOD HISTORY WITHIN THE CULTURE

The Dutch are not known for their culinary creativity; their relationship with food is one of pragmatism and necessity (Allart, 1797). The French philosopher Sartre described Dutch cooking as follows: "butter, cheese, and salt meat are not foods which demand a great deal of attention . . . their meat-broth is nothing more than water full of salt or nutmeg, with sweet breads and minced meat added, having not the slightest flavor of meat . . ." (Zumthor, 1963, p. 68). While other countries used spices frugally, the Dutch used these with abandon.

In many families, cooking was done once a week and these dishes were reheated for the rest of the week (Allart, 1797; Zumthor, 1963). Zumthor (1963, p. 64) describes the traditional meal scene during the 1600s: "a table was covered with a cloth which was sometimes finely embroidered . . . along the table were ranged goblets of plain or cut glass, dishes and pots of pewter or silver, earthenware plates and a wooden trencher on which bread or meat was carved." The Dutch ate with their hands aided by a knife and wiped their fingers on napkins. Spoons existed but were considered precious and collected rather than used, and forks were not used until the 1700s (Prak, 2002; Zumthor, 1963).

As with other cultures, food patterns and dietary habits change after exposure to different customs (non-native ingredients, eating habits, fast-food restaurants) and as a result of modernity (e.g., more women working, less time to prepare food, travel, and changing gender roles). Eastern ingredients that influenced Dutch cuisine include most notably rice and spices such as nutmeg and ginger. Social distinctions, while evident in housing and clothing, were relatively nonexistent in dietary composition. Nearly everyone consumed turnips, fried onions, bread, and beer. Those living near the coast ate fish, gruel, and cheese. The national dish was called *Hutsepot*, which to this day is still consumed (Allart, 1797; Prak, 2002). The Netherlands' cereal (grains) production and subsequent meager harvests

meant that fine wheat bread was considered a delicacy consumed only on Sundays or religious holidays (Zumthor, 1963); instead, their daily bread was black, soft, and sticky—consisting of a mixture of rye, barley, buckwheat, oats, and even beans—which was well documented to be inedible (Prak, 2002).

MAJOR FOODS

Even in a country as small as Holland, there are regional variations in food preferences. This chapter limits its discussion to the mainstream culinary tradition associated with the urban Dutch-speaking population.

Protein Sources

In Rembrandt's time, Dutch citizens from most socio-economic strata could be considered vegetarian as their diets consisted largely of eggs and fish; meat was rarely consumed. Large chicken farms were in the northern part of Holland and as such eggs were readily available and affordable (Zumthor, 1963). Today, the picture is very different.

Chicken, beef, and some lamb are the preferred meat sources, accounting for approximately 30% of the daily protein intake (FAO, 2005). The other main protein source for the Dutch comes from dairy products, especially milk consumption, which accounts for nearly 30% of the average daily protein intake (FAO, 2005). Despite the fact that Holland has a robust fishing industry, domestic fish consumption is relatively low, accounting for 7.3% of the average daily protein intake (FAO, 2005). Although a wide variety of fish are consumed, herring and salmon are among the most popular. Herring is eaten raw (salted), smoked, or pickled, and there are fish kiosks in every town and city, which often provides a midday snack. Herring is considered a national symbol: the new season's first barrel is always presented to the Queen. Seafood, such as mussels, shrimp, oysters, and crabs, are consumed boiled or fried. On average, 24.5 kg per person of fish are consumed annually (FAO, 2005).

Starch Sources

Wheat, barley, maize, rye, and oats are the main sources of starch for the Dutch (Bol, 2007; FAO, 2008). The latest data available indicate that Holland produced over 1.75 million metric tons of cereals (wheat, barley, maize, rye) in 2000, up from 1.36 million metric tons in 1990

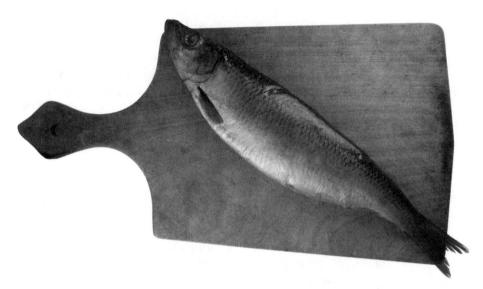

Herring is considered a national symbol; the new season's first barrel is always presented to the Queen.

(FAO, 2008). Bread forms the staple of most meals and has come a long way since the black sticky bread served during the Middle Ages (OECD, 1973; Prak, 2002; Zumthor, 1963). The selection of bread is well varied from light wheat to dark and dense pumpernickel and rye breads. Compared with historical yields, current cereal harvests have increased substantially; nevertheless, supply cannot keep pace with demand (OECD, 1973). Holland imports cereals from eastern Europe in order to meet the growing demand (FAO, 2008).

 ## Fat Sources

The Dutch diet consists of both saturated and unsaturated fat originating mostly from their beef and fish protein sources. Even though fish is in abundance, the Dutch have a high mortality rate that correlates to cardiovascular disease. The Dutch consume insufficient fruit and fiber, thus may secondarily affect heart disease.

 ## Prominent Vegetables

Due to limited cereal production, vegetables still make up most of the Dutch diet. Vegetable consumption is dependent on climate, geography, and soil conditions; in Holland all three factors were, and are, conducive to growing an array of vegetables (Bol, 2007; OECD, 1973; Zumthor, 1963). Holland's vegetable production has more than doubled during the past decades, due in large part to advances in agriculture and horticulture techniques. Throughout history, and today, the

most significant vegetable crops grown include peas, beans, cabbages, carrots, turnips, onions, cucumbers, cauliflower, artichokes, and asparagus (Bol, 2007). One popular yet simple dish is bread with fried onions. Interestingly, the potato, which is an integral part of today's diet, was considered poisonous and grown solely as a decorative plant (Zumthor, 1963).

 ## Prominent Fruits

As with other produce, fruit production is dependent on geography. Holland's climate is conducive to growing a wide range of fruits. Fruits were not always eaten raw traditionally but instead were cooked together with vegetables. Some traditional dishes include pea soup with prunes flavored with ginger, white beans with prune syrup, and minced ox tongue with green apple (Allart, 1797; Zumthor, 1963). Today, fruits are mostly consumed raw. Fruits are usually enjoyed fresh as a dessert or as snacks throughout the day. The fruits grown most efficiently include strawberries, blackberries, raspberries, gooseberries, red and black currants, prunes, plums, apples, and pears.

 ## Spices and Seasonings

Since the days of the Dutch East Indian Company, spices have been used in Dutch cooking. Despite their expense, the Dutch used spices with liberty—what some have described as a technique to mask their inability to cook! The most commonly used seasonings include cinnamon, cloves, nutmeg, paprika, and ginger.

Herbs that are commonly used include parsley, chives, and scallions. Traditional Dutch dishes were not spicy; however, as a direct result of their colonial pursuits in eastern Asia and Africa, spices became readily available, which translated into a subsequent increase in spicy dishes.

 Beverages

Historically, beer was the most common drink and served on every occasion, from breakfast to late evening. Records show that during the 1600s, the town of Haarlem consumed more than 5 million gallons of beer (Zumthor, 1963). Milk was and is still a popular drink. Sweetened wine and brandy were also popular (Zumthor, 1963). Spiced wine is often served during the winter months, and the most basic recipe is sweetened wine diluted with water, with the addition of cinnamon, ginger, and cloves. While the Dutch still consume a lot of beer, these days it is reserved for the evening hours. In 2004, the Dutch consumed over 1.3 billion liters of beer (Statistics Netherlands, 2005).

 Desserts

As mentioned previously, fresh fruits are often served as dessert. Yogurt, custards, and puddings can also be served. Depending on the season, puddings or custards are either served hot or cold. Two distinct Dutch puddings are *krentenbrij* (made with pearl barley, raisins, currants, and black currant juice) and *karnemelksepap* (made with pearl barley and buttermilk).

What the Dutch lack in cooking artistry they redress with their baking talents. A wide variety of cakes and pastries are regularly made for no special occasion; many are made with apples, raisins, currants, and almonds. A simple apple pie is at least 2 inches high and consists of apples, raisins, and currants, and is flavored with cinnamon (occasionally cloves), giving it closer resemblance to a torte than a fruit pie. For New Year's Eve celebrations, it is customary to eat *oliebollen*, deep-fried dough either plain or with chunks of apple and raisins, sprinkled with powered sugar. Christmas would not be complete without a *banket staaf*, a flaky pastry crust filled with almond paste shaped into straight baguettes or letters.

 TYPICAL DAY'S MENU

A typical day starts with a breakfast of bread, butter, cheese, and a variety of fruit spreads, served with milk, tea, or coffee, although heartier breakfasts, such as oatmeal and wheat germ, are consumed regularly during the winter months and, compared with the breakfasts of urban dwellers, more frequently in rural areas. Lunch is a light meal that consists of bread with cheese and cold meats, and occasionally soup. Dinner, called the *warme maalitijd* or warm mealtime, is the main meal and consists of potatoes, meat, and a cooked vegetable or salad (Waijers et al., 2006). Yogurt, custards, puddings, or fruit follow as dessert. Between meals, the Dutch snack on fruits, chocolates, black salted licorice, and cakes with coffee or tea.

 HOLIDAY MENUS

Holland's sole national holiday is the Queen's Day, when everyone enjoys the day off from work and school. No special menu accompanies this day. It is more likely that the family will spend the day enjoying festivities in town/city centers, feasting on kiosk delicacies such as French fries served with mayonnaise, a variety of smoked and raw fish, and deep-fried dough sprinkled with icing sugar.

Christmas dinner is the only notable holiday menu. The menu varies regionally and according to traditional family status. Today, the Christmas menu is more likely to be influenced by the families' travels rather than tradition. The Christmas menu typically includes roast beef, duck, rabbit, pheasant, or roasted ham served with a variety of vegetables such as green beans, cauliflower, potatoes, and a variety of salads (e.g., potato salad, red beet salad, green salad). An almond pastry dessert usually follows the meal.

 HEALTH BELIEFS AND CONCERNS

The Dutch believe that ill health is a direct consequence of germs and microbes, lack of exercise, and poor eating habits (Aarts, Paulussen, & Schaalma, 1997; Oenema, Brug, & Lechner, 2001). The Dutch pragmatically focus on scientific reasoning rather than spiritual beliefs in matters related to health and disease; thus, they tend to follow biomedical and scientific approaches to health management and treatment (Oenema et al., 2001; van Wieringen, Harmsen, & Bruijnzeels, 2002). For those who are religious, prayer is often believed to assist in the healing process, if not to cure per se, more precisely in order to provide strength to the patient and his or her family (Waijers et al., 2006). Prayer is used in conjunction with biomedical treatments. It is important to realize that the ethnocultural minorities living in Holland are shaped by their cultural traditions as well as interpretations of disease and well-being.

GENERAL HEALTH AND NUTRITIONAL INDICATORS SUMMARY

Optimal health and well-being is influenced by nutrition that can be monitored and evaluated through a variety of demographic and health indicators. The United Nations Development Programme established the Human Development Index (HDI) to assist in evaluating where countries rank in terms of human progress and development. The HDI is a composite measure of three dimensions of human development: life expectancy, adult literacy, and standard of living in economic terms. The HDI for the Netherlands is 0.958, or high human development. While the HDI does provide a general indication of the population's well-being it is important to note that indicators for gender and income equality, human rights, or political freedoms are not included (UNDP, 2008).

The Dutch live an average of 79 years. The country has a birth rate of 187/1000 and a crude death rate of 9/1000 (UNICEF, 2007). The infant and under-5-years mortality rates are 4/1000 and 5/1000, respectively, and Holland has a relatively low maternal mortality rate of 16 deaths per 100,000 births (UNICEF, 2007). In Holland, 77% of adults are literate. No data are available for the percentage of low-birth-weight babies, and the percentage of children who are stunted (height for age), underweight (weight for age), and/or wasted (weight for height) (UNICEF, 2007).

One consequence of inadequate nutrition, specifically iron deficiency, is anemia. Anemia occurs when there are insufficient red blood cells or when the red blood cells do not contain sufficient hemoglobin (WHO, 2008). While not the sole cause of anemia, iron deficiency is by far the most common. The prevalence of anemia in children under 5 years of age is 9% (approximately 84,000 children). For nonpregnant women the prevalence of anemia is 14%, which translates into slightly more than half a million women with anemia. Interestingly, the prevalence of anemia decreases to 12% (approximately 22,000) for pregnant women (WHO, 2008).

COMMUNICATION AND COUNSELING TIPS

The Dutch people are modest, tolerant, self-reliant, and entrepreneurial (Donald, 1974). They value hard work and education and are averse to the nonessential. Accumulating money is fine, but spending money (especially overtly) is considered a vice and in bad taste (Schama, 1987). A trait frequently bestowed on the Dutch is their extremely pragmatic nature; the majority of decisions are methodically deliberated based on sensibility and realism.

The Dutch are characteristically direct and straightforward. Although this directness may be misinterpreted as rudeness, when read through the lens of pragmatism the Dutch simply want to get to the heart of the matter immediately. Also, they are quick to criticize; no criticism generally means one has received a compliment, albeit passively, as direct compliments are offered sparingly. Their sense of humor is dry, often a play on words, sarcastic, and/or sardonic. Small talk is not customary and is not required in every social context. The Dutch expect eye contact while speaking with someone; looking away is considered impolite and could be perceived as being deceitful.

When counseling a Dutch person, it is best to be direct, provide all the facts in a straightforward manner, and to expect that there will be numerous clarification questions and that the deliberation process will be lengthy.

TABLE 12-1 Primary Language of Food Names with English and Phonetic Translation

Food*	English Translation	Phonetic Translation	Food*	English Translation	Phonetic Translation
Apple	Apple	A-pEl	Kool	Cabbage	koUl
Dadel	Date	da-dEl	Wortel	Carrots	vor-tEl
Fijg	Fig	fEIx	Erwt	Pea	Ervt
Sinasappel	Orange	sin-As-a-pel	Kaas	Cheese	Kas
Pruim	Plum	pr-WYm	Melk	Milk	mElk
Kers	Cherry	kErs	Yogurt	Yogurt	jo-Q-Yrt
Krent	Currant	KrEnt	Schaap	Sheep	sQa-ap
Druif	Grape	dr-WYf	Geit	Goat	X-Elt
Abrikoos	Apricots	a-bri-koUs	Rundvlees	Beef	rYnd-vleIs
Aardbij	Strawberry	ard-bEl	Kip	Chicken	Kip
Komkomer	Cucumber	kom-kom-mEr	Kofie	Coffee	ko-fi
Tomaat	Tomato	to-mat	Thee	Tea	theI
Ui	Onion	WY	Bier	Beer	Bir
Knoflook	Garlic	knof-loUk	Soep	Soup	Sup
Aardappel	Potato	ard-A-pEl	Brood	Bread	broUd
Boon	Beans	boUn	Pannekoek	Pancake	pAn-ne-kuk
Spinazie	Spinach	spi-na-zee			

*All names are in Dutch.

FEATURED RECIPE

Snert (Pea Soup)

6 cups water

3 cups dried split green peas, rinsed

1 smoked ham hock

2 potatoes, peeled and cubed

1–2 leeks, thinly sliced

1 small onion, thinly sliced

3–4 celery stalks, sliced

1 tsp. nutmeg

1 tbsp. lemon juice

Salt and pepper

1. Bring the water to a boil in a large heavy pot and add the peas and ham hock.
2. When the water begins to boil again, reduce heat and simmer for 2 hours, stirring occasionally.
3. Add the potatoes, leeks, onion, celery stalks, nutmeg, and lemon juice. Simmer for 30 minutes, stirring occasionally.
4. Remove and cut the ham hock, then return it to the pot. Simmer for 10 minutes.
5. Serve with dark pumpernickel or rye bread.

More recipes are available at http://nutrition.jbpub.com/foodculture/

Pea Soup

REFERENCES

Aarts, H., Paulussen, T., & Schaalma, H. (1997). Physical exercise habit: On the conceptualization and formation of habitual health behaviours. *Health Education Research, 12*(3), 363–374.

Allart, J. (1797). *Nieuwe Vaderlandsche Kookkunst (New national cooking art)*. Retrieved on March 27, 2008, from http://users.pandora.be/willy.vancammeren/NVK/index.htm/

Bol, R.P.L. (2007). *Facts and figures of the Dutch agri-sector.* Retrieved March 23, 2008, from http://www.minlnv.nl/portal/page?_pageid=116,1640360&_dad=portal&_schema=PORTAL&p_file_id=14741/

CIA World Factbook. (2008). Retrieved March 21, 2008, from https://www.cia.gov/library/publications/the-world-factbook/geos/ir.html/

Donald, C. (1974). *Holland: The land and the peoples.* South Brunswick, NJ: A.S. Barnes and Company.

Food and Agriculture Organization (FAO). (2005). *Fishery country profile: The Netherlands.* Retrieved March 20, 2008, from http://www.fao.org/fi/fcp/en/NLD/profile.htm/

Food and Agriculture Organization (FAO). (2008). *Country profile: The Netherlands.* Retrieved March 20, 2008, from http://www.fao.org/es/ess/yearbook/vol_1_2/pdf/Netherlands.pdf/

Hooker, M.T. (1999). The history of Holland. In F.W. Thackeray & J.E. Findling (Eds.), *The Greenwood histories of the modern nations.* Westport, CT: Greenwood Press.

Huning, M. (2008). *Dialects.* Retrieved June 15, 2008, from http://www.ned.univie.ac.at/Publicaties/taalgeschiedenis/en/dial.htm/

Oenema, A., Brug, J., & Lechner, L. (2001). Web-based tailored nutrition education: Results of a randomized controlled trial. *Health Education Research, 16*(6), 647–660.

Organization for Economic Cooperation and Development (OECD). (1973). *The state of Dutch agriculture. Agricultural policy in the Netherlands* (pp. 7–30). Paris: OECD.

Prak, M. (2002). *The Dutch republic in the seventeenth century: The golden age.* (D. Webb, Trans.). Cambridge, England: Cambridge University Press.

Schama, S. (1987). *The embarrassment of riches: An interpretation of Dutch culture in the Golden Age.* New York: Vintage Books.

Statistics Netherlands. (2005). *Beer consumption declining in the Netherlands.* Retrieved March 27, 2008, from http://www.cbs.nl/en-GB/menu/themas/industrie-energie/publicaties/artikelen/archief/2005/2005-1773-wm.htm/

United Nations Children's Fund (UNICEF). (2007). *Women and children: The double dividend of gender equality. The state of the world's children 2007.* Retrieved April 14, 2009, from http://www.unicef.org/sowc07/statistics/tables.php/

United Nations Development Programme (UNDP). (2008). *Fighting climate change: Human solidarity in a divided world.* Human Development Report 2007–2008. Retrieved April 14, 2009, from http://hdr.undp.org/en/

United States Census Bureau. (n.d.). *Country summary: The Netherlands.* Retrieved March 20, 2008, from http://www.census.gov/ipc/www/idb/

van Wieringen, J.C.M., Harmsen, J.A.M., & Bruijnzeels, M.A. (2002). Intercultural communication in general practice. *European Journal of Public Health, 12,* 63–68.

Verheijden, M.W., van der Veen, J.E., Zadelhoff, W.M., Bakx, C., Koelen, M.A., van den Hoogen, H.J.M., et al. (2003).

Nutrition guidance in Dutch family practice: Behavioral determinants of reduction of fat consumption. *American Journal of Clinical Nutrition, 77*(4), 1058–1064.

Waijers, P., Ocke, M.C., van Rossum, C.T.M., Peeters, P.H.M., Bamia, C., Chloptsios, Y., et al. (2006). Dietary patterns and survival in older Dutch women. *American Journal of Clinical Nutrition, 83*, 1170–1176.

World Health Organization (WHO). (2008). *Worldwide prevalence of anemia 1993–2005: WHO global database on anemia.* Retrieved April 14, 2009, from http://whqlibdoc.who.int/publications/2008/9789241596657_eng.pdf/

Zumthor, P. (Ed.). (1963). The Dutch interior. In S.W. Taylor, Trans., *Daily life in Rembrandt's Holland* (pp. 37–78). New York: MacMillan.

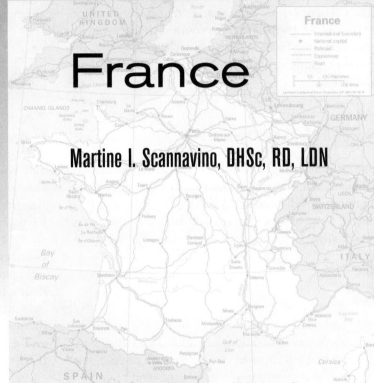

CHAPTER 13

France

Martine I. Scannavino, DHSc, RD, LDN

CULTURE AND WORLD REGION

According to the Library of Congress, as of May 2007 the estimated population of France was 60,876,136 with nearly three quarters of the population living in urban settings. France is recognized among European nations for having one of the most ethnically diverse populations. This diversity dates back to France's earliest history when the nation was populated by a blend of European ethic groups. France's current diverse population reflects her history of significant immigration trends over the past two centuries. Nearly 40% of France's inhabitants include those with ethnic ties to southern Europe, eastern Europe, Arabic, North African, Asian, and sub-Saharan African origins.

It is estimated that nearly 90% of France's population is Roman Catholic. The estimated Muslim population ranges between 5 and 6 million, greater than that of any other European nation. An estimated 1% is Jewish and 2% are Protestant. France is dedicated to the principle of religious neutrality and does not collect data on religion in its census; therefore, accurate statistical data for religious affiliations of the French population are not available.

Hall and Hall (1990, p. 96) explain that within the traditional French culture relationships begin within the immediate family. The French social construct is made up of a close group that may include grandparents, aunts, uncles, and cousins, and may extend to include a few classmates and long-time family friends. This close-knit group offers support, acceptance, and personal connections throughout life, although over the past few decades there have been dynamic changes resulting in a noted disintegration of the traditional family structure. These changes are reflected in the decline of elderly family members living with younger generations and an increase in divorce rates. The French marriage rate has declined by more than 30%.

France is located in western Europe. It is the largest western European nation and is often referred to as the "hexagon" due to its six-sided shape. Three sides of France are bordered by water: the English Channel and North Sea to the north, the Atlantic Ocean and Bay of Biscay to the west, and the Mediterranean Sea to the south (Library of Congress Federal Research Division, 2007). There are seven countries that border France: Spain and Andorra border the southwest; to the northeast Belgium, Luxembourg, and Germany; and the eastern regions of France are bordered by Switzerland and Italy.

 LANGUAGE

The primary language spoken in France is French. There are a number of dialects spoken throughout the many regions that include Alsatian, Corsican, and Provençal; however, there is a noted decline in the use of these dialects.

 CULTURE HISTORY

The food practices and culture of France today is a culmination of generations of cultural and ethnic influences and advances in agriculture and trade. Looking back at the early food ways of the land region we now know as France, we can compose a timeline that illustrates ethnic, regional, agricultural, and geographical influences in the current food traditions. Gastronomic history has felt the impact of the diverse cultures that inhabited France including the Phocaeans (Greeks who founded Massilia, later to be called Marseille) in the 6th century BCE, the Celts during the 7th century BCE, and the Romans during the 5th century BCE. Trade throughout Asia and the discovery of the New World (the Americas) brought new and unusual foods to France, such as chocolate, potatoes, rice, corn, and spices.

The Phocaeans brought olive trees, wheat, and grapevines to the Provençal region of France. With the Phocaeans also came many new pulses such as lentils, fava beans, and chickpeas, and staple vegetables that included onions and garlic. The Celts were tribes of Indo-Europeans whose civilization was deeply rooted in agriculture. The Celts were sophisticated metal workers who revolutionized farming through the introduction of iron farming tools. The Celtic diet was diverse and rich in meats from domesticated animals such as cattle and pigs, as well as grains, dairy, and ale. The Romans, lead by Julius Caesar, conquered the

Celts (they called them Gauls) in the 5th century BCE. The new Gallo-Roman culture developed food practices that drew on Greek etiquette and gastronomic specialties from across the Roman Empire that had trade routes throughout India and China as well as the agricultural riches of Gaul.

 FOOD HISTORY WITHIN THE CULTURE

French culinary expertise has evolved over the centuries, dating back to the early origins of a national cuisine in the Middle Ages. While the much-admired and respected specialties of regional cooking have their place in the French culinary tradition, fine cuisine (*haute cuisine*) came about in the 17th century in Paris. Chefs to royal courts perfected this fine style of cooking and documented their work in the first noted culinary texts of France. Chefs began to warrant recognition and were considered national treasures. Some of their names, such as La Varenne and Escoffier, are still recognized today. This style of cooking evolved from the use of complex preparation methods, rich sauces, and elaborate presentations. Until the 20th century there were two recognized schools of thought in the culinary tradition: *haute cuisine* and the more common country style of cooking, Provençal. In the mid- to late 20th century *nouvelle cuisine* (new cuisine), a movement made popular by chefs in the 1960s, whose preparations and presentations reflected a new and simple style in rebellion to the *haute cuisine* of Escoffier, became popular and remains so today.

 MAJOR FOODS

Food consumption patterns throughout France parallel the diverse geography and ethnic influences. Over the past 24 years there has been a steady increase in the per capita daily calorie consumption for the French population. In 1979, the average French citizen consumed 3390 calories per day; in 2003 that number had risen to 3640. Within this time protein consumption remained pretty consistent at about 120 g per day, while fat consumption rose from 150 g/day in 1979 to 175 g/day in 2003. (FAO, 2004b). Throughout Europe, France is second to Spain in overall meat consumption.

France is divided into 22 regions and 96 departments of metropolitan France. A multitude of culinary specialties hail from each of these regions, each reflecting the foods most suited to the geography, climate, and ethnic/historical influences to the region. The coastal regions of Nord Pas de Calais and Picardy as well as Normandy and Brittany, and of course, Provence and Côte d'Azure, which is renowned for its *bouillabaisse*, are most noted for their fish and seafood dishes. The region of Toulouse is known for producing the finest sausage, which is used to make a specialty of the region, *cassoulet*, a hearty stew of *haricot blancs* (a white bean), pork, duck, goose, or lamb and sausage in a tomato-based sauce that is slow cooked over many hours.

Cheese and wine are integral to the French diet and their production is well regulated to ensure the finest products. Recognizing that foods produced in different regions will reflect the quality of the soil, as well as the quality of the air and climate, the French have implemented regulations that demand that certain food products be made only in their region of origin. These laws are called the *Appellation d'Origine Controlée* (AOC: "Appellation of Controlled Origin").

Alternate distinction of diet and food-consumption habits exist, including that of Waverly Root (1966) who divides France into three domains: butter, fat, and oil. The Domain of Butter includes Touraine, "The Golden Crescent" (Ile-de-France, Poitou, Anjou, Orléanais), "The Flat Lands" (Picardy, Champagne, Artois, Flanders), Normandy, Brittany, The Bordeaux Country, Burgundy, and "The Mountains" (Franche-Comté, Jura, Savoy, and Dauphiné). The Domain of Fat encompasses Alsace–Lorraine, "The Central Plateau" (Périgord, Auvergne, Marche, Limousin, Guienne), and Langdoc. The Domain of Oil includes Provence, Côte d'Azur, Nice, and the island of Corsica. Each of these domains mirrors the geography, climate, ethnic influences, and culinary styles of these regions.

 Protein Sources

France is the primary meat producer in the European Union. The traditional French diet dating back to the Celts has been rich in animal proteins. French cuisine, although reputed for being rich and elegant, has deep roots in the frugal and innovative culinary skills of French cooks. Many exquisite dishes have been created making use of virtually all parts of the animals (including offal); for example, *ris de veau* (veal sweetbreads; the thymus gland of the calf), *rognons* (kidneys), *cervelle(s)* (brains of lamb or calf), *andouille (andouillette)* (a sausage made of tripe), and *tripes à la mode de Caen* (beef tripe, with vegetables cooked in

water, cider, and Calvados (apple brandy), a specialty of Normandy. The more unusual protein sources consumed by the French include very rich dishes, for example, *foie gras d'oie* or *foie de canard* (liver of fattened goose or duck), *escargot de Bourgogne* (land snails prepared with butter, garlic, and parsley), and *cuisse de grenouille* (frog legs).

The types of meats in the French diet include beef, primarily from the beautiful white Charolais cow, veal, lamb, venison, and goat. Horse meat, once popular, is still consumed, although it has lost favor over generations. Pork is very popular and virtually every part of the pig is consumed (pig feet, bacon, sausages, and hams), both fresh and cured, and of course the pork meat and pork liver used in numerous terrine and pâté preparations. Pig meat provides the majority of the calories consumed from animal meat in the French diet.

The French love fish and seafood, although they are rarely prepared in the home but instead are consumed in restaurants in quantities equal to that of meats (Abramson, 2007, p. 51). Fish selections include monk fish, cod, salmon, turbot, and sole. Shellfish are also prized by the French; the exquisite Belon oyster from Brittany is world renowned for its silky texture and briny flavor. Clams and oysters are often eaten raw on the half shell but may also be served cooked. Mussels are also very popular and are always served cooked. Shrimp, lobsters, sea urchin, crayfish, squid, eel, and octopus are also consumed with great gusto.

Poultry plays a notable role in the French diet. Many regional specialties reflect the importance of poultry and fowl. *Coq au vin* (chicken in wine sauce) from the Burgundy region reflects the use of poultry and the fine wines produced in the region. *Confit de canard* (duck preserved by salt curing and slow cooking and then stored in its own fat) originates from the southwest regions of France and is very versatile in its uses. Game birds, such as quail and partridge, are eaten for special occasions. Turkey and goose are quite popular at Christmas. Rabbit is consumed more often in France than in the United States. Legumes are well represented in the diet: lentils, chickpeas, and fava beans are used in soups, baked in casseroles, and served in cold salads.

One cannot complete the discussion of protein sources in the French diet without addressing the significant role of cheese. The cheeses of France hold as prestigious a place in culinary appreciation as does wine. Cheeses are most often named for the region in which they are produced and are strictly regulated by the *Appellation d'Origine Controlée*. Cheese may be made from the milk of cows, goats, or sheep, and come in an astounding array of styles and textures. Some familiar cheeses of France include *roquefort* (a blue-veined, sheep's milk cheese) and *chèvre* (goat's milk cheese), which come in numerous shapes and consistencies; smooth and creamy, crumbly or firm. In addition, there are the popular *brie de meaux* and *gruyère de comté*. Cheese is eaten as part of a meal, used in cooking, and served as part of the dessert course.

 ## Starch Sources

Who can resist the crisp crust and chewy center of a fresh-baked *baguette*, the golden crispness of freshly fried *pommes frites* (French fries), or the savory richness of *gratin savoyard* (casserole of sliced potatoes with cheese and butter)? These are just a few common examples of the starches that are found in the French diet. Bread plays an integral role in the French diet; a meal is not complete without the inclusion of some form of bread. The vast array of shapes and sizes, as well as the many types of breads consumed, is well represented at any of France's local *boulangeries* (bakeries). The quality and artistry of artisan bakers is well respected throughout France.

Pasta, potatoes, rice, and an assortment of grains consumed in France reflect the diverse ethnic influences in the culinary traditions today. Pasta has been a part of the French culinary tradition for centuries. *Riz de Camargue* is a fragrant, nutty rice that is grown in the Camargue region of the South of France. French people do not eat much rice (about 7 kg/person per year). Despite this limited consumption, France must import rice yearly to meet local demand (FAO, 2004a). Rice is used in dessert preparations and as accompaniments to *entrées* and cold salads. Corn is not a commonly consumed starch in France. For many French people, corn is considered food for livestock. The Foreign Agricultural Service of the United States Department of Agriculture (FASUSDA; 2001) reports that France is the leading producer of processed sweet corn in Europe, although there has been a noted decline in consumption by the French due to growing concerns of genetically modified corn in the food supply. Couscous, a Moroccan wheat-based pasta, is very popular and consumed much in the way rice or pasta may accompany a meal.

Each year, per capita consumption of fresh potatoes by the French nears 30 kg (FASUSDA, 2008). The *pomme de terre* (potato) was introduced from the New World to France in the 17th century with little accep-

tance. In the 18th century a French chemist named A.A. Parmentier recommended its use as a solution to the ensuing famines devastating France at that time (FASUSDA, 2008). Since then, in their culinary zeal the French have created numerous preparations of the potato including the popular *pommes frites*, *croquettes*, *dauphinoise* (a gratin of sliced potatoes baked with cream, garlic, cheese, and egg), and *lyonnaise* (potatoes sautéed with onions).

 ## Fat Sources

The French diet is rich in variety in terms of fruits, vegetables, grains, and lean meats. Fat consumption is quite high in France. Bellisle (2005, p. 1870) remarks on the relationship between the "high intake of dietary fats (35–40% of total calories per day) and the surprisingly low rate of cardiovascular mortality compared with the other developed countries of Europe and the United States." The type of fat consumed is often particular to the region of France and the traditional preparation method of a food that originates from a specific region. Olive oil consumption is more prevalent in the southern regions, while animal fats (butter and lard) are more common in the western and northern regions. Some of the finest butters are produced in the northern regions of Brittany and Normandy. The term *cuisine au beurre*, the traditional butter-enriched style of cooking, illustrates the importance of butter as a cooking ingredient. While this rich style of cooking is less popular today, butter is still a staple ingredient in the fine and delicate pastries of France. Provençal often refers to dishes that are cooked with ingredients distinct to Provence, such as tomatoes and garlic, but most notably implies the inclusion of olive oil in the preparations. Duck fat, lard, and goose fat are found in the many dishes traditional to the northern and western regions, such as *cassoulet* and *confit de canard*. Canola oil is a common everyday cooking oil, and nut oils, such as hazelnut or walnut oil, are used to add a delicate nut flavor to cold-dressed dishes.

 ## Prominent Vegetables

Vegetables play a substantial role in the French diet. The World Health Organization's (WHO) Highlight on Health in France (2004) recommends a fruit and vegetable intake of more than 400 g per person per day, but the average intake in France in 1997 was 437 g/day. Vegetables are consumed as accompaniments to *entrées*, cooked within food preparations, served as an individual course, and eaten raw in salads. The use of herbs is integral to the subtle nuances of many dishes. Roots, leaves, flowers, stalks, and fruits of vegetables may appear throughout a meal. To identify the many different vegetables found in the typical French diet, one need only consider the regional specialties and seasonal offerings. In the South of France tomatoes, garlic, artichokes, zucchini (both the vegetable and the blossom), fennel, *haricot vert*, Swiss chard, and eggplant all play a prominent role in the diet. The warm climate and fertile land provide a year-round abundance of fresh vegetables. In the northern regions cabbage is prominent, either eaten in soups, stuffed, salted, or pickled in the Alsatian style. Most often, vegetables are eaten cooked unless served as part of a mixed salad or *crudités* (an arrangement of individually dressed raw vegetables). The variety is impressive and includes carrots, beets, cauliflower, fresh green beans, celery, sweet peppers, asparagus, salsify and celeriac, and a vast assortment of salad greens that may include *maché* (lambs lettuce), sorrel, spinach, romaine lettuce, *roquett* (arugula), and endive (curly and Belgian).

The discussion of vegetables in the French diet is not complete without paying homage to the mushroom. France is the one of the world's largest producers and exporters of cultivated mushrooms (Economic Research Service of the United States Department of Agriculture, 2004). Mushrooms used in cooking may be the cultivated *Champignons de Paris* or any of the numerous wild mushrooms such as the chanterelle or morel. Truffles are prized and very expensive, costing upward of $1000/kilo in French markets. The black truffle comes from Périgord and is foraged in the wild, usually under oak trees, with the assistance of either pigs or dogs especially trained for the task.

 ## Prominent Fruits

Fruit is abundant in the traditional French diet. Fruit is eaten fresh as snacks or at the end of a meal for dessert. Fruit is used for making some of the most sumptuous pastries, beverages, *confiture* (jams), liquors, and brandies. The grape, of course, is used to make some of the world's finest wines. Apples account for the largest share (22%) of fruit consumption in France (FA-SUSDA, 2000). Apples are central to the culinary style of Normandy, famous for its apple brandy called Calvados, fine apple cider, and apple-based desserts such as the classic *tarte tatin*. Introduced from Asia by the Romans, cherries and apricots are favorites. Peaches, pears, plums, and black currants, as well as a vast assortment of berries including strawberries, raspberries,

and the prized *fraises du bois* (wild strawberries), are consumed often when seasonally available or preserved as *confiture*. Citrus fruits are enjoyed fresh or as juice. The warm climate and intense sun of Provence make them ideal for growing figs, pomegranates, and olives.

 ## Spices and Seasonings

Subtle blending of flavors and use of spices and herbs as enhancements to flavor are established rules in French cooking. Herbs and spices should never overpower the flavors of the foods with which they are cooked. Salt is used judiciously and has a long history in France. Salt is harvested in Breton, Ile de Ré, and Aigues-Mortes. These salts have distinct flavors; the popular *fleur de sel* and *sel gris*, with its gray hue, are just two examples. The importance and use of salt in the French diet dates back to France's earliest history and its use as a preservation method for meats.

Herbs and spices are used individually to complement flavors and are often found in traditional combinations that are used repeatedly in preparations. Examples of common herbs and spices include (1) *quatre épices*, a mix of pepper, cinnamon, nutmeg, and cloves; (2) *herb de Provence*, a southern specialty that may include rosemary, marjoram, basil, bay leaf, thyme, and lavender flowers; (3) *fines herbes*, a standard combination of northern origin that consists of parsley, chervil, tarragon, and chives; and (4) the *bouquet garni*, which is used to flavor soups and sauces and is traditionally tied in a small pouch and removed after the flavors have been steeped into the dish, and is composed of thyme, parsley, and bay leaf.

Mustard and vinegar play key roles as both condiments and cooking ingredients. Vinegar is made from wine grapes (either red or white) and can be flavored with herbs. It is used in salad dressings, as marinades, and for adding an acidic tang to cooked dishes. Mustard comes in different styles and may be smooth and mild or hot and grainy. It is used to make sauces and marinades for poultry as well as served as a condiment.

 ## Beverages

Coffee is one of the most popular beverages in France. The traditional French coffee is a dark roast similar to Italian espresso and served either black (*café noir*) or with hot milk (*café au lait*). *Café au lait* is consumed with the morning meal from a large bowl (breakfast cup) and is considered a nourishing beverage because of the large quantity of milk consumed. Black coffee, served in small cups (*demitasse*), may finish a meal or provide a midday boost. Tea is also very popular; the health benefits of teas have been recognized and tea consumption is on the rise in France. Herbal teas, also known as tisanes, are infusions of herbs and flowers, such as chamomile, and are often served after meals or to the infirmed for its traditional healing qualities.

France has about the lowest per capita consumption of milk in Europe. After infancy and childhood, milk rarely serves as a beverage. Milk is used to make hot chocolate, *café au lait*, is used in cooking preparations and rich desserts (whole milk, cream, and *crème fraiche*), and is used in breakfast cereals.

French bottled waters hold a very prestigious and profitable share of the bottled-water market with notable brands, such as Evian®, Volvic®, and Perrier®, being popular worldwide. In France per capita consumption of bottled water has jumped from 27.3 gallons in 1997 to 37.7 gallons in 2002. (Global Bottled Water Market, n.d.). While bottled-water consumption has increased, tap water remains the primary drinking-water source in France.

Soft drinks are gaining in popularity throughout France. Mirroring global consumption trends, soda consumption in France is on the rise. Soft drinks other than bottled sodas may include sweet fruit, herbal, almond, or mint-flavored *sirops* (syrups), which are added to water for a light, flavorful beverage.

The legal age for alcohol consumption in France is 16 years. Many parents do not allow or approve of their teenage children drinking outside of the home; however, wine is often consumed at home with meals, and children may be introduced to wine at a young age. To foster a sense of unity it is common practice to add a spoonful of wine to the water glass of the children at the table.

Beer has a long history in France dating back to the ale consumed by the Gauls. Per capita beer consumption nears the bottom of the list for all European Union nations. Beer consumption is highest in the leading beer-making regions of France: Nord, Pas de Calais, Alsace–Lorraine, and Brittany.

A fine hard cider hails from the northwestern regions, which are recognized for their bountiful apple production. While cider is not as popular throughout the rest of France, it is a traditional and frequently consumed alcoholic beverage in Normandy and Brittany.

The French are renowned for their fine wines. The history and tradition of wine making is synonymous with the regions of France where wines are produced. Wine is consumed daily with meals and used in a multitude of cooking preparations. Wine-producing locals

are identified by more than 100 *terriors*, a term reflecting a group of vineyards from a particular region, and a specific appellation, having the same quality soil, climate conditions, grapes, and vintner, which result in a specific and highly regulated quality of the wine. Some of the more prominent wine-producing regions in France include Alsace, Burgundy, Bordeaux, the Loire Valley, and Champagne. French wines are often the standard by which other wines of the world are judged.

France is celebrated for its fine cognacs and fragrant *eaux-de-vie* (water of life, a distilled alcohol made from fruits such as pear, raspberry, and plums). *Pastis* is an anis-flavored liquor that gained popularity after the prohibition of absinthe, which also had an anis flavor. Many of the distinct liquors, brandies, and cordials have a history within monastic sects, such as Chartreuse, Benedictine, and Cointreau.

 Desserts

The French are legendary for their rich and delicate dessert specialties. While sweets and desserts do not play a very prominent role in the daily meal plans of the French, there is great appreciation and pride for the delectable specialties that are prepared or purchased from the local *boulangerie* and *patisserie* (pastry shops). After the introduction of sugar and chocolate to France, the confectioners, patissier, and chocolatiers became notable artisans. French chocolates are ranked as some of the world's finest. Popular artisan candies include nougats, pralines, and exquisite hand-blown sugar confections that look like glass sculpture.

The making of cakes and fine pastries is an art form and a valued profession. Breakfast pastries include brioche, croissant, *pain au chocolat* (a croissant filled with dark chocolate), and apple turnovers. Special occasions may warrant the preparation or purchase of a cake. *Mousse au chocolat*, *crème caramel*, or *crème brûlée* (a rich cream-and-egg custard topped with caramelized sugar), fresh fruit tarts, or the *Saint Honoré* (choux pastry filled with a rich pastry cream) are all favorites.

The rustic and simple *tarte tatin* (apple tart) or *clafoutis* (a fruit-and-custard baked dessert) may end a weekend meal with friends. Frozen treats are much loved. *Sorbet* (ices made from puréed fruits and sugar) and *glace* (ice cream) come in a vast assortment of flavors such as chocolate and vanilla as well as honey, lavender, and numerous fruit flavors.

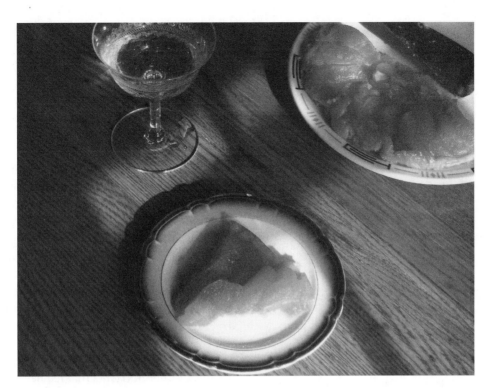

Tarte Tartin
Courtesy of the author

FOODS WITH CULTURAL SIGNIFICANCE

Eating foods that are well prepared and from the freshest ingredients is very important to the French. Wine and bread carry special significance. Bread is a dietary staple and has also carried strong religious connotations for the French throughout history. A meal is not considered complete without bread. Wine has a long and complex history in France and is considered restorative, strengthening, and nourishing.

TYPICAL DAY'S MENU

Snacking is very uncommon in France, although it has gained some acceptance among the younger generations. The traditional French meal plan is three meals a day without snacks, or perhaps a small snack with coffee or tea late in the day. The meal is made up of different components that may include the *entrée* (first course) of soup or *crudités*, followed by the *plat principal* (main dish) and then a salad course, and end with some cheese, fruit, and coffee. Bread and wine accompany the meals. The first meal of the day is *petit déje-*

uner (breakfast), the basis for the continental breakfast that consists of *café au lait* and bread spread with jam and butter. Children often drink hot chocolate with breakfast, and breakfast cereals have gained in popularity. Lunch is a 2-hour event and a full multicourse meal is often consumed. Leisurely meals are integral to the French way of life. Dinner is often a simply prepared meal at home that may include a simple starter of soup or *crudités*, and a main course of meat or fish accompanied by a vegetable and either a grain or potato. Weekend meals are somewhat more elaborate and provide an opportunity for socializing.

HOLIDAY MENUS

There are a number of public holidays on the French calendar: New Year's Day, Easter Monday, Labor Day, Ascension Day, World War II Victory Day, Bastille Day, Assumption, All Saints Day, Armistice Day, and Christmas Day. Special holiday or celebratory meals or dishes may be served for each of these occasions. Holidays and special occasions are opportunities to prepare traditional and regional fare. For Christmas the food choices differ by region, but it is common to celebrate the day with *le réveillon* (awakening), a festive late-night meal shared by the family. This is the culinary highlight of the Advent season. Turkey or goose may be served as the center of the meal and traditional blood pudding (*boudin noir*) may be prepared. Special desserts are offered and may include *la bûche de Noël*, a cake roll traditionally made of chocolate and chestnut, shaped and decorated to look like a log. In the South of France *le pain calendeau* (a Christmas loaf) is served, and tradition holds that a part of this loaf should be given to a person less fortunate than oneself. The meal is accompanied by the best wines, and champagne is served with dessert.

 ## HEALTH BELIEFS AND CONCERNS

The French believe that to be healthy one must live life by three principles: balance, moderation, and pleasure. Eating is just one of the many ways the French express a life of these three principles. Eating a diet based on variety and small portions allows for enjoyment of rich energy-dense foods balanced with light nutrient-dense foods. The nutritional quality of a meal is only part of the equation; appreciation of the expertise of preparation, marriage of flavors and textures, and, of course, the company with whom a meal is shared is integral to the French dining experience. Meals are rarely rushed: the French "lunch hour" is actually a 2-hour respite that allows families and friends to gather for the midday meal either at home, at a café, or at the company restaurant. An active lifestyle where one can maintain a balance of work life and recreation is of great importance. To ensure this balance France mandates a 35-hour work week and a minimum of 5 weeks paid vacation. France prizes the health and well-being of its population. In 2000 the WHO issued a first-ever comparative analysis of 191 of the world's healthcare systems. The WHO ranked the French healthcare system as the "best in the world" (Library of Congress Federal Research Division, 2007, p. 11).

 ## GENERAL HEALTH AND NUTRITIONAL INDICATORS SUMMARY

When compared with other industrialized nations, France ranks among the best for health and mortality indicators (Library of Congress Federal Research Di-

vision, 2007). A review of the UNICEF Basic Health Indicators for the Country of France (UNICEF, 2007b) reveals that France ranks 173rd (of 189) worldwide for under-5-years infant mortality rate. The Population Reference Bureau (n.d.) reports a life expectancy at birth for both sexes to be 81 years, which is among the highest in the world.

In the European Nutrition and Health Report 2004 Executive Summary, Elmadfa and Weichselbaum (2004) detail reported intake data of selected nutrients in European adults ages 19–64 years for 13 European countries including France. The intake data are compared with recommended values using both Eurodiet 2000 and Scientific Committee for Food 1993. The report reveals that the average protein intake as a percentage of total calories was above the recommended upper level of 15% of total calorie intake. Carbohydrate intake for men and women was 38–53% of total calorie intake, below the recommended >55%. The average dietary fiber intake was also lower than recommended. Other nutrients that fell below recommended intake levels included folate and calcium. On average, fat intake, particularly total fat, saturated fat, and cholesterol, was high. The authors note that France and Hungary have the highest average cholesterol intake for both men and women of reviewed nations. Reported sodium intake was also markedly above recommended values.

There has been much attention paid to the "French Paradox." Bellisle (2005, p. 1870) addresses the question as to why "despite a high intake of dietary fats (35–40% of daily energy), cardiovascular mortality in France appears surprisingly low compared with other developed countries of Europe and the United States." Popular speculation includes the practice of daily intake of red wine and the "Mediterranean diet" intake pattern; however, while a diet rich in fruits and vegetables, fish, and vegetable oils proves health promoting, and moderate intake of wine has been associated with beneficial health effects, it is important to recognize that local dietary patterns correlate to overall health outcomes. Higher rates of cardiovascular disease (CVD) are reported in the northern regions of France where diets are higher in saturated fat and cholesterol. Conversely, in the southern regions, where a Mediterranean diet is consumed, lower rates of CVD are reported.

Recent trends show an increase in the prevalence of overweight and obesity in France, with rates reported to be higher for men than women. The International Diabetes Federation (n.d.) reports the prevalence of diabetes (types 1 and 2) in French adults (male and female) for 2007 to be 8.4% of the total population and a projected increase to a prevalence of 10.5% of the total population by 2025. Increased rates of CVD, diabetes, hypercholesterolemia, and obesity rates for adults and children have been reported. These data illustrate the anticipated increase in comorbidities associated with the rising rates of obesity and overweight as well as westernization of the diet and intake habits for the population.

In 2000, according to the WHO, the French healthcare system ranked high in overall population health, health system responsiveness, and distribution of services (Library of Congress Federal Research Division, 2007). Remaining true to their commitment to the health and well-being of the population, in 2001 the French Ministry of Health launched the *Programme National Nutrition Santé* (PNNS) to investigate and address dietary intake and associated health parameters. Findings by Estaquio et al. (2008) confirm that healthy diet and lifestyle are associated with a lower risk of chronic diseases, particularly in men, thereby verifying the importance of the PNNS and subsequent French nutritional recommendations. Hercberg, Chat-Young, and Chauliac (2008) explain the PNNS, the rationale for its inception, the ideology of its principles, and current results. The PNNS addresses nine priority objectives for the population. Hercberg et al. (2008) identify the following programmatic objectives: five objectives focus on dietary intake of fruit and vegetables, calcium, vitamin D fat intake, carbohydrates, and fiber and alcohol consumption; three objectives relate to three nutritional markers (cholesterol, blood pressure, and obesity); the ninth objective addresses physical activity. The ideology of the PNNS reflects the rich culinary traditions of the culture in its recognition and inclusion of cultural, physiological, and social aspects of eating, highlighting freedom of individual food choice, pleasure, hospitality, and gastronomy in the dietary recommendations and educational approach. The methodology is a positive behavioral approach stressing healthful inclusion rather than dietary restriction. The overall concept of PNNS is to promote the idea that health is compatible with pleasure.

Prior to the initiation of PNNS, France had no existing nutrition policies in place. Hercberg et al. (2008, p. 76) report that France's PNNS is "considered one of the most advanced public health nutrition programs in Europe."

COMMUNICATION AND COUNSELING TIPS

Hall and Hall (1990) describe the French as high-context communicators who prefer subtlety and discretion to bluntness and detail. The French are known to talk around an issue. In a counseling setting it is important to listen for nuances and hidden messages in their communications. It is very important to allow a fair amount of time for customary conversation before getting to business; this enhances the comfort level and allows for more openness. Hall and Hall (1990) also describe the French communication style as one that is multisensory (the use of body language is apparent), and direct eye contact is of great importance.

The French tend to live in the here and now. Hall and Hall (1990, p. 89) explain that long-term planning is especially difficult for the French. The French are also a pragmatic and logical people who have a keen understanding of "what will work and won't, they like strategies that produce results" (Hall and Hall, 1990, p. 104); therefore, in a counseling situation, setting short-term, achievable goals with clear and concise plans of action would be the most appropriate with this population.

TABLE 13-1 Primary Language of Food Names with English and Phonetic Translation

French Term	Phonetic Translation	English Translation
Une baguette	Oon bah-get	A baguette (long thin loaf of bread)
Un petit pan	uh ptee pan	A bread roll
Une glace	Oon glahss	An ice cream
Le café	Ler Cah-feh	The coffee
Le fromage	Ler Froh-mahsh	The cheese
L'huile	Lweel	The oil
La confiture	Lah Cohn-fee-toor	The jam
Le lait	Ler leh	The milk
La viande	Lah Vee-ahnd	The meat
Le sel	Ler sel	The salt
Le pain	Ler pan	The bread
Le beurre	Ler ber	The butter
Le vin	Ler van	The wine
Les œufs	Leh-zerf	The eggs
Les fruits	Leh frwee	The fruits
Les pâtes	Leh paht	The pasta
Saucisson à l'ail	Soh-see-sohn ah lye	Garlic sausage
Pâté	Pah-teh	Paté
Les légumes	Leh leh-goom	The vegetables
Rôti de bœuf	Roh-tee der berf	Roast beef
Rôti de porc	Roh-tee der por	Roast pork
Bœuf aux champignons	Berf oh shahm-pee-nyohn	Beef stew with mushrooms in wine sauce
Bœuf en daube	Berf ahn dohb	Cut beef cooked in a thick wine sauce
Tarte à l'oignon	Tart ah loh-nyohn	Onion pie
Pommes de terre	Pom der tair	Potatoes

Compiled from Ellis, D.L. (2005).

FEATURED RECIPE

Crème Caramel

½ cup of sugar (for the caramel)   3 whole eggs

⅓ cup of sugar   2 egg yolks

1 cup milk   1 tbsp. cognac

1 cup heavy cream

1. Preheat the oven to 325°F.
2. In a small heavy-bottom sauce pan, melt the ½ cup of sugar until it becomes a golden rich caramel color.
3. Pour a thin layer of caramel into the bottom of six ovenproof ramekins, and allow to cool completely.
4. In a large bowl stir together the ⅓ cup of sugar, milk, heavy cream, eggs, egg yolks, and cognac. Strain through a fine sieve and fill ramekins to within ¼ inch of the top.
5. Bake the *crème caramels* in a water bath for 30–40 minutes. Allow to cool completely, then chill for at least 1 hour.
6. To serve, loosen the *crème caramel* by running a thin knife around the inside of the ramekin, and invert on a dessert plate.

More recipes are available at http://nutrition.jbpub.com/foodculture/

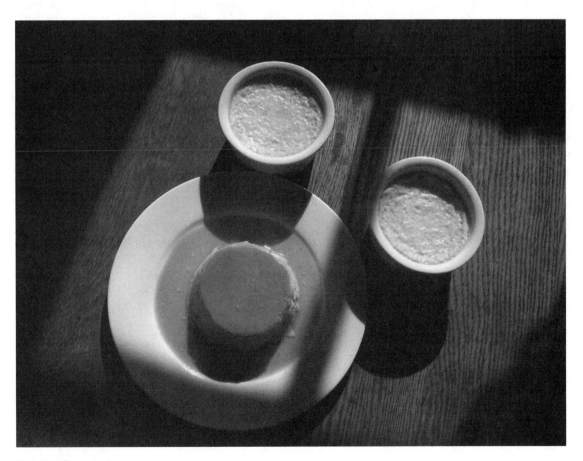

Crème Caramel
Courtesy of the author

REFERENCES

Abramson, J. (2007). *Food culture in France*. Westport, CT: Greenwood Press.

Bellisle, F. (2005). Nutrition and health in France: Dissecting the French paradox. *Journal of the American Dietetic Association, 105*, 1870–1873.

Economic Research Service of the United States Department of Agriculture. (2004). *Mushrooms: U.S. import-eligible countries; world production and exports.* http://www.ers.usda.gov/Data/FruitVegPhyto/Data/veg-mushroom.xls

Ellis, D.L. (2005). *Just enough French: How to get by and be easily understood.* (2nd ed.). New York: McGraw-Hill.

Elmadfa, I., & Weichselbaum, E. (2004). European Nutrition and Health Report Executive Summary. *Annals of Nutrition & Metabolism, 48*(2), 1–16. http://www.univie.ac.at/enhr/downloads/enhr04sum.pdf/

Estaquio, C., Castetbon, K., Kesse-Guyot, E., Bertrais, S., Deschamps, V., Dauchet, L., et al. (2008). The French national nutrition and health program score is associated with nutritional status and risk of major chronic diseases. *Journal of Nutrition, 138*(5), 136. http://jn.nutrition.org/cgi/reprint/138/5/946/

Food and Agriculture Organization of the United Nations (FAO). (2004a). *International year of rice.* Retrieved February 22, 2008, from http://www.fao.org/rice2004/en/p5.htm/

Food and Agriculture Organization of the United Nations (FAO). (2004b). *Statistical yearbook (FAOUNSY). Country profile: France.* Retrieved March 1, 2008, from http://www.fao.org/ag/againfo/resources/en/pubs_sap.html/

Foreign Agricultural Service of the United States Department of Agriculture (FASUSDA). (2000). *Organic updates: Fresh organic deciduous fruit production overseas.* Retrieved March 14, 2008, from http://www.fas.usda.gov/htp2/circular/2000/00-11/organics.htm/

Foreign Agricultural Service of the United States Department of Agriculture (FASUSDA). (2001). *Processed sweet corn in selected countries.* Retrieved February 19, 2008, from http://www.fas.usda.gov/htp/Hort_Circular/2001/01-12/Stats/procwc.pdf/

Foreign Agricultural Service of the United States Department of Agriculture (FASUSDA). (2008).

Global Bottled Water Market. (n.d.). *The 2002 statistics.* Retrieved March 23, 2008, from http://www.bottledwater.org/Feature_Stats1.doc/

Hall, E.T., & Hall M.R. (1990). *Understanding cultural differences: German, French, and Americans.* Yarmouth, ME: Intercultural Press.

Hercberg, S., Chat-Young, S., & Chauliac, M. (2008). The French national nutrition and health program: 2001–2006–2010. *International Journal of Public Health, 53*, 68–77.

International Diabetes Federation. (n.d.). *Diabetes atlas.* Retrieved April 27, 2009, from http://www.eatlas.idf.org/index80fd.html/

Library of Congress Federal Research Division. (2007). *Country profile: France (2007).* Retrieved March 3, 2008, from http://lcweb2.loc.gov/frd/cs/profiles/France.pdf/

More, M. (2006, November 21). *More longtime couples in France prefer l'amour without marriage.* Washington Post, A22. http://www.washingtonpost.com/wpdyn/content/article/2006/11/20/AR2006112001272 ml/

Population Reference Bureau. (n.d.). *Data by geography: France.* Retrieved April 30, 2009, from http://www.prb.org/Datafinder/Geography/Summary.aspx?region=190&region_type=2/

Root, W.L. (1966). *The foods of France.* New York: Vintage Books.

UNICEF. (2007a). *The state of the world's children. Women and children, the double dividend of gender equality.* Retrieved April 14, 2009, from http://www.unicef.org/sowc07/statistics/tables.php/

UNICEF. (2007b). *At a glance: France—statistics.* Retrieved April 30, 2009, from http://www.unicef.org/infobycountry/france_statistics.html?q=printme/

World Health Organization (WHO). (2004). *Highlight on health in France: 2004.* Retrieved February 13, 2008, from http://www.euro.who.int/document/E88547.pdf/

Greece

Elizabeth Metallinos-Katsaras, PhD, RD

 CULTURE AND WORLD REGION

A classic view of Greece is "the birthplace of democracy," although Greek Americans often quip "We gave the light to the world and then we lost it." This reflects the contrast in views and perceptions between people who are Greek, or of Greek descent, and those who are not of Greek descent. This chapter describes the traditional and contemporary food habits of Greeks, factors that influence them, the health and nutritional status of Greeks, and communication styles and counseling strategies that are sensitive to the influence of Greek culture. Because people of Greek descent living outside of Greece comprise a large percentage of those worldwide, this chapter incorporates, when relevant, research on both Greeks living in Greece and those of the Greek diaspora.

Traditionally, Greece has been patriarchal, with the men working outside of the home and the women serving as the homemakers (i.e., cooking, cleaning and dec-

orating the home, taking care of the children), and has been group- rather than individual oriented. Moreover, traditional Greek culture has been greatly influenced by its Greek Orthodox religion. The attitude of traditional Greeks is that the well-being and needs of immediate and extended family are extremely important, more important than those of the individual. Children are valued and indulged. Parents view sacrifice for their children's well-being as their responsibility often even when the children are adults. Education is highly valued. Although traditionally this implied the education of boys and men, girls' and women's education has become a priority. Elders are valued and respected.

One word that describes an overarching principle of Greek culture is *philotimo* (pronounced feel-o-tee-mo) whose literal translation is love of honor. One's *philotimo* is fundamentally reflected in one's actions, particularly with respect to recognition of obligation to others and reciprocating appropriately. It is a pervasive value that frequently determines many individual and family actions. Being *philotimo* is important even if one has an indirect obligation. For example, if you have a friend who goes to Greece and you refer them to a friend of yours there who shows your friend around (and perhaps invites him or her to dinner), then *you* are also indebted, not just the recipient of the Greek person's hospitality. There are many facets of everyday life that are influenced by *philotimo*.

Hospitality is also greatly valued in Greek culture. Showing hospitality is reflected in people's willingness to welcome people into their homes, provide refreshments, and be gracious even if the guests are not particularly agreeable. Being hospitable also means that even if one has an appointment, an uninvited guest is never turned away. Traditionally, people do not call before visiting; however, this is changing.

Greek culture is one of many cultures that are relationship oriented rather than time oriented. Moreover, relationships are valued over accomplishments. Time, and being on time, are not as important as making certain one is respectful, showing *philotimo*, being hospitable, and taking care of family. Greek culture does not place great value on punctuality, although, in westernized countries, where being on time is greatly valued, there has been some adaptation by Greeks, particularly if one is a professional or has an appointment with a professional (e.g., a doctor); however, in the social context, one may invite a Greek family for dinner at 6 PM and they may arrive 1 or 2 hours later.

Although the Greek census does not collect data on ethnicity, there are data to suggest that the majority of people living in Greece are of Greek descent, with only 10% of the population being immigrants. The main religion practiced by Greeks is Eastern Orthodox Christianity; approximately 98% of Greeks living in Greece are Greek Orthodox (U.S. State Department, 2008). Muslim, Jewish, Catholic, Protestant, and other religious communities comprise about 1.3% of the population living in Greece (U.S. State Department, 2008). In the United States 0.6% of the adult population is affiliated with the Christian Orthodox Church, although only 0.3% are Greek Orthodox (Pew Research Center, 2008). The word "Orthodox" comes from the Greek words *orthos*, meaning correct, and *doxa*, which means "worship." The Greek Orthodox Church has greatly influenced the food habits and patterns of Greeks throughout its history because of the great number of dietary restrictions during periods of fasting. According to the Greek Orthodox Church, "fasting" is not only abstinence from food but also from bad habits and sin. (Metropolitan Maximos, 2008).

Between 180 and 200 days per year are "fasting" days. Fasting in the Greek Orthodox Church is a selective fast, meaning that complete abstention from food is not required. On fast days all animals, their products, and frequently fish are excluded from the diet. This includes meat, poultry, eggs, all animal fats (i.e., butter or lard), dairy, and oil, although the latter is often not observed by laity. Fish is sometimes allowed during specific fasting periods (noted below). Shellfish is also allowed on many fasting days. As given by Mastrantonis (n.d.), the major official fasting periods of the Greek Orthodox Church are as follows (degree of adherence to these rules varies greatly; some may decide to eat oil throughout Great Lent, for example):

- Wednesdays and Fridays every week of the year, except the week after Christmas, Easter, and Pentecost.
- Great Lent (48 days preceding Easter): On the annunciation (March 25) and Palm Sunday, fish is allowed. Shellfish, wine, and oil are allowed on Saturday and Sundays.
- Fast of the Apostles: This fast ranges from 1–6 weeks depending on the year. Fish consumption is allowed.
- Fast of the Dormition of the Theotokos (Virgin Mary): This fast is from August 1 to 15.
- Christmas fast (40 days preceding Christmas): Fish consumption is allowed.

There are few data on the prevalence of fasting among those affiliated with the Greek Orthodox Church. One estimate suggests that one in three individuals in Greece score high on their adherence to religious practices promoted by the Greek Orthodox Church (Chliaoutakis et al., 2002). These practices include religious fasting, although many other components of religiosity were included, such as attending church and praying; thus, the prevalence of religious fasting is likely lower than the one third reported. Researchers have noted that many of the health-conferring properties of the traditional Greek diet may largely be due to the Orthodox Church's dietary recommendations (Sarri, Tzanakis, Linardakis, Mamalakis, & KaFatos, 2003; Sarri, Linardakis, Bervanaki, Tzanakis, & KaFatos, 2004). In a study of a small sample of adults living on the island of Crete, Greek Orthodox fasting practices were associated with significant declines in energy intake, dietary cholesterol, total fat, saturated fat, trans fat, and protein during times of fasting (Sarri et al., 2004) with concomitant declines by the end of the fasting period in total cholesterol, low-density lipoprotein (LDL) cholesterol, LDL/HDL ratio, and body mass index (BMI) (Sarri, Linardakis, Codrington, & Kafatos, 2003), but not in blood pressure (Sarri, Linardakis, Codrington, & Kafatos, 2007).

Greece is a small country located in southern Europe that borders the Aegean Sea, the Ionian Sea, and the Mediterranean Sea, and lies between Albania and Turkey. According to a 2005 estimate the population of Greece is 11,104,000 (U.S. State Department, 2008). Greece attained its independence from Turkey in 1830. Greece's government has been democratically elected, although there have been short periods of autocratic rule in its history. The following are the major political parties in Greece representing in turn, the far right, center, and far left: New Democracy (ND), Panhellenic Socialist Movement (PASOK), Communist Party of Greece (KKE), Coalition of the Left (SYNASPISMOS), and Popular Orthodox Rally (LAOS) (U.S. State Department, 2008). Greek education is free, and educational attainment is relatively high with 9 years of schooling compulsory and 97.5% literacy (U.S. State Department, 2008).

 ## LANGUAGE

The primary and official language spoken in Greece is Greek. Modern Greek preserves many of the elements of ancient Greek; the latter's roots date back at least 3500 years. Albanian is spoken by about 700,000 people in Greece, and English is the most commonly spoken second language (U.S. State Department, 2008).

 ## CULTURE HISTORY

Greek culture's roots date back 3500 years (U.S. State Department, 2008). The maritime empire of the Minoans existed on the island of Crete during the second millennium BC. The Minoans were replaced by the mainland Greek Mycenaeans whose language was based on an ancient Greek dialect. The population of Greece became more ethnically diverse after the Roman, Byzantine, and Ottoman Empires (U.S. State Department, 2008).

Greek society, even today, has been influenced by its history of occupation by the Ottoman Turks. Constantinople (present-day Istanbul) fell to the Ottoman Turks in 1453; prior to that time, this part of Turkey was part of Greece. Other parts of Greece, including some of the islands, became occupied soon afterward.

It was not until the early 1830s, after almost 400 years of Turkish occupation, that Greece attained its independence, although parts of modern Greece did not officially become a part of Greece until the 20th century (Clogg, 2001). According to historians, the Ottoman rule altered the evolutionary trajectory of Greek society in comparison with that of western Europe, because it isolated the Greeks from the following important historical movements: the Renaissance, the Reformation, the scientific revolution, the Enlightenment, the French Revolution, and the Industrial Revolution (Clogg, 2001). It also segregated Greek Orthodoxy from the expansion of the then Catholic Church.

The enmity between Greece and Turkey, which has its roots in that time, continues to this day, although there have been many instances in recent history of Turkish and Greek collaboration. For example, their relationship improved considerably when both Greece and Turkey sent assistance to one another during recent earthquakes (Clogg, 2001), and Greek and Turkish musicians have recently collaborated on artistic projects (e.g., "The Music of Cyprus"). It is quite apparent to Greeks and Turks alike that there are many similarities between the two cultures particularly in cuisine and music.

Throughout their history Greeks have immigrated to other countries (Clogg, 2001). This historical emigration underlies their description as "a people of the Diaspora." Depending on the source, it is estimated that between 3 and 7 million people of Greek descent live outside of Greece. Countries to which a significant number of Greeks emigrated during the 19th and 20th centuries include Egypt, southern Russia, the United States, Australia, and Germany (Clogg, 2001). The United States has one of the largest populations of Greeks living outside of Greece. According to the 2000 U.S. Census figures, there were 1,153,307 people of Greek descent living in the United States at that time (U.S. Census Bureau, 2004); however, other estimates note that 3 million U.S. residents claim Greek descent (U.S. State Department, 2008). The highest population of people of Greek descent live in the following five states: New York, California, Illinois, Massachusetts, and Florida. Large populations of Greek descent also live in Cyprus, the United Kingdom, and Australia.

 ## FOOD HISTORY WITHIN THE CULTURE

The precise components and composition of the traditional Greek diet is to some degree debatable, because it appears to depend on the region (Ferro-Luzzi, James, & Kafatos, 2002; Kochilas, 2001; Kromhout, 1989) and the time period (Matalas, 2006) in which Greeks lived. In addition, most information available on the "traditional Greek diet" was originally derived from research by Ancel Keys in the Seven Country Study in the 1960s (Kromhout, 1989) on a small sample of men who lived on two islands in Greece (Corfu and Crete). In that study, Greece became known for its low rate of cardiovascular disease (Keys, 1980); however, some researchers have noted that the dietary information derived from that study may not be accurate, particularly with respect to total dietary fat (Ferro-Luzzi et al., 2002). Specifically, there is some discrepancy as to the actual fat content of the diet; the chemical analysis of the Cretan sample estimated that 36–38% of energy came from fat (primarily olive oil), and the analysis based on food composition tables yielded a value of 42% of energy from fat.

What, therefore, constitutes the traditional Greek diet? Some evidence from historical data suggests that in 19th-century rural Greece, cereals (e.g., wheat, barley, rye, and corn), probably in the form of bread, and legumes, cheese, olive oil, and fruits and vegetables (although the latter two could not be quantified), comprised the rural Greek diet. Some meat and fish were also consumed, but in small quantities (Matalas, 2006). It is noteworthy that much of the "bread" consumed is in the form of dried bread known as rusks. (Drying the bread preserves it from spoiling; throwing away bread has traditionally been considered sacrilegious.) Data from pre-World War II Greece (i.e., about the 1930s) suggest that these same foods were dietary staples, but potatoes also became an important component with a concomitant decline in legumes. In addition, meat consumption appeared to increase somewhat (Matalas, 2006). During those two time periods, olive oil was the primary added fat to the diet, but estimated quantities were much lower than those derived from the Keys research in the 1960s, suggesting that the traditional Greek diet did not contain as much added olive oil as suggested by the research primarily in Crete (Ferro-Luzzi et al., 2002; Matalas, 2006).

Regional differences also exist (Kochilas, 2001; Kromhout, 1989). For example, based on the Seven Countries study in the 1960s, more fish was consumed in Corfu, and more milk in Crete (Kromhout, 1989). In the mountainous regions of Greece (i.e., regions of Epirus, Roumeli, and Thessaly), milk, cheese, and yogurt comprised a very important part of the diet (Kochilas, 2001).

Traditional Greek diet (again, based primarily on the Cretan diet) is also described as consisting of fruits and vegetables (comprised in large part of wild plants), cereals (mostly in the form of bread), fish, cheese/yogurt, olive oil and olives, eggs, nuts, and moderate wine consumption (Simopoulos, 2001). The consensus derived from research that describes the traditional Greek diet is that it is rich in fruits and vegetables (including wild plants), cereals (primarily eaten in the form of wholegrain bread), olives, olive oil as the primary added fat, low to moderate dairy (mostly in the form of cheese or yogurt), and, according to data from the 20th century onwards, potatoes. The extent to which fish and milk products contribute to the traditional Greek diet appears to vary by region as does the amount of added olive oil.

Many commonly eaten Greek dishes, even today, are cooked on the stovetop and not in the oven. Until recently (i.e., the past 20–30 years) Greeks did not have their own ovens; therefore, for many people cooking on the stovetop was much more convenient. Prior to the acquisition of ovens by the majority of the population, many Greeks took their prepared (uncooked) dishes to the local privately owned ovens; these were often bread shops that charged for use of their ovens. One would drop off the dish in the morning and pick it up around noon or shortly thereafter. If there was anything to add to the dish, it would be provided to the baker and he would add it.

Although the traditional Greek diet has been touted, with good reason, as health promoting (Simopoulos, 2001), the plethora of evidence in support of its retention has failed to prevent the dramatic changes, over the past two decades, in the diets of many Greeks living in Greece and of the Greek diaspora. The dietary patterns of Greeks in the 21st century vary not only by the country and region (i.e., urban vs rural) of residence, but also by age, generation, and degree of adherence to religious fasting. Contributing to the evolving Greek diet is the documented drastic shift from the traditional rural way of life to the postindustrial era. This shift in a country's way of life has taken 150 years in many other countries; however, in Greece, this occurred over a much shorter period of time (Softas-Nall & Baldo, 2000). There is evidence that there have been drastic shifts in the dietary habits of Greeks living in Greece over the past 30–40 years (Kafatos, Verhagen, Moschandreas, Apostolaki, Van Westerop, 2000); westernized food habits have become incorporated into the food habits of Greeks, especially in the younger generation.

Kafatos et al. (2000) illustrated this shift quite dramatically by depicting typical diets for a 7-day period based on the research by Keys in the 1960s and data collected on adolescents in 1994. The diets included three meals (breakfast, lunch, and dinner) as well as a mid-morning and mid-afternoon snack. Table 14-1 was derived from the menus published by Kafatos et al. (2000) by summing the total frequencies of some of the major food groups and other food categories. What is truly astounding is the contrast in the dietary patterns between the 1960s male sample and the adolescents living on the same island in 1994. Frequency of consumption of healthful food groups or types, such as fruits and vegetables, whole grains, and fish, is much lower in the 1994 adolescent menu than in that of the adults in the 1960s, with concomitantly higher frequency of less-healthful food groups or types such as sweetened beverages, foods with added sugar, French fries, and red meat. A case in point is fruit and vegetable consumption. According to the menus published by Kafatos et al. (2000), Cretan males in the 1960s ate fruits and vegetables (excluding potatoes) 39 times a week (or almost 6 times a day). In contrast, adolescents in the 1990s consumed them 10 times a week (or about 1.5 times a day). Similarly, whole-grain products were consumed typically 11 times

a week in the menus of the 1960s, whereas among adolescents in the 1990s whole-grain products did not appear even once in the 7-day menus.

Research on a nationally representative sample (28,034 adults), based on the Greek cohort of the European Prospective Investigation into Cancer and Nutrition (EPIC study), support the contention that the diet of Greeks living in Greece has changed (Costacou et al., 2003). Results showed that only about 45% of adults adhered to a dietary pattern (determined by cluster analysis) that was similar to the traditional Greek/Mediterranean diet, while the remaining 65% had dietary patterns that exhibited low consumption of vegetables, legumes, fish, and olive oil, and high consumption of meat, eggs, butter, margarine, and sugar products. Characteristics associated with having a Mediterranean pattern (based on factor analysis) were being female, older, better educated, having higher physical activity, and higher BMI.

Similarly, the ATTICA study, an epidemiologic study of a random sample ($n = 3042$) of adults living in the province of Attica (includes greater Athens), provided evidence that the contemporary Greek diet

TABLE 14-1   Frequency of Various Categories of Foods Derived from Seven-Day Menus for Two Different Time Periods in Crete, Greece

Food Category	Diet Based on 1960s Practices of Adult Males		Diet Based on 1994 Practices of Adolescents	
	Weekly frequency	Daily average	Weekly frequency	Daily average
Red meat (i.e., beef or pork)	0	0	9	1.3
Chicken or rabbit	2	0.3	1	0.1
Fish	4	0.6	0	0
Whole-grain wheat, barley products (mostly bread or dry bread)*	11	1.6	0	0
Fruit	23	3.3	5	0.7
Vegetables (excluding potatoes)	16	2.3	5	0.7
Legumes (e.g., beans)	4	0.6	1	0.1
Foods or milk with added sugar	6	0.9	15	2.1
Soda or sweetened juices	0	0	13	1.9
French fries	0	0	3	0.4

Compiled from menus given by Kafatos et al. (2000).

*Counted as whole grain if the food specifically stated whole wheat or whole grain.

is relatively high in red meat (four and five times/week, respectively, for women and men) and sweets (about five times/week). The average Mediterranean-diet-adherence score was relatively low (26 out of a maximum of 55) in both men and women, although women scored higher than men (Arvaniti, Panagiotakos, Pitsavos, Zampelas, & Stefanadis, 2006). Nevertheless, some of the hallmarks of the traditional Greek diet remain. Illustrative is the reported average intake of fruits, vegetables, and legumes. Average weekly fruit consumption was 28 servings for women and 26 servings for men, while for vegetables (not including potatoes) it was 35 servings for women and 34 servings for men. This translates into eating 4 servings of fruit and 5 servings of vegetables per day. Fat intake and energy intake were also quite high: 45% of calories in men (mean caloric intake = 2595) and 47% in women (mean caloric intake = 2132).

The study, however, that provides a frightening window to the future evolution of the Greek diet was recently conducted on a nationally representative sample of Greek preadolescent and adolescent children 11–15 years of age in Greece (Yannakoulia, Karayiannis, Terzidou, Kokkevi, & Sidossis, 2004). It suggests that drastic changes are occurring in the diets of younger Greeks. Using a Food Frequency Questionnaire, the researchers obtained dietary data on 4211 children. Similar to the study by Kafatos et al. (2000), children in this study had a higher consumption of sweets, sodas, hamburgers, hot dogs, and sausages, and a much lower consumption of vegetables and bread (refined and unrefined). Specifically, although between 75 and 87% (depending on the age and sex) of subjects reported eating fruit at least once a day (this was the highest figure for any category reported in the study), only between 38 and 44% reported a daily consumption of vegetables and 25–39% reported a daily consumption of bread; the latter was less than the 33–61% who reported a daily consumption of sodas. The researchers devised an index of unhealthy eating, coined the Unhealthy Food Choices Score (UFCS), which had values from 9 (least unhealthy) to 45 (most unhealthy); averages by age and sex ranged from about 23 to 26, suggesting, on average, that their diets were moderately unhealthy. Boys and older children had more unhealthy diets than girls and younger children (Yannakoulia et al., 2004).

Another study of adolescents in northern Greece, although not representative, also noted evidence of a westernization of the Greek diet, and that there were health repercussions. In that study overweight ado-

lescents had a higher consumption of snacks (potato chips, chocolate bars, pizza, cheese pie, and cream pie), sugar, jam, and honey, and a lower consumption of legumes, vegetables, and fruits, than their non-overweight counterparts (Hassapidou, Fotiadou, Maglara, & Papadopoulou, 2006).

Little research has been conducted on changes in the traditional Greek diet among the immigrants that comprise the Greek diaspora. It has been reported that people of Greek descent living in the United States continued to use olive oil as a major oil (Valassi, 1962). Another study of Greeks living in Australia showed that those born in Greece, compared with their Australian-born counterparts (i.e., descendents from the British Isles and Holland or Germany), had higher household expenditures on fruits, vegetables, cereal products, and fish, and substantially less on alcohol (Powles, Hage, & Cosgrove, 1990).

 MAJOR FOODS

Generally, preparation of Greek dishes is time-consuming, includes multiple food groups, and food is cooked slowly. Foods are also cooked thoroughly and fresh ingredients are valued and sought.

 Protein Sources

The major protein sources of the Greek diet were traditionally legumes in combination with bread, eggs, cheese, and yogurt. In certain regions of Greece, particularly by the coastline or on the islands, fish is also an important source of protein and a dietary staple. Dried or salted fish is also eaten especially when fresh fish is not available. Given the westernization of the Greek diet, however, more frequent consumption of chicken, beef, and pork have now made them important sources of protein.

 Starch Sources

The major source of starch in the Greek diet is bread; it is also a dietary staple. Bread is generally bought at a bread shop (called an *artopioion*) and usually is not sliced, although more recently sandwiches are being made with sliced bread. Bread always accompanies meals irrespective of whether there are other sources of starch. In addition, potatoes are frequently consumed, either roasted, fried (homemade), or in a vegetable stew. Rice and pasta are also starch sources, although they are consumed less frequently.

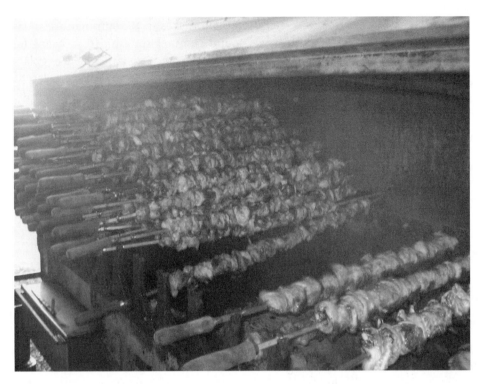

Souvla
Courtesy of Agni Thurner

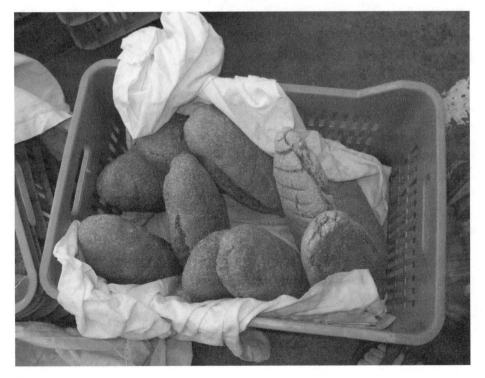

Breads
Courtesy of Agni Thurner

Fat Sources

Traditionally, the major fats in the Greek diet were provided by olive oil and olives. Butter was mostly used in desserts, but not in other types of dishes; however, in certain regions of Greece (mountainous areas in which sheepherding was the major occupation), more recipes include butter (Kochilas, 2001, p. 2). Given the westernization of the Greek diet, more corn and canola oil is used, as well as margarine and butter. In addition, meats have become a significant source of fat in the Greek diet.

 Prominent Vegetables

Usually, vegetables are eaten in season, so the prominent vegetables vary by season. Moreover, many vegetables comprise main dishes; thus, those dishes also vary by season. In the late spring, summer, and early fall, tomatoes and cucumbers are eaten almost daily in the form of the famous "Greek salad." Wild greens (generically called *hórta* in Greek), including dandelion greens, purslane, and other local wild greens, are cooked and topped with lemon and oil, and accompany the meal. Other prominent vegetables eaten as cooked main dishes in the summer are squash (e.g., zucchini and summer squash), fresh beans (e.g., string beans, long beans), eggplant (fried eggplant with a tomato sauce), and okra. Some vegetables, such as tomatoes, eggplant, squash, and peppers, are stuffed and baked. Stuffing usually consists of rice, seasonings, and olive oil, although some people also include ground beef or lamb. In the winter months, prominent vegetables used in salads are lettuce and cabbage. Vegetables used in main dishes in the winter are spinach (spinach and rice) or spinach pie, cabbage (frequently stuffed with rice and ground beef or lamb), and artichokes.

 Prominent Fruits

Fresh fruit is also traditionally eaten in season and is typically eaten for dessert. From mid-fall through winter, apples and oranges are predominantly eaten; tangerines are eaten beginning in early spring. Dried figs and raisins are also eaten. In late spring and summer, commonly eaten fruit includes watermelon and other melons, peaches, nectarines, grapes, and figs (August and September). Pomegranates are also eaten in early fall. Preserved fruits are often eaten in the winter; however, they contain a high amount of sugar

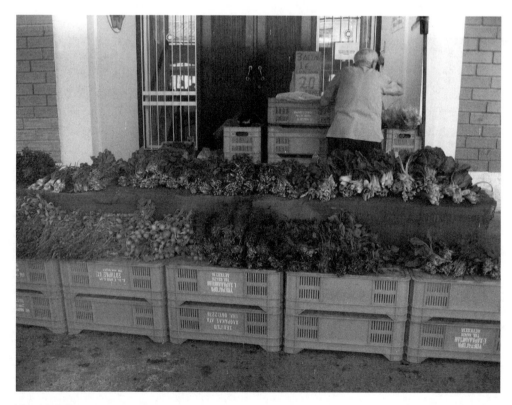

Vegetables
Courtesy of Agni Thurner

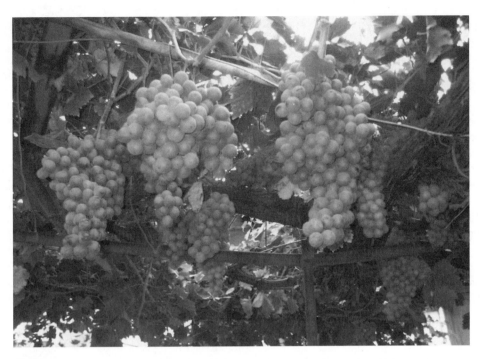

Grapes
Courtesy of Agni Thurner

and therefore would be more appropriately classified under sweets.

Spices, Seasonings, and Herbs

The herbs and seasonings used in Greek cuisine that provide its distinctive flavors are onions, garlic, oregano, and lemons. Mint and dill are used to a lesser extent. Cinnamon and nutmeg are used primarily in desserts. Basil is not used in cooking but rather in religious ceremonies.

Beverages

The main beverages consumed by adults are coffee and wine. Greek coffee is widely consumed for breakfast and in the late afternoon/early evening. Another type of coffee that is popular among the younger generations and adolescents in Greece is Nescafe® Frappe (iced coffee using instant Nescafe® coffee). Depending on tastes, milk is added; otherwise, little milk is consumed by adults. Children drink milk, although consumption of sweetened beverages, such as juice and soda, has increased in this group. Wine and beer are consumed with meals. Other alcoholic beverages, such as ouzo, raki, and metaxa (Greek cognac), are less commonly consumed, but again, when they are offered, they are accompanied by some food.

Desserts

It is noteworthy that traditionally sweets are not eaten after a meal, unless it is a special occasion, one has guests, or it is a holiday. This may be changing somewhat; however, sweets are still more commonly eaten with coffee in the late afternoon/early evening. It is also noteworthy that Greeks consume desserts specifically for the Lenten or fasting periods that have no animal products (i.e., eggs or butter).

There are numerous Greek desserts that are popular in Greece and internationally. A hallmark of Greek desserts is that they are very sweet. There are sweets that use phyllo dough and are topped with syrup. Two such popular Greek desserts include *baklava*, which is layers of phyllo dough filled with walnuts, almonds, or a combination of both, and *galaktobouriko* (custard pie). In addition, *kadaifi* is a wheat-based (i.e., like shredded wheat) dessert filled with nuts and topped with syrup. There are also syrup-topped cakes such as *karidopita* (walnut cake) and *ravani* (a golden cake made with semolina and flour). *Kourambiedes* are butter cookies (often crescent shaped) topped with powdered sugar; traditionally made at Christmas, they are now eaten year-round. *Melomakarona* are syrup-soaked Lenten cookies made with olive oil that do not contain any eggs or butter. There are also cookies that are served with coffee, which are not as sweet; these

Observations from the Author (Elizabeth Metallinos-Katsaras)

One aspect of traditional Greek food preparation that I first noticed when living in Greece was an inherent difference between my Americanized notion of what is considered an appropriate degree of "doneness" and that of traditional Greek cuisine. Greeks are very particular about meats, vegetables, and pasta being "cooked enough." The definition of "cooked enough" from the Greek perspective was quite different from mine. One of the first times I ate cooked broccoli in Greece, I noticed that it had no texture left. To my mind, it was extremely overcooked, almost like mush, which would be great for baby food but was unappealing to me. After that, I noticed that every cooked vegetable, from cauliflower to carrots, was not considered "cooked" unless there was the ability to mash it; in other words, it had to have a "melt in your mouth" feel. The same is true for pasta. The concept of cooking pasta to the "al dente" stage does not fit with the traditional Greek food habits, and if one deigns to "undercook" it in this way, Greeks call it "raw" pasta. Finally, when living in Greece I had to forget the notion of cooking beef to the rare, medium-rare, or medium stages, because unless meat is well done, it is considered raw. First-generation Greeks in the United States also generally demand that their meat be well done. One time I went to a wedding reception in which prime rib was served. Most of the Greeks at my table sent back their prime rib because it was not well done. The lesson here is that if one caters a "Big Fat Greek Wedding," one should be cognizant of what is acceptable in terms of the degree to which both meat and vegetables should be cooked so that the guests are satisfied with their meal.

are *koulourakia* and *paximadia* (hardened cookies similar to a biscotti).

FOODS WITH CULTURAL SIGNIFICANCE

There are several foods that have notable cultural significance because of their religious symbolism and use. A major nondietary use of olive oil among Greeks is in votive candles, in which the primary fuel for the flame is olive oil. Churches, shrines, cemeteries, and homes keep these votive lights burning using olive oil. In addition, olive oil is used for anointing and blessing during certain religious Greek Orthodox ceremonies. Wheat and bread also have religious significance; bread is used for Holy Communion and wheat kernels are used to make *kolyva* that is presented to the church and blessed during memorial services for the deceased. Finally, wine also has religious significance because of its involvement in the first miracle that Christ carried out (transformation of water into wine) and is part of Holy Communion.

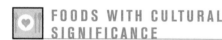

A TYPICAL DAY'S MENU

A typical day's menu would depend on whether it is Wednesday or Friday (i.e., fasting days), other days, or Sunday. It also depends on the season. Table 14-2 depicts a typical day's menu for fasting days, nonfasting

days, and Sunday, for summer and winter. The menu is also largely dependent on whether one is working or on vacation (Greeks in Greece generally get 4 weeks of vacation per year). The main meal is the midday meal, which, depending on work schedules, may be eaten anytime between 1 PM (for those not working) to 3–4 PM for those who do work. After this large midday meal, many take an afternoon nap. Then they have their coffee or snack in the early evening (5–7 PM). Dinner is generally lighter and later in the evening (9–11 PM).

HOLIDAY MENUS

Holiday menus vary somewhat by region because there are often regional festive foods; however, one overarching principle of holiday menus is to maximize the variety of dishes and make enough food to feed an army. Every Greek holiday is like the American Thanksgiving. The major holidays are New Year's Day (commemoration of Saint Basil the Great), Clean Monday (the beginning of Lent), Easter, the Dormition of the Virgin Mary, and Christmas. Easter is considered the most important holiday and a traditional menu is as follows:

- *Mayeritsa* (the meal after the midnight Easter service, between 1 and 3 AM). This is the traditional Easter-egg lemon soup made from lamb intestines and other organ meats, dill, and green onions. Regional differences exist as to how this soup

TABLE 14-2   Sample Fasting and Nonfasting Menus for Summer and Winter

	Summer	Winter
Fasting days*	Breakfast: Greek coffee, tahini, rusks	Breakfast: Greek coffee, tahini, rusks
	Snack: grapes	Snack: an orange
	Lunch: fresh green beans, zucchini, potato stew (seasoned with olive oil, onions, parsley, and tomato sauce or paste), bread, olives, fresh figs	Lunch: tahinosoupa (soup with tahini and orzo), bread, olives, peeled and sliced apples with cinnamon
	Early evening: Greek coffee, bread and marmalade	Early evening: Greek coffee, raisins, almonds
	Dinner: fresh green bean stew (smaller portion), bread, olives, a peach	Dinner: tahinosoupa (smaller portion), olives, bread, an orange
Nonfasting days (weekdays)	Breakfast: Greek coffee and milk, barley rusk, Graviera cheese	Breakfast: Greek coffee and milk
	Snack: fresh fruit (watermelon)	Snack: ham and cheese panini
	Lunch: fried fish, bread, tomato, cucumber and pepper salad with oregano and olive oil, olives, feta cheese, bread, sliced watermelon	Lunch: fasolada (bean soup with white beans, onions, celery, carrots, olive oil, sometimes with tomato paste or sauce and sometimes with lemon), bread, olives
	Early-evening snack (at the outdoor café): Nescafe frappe with evaporated milk, koulourkia (Greek cookies)	Early evening: Greek coffee, baklava (at a friend's house)
	Dinner (light): yogurt with honey, fresh apricots	Dinner: fasolada (smaller portion), bread, olives, an apple
Sunday	Breakfast: none, because no eating or dinking anything except water before church	Breakfast: none, because no eating or dinking anything except water before church
	Late-morning snack (after church): Greek coffee, koulourakia	Late-morning snack (after church): Greek coffee, koulourakia
	Lunch: lamb in the oven with orzo, tomato sauce, and olive oil base, grated cheese, tomato, cucumber and pepper salad, cheese pie; assorted fruits: cantaloupe, grapes, watermelon	Lunch: chicken egg-lemon soup, potatoes, boiled wild greens (on the side) with lemon and olive oil, bread, cheese, spinach pie; assorted fruits: tangerines, apples
	Early evening: Nescafe frappe, ice cream	Early evening: Greek coffee and galactoboureko (custard pie)

*The summer menu includes olive oil, whereas the winter menu is reflective of more strict adherence of the fast, with the omission of olive oil.

is made, but the basic ingredients are the same: roast lamb and hard-boiled eggs dyed red. There are also many side dishes, such as cheese pie, spinach pie, *keftedes* (Greek meatballs), *tzatziki* (yogurt, garlic dip), and assorted salads. Wine is served as well, as are Easter cookies and regional desserts specific to Easter. For example, on the island of Tinos, two types of sweets with cheese and homemade phyllo dough are made specifically for Easter.

- For the midday meal, roast lamb on the spit, roast entrails on the spit (called *kokoretsi*), other meats, roast potatoes, Greek Easter bread (*tsoureki*), assorted cheeses, red-dyed boiled eggs, assorted salads, wine, beer, *tzatziki* (yogurt, garlic dip), cheese pie (*tyropita*), spinach pie (*spanakopita*), bread, and assorted Greek sweets are served.

 HEALTH BELIEFS AND CONCERNS

A belief in the germ theory of disease is lacking by many less-educated older Greeks, and therefore many illnesses are attributed to other causes. Keeping warm is considered an important measure to prevent illnesses such as colds or flu. If one contracts a cold, it is often attributed to going outside without sufficiently warm clothing or going outside too soon after taking a bath or washing one's hair. Eating well and enough is also thought to be important for health maintenance, especially for children. Unfortunately, the perception of "enough" may be too much from the perspective of a health professional. One classic picture of a Greek mother would be a woman with a very large spoon waiting outside the schoolyard in order to ensure that her child eats his or her snack. (This is not an exaggeration!) A child who is not plump is perceived by many older Greeks in particular as not being healthy.

Many traditional Greeks also have a belief that God determines one's longevity, and that many important events of one's life course are predetermined. This fatalistic attitude has implications for the degree to which traditional Greeks believe that they have control over their lives, including their health. This also has implications in terms of counseling Greeks, especially elderly Greeks.

Finally, like many other cultures, Greeks believe in the "evil eye." In simple terms, it is defined as misfortune that befalls a person or family that Greeks attribute to another person's envy (either deliberate or subconscious).

Many changes have occurred in the past 50–60 years in the health status of Greeks. Post–World War II (1956–1985) changes in food availability with concomitant increases in energy (27%), lipid (67%), and protein intake (24%) appeared to result in beneficial effects on child growth as evidenced by average increases of approximately 7 cm (2.8 in.) in height and approximately 4 kg (8.8 lbs.) in weight of military recruits (Trichopoulou & Efstathiadis, 1989). Food scarcity, particularly foods of animal origin, likely constrained child growth earlier in the 20th century and particularly during the famines that occurred during World War II. Based on mortality statistics and research in selected areas of Greece in the 1960s, Greece had low mortality rates of coronary heart disease (CHD), colon cancer, and breast cancer (Trichopoulou & Efstathiadis, 1989). In particular, the low rates of CHD reported by Keys in the Seven Countries Study captured the world's attention (Keys, 1980), and much of this difference has been attributed to diet (Simopoulos, 2001), although other lifestyle factors were also drastically different between these Greek populations and the other countries to which Greece was compared. One such factor was that in the 1960s Greek society was much more agrarian (Clogg, 2001). Not only were physical-activity levels much higher, but other lifestyle factors, such as eating patterns, social interactions and support, perceived stress levels, and sleeping patterns, were much different than those of comparison countries. Such lifestyle factors are inextricably tied to dietary patterns, thus making it difficult to separate the effect of dietary changes from other lifestyle differences. Nevertheless, some experimental studies (e.g., the Lyon Diet Study) have lent credence to the assertion that the traditional Greek diet confers health-promoting and disease-preventing properties, in part due to its high omega-3 fatty acid levels (Simopoulos, 2001).

With respect to general indicators of a population's health in the 21st century, based on current World Health Organization's (WHO) health statistics, Greece has one of the lowest rates of under-5-years mortality (4/1000 live births) in Europe (World Health Association, 2006) and a fairly high life expectancy at birth (77 and 82 years for males and females, respectively) (WHO, 2006). Greece also has a moderately high healthy-life expectancy at birth (69 and 73 years for males and females, respectively) (World Health Organization, 2003); however, in the past 20 years, overweight and obesity among adults and children has risen dramatically. It is at an all-time high (Kapantais et al., 2006; WHO, 2008) with estimates (depending on age and study sample) indicating that between 38.1 and 61.3% of women, and between 66.1 and 75.7% of men, are either overweight or obese (BMI ≥ 25); moreover, abdominal obesity is common, with an estimated 35.8% of women and 26.6% of men exhibiting this type of obesity (Kapantais et al., 2006). These alarming statistics will likely affect the future health of the Greek population.

Children in Greece are also experiencing high rates of obesity;[1] this includes all age groups. A 15-country (13 European countries, the United States, and Israel) comparative study of school-aged children ranked Greece as having the highest prevalence of overweight among adolescent children (13- and 15-year-olds) in Europe, second only to the United States. About 29% of 13- and 15-year-old boys, and 18.9% of 13-year-old girls and 16.4% of 15-year-old girls, were classified as either at risk for overweight or overweight (BMI for age ≥ 85th percentile) (Lissau et al., 2004); these were based on self-reported weights and heights, so they may underestimate prevalence. Similarly, very young children are also experiencing high risk of overweight: a representative study of five counties in Greece showed that about 16% of those 1–5 years of age were found to be overweight and another 16% were at risk for overweight, bringing the total over 30% for children either at risk of overweight or overweight (Manios et al., 2007). Abdominal obesity also appears to be high in children (Tzotzas et al., 2008). Accelerating childhood overweight is not limited to Greeks living in Greece; high overweight prevalence was also found for preadolescent children and adults in Cyprus (Lazarou, Panagiotakos, Panayiotou, & Matalas, 2008). These changes may in part be attributable to changes in diet, but also to increases in sedentary behavior (e.g., TV watching) and declines in physical-activity levels; by 4–5 years of age, children were reported to watch an average of over 2 hours of TV per day (Manios, 2006). In addition, energy intakes of children who were overweight or at risk for overweight were higher than their normal-weight counterparts (Manios et al., 2007).

In addition, other indicators of disease risk (and disease itself) have been increasing. Between 1982 and 2002, adverse changes in CHD risk factors, such as total cholesterol, LDL cholesterol, HDL cholesterol, and triglycerides, were shown in a small sample of Greek children. Overweight in these children was associated with these adverse changes in lipid profiles (Manios, Magkos, Christakis, & Kafatos, 2005). There is also evidence that the prevalence of metabolic syndrome in Greek adults is also quite high; one study indicates that the age-adjusted prevalence is 23.8% (Athyros et al., 2005).

The prevalence of hypertension is relatively high with national studies estimating that 13.3% of men and 13.5% of women are hypertensive (Matalas, 2006). Among the elderly it appears to be much higher; one study of elders (≥ 65 years) living in the Mediterranean islands estimated, using clinical and biochemical measurements, that 57% of men and 64% of women had hypertension, 36% of men and 59% of women had high-serum cholesterol, and 17% of men and 20% of women had diabetes (Panagiotakos, Bountziouka, Zeimbekis, Vlachou, & Polychronopoulos, 2007).

A study in the province of Attica (the greater Athens area) suggests that the prevalence of high cholesterol is 46% in men and 40% of women (Panagiotakos, Pitsavos, Chrysohoou, Skoumas, & Stefanadis, 2004); almost half of those with high cholesterol were unaware of it. In addition, 28% of men and 13% of women had triglyceride levels > 150 mg/dl.

Smoking rates are also relatively high among Greeks living in Greece, although the statistics show that many are former smokers; one national study indicated that 48.2% of males and 35.1% of females were current smokers, whereas 23.1 and 11%, respectively, were former smokers (Matalas, 2006).

 ### GENERAL HEALTH AND NUTRITIONAL INDICATORS SUMMARY

Greece has one of the lowest rates of infant mortality (4/1000 live births in 2005) and under-5-years mortality rates (4/1000 live births) in Europe. Similar to the United States, Greece has only a moderately low rate of low birth weight (8% of births) (UNICEF, 2007); thus, Greece still has work to do to improve this rate. The Greek population has a 96% literacy rate, which is very high. This is likely due to the high rates of primary and secondary school enrollments, which are about 100% and 96% of age-eligible children, respectively (UNICEF, 2007).

Undernutrition is not a major problem in Greece; however, in the past 20 years, overweight and obesity among adults and children has risen dramatically: they are at an all-time high (Kapantais et al., 2006; WHO, 2008), with estimates (depending on age and study sample) indicating that between 38.1 and 61.3% of women, and between 66.1 and 75.7% of men, are either overweight or obese (BMI > 25). Child obesity is

---

[1] Note that the definition of overweight and obesity in children varies by study. Some use the IOTF's cut-offs of BMI ≥ 25 as overweight and ≥ 30 as obese, whereas others use the CDC growth reference data of overweight, which is defined as BMI for age ≥ 95 and at risk for overweight ≥ 85 to < 95.

also high, with about 29% of 13- and 15-year-old boys, and 18.9% of 13-year-old girls and 16.4% of 15-year-old girls, classified as either at risk for overweight or overweight (BMI for age > 85th percentile) (Lissau et al., 2004).

COMMUNICATION AND COUNSELING TIPS

Greek communication style is expressive and frequently loud. Often, many people speak simultaneously in their eagerness to participate in a conversation. Hand gestures are used quite extensively when speaking, and personal space is much smaller than that expected in many Western countries (Remland, Jones, & Brinkman, 1995). Hand shaking is common when greeting, even among relative strangers. Among friends and relatives, kissing on both cheeks is preferred, even between sexes.

It is noteworthy that among the Greek diaspora and younger-generation Greeks, some of these traditional views and perceptions are constantly changing and becoming more westernized. This is also dependent, to a large degree, on the educational level of the individual; thus, the traditional worldview and communication style may not describe more educated younger Greeks in Greece and those who are second and third generation, or higher, among the Greek diaspora. Nevertheless, being cognizant of the traditional values and beliefs of Greek culture can significantly improve effectiveness when interacting with them, although one should not assume that such beliefs and practices apply to all individuals.

When counseling Greeks, particularly Greeks from Greece, one should consider the value they place on building and maintaining relationships. Asking about a client's family, children, grandchildren, and significant life events prior to counseling sessions or at the beginning of an appointment implies that the provider cares about his or her client. This will take a few more minutes but will contribute greatly to building a trusting relationship and will improve receptivity to advice the provider may provide. In addition, the client may bring other family members to the appointment; privacy of medical and health information may not be considered when doing so. Sometimes family members accompany a client in order to interpret the complex medical information that the provider may supply; other times, family members simply come so that the client feels supported.

Greek culture values the medical profession; however, media sensationalism, which has publicized alleged malpractice among Greek health professionals in Greece, media misinformation, or even simply selective hearing or misunderstanding about health issues discussed by the media, has altered the public's perceptions of the health professions. Low educational attainment of some of the older generations of Greeks contributes to this misunderstanding. An example of this is described below by a dentist for whom Greeks comprise a large proportion of his client pool:

> "When I told one of my patients to take antibiotics, she said she had heard that taking antibiotics could be damaging. When I asked her to explain why she believed this she said that she had heard that not finishing an entire course of antibiotics could be damaging to the body. She had basically retained the 'damaging to your body' and not the qualifying statement." (A. Katsaras, personal communication, 2008)

Greeks are extremely proud of their heritage. When providing dietary counseling one should utilize a strategy that capitalizes on this "Greek pride" by emphasizing the many food habits of the traditional Greek diet that are healthful. There are also many misconceptions about dietary constituents, such as fat. While acknowledging that fat contributes to excess calories in the diet, many people believe that olive oil is exempt. In fact, the message about olive oil's healthful fatty acid composition has been resoundingly heard, which has translated into an almost indiscriminate use of olive oil and a reluctance to reduce the quantity of it in both cooked foods and raw foods such as salads. Criticizing olive oil is not culturally acceptable; therefore, one needs to be sensitive to this attitude and emphasize it as an appropriate oil to use (to replace other fats), but not without stating that it should be used in moderation. Using the Greek saying, "pan metron ariston," which means "everything in moderation," can be used to support this message.

As noted previously, traditional Greeks are somewhat fatalistic. This sometimes can be a barrier to preventative care as well as clinical treatment. People often say that the length of their lives is "written" or already determined. One tact that may avert direct opposition to this statement is to discuss the goals of staying strong and functional as one grows older, and of not becoming a burden to one's children.

TABLE 14-3 Phonetic Pronunciation of Common Greek Foods

Food	Phonetic Pronunciation	Food	Phonetic Pronunciation
Bread	Psomeé	Potatoes	Patátes
Olive oil	Eleólatho	Beans	Fasólea
Vegetables	Lahaneeká	Fruit (plural)	Froóta
Cooked greens	Hórta	Rice	Reézee
Dishes with vegetables, grains, and pulses that are fasting dishes and cooked with olive oil	Latherá	Cheese pie	Teéropitta
		Spinach pie	Spanakópita
Salad	Saláta	Water	Neró
Tomatoes	Ntomátes	Coffee	Kafé
Meat	Kreas	Milk	Gála
Chicken	Kotpóulo	Sugar	Záharee

Note: Two e's are pronounced long and one is short.

FEATURED RECIPE

White Bean Soup (*Fasolada*)

1 lb. dry great northern beans

2 medium onions, chopped finely

4 medium carrots, halved and sliced

1½ cups chopped celery

½ cup extra virgin olive oil

½ cup tomato sauce or 3 tbsp. tomato paste

Salt and pepper to taste

1. Soak the beans overnight in a large pot. Drain the beans and add about 8 cups of water. Bring to boil and simmer for about 30 minutes.
2. Add onions, carrots, and celery. Cook for another 25 minutes, then add olive oil, tomato sauce or paste, and simmer for another 20 minutes or until beans and vegetables are tender.

More recipes are available at http://nutrition.jbpub.com/foodculture/

REFERENCES

Arvaniti, F., Panagiotakos, D.B., Pitsavos, C., Zampelas, A., & Stefanadis, C. (2006). Dietary habits in a Greek sample of men and women: The ATTICA study. *Central European Journal of Public Health, 14*(2), 74–77.

Athyros, V.G., Bouloukos, V.I., Pehlivanidis, A.N., Papageorgiou, A.A., Dionysopoulou, S.G., Symeonidis, A.N., et al. (2005). The prevalence of the metabolic syndrome in Greece: The MetS-Greece multicentre study. *Diabetes, Obesity & Metabolism, 7*(4), 397–405.

Benetou, V., Trichopoulou, A., Orfanos, P., Naska, A., Lagiou, P., Boffetta, P., et al. (2008). Conformity to traditional Mediterranean diet and cancer incidence: The Greek EPIC cohort. *British Journal of Cancer, 99*(1), 191–195.

Clogg, R. (Ed.). (2001). *A concise history of Greece* (2nd ed.). Cambridge, UK: Cambridge University Press.

Chliaoutakis, J., Drakou, I., Gnardellis, C., Galariotou, S., Carra, H., & Chliaoutaki, M. (2002). Greek Christian orthodox ecclesiastical lifestyle: Could it become a pattern of health-related behavior? *Preventive Medicine, 34*(4), 428–435.

Costacou, T., Bamia, C., Ferrari, P., Riboli, E., Trichopoulos, D., & Trichopoulou, A. (2003). Tracing the Mediterranean diet through principal components and cluster analyses in the Greek population. *European Journal of Clinical Nutrition, 57*(11), 1378–1385.

Ferro-Luzzi, A., James, W.P.T., & Kafatos, A. (2002). The high-fat Greek diet: A recipe for all? *European Journal of Clinical Nutrition, 56*(9), 796–809.

Hassapidou, M., Fotiadou, E., Maglara, E., & Papadopoulou, S.K. (2006). Energy intake, diet composition, energy expenditure, and body fatness of adolescents in northern Greece. *Obesity 14*(5), 855–862.

Kafatos, A., Verhagen, H., Moschandreas, J., Apostolaki, I., & Van Westerop, J.J. (2000). Mediterranean diet of Crete: Foods and nutrient content. *Journal of the American Dietetic Association, 100*(12), 1487–1493.

Kapantais, E., Tzotzas, T., Ioannidis, I., Mortoglou, A., Bakatselos, S., Kaklamanou, M., et al. (2006). First national epidemiological survey on the prevalence of obesity and abdominal fat distribution in Greek adults. *Annals of Nutrition & Metabolism, 50*(4), 330–338.

Karayiannis, D., Yannakoulia, M., Terzidou, M., Sidossis, L.S., & Kokkevi, A. (2003). Prevalence of overweight and obesity in Greek school-aged children and adolescents. *European Journal of Clinical Nutrition, 57*(9), 1189–1192.

Keys, A. (1980). Wine, garlic, and CHD in seven countries. *Lancet, 1*(8160), 145–146.

Kochilas, D. (2001). *The glorious foods of Greece: Traditional recipes from the islands, cities and villages.* New York: HarperCollins Publishers.

Kremmyda, L., Papadaki, A., Hondros, G., Kapsokefalou, M., & Scott, J.A. (2008). Differentiating between the effect of rapid dietary acculturation and the effect of living away from home for the first time, on the diets of Greek students studying in Glasgow. *Appetite, 50*(2–3), 455–463.

Kromhout, D. (1989). Food consumption patterns in the seven countries study. Seven Countries Study Research Group. *Annals of Medicine, 21*(3), 237–238.

Lazarou, C., Panagiotakos, D.B., Panayiotou, G., & Matalas, A. (2008). Overweight and obesity in preadolescent children and their parents in Cyprus: Prevalence and associated socio-demographic factors—the CYKIDS study. *Obesity Reviews: An Official Journal of the International Association for the Study of Obesity, 9*(3), 185–193.

Lissau, I., Overpeck, M.D., Ruan, W.J., Due, P., Holstein, B.E., & Hediger, M.L. (2004). Body mass index and overweight in adolescents in 13 European countries, Israel, and the United States. *Archives of Pediatrics & Adolescent Medicine, 158*(1), 27–33.

Manios, Y. (2006). Design and descriptive results of the "growth, exercise and nutrition epidemiological study in preschoolers": The GENESIS study. *BMC Public Health, 6*, 32.

Manios, Y., Costarelli, V., Kolotourou, M., Kondakis, K., Tzavara, C., & Moschonis, G. (2007). Prevalence of obesity in preschool Greek children, in relation to parental characteristics and region of residence. *BMC Public Health, 7*(147), 178.

Manios, Y., Magkos, F., Christakis, G., & Kafatos, A.G. (2005). Changing relationships of obesity and dyslipidemia in Greek children: 1982–2002. *Preventive Medicine, 41*(5–6), 846–851.

Mastrantonis G. (n.d.) *Fasting from iniquities and foods.* Retrieved August 21, 2008, from http://www.goarch.org/en/ourfaith/articles/article8125.asp/

Matalas, A. (2006). Disparities within traditional Mediterranean food patterns: An historical approach of the Greek

diet. *International Journal of Food Sciences and Nutrition, 57*(7–8), 529–536.

Panagiotakos, D., Bountziouka, V., Zeimbekis, A., Vlachou, I., & Polychronopoulos, E. (2007). Food pattern analysis and prevalence of cardiovascular disease risk factors among elderly people from Mediterranean islands. *Journal of Medicinal Food, 10*(4), 615–621.

Panagiotakos, D.B., Pitsavos, C., Chrysohoou, C., Skoumas, J., & Stefanadis, C. (2004). Status and management of blood lipids in Greek adults and their relation to socio-demographic, lifestyle and dietary factors: The ATTICA study. Blood lipids distribution in Greece. *Atherosclerosis, 173*(2), 353–361.

Pew Research Center. (2008). *U.S. Religious Landscape Survey, religious beliefs and practices: Diverse and politically relevant.* Retrieved August 23, 2008, from http://religions.pewforum.org/pdf/report2-religious-landscape-study-full.pdf/

Pitsavos, C., Milias, G.A., Panagiotakos, D.B., Xenaki, D., Panagopoulos, G., & Stefanadis, C. (2006). Prevalence of self-reported hypertension and its relation to dietary habits, in adults; a nutrition & health survey in Greece. *BMC Public Health, 6*, 206.

Powles, J., Hage, B., & Cosgrove, M. (1990). Health-related expenditure patterns in selected migrant groups: Data from the Australian household expenditure survey, 1984. *Community Health Studies, 14*(1), 1–7.

Remland M., Jones T.S., & Brinkman H. (1995). Interpersonal distance, body orientation, and touch: Effects of culture, gender, and age. *The Journal of Social Psychology, 135*(3), 281–297.

Sarri, K., Linardakis, M., Codrington, C., & Kafatos, A. (2007). Does the periodic vegetarianism of Greek orthodox christians benefit blood pressure? *Preventive Medicine, 44*(4), 341–348.

Sarri, K.O., Linardakis, M.K., Bervanaki, F.N., Tzanakis, N.E., & Kafatos, A.G. (2004). Greek Orthodox fasting rituals: A hidden characteristic of the Mediterranean diet of Crete. *British Journal of Nutrition, 92*(2), 277–284.

Sarri, K.O., Tzanakis, N.E., Linardakis, M.K., Mamalakis, G.D., & Kafatos, A.G. (2003). Effects of Greek Orthodox Christian Church fasting on serum lipids and obesity. *BMC Public Health, 3*, 16.

Simopoulos, A.P. (2001). What is so special about the diet of Greece? The scientific evidence. *World Review of Nutrition and Dietetics, 95*, 80–92.

Softas-Nall B.C., & Baldo, T. (2000). Dialogues within a Greek family: Multicultural stories of a couple revisited. *Family Journal: Counseling and Therapy for Couples and Families, 8*(4), 396–398.

Trichopoulou, A.D., & Efstathiadis, P.P. (1989). Changes of nutrition patterns and health indicators at the population level in Greece. *American Journal of Clinical Nutrition, 49*(5), 1042–1047.

Tzotzas, T., Kapantais, E., Tziomalos, K., Ioannidis, I., Mortoglou, A., Bakatselos, S., et al. (2008). Epidemiological survey for the prevalence of overweight and abdominal obesity in Greek adolescents. *Obesity 16*(7), 1718–1722.

UNICEF. (2007). *The state of the world's children 2007: Women and children, the double dividend of gender equality.* Retrieved April 14, 2009, from http://www.unicef.org/sowc07/statistics/tables.php/

U.S. Census Bureau. (2004). *Ancestry: 2000, census 2000 brief.* Retrieved August 23, 2008, from http://www.census.gov/prod/2004pubs/c2kbr-35.pdf/

U.S. State Department. (2008). *Greece (05/08).* Retrieved August 23, 2008, from http://www.state.gov/r/pa/ei/bgn/3395.htm/

Valassi K. (1962). Food habits of Greek Americans. *American Journal of Clinical Nutrition, 11*, 240–248.

World Health Organization. (2003). *Core health indicators.* Retrieved August 21, 2008, from http://www.who.int/whosis/database/country/compare.cfm?country=GRC&indicator=HALE0Male,HALE0Female&language=english/

World Health Organization. (2006). *Core health indicators.* Retrieved August 23, 2008, from http://www.who.int/whosis/database/country/compare.cfm?country=GRC&indicator=LEX0Male,LEX0Female&language=english/

World Health Organization. (2008). *Global InfoBase. InfoBase country page.* Retrieved August 21, 2008, from http://www.who.int/infobase/report.aspx?rid=111&iso=GRC/

Yannakoulia, M., Karayiannis, D., Terzidou, M., Kokkevi, A., & Sidossis, L.S. (2004). Nutrition-related habits of Greek adolescents. *European Journal of Clinical Nutrition, 58*(4), 580–586.

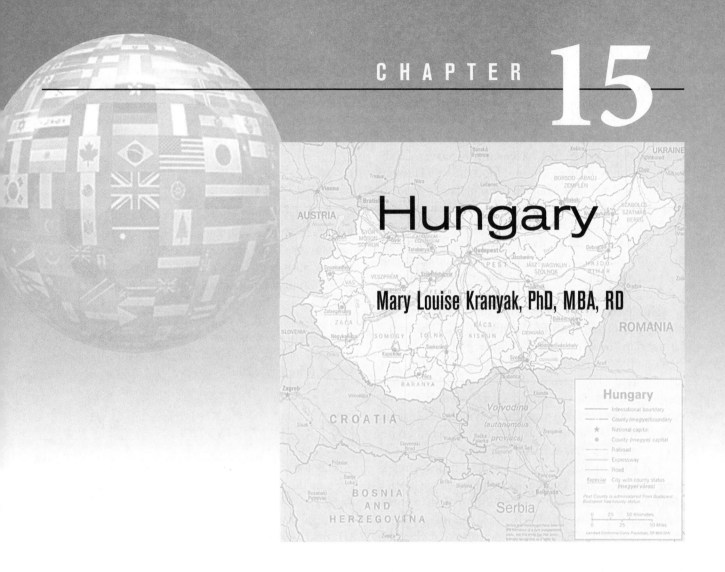

CHAPTER 15

Hungary

Mary Louise Kranyak, PhD, MBA, RD

CULTURE AND WORLD REGION

Hungary is fairly homogeneous ethnically, with Hungarians representing nearly 90% of the total population while the remainder consists of several minorities (Hungary, 2001). The largest minority is the Roma, who make up approximately 5% of the inhabitants (Ember & Ember, 2001). The Roma are also known as Gypsies, because in some places they were thought to be Egyptian pilgrims (MFA, 2007). The second largest minority are the Germans and the remainder include mostly Slovaks, Croatians, Romanians, and Serbs (Ember & Ember, 2001; Hungary, 2001).

Among the Hungarians who have declared a religious affiliation, 68% are Roman Catholic, 21% are Reformed (Calvinist) Protestant, 6% are Evangelical (Lutheran) Protestant, 3% are Eastern Orthodox, and less than 1% are Jewish (Budapest Hotels, 2008; Levinson, 1998).

Nearly all adults in Hungary are literate. Education is compulsory until the age of 16 years, with schools providing 8 years of primary education and 4 years of secondary education. (Hungarians, 1998).

In Hungary the family is the center of the social structure and imparts both emotional and financial support to its members. Often generations of extended family live together, with the grandparents participating in raising their grandchildren (KCCS, n.d.). Hungarians value openness of thought and expect their friends to share private and intimate details of their personal lives (eHow, 2008; KCCS, n.d.).

Hungarians pride themselves on the use of proper etiquette in all situations and expect the same of others (KCCS, n.d.). When greeting each other, close friends may kiss one another lightly on both cheeks, beginning with the left cheek (KCCS, n.d.; Martire & Kelly, 2005). Hungarians remove their shoes when entering their homes and may request that their guests do the same (Professional Travel Guide, 2008). Hungarians are very hospitable and open-hearted (TJC Global, 2007). When having guests, it is a Hungarian custom to make more food than can be eaten, since hospitality is measured by the quantity and variety of food served (Farkas, 1998; KCCS, n.d.). According to Sasvari (2005, p. 7), "No one confuses love and food the way Hungarians do, and when a Magyar cook places in front of you a steaming bowl of *gulyás*, what he or she is really offering you is comfort and affection and a safe refuge from the harsh realities of life." This is understandable, given the austerities the Hungarians endured during the many foreign invasions and dominations that often led them to flee their homeland (Sasvari, 2005).

Hungarian food preparation and preferences are closely associated with family history and traditions. Hungarian food traditions are inherited and are carried on with vehemence. Moreover, Farkas (1998, p. 9) affirms that "Hungarians very jealously guard their recipes and if a Hungarian trusts you with her recipe you can trust her with your life. Giving your favorite recipe away is the ultimate bonding experience between women; it makes friends for life."

For Hungarians, dinner is a special time for relaxation (eHow, 2008). Quietness during meals is both a cherished tradition and a reflection of their Central Asian heritage (Sasvari, 2005). Table manners are formal (KCSS, n.d.). Elbows are not permitted on the table and hands must be visible at all times (eHow, 2008). The fork is held in the left hand and the knife is held in the right hand (KCCS, n.d.). Conversation is generally devoid of politics and religion (eHow, 2008).

A landlocked country, Hungary is located in the Carpathian Basin in Central Europe, where it is bound by seven countries. To the north is Slovakia, to the northeast is Ukraine, to the east is Romania, to the south is Serbia and Croatia, to the southwest is Slovenia, and to the west is Austria. By comparison, the 93,030 square kilometer area occupied by Hungary is slightly smaller than Indiana in the United States (Hungary, 2001). Hungary is surrounded by the Alps, the Carpathian Mountains, and the Dinaric Alps. There are two major rivers that flow through Hungary, the Tisza and the Danube, which divide Hungary along the midsection and also bisects Budapest, the capital (Hungary, 2001; Sasvari, 2005). Budapest actually consists of three cities: Buda, Óbuda, and Pest, which were linked in 1873 to form Budapest (Sasvari, 2005). In the central-western part of Hungary is Lake Balaton, the largest freshwater lake in Europe, and within 6 km is Lake Hévíz, the largest medicinal thermal lake

in Europe and one of the natural wonders of Hungary (Freeman, 2004; MFA, 2007). Hungary has four distinct seasons with yearly temperatures ranging from 7°F to 97°F (Ember & Ember, 2001; Hungary, 2001).

LANGUAGE

The official language of Hungary is Hungarian, also known as Magyar (Hungary, 2001). Linguistically, it belongs to the Ugor branch of the Finno-Ugric language family (Ember & Ember, 2001). Along with the letters of the English language, the Hungarian language also has the following letters and combinations of letters: á, é, í, ó, ö, ő, ú, ü, ű, cs, dz, dzs, gy, ly, ny, sz, ty, and zs. Additionally, Hungarian (Magyar) is represented by a mixture of Turkish, Slavic, German, Latin, and French words (Hungary, 2001).

CULTURE HISTORY

Archeological findings of the earliest occupants of present-day Hungary date back 250,000 to 500,000 years ago. The area was occupied by Celtic tribes prior to the invasion by the Roman legions around 1 BC (Hungary, 2001; Sasvari, 2005). The Romans brought grapevines and winemaking to the area. Around 420 AD the Huns began raiding the area and in 441 AD their warrior prince, Attila, and his brother led the attacks on the Romans that ended in their victory and expulsion of the Romans. The process of rebuilding began; however, after the death of Attila, his followers revolted against his sons and welcomed the Romans back. This sequence of events—invasion, occupation, rebellion/uprising/war, a country in ruins followed by reconstruction—proved to be the country's "template" for the next 1500 years (Sasvari, 2005).

In 896 AD, the Carpathian Basin was invaded by the Magyars (Hungarians). They had originated from western Siberia, where they belonged to a group of tribes that spoke a language now called Finno-Ugric. Around 2000 BC, they had begun a slow and continuous migration south and west that lasted over 28 centuries. During this time, they lived under the influence of many different domains, including that of Russia, Kazakhstan, Bulgaria, and the Turks, from which new habits and practices were acquired. These practices included winemaking, agriculture, handicrafts, commerce, cooking techniques, and language development

(Lang, 1994; Sasvari, 2005). After passing through the Ukraine, they reached the Carpathian Mountains, which encircled a geographical landform called the Carpathian Basin. There they waged merciless wars to conquer the powers that occupied the area, including the Byzantines, the Bulgars, and the Franks (Sasvari, 2005). This was the last stage of their migration. They named the nation Magyar, which was originally the name of the dominant ruling tribe (Lang, 1994).

Although the Magyar tribes had reached their final destination, they continued to invade other territories across Europe (Lang, 1994). They reigned until they were defeated at Augsburg in 955 AD by Otto the Great, King of Germany (and later Holy Roman emperor), who forced them to abandon their western attacks. Eventually, this coerced the pagan Hungarians to convert to a civilizing Christianity under the reign of King Stephen I (1001–1038), who created the Kingdom of Hungary as its first king (Lang, 1994; MFA, 2007). Monasteries were built and had the responsibility of providing lodging and food for travelers. Simultaneously, certain landowners received a royal grant to sell wine and lodge guests within the boundaries of their property. This was the advent of the tavern-and-inn concept (Lang, 1994). In 1083, King Stephen I was canonized and the Holy Crown of St. Stephen became the national symbol (Hungary, 2001).

The successors of St. Stephen continued to embrace western culture and establish medieval Hungary as an international power (MFA, 2007). Indeed, Hungary became an important defensive bastion of Western Christendom as its eastern and southern borders were the boundaries of the Western world; however, medieval Hungary endured many invasions, primarily from the east. As a result, many groups and nationalities that were not ethnically Hungarian lived in the nation (Ember & Ember, 2001; MFA, 2007).

In 1456, the Hungarians repelled the first Turkish invasion. This was followed by the peaceful reign of King Matthias I, who introduced Renaissance culture to Hungary (Sasvari, 2005); however, in 1526, the Turks successfully invaded Hungary. By 1541, the country was split into three parts where the Turks ruled the middle, the Austrian Hapsburgs ruled in the west, and in the east the Ottomans made Transylvania a semi-independent state (Sasvari, 2005). The Turkish occupation that lasted 158 years was an especially brutal period, with many battles and bloodshed that killed more than half of the Hungarian population. The land that was the most fertile in Europe became barren and devastated (Sasvari, 2005).

In 1526, a young Hungarian king was defeated in a battle with the Ottoman Turks. Consequently, a marriage contract permitted the Habsburg kings of Austria to claim the Hungarian throne. This resulted in many unsuccessful Hungarian uprisings against the Habsburgs over many years. Nonetheless, after the Habsburgs conquered the Ottomans in 1686 and 1712, Hungary was bound to Austrian rule (Ember & Ember, 2001; Hungary, 2001). Subsequently, the Austrians declared German as the national language and encouraged people to leave overcrowded parts of Germany and relocate to Hungary and rebuild its population (Sasvari, 2005).

It was not until the first half of the 19th century that Hungary experienced an upsurge of Magyar nationalism, beginning with the language reform movement that changed the national language back to Hungarian (Hungary, 2001; Sasvari, 2005). On March 15, 1848, a Hungarian revolution took place in demand of democratic reforms and more independence from Austria. This marked the first time that the general population sustained a sense of national unity; however, only a few of the nationalities shared the experience while most turned against the Hungarians (Ember & Ember 2001; Sasvari, 2005). Although Austria defeated the revolution and continued to dominate, the Hungarians continued to resist. Eventually Austria gave into Magyar national aspirations and the Austrian tyranny ended with the 1867 Austrian–Hungarian Compromise. The Austro-Hungarian monarchy was formed, allowing for some Magyar self-government. During the next 50 years, the dual monarchy improved life for most of the people and allowed Hungary to become one of the most advanced countries in Europe (Sasvari, 2005); however, this monarchy ended after World War I with the Trianon Treaty of 1920, which altered the territorial integrity of Hungary. Approximately 70% of its historical territory and 58% of its former population were relinquished to neighboring countries (Sasvari, 2005). The border changes devastated the economy of Hungary, which then became a landlocked country as Croatia became part of Yugoslavia, thus depriving Hungary of its access to the sea. Hungary's shipping industry for goods was dismantled as was much of its banking industry. Hungary lost two thirds of its roads and railroads, nearly two thirds of its arable land, 90% of its timber, and more than half of its industrial plants as these became part of other countries. Consequently, Hungary was left with no allies and was surrounded by enemies. It was lodged between two superpowers with Stalin and Communism in the east and Hitler and Fascism in the west. Despite this, throughout the 1930s the economy improved, crime was down, the government was democratically elected, and fairly rational discussions were taking place in the parliament. In addition, some of the land, mainly part of Transylvania, was returned (Sasvari, 2005); however, at the end of World War II, Hungary was relinquished to Soviet occupation and Moscow leadership (Ember & Ember, 2001).

The standard of living in Soviet-occupied Hungary plummeted and both tension and dissatisfaction escalated. In 1956, a Hungarian uprising and subsequent revolt occurred. Consequently, approximately 200,000 Hungarians fled from Hungary to any country that would accept them, including the United States, Canada, the United Kingdom, France, Germany, Switzerland, Australia, and New Zealand. This exodus consisted primarily of young people, skilled workers, white-collar workers, professionals, and intellectuals (Ember & Ember, 2001; Sasvari, 2005).

On October 23, 1989, Hungary declared itself a republic and the Communist regime ended in Hungary. Soon after, Hungary became the first Socialist-Bloc country to dismantle its section of the Iron Curtain (Hungary, 2001; Sasvari, 2005). Subsequently, on November 9, 1989, the 155-km Berlin Wall constructed in 1961 between East and West Germany was dismantled (Sasvari, 2005). In March 1999, Hungary became a member of the North Atlantic Treaty Organization (NATO). The Republic of Hungary began the process of integration into the European Union and, on May 1, 2004, became a member state. Accordingly, Hungary's integration process into the European Union continues to progress (MFA, 2007).

FOOD HISTORY WITHIN THE CULTURE

There are two major facets that contributed to the originality of Hungarian cuisine. One factor was the adjacency and blending of many different cultures through the centuries; the other was the extended isolation of much of Hungary from the west. Although these two aspects may appear paradoxical, they actually worked harmoniously to influence and preserve traditional ways (Derecskey, 1972).

The history of Hungarian food begins with a soup kettle, or *borgrács*, the vessel used by the Magyars hundreds of years before they settled into the Carpathian Basin and is still used today. It is the vessel from which all the Hungarian signature dishes emerged, including *gulyás, pörkölt, paprikás,* and *halászlé*. The Magyars were best known for their herds of cattle, such as the Hungarian gray cattle (also known as *szürkamarha*), which were very hardy with sleek gray coats, long horns, and lean, flavorful flesh. The herdsmen learned to cook because they were away for long periods of time as they drove the cattle across the plains to large cattle markets. Along their journey, they would slaughter one of the beasts and use the meat to make a *gulyás* that would last for several days (Sasvari, 2005). During this era, a variety of preservation techniques were utilized that allowed the meat to be transported. One method was to cook the meat until it was completely dry; when ready for use, water was added and the mixture was brought to a boil (Lang, 1994).

It was not until after the Magyars reached the Carpathian Basin that they began to eat pork. This is because they were previously associated with Muslims and with the Khazar Kingdom, which was converted to Judaism in 740 AD. Indigenous to Hungary is the Mangalica pig, which required little tending and was left to forage alone. The fat and meat of this species is extremely low in cholesterol. Traditional Hungarian cuisine relied on its fat and bacon in preparing both meat dishes and the famed Hungarian paprika sausage (MFA, 2007). The Mangalica pig was the most important breed in Hungary until the mid-1950s when modern commercial pig breeds began to proliferate. Recently, however, the value characteristics of the Mangalica pig, including disease resistance and meat quality, have once again been sought. Efforts are being made to save and propagate the breed (ASD, 2008).

Bread became a fundamental part of Hungarian cuisine. During the Middle Ages, three kinds of bread were available at the marketplace, each sold by bakers of three different ranks. The master baker made white rolls and bread. The "middle" baker made the everyday bread and the "black-bread" baker made the cheapest, unrefined loaves. Both the master and middle bakers were allowed to sell their products on a table or bench; however, the black-bread baker could sell his bread only from the ground. By the 16th and 17th centuries bread was served as a part of every meal (Lang, 1994). In the middle of the 17th century, iron rollers were introduced for milling wheat, which forced the wheat germ to be extricated without crushing. This resulted in the whitest milled flour available anywhere and the breads, cakes, and pastries baked with this new white flour rapidly became a status symbol (HFC, 2008).

Pasta is a favorite Hungarian food. The most rustic form of Hungarian pasta is the pellets called *tarhonya*.

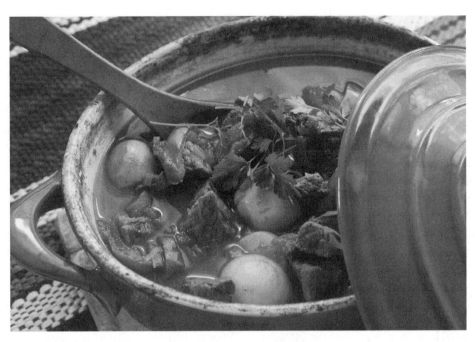

Hungary's first signature dishes, including gulyás, pörkölt, paprikás, and halászlé, were prepared in soup kettles.

It is believed that this came with the Magyars from Asia, although it is also suspected that it was a gift of the Turks (Sasvari, 2005). *Tarhonya* is kneaded from eggs and flour and granulated into small pellets, dried, and may be stored in the dry condition for extended periods. When needed, it is cooked in water and served as an accompaniment to meat dishes (Venesz, 1982). Nevertheless, what is considered as authentic pasta was brought from Italy by the Italian princess Beatrice who married King Matthias I in 1475. It was King Matthias who introduced fine dining to Hungary. Beatrice also brought a variety of other foods to Hungary including cheeses, pastries, ice creams, chestnuts, figs, anise, dill, capers, onions, and garlic (Lang, 1994; Sasvari, 2005). The onion became an important ingredient in Hungarian cuisine, as it is the base for Hungary's famous soups and stews (Sasvari, 2005). Additionally, King Matthias requested from the Duke of Milan a variety of domestic fowl and a caretaker for them. These birds acclimated themselves to the extent that the fame of Hungarian geese, ducks, hens, and other birds slowly spread over Europe and today are considered as the most choice on the continent (Lang, 1994).

Although the Turks exploited the area, they brought with them what eventually became many of the country's favorite foods, including paprika, sour cherries, corn, and tomatoes. The Hungarians are in such awe of tomatoes that they call them *paradicso*,

or paradise (Lang, 1994; Sasvari, 2005). The Turks introduced a variety of rice pilafs as well as *pitah*, which remained as *lángos*, the ancestor of the pizza (Lang, 1994). The Turks also brought a new beverage called coffee, which was discovered in Ethiopia and gradually made its way north to the Turks. Hungarian *kávé* has a dark, rich flavor and today is considered the true Hungarian drink, more important even than wine, *pálinka*, or soda water, which was a local invention (Sasvari, 2005). In addition, the Turks brought their filo pastry invention. (The word "filo" or "phyllo" comes from the Greek word for leaf.) However, unlike the Turks and the Greeks, who usually layered the filo with fillings in a dish, the Hungarians rolled the filo around a filling, such as fruit and/or nuts or raisins, to create a tender, flaky log of pastry called strudel (Sasvari, 2005).

When the Habsburgs assumed control over Hungary in the 17th century, they attempted to Germanize all walks of life, including the expressions and style of cooking (Lang, 1994). During the 18th century, the Habsburgs used Hungary as the agricultural part of their empire and prohibited the development of industry. This actually had a positive effect on the cuisine, which became the main occupation of the entire nation. The vineyards were replanted and the quantity, quality, and variety of wines were vastly increased and improved. Restaurants and pastry shops opened up, and along the Danube little boutiques (*butiks*) sold ice cream, lemonade, fruit, and other refreshments. *Pálinka* (fruit brandy) became a popular drink (Lang, 1994). It is likely that the Germans also brought a vast selection of dumplings or *nokedli* (Sasvari, 2005).

Although the Hungarians had been making sausage for centuries, the Germans brought their sophisticated smokehouse traditions for making sausage, one of the world's first convenience foods. Hungary was soon producing a multitude of sausage varieties, from pork, beef, goose, game, fish, and organ meats that were flavored with salt, paprika, garlic, and pepper, as well as more exotic ingredients such as truffles, marjoram, cumin, horseradish, and lemon rind. The German smokehouses allowed the Hungarians to develop bacon, another great Hungarian foodstuff. There are more than 20 types of bacon in Hungary, including cured, salted, smoked, sweet, plain, and spicy (Sasvari, 2005).

The Austrians gave Hungary the *virsli* (wiener) and the wiener schnitzel, known as *bécsi szelet* in Hungary. In addition, the Austrians provided Hungary with the fine art of pastry making. Both countries enjoy a torte made with eggs and nuts. In Hungary, the base of this torte was used to make *Dobos torta*, which became a national cake (Sasvari, 2005).

Throughout the history of Hungary, the borders in the region frequently shifted and the people moved around and often intermarried. As a result, Hungary shares many culinary traditions with her neighboring countries. For example, although the cabbage roll or stuffed cabbage is a part of every cuisine in Central Europe, it is closely associated with Hungary (Sasvari, 2005). According to Sasvari (2005, p. 57), there was supposedly a saying in the 18th century that "Meat and cabbage are the coat of arms of Hungary." The meat fillings for the cabbage rolls and other stuffed dishes came from the Balkan cultures that, in turn, learned it from the Turks. Hungarians traditionally serve cabbage rolls with sour cream, unlike other cuisines that make them with a tomato-based sauce (Sasvari, 2005).

Along with the 19th-century reformation, a culinary renaissance occurred. The "national" dishes, such as *gulyás*, which previously existed only in the cooking vessels of the peasants, began to be served on the tables of the nobility. For the first time, the five elements of Hungarian cuisine were united. It had begun with the culinary techniques of Hungary's Asiatic ancestors, grew with the Italian Renaissance influences of King Matthias, expanded with the ingredients brought by the Turks (including corn, cherries, coffee, and strudel), and finally was provided a sophistication, finesse, and lightness of touch by the French chefs who arrived

via Austria. (Sasvari, 2005). The French, who believe restraint is virtuous, retained the national Hungarian cuisine while reducing the heaviness of foods and using spices more judiciously (Lang, 1994).

Hungary is a land of romance, wine, gypsy music, and pastry lovers. At the beginning of the 19th century, Hungarians learned of tortes and tarts from the French, and from the Austrians they learned of home-style cakes and pastries. Nonetheless, the origins of Hungarian pastry-making crafts have been lost in the Middle Ages. Records from the 15th century indicate that a guild existed in which its members had permits to make medicine, spiced drinks, candies, and pastries. Chocolate making was learned from Italian traveling candy makers. From the Turks they learned the art of honeyed sweetmeats and Near Eastern specialties. The first pastry shop was opened in Hungary in the middle of the 18th century. With few exceptions, pastries are found in pastry shops and espressos, but not in restaurants in Hungary. Restaurants are allowed to make their own type of hot-noodle dessert. A *csárda* (inn or tavern) may possibly have strudel, but no other sweets. Pastry shops are thought to be a haven against the cruelty of the outside world, offering assorted consolations of cake and coffee, lace and legend (Lang, 1994).

In the 16th century, during Turkish occupation, there were kahva hanes (coffeehouses) in several sections of Buda, Óbuda, and Pest; however, the first Hungarian coffeehouse opened in Buda in 1714. Unlike the Turkish coffeehouses, which were noisy and filled with smoke and bargaining merchants, the first Hungarian coffeehouse offered not only coffee and tobacco, but also a place to play chess, an early form of billiards, and various card games. Gradually, the bill of fare was extended to include tea, hot chocolate, sweet wafers, and ice cream. Later, the ambiance expanded as well. During the warm weather, a wall was removed to create the garden coffeehouse. With the addition of gypsy musicians, the coffeehouse tradition grew and became closely intertwined with the cultural, political, and literary life of Hungary. In 1827 they began serving cold meats, sausages, cheeses, and pâtés, and eventually they also served supper dishes, thus competing with restaurants (Lang, 1994).

Hungary is one of the historic wine-growing areas of the Old World and produces many fine wines (Derecskey, 1972; HFC, 2008). Viticulture in the Carpathian Basin preceded the arrival of the Magyars. It was actually a relatively indistinct Roman emperor named Probus from the 3rd century who ordered his legions to plant and cultivate grapes in the area (Derecskey, 1972).

Miraculously, viticulture survived in Hungary through the centuries that included both historic and natural disasters (Derecskey, 1972). Viticulture is particularly evident around the hills of Tokaj in northern Hungary, characteristically known as the Hungarian wine-growing district (Lang, 1994). *Tokaj*, the most famed Hungarian wine, is sweet and unlike any other wine in the world (Advameg, 2007; MFA, 2007). According to Lang (1994, p. 104), after centuries of controversy, 25 villages of the *Tokaj-Hegyalja*, which means "at the feet of the hill," were granted the right to call their wines *Tokaj*, also known as "Tokay" outside of Hungary.

 MAJOR FOODS

According to Sasvari (2005, p. 8), traditional Hungarian food is "rich, fattening, deep-fried, and frequently loaded with sour cream, potatoes, lard and lots and lots of onions," yet it is also "cheap and hearty and flavorful" (Sasvari, 2005, p. 8). Hungarians cook economically, waste nothing, and capitalize on seasonal produce (Ender, 1986). In addition, Hungarian cuisine is beset with new endeavors. A Hungarian cook uses a recipe as a starting point and then goes beyond the recipe to carry out a new experiment (Asturias & Neruda, 1969).

 Protein Sources

The most popular meats in Hungary are pork and veal, followed by beef. These meats are the basis of stews and many casseroles. Chicken is still considered as a special-occasion meal and Hungarians seldom eat lamb (Derecskey, 1972). Salami, smoked sausages, bacon, and other by-products of pig butchering are an integral part of Hungarian life (Derecskey, 1972; Farkas, 1998; MFA, 2007). All types of offal and variety meats are used in sausages, stews, soups, and casseroles with vegetables (HFC, 2008).

Fish is not consumed in great amounts. Because of the country's geography, only freshwater fish is available domestically, originating from the country's rivers and lakes. These fish include *sterlet*, a small sturgeon, *pike-perch* or *fogas*, as well as carp, trout, *silure* or *catfish*, and small amounts of tiny crabs and crayfish (HFC, 2008; Venesz, 1982). Hungarians are very particular about the freshness of their fish and prefer to consume locally caught fresh fish rather than imported varieties. Fish is made into a soup or prepared as a main dish (Derecskey, 1972).

Eggs are considered to be most suitable as a starter, although they can also be served as the main dish. Cheese, including cottage cheese, is often eaten raw but is also served cooked in a variety of dishes (Venesz, 1982). Although legumes and dried beans are occasionally used in soups or in a bean casserole called *somogyi*, they are not an important part of the Hungarian diet (Ender, 1986; HFC, 2008).

 Starch Sources

Wheat and rye, as well as other types of cereal grains, are considered as the staff of life in Hungary (Lang, 1994). Moreover, Hungarian wheat, *bankoti*, has a high gluten content and is considered one of the finest in the world (Berkoff, 2002; MFA, 2007). A Hungarian table is seldom set without a variety of bread and rolls, with white loaf bread being a favorite (HFC, 2008; Lang, 1994). Noodles (*metelt*) are widely used and encompass a vast variety in Hungary with every household and restaurant having its own technique for mixing flour and water together to make them (Berkoff, 2002; HFC, 2008). The most popular noodles are *galuska*, soft noodles made by dipping thin pieces of bread dough into simmering water. They are usually served with stews such as *pörkölt* and *paprikás* (Berkoff, 2002; Savari, 2005). There are many other dumplings, including the large, savory liver dumpling used in soups. There are also the filled-potato dumplings known as *gombóc*, which are similar to the perogy but with a lighter dough with more varied fillings, such as fruit, *túro* (a smooth cottage cheese), or meat. The most popular dumpling is the *szivás gombóc*, which is stuffed with plums and sugar, boiled, and then quickly fried with bread crumbs (Sarvari, 2005). *Tarhonya* is a type of egg barley that is made from flour and eggs and grated into boiling water (Berkoff, 2002). Cereals, such as dried breakfast flakes or cooked porridge, are not traditionally used (HFC, 2008).

 Fat Sources

Lard has been the primary fat in Hungarian cookery, although the use of oil is becoming more prevalent (Biró, 2007; Ender, 1986). Butter is also used for flavor and in baked goods. Because the quality of the available margarines and oils has been considered inferior, they have not been traditionally used (HFC, 2008). Other fat sources include bacon with a large percentage of fat, sour cream, sweet butter, and cream (Advameg, 2007; Derecskey, 1972; Ender, 1986; Water and Fire, n.d.). Hungarian sour cream has a thinner consistency and its flavor is more tart than the American product (Derecskey, 1972). Cream is often used for desserts (Water and Fire, n.d.).

 ## Prominent Vegetables

Many or most of the vegetables consumed in Hungary are of the nongreen variety. Vegetables are rarely served raw or simply steamed, boiled, or sautéed, because such processes would merely be a first step in the preparation process (Berkoff, 2002; EHFD, 2008; Lang, 1994). The consumption of plain, boiled vegetables is incomprehensible to a Hungarian (Lang, 1994). After being braised, baked, or boiled, vegetables are drained and blended in a variety of methods including with a roux or thickened with sour cream, blended with a sauce of onions, paprika, and sour cream, or topped with buttered crumbs. They may also be prepared as stuffed vegetables, vegetable puddings, vegetable souflés, or fresh vegetable soups, and thus may be included in different parts of the meal (HFC, 2008; Lang, 1994; Venesz, 1982).

The vegetables that are considered to be the staples of Hungarian cuisine and the most popular are cabbage, peppers, tomatoes, potatoes, onions, and cucumbers. These vegetables are typically the basis for stews and soups, and are also stuffed or pickled (Berkoff, 2002; HFC, 2008). Sauerkraut or pickled white cabbage is preferred to ordinary raw cabbage for many combination dishes. White cabbage is used for stuffed cabbage (Ender, 1986). A variety of sweet peppers are used. Red peppers are preserved and used for flavoring dishes or may be used raw in salads. A special horn-shaped red pepper is grown for making paprika. Green bell peppers are used raw in salads but are never used for cooking due to their bitter flavor. Both the pale green (almost white), elongated peppers and yellow peppers are stuffed. The tiny, round, red cherry peppers are usually strung together and dried; they are often used to spice up soups, especially the fiery fish soups (Ender, 1986). Onions are chopped and slowly stewed in hot fat until they turn soft, which is a fundamental technique of Hungarian cooking (Derecskey, 1972). Other useful vegetables include *kohlrabi*, or parsley roots, which are used in conjunction with carrots to give flavor to soups and stews, as well as celeriac, which is used in place of celery (Ender, 1986; Venesz, 1982).

The classical Hungarian salad consists of a vegetable that has been immersed in a sweet–sour vinegar solution. Salads are consumed in moderation to assist in the digestion of food, particularly meat dishes (to help digest the fat). Salads are not consumed as appetizers before the main course (Farkas, 1998).

 ## Prominent Fruits

Apricots, plums, peaches, cherries, and sour cherries are grown in Hungarian orchards. They are used as strudel fillings and for chilled fruit soups (Ender, 1986). Apples, plums, apricots, and melons are consumed fresh and are also made into preserves and brandies (HFC, 2008).

 ## Spices, Seasonings, and Herbs

Onions, garlic, and paprika are most often used to flavor meals (Water and Fire, n.d.). Paprika is the most commonly used spice, following salt (Farkas, 1998). Paprika provides Hungarian food with its characteristic taste and color by enhancing flavor rather than dominating it (Magyar, 1989). Paprika has very little aroma and no flavor of its own; however, when heated in a liquid, it has a peppery flavor with a range from mild and sweet to fiery hot (Sasvari, 2005). Paprika is made from sweet red peppers that have been dried and pulverized. It is available in hot and sweet varieties (Sasvari, 2005). Generally, mild paprika is used for cooking and hot paprika is sprinkled on food at the table (Ender, 1986). Other herbs that are used include fresh dill, parsley, marjoram, tarragon, and basil (Ender, 1986; Magyar, 1989).

Nuts and poppy seeds are important for flavoring and are used in cakes, tortes, strudel, yeast pastries, and breads. They are also tossed with buttered noodles and consumed as a side dish, snack, or dessert (Berkoff, 2002; Magyar, 1989). Poppy seeds are used cooked or raw. They are often used in ground form, sweetened with sugar, and used for filling pastries (Venesz, 1982). In addition, caraway seeds are used in simple soups and vegetable sauces (Magyar, 1989).

 ## Beverages

The main Hungarian beverages are coffee, wine, and brandy. Coffee is served in different ways depending on the time of day it is consumed. Breakfast coffee is served with hot milk, whereas afternoon coffee is often served with whipped cream, and dinner coffee is served black (Berkoff, 2002). The ambience of a Hungarian meal is considered deficient without wine (Derecskey, 1972). *Pálinka* is a fruit brandy that has an alcohol content higher than 40%. The most popular Hungarian flavors are apricot, plum, and cherry (Sasvari, 2005). Although fresh milk is seldom used as a beverage, it is incorporated into many dishes, including puddings, custards, and milk soups (HFC, 2008). Mineral water is considered one of the best natural resources of Hungary (TJC Global, 2007).

 ## Desserts

Hungarians have a national preference for cakes, cookies, and pastries, rather than candy (Berkoff, 2002; HFC, 2008). Sweet baked goods are consumed as a snack with coffee and as dessert (HFC, 2008). Hungarian meals usually end with something sweet (Derecskey, 1972).

Strudel or *rétés* is a favorite with coffee (Sasvari, 2005). *Dobos torta*, invented in 1884 by József Dobos, consists of six layers of sponge torte, with a vanilla and chocolate buttercream layered in-between them and topped with a hard layer of caramel (MFA, 2007; Sasvari, 2005). Gundel pancake was created by Károly Gundel in the late 19th century. The pancake is filled with cottage cheese that has been mixed with rum-soaked raisins, lemon peel, and ground walnuts, and topped with warm vanilla-and-chocolate sauce (MFA, 2007). Palacsinta are very thin pancakes that are most often used for sweet dishes. Traditionally, they are filled and served rolled up and eaten with a fork and knife. Fillings include fruit preserves, with apricot jam being most popular, cottage or cream cheese, and chopped nuts (Berkoff, 2002; Derecskey, 1972).

 ## FOODS WITH CULTURAL SIGNIFICANCE

Hungarians typically prefer rich and spicy sauces and stews, rather than dishes that do not contain liquid. They freely use red pepper, fresh green peppers, tomatoes, sour cream, and lard. Although lard and goose fat are still used for cooking, the use of vegetable oils has become more popular. Hungarians also use pastas for desserts, such as noodles with cottage cheese or *túróscsusza*, egg squares with fried cabbage, or *káposztáskocka* (Water and Fire, n.d.).

Soup is considered to be the soul of Hungarian cuisine. There is a soup for every occasion and for every menu (Derecskey, 1972). Hungarians are said to be able to make a soup from almost anything (HFC, 2008). Traditionally, no Hungarian meal is acceptable without soup as a first course (Farkas, 1998). Fish soup or *halászlé* is a national dish (Advameg, 2007). Soups are served piping hot in soup plates that have a wide rim. The soup spoons used in Hungary are deep and larger than the typical "soup spoons" found in American flatware sets (Farkas, 1998).

The most famous Hungarian dish is *gulyás* (goulash), a thick, spicy soup that is most often made with beef that has been cut into cubes up to 1 inch in size, browned with onions, and cooked in a lot of stock until tender. It also contains potatoes, other vegetables, and is seasoned with paprika (Derecskey, 1972; Farkas, 1998; Hungarians, 1998).

One of the most notable characteristics of Hungarian cooking is the braising of meat on a base of onions seasoned with paprika for certain meat dishes such as *gulyás* (Venesz, 1982). *Pörkölt* is a stew made with either pork or veal, not usually with beef. The meat is cut into cubes at least 1 inch in size, browned, and then braised

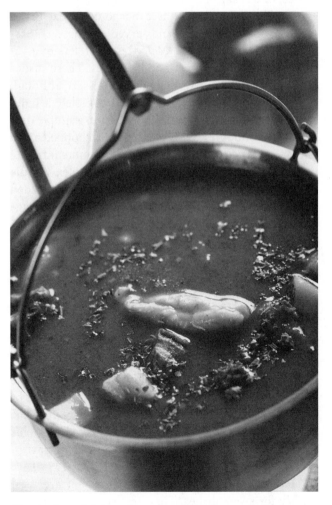

Goulash, a thick, spicy soup that is most often made with beef, is Hungary's most famous dish.

in a small amount of stock or water. (Derecskey, 1972; Hungarians, 1998). *Paprikás* is a *pörkölt* or stew with sour cream added at the end of the cooking process. The best *paprikás* is made with veal or chicken (Derecskey, 1972; Hungarians, 1998).

Lesco is a commonplace staple that consists of onions, green peppers, garlic, and tomatoes that are simmered to meld the flavors. It is served as a side dish and is also used as a flavoring agent for soups and stews (Berkoff, 2002; Derecskey, 1972).

The classical Hungarian salad is a vegetable, such as cucumber, immersed in a sweet–sour vinegar solution and consumed in moderation to assist in the digestion of food, particularly the fat from meat. Salads are not consumed as appetizers before the main course (Farkas, 1998).

There are a multitude of noodle dishes in Hungarian cuisine, with each dish designed for a specific noodle. Various noodles can be used in soup, as side dishes, or as easy main courses using inexpensive vegetarian ingredients such as cabbage or wheat germ, whereas others are sweet and served as a dessert (Sasvari, 2005; Venesz, 1982). *Meleg tesztak* refers to a variety of Hungarian sweet noodle dishes. These dishes are always served hot and usually as a dessert, although they often follow a soup entree and complete a light, satisfying meal. *Meleg tesztak* varies from a simple dish of buttered noodles tossed with sugar, chopped nuts, cinnamon, and possibly poppy seeds, to more intricate noodle-type puddings. These more complex noodle dishes are baked and consist of noodles lightly folded with beaten separated eggs as well as sieved cottage cheese, nuts, raisins, and fruit preserves (Berkoff, 2002; HFC, 2008).

Hungarians are renowned for their elegant pastries and cakes. *Rétes*, the Hungarian version of strudel, can be sweet or savory. Strudel shops in Budapest offer prune, plum, poppy seed, and apricot fillings, as well as savory fillings of potatoes and cheese (Berkoff, 2002).

One of the oldest Hungarian crafts is the honey-bread craft. Originally known by the Latin term *dulciariorum*, this was changed around the end of the 19th century to the literal translation of *mézeskalács* or *mézesbábos*, which means honey cake, honey puppets, or honey dolls (Lang, 1994). They are baked in molds that craftsmen used to hand carve and are a part of every village fair and holiday festival (Lang, 1994).

Palacsinta are very thin pancakes that are used mostly for sweet dishes. They are served with dessert fillings, such as fruit preserves, cream cheese, and chopped nuts (Berkoff, 2002).

TYPICAL DAY'S MENU

The Hungarian meal pattern consists of an early but light breakfast followed by a more substantial, satisfying breakfast, called *Tizórai*, at 10 AM. Next is the noon meal, which is usually the main meal of the day. This is followed by a snack in the middle of the afternoon, usually coffee with a piece of rich pastry or coffee cake. Supper is typically lighter than the noon meal. Beverages that accompany meals include primarily coffee, beer, or Tokay wine. Coffee is served plain, diluted with milk, or topped with a generous mound of whipped cream (de Proft et al., 1955).

Breakfast consists of coffee with hot milk, rolls, and preserves (Berkoff, 2002; HFC, 2008). *Tizórai* or mid-morning snack may consist of a small bowl of *gulyás* or bread and onions, or something similar to breakfast such as coffee with bread or rolls (HFC, 2008).

The noon meal is usually the largest meal of the day. It typically consists of three parts: a starter, a main dish, and dessert (Water and Fire, n.d.). The usual Hungarian starter is soup. The main dish that follows is generally a type of meat and a garnish (Water and Fire, n.d.). Either cabbage, potatoes, or noodles are incorporated with the meat dish or served as a side dish. The meal is habitually completed with dessert, such as stewed fruits, thin dessert pancakes or *palacsintak*, dumplings served with sweet sauces, fritters or noodle desserts, soufflés, custards, or puddings; however, for a poor household, this noon meal may consist of only soup and bread (HFC, 2008). Beverages, usually water, or seltzer during the summer, are served midway through dinner or after the meal (Farkas, 1998).

Starters or entrees are served before or after the soup, but always before the main course. They are light dishes and combinations of various dishes and may be either hot or cold. Their purpose is to whet the appetite and provide nutritive value. A light starter can be served before a heavy meat course, or a more substantial starter can be served when the main course is not so rich. They can be prepared with a variety of vegetables or various kinds of meat, fish, and eggs (Venesz, 1982). Appetizers are served only in restaurants or aristocratic homes (HFC, 2008).

The afternoon snack consists of honey cake or coffee cake, and coffee served with whipped cream (Berkoff, 2002; HFC, 2008). When there are guests, the snack may be more elaborate, with a choice of pastries, cakes, strudel, and *torta*, which may be consumed at a coffeehouse (HFC, 2008).

The evening meal is eaten between 7 and 9 PM and usually consists of a light supper. This may be leftovers from the noon meal, such as soup and dessert, or it may consist of soup with bread or light dishes made from eggs (HFC, 2008).

HOLIDAY MENUS

In Hungary the most important religious holiday is Easter. Dinner on Good Friday consists of wine-flavored soup, stuffed eggs, and baked fish (HFC, 2008). The Easter Eve feast is the biggest and most important Hungarian meal of the year. It consists of a rich chicken soup served with dumplings or noodles and is followed by roasted ham, hard-boiled eggs, horseradish, and red and yellow pieces of aspic. Pickled vegetables and stuffed cabbage rolls may also be included (Magyar, 1989). The meal is completed with a selection of sweet cakes, including walnut and poppy-seed rolls and black coffee (HFC, 2008; Magyar, 1989). On Easter Sunday, the feast continues with a traditional main dish of roast lamb and "blessed" ham. The meal begins with clear soup with liver dumplings followed by stuffed cabbage and subsequently with more cakes and pastries (HFC, 2008; Magyar, 1989).

Christmas Eve day is a fasting day in Hungary. This means that Hungarians abstain from eating meat. The Christmas Eve meal is fairly simple: fish and potatoes followed by cakes and tortes made with nuts and poppy seeds (HFC, 2008). Christmas dinner is usually consumed in the early or mid-afternoon. It typically begins with apricot brandy followed by a soup, such as carp-fish soup or turkey-giblet soup. The main meal is celebrated with roast turkey stuffed with chestnut dressing, followed by walnut rolls and poppy-seed rolls and wine (Cleveland Heritage Museum, 2007; Magyar, 1989).

On New Year's Eve, *krambambuli*, a spicy punch, is served. The ingredients include chopped fruit, candied orange peel, walnuts, sugar, rum, and brandy. On New Year's Day, eating roast pig is thought to bring good luck (Advameg, 2007).

HEALTH BELIEFS AND CONCERNS

In 2005, life expectancy in Hungary at birth for males and females was 69 and 77 years, respectively; however, healthy life expectancy at birth was lower for both males and females at 62 and 68 years, respectively. Regarding their general state of health in 2000, 23% of males and 25% of females in Hungary reported feeling restricted in their usual activities. In the same year, only 48% of men self-assessed their health as being good, while only 39% of women self-assessed their health as being good or very good (NISHR, 2005); however, the deterioration of health among Hungarians has been more evident among men than women in the past decade (Skrabski, Kopp, Rózsa, Réthelyi, & Rahe, 2005). The results of a nationally representative Hungarian study by Skrabski et al. (2005) showed that meaning in life is a positive psychological resource that enhances health in the Hungarian population. Specifically, life meaning was correlated with several positive psychosocial factors, including self-efficacy, problem-focused coping, religiousness, and high levels of social support. In addition, they found life meaning to be relatively independent of age, gender, and education (Skrabski et al., 2005).

The leading causes of morbidity and mortality are noncommunicable diseases, with a prevalence of lifestyle risk factors; namely smoking, an unhealthy diet, and a lack of physical activity. Of particular concern is the high mortality rate among men ages 30–65 years. Hungarian males have the highest mortality rate in the world from lung cancer. In women, cancers of the respiratory tract that are attributable to smoking have increased since the 1980s (WHO, 2008). In fact, Hungary has one of the highest smoking rates in Europe (Hungary, 2001). In the year 2000, 38.3% of males and 23% of females reported being "regular smokers" (NISHR, 2005).

Standardized mortality rates for cardiovascular disorders in Hungarians less than 65 years are three times higher than the European average (Skrabski et al., 2005). In 2005, ischemic heart disease and cerebrovascular disease accounted for 37.8% of the total deaths in Hungary. Hypertension affects more than 50% of Hungarians in the age range of 25–64 years and type 2 diabetes affects approximately 10% of Hungarians (WHO, 2008). Moreover, obesity, hypertension, and nutritional deficiencies in the Hungarian population are attributable to an unhealthy diet. Hungarians have high intakes of animal fat, cholesterol, and salt, and inadequate intakes of vegetables, minerals, and dietary fiber. These factors are further accentuated by low levels of physical activity (WHO, 2008). Although the average total fat consumption has remained relatively unchanged since 1990 (38% of total calories), the consumption of lard has decreased by 30% since 1980 and the use of sunflower oil and other plant oils has increased (Biró, 2007; Rodler & Zajkás,

2002). Hungarian vegetable and fruit purchase patterns have remained unchanged since the 1970s and are among the lowest among European countries (Rodler & Zajkás, 2002). In 2005, only about 21% of males and 14% of females in the 15- to 64-year age range actually exercised regularly. Indeed, in 2005, two thirds of Hungarian men and half of the Hungarian women were overweight or obese (WHO, 2008). Rurik's (2006) study with elderly Hungarians indicated that none of the males >65 years of age nor the females >60 years of age engaged in regular exercise. Furthermore, their body weight had continuously increased over their lifetime, with higher increases in the women than in the men, and dieting attempts were made by 8% of the men and 30% of the women.

In Hungary, cancer was the cause of every fourth death in 2005, a rate that is among the highest in international comparisons and twice as high as the European average (Skrabski et al., 2005; WHO, 2008). In comparison with the rest of Europe in 2005, Hungarians had the highest death rates for cancer of the lip, colon, rectum, larynx, trachea, bronchi, and lung (WHO, 2008). One risk factor for the development of certain cancers is alcohol consumption. Based on 1999 purchase statistics, the average alcohol–energy percentage of the daily dietary intake was 6.5% (Rodler & Zajkás, 2002). Moreover, in the year 2000, only 10.1% of males and 36.5% of females reported that they did not consume alcohol (NISHR, 2005). A study by Rurik (2006) found that Hungarian males >65 years of age consumed greater quantities of alcoholic beverages and at a higher frequency than did Hungarian females >60 years of age. In addition, excessive alcohol consumption is likely to be the main cause of high male mortality from cirrhosis of the liver (WHO, 2008).

Kósa et al. (2007) compared the health of adults in the general Hungarian population with that of people living in Roma settlements, which tend to be on the outskirts of towns and villages. The results showed that the Roma were less educated and less likely to be employed, had worse living conditions, much lower income, and weaker social support, as compared with the general population. The self-reported health status of the Roma was found to be much worse than it was for the general population. Furthermore, a much smaller proportion of Roma thought that they could do much or very much to promote their own health than did people in the general population. In addition, the use of health services by the Roma population was similar to that in the lowest-income quartile of the general population. Furthermore, a clear contrast was seen in the dietary intake of the two populations. The proportion of persons who ate fresh fruits and vegetables daily and tended to use vegetable oil in cooking was much higher in the general population, even in comparison with people in the lowest-income quartile. Nevertheless, although the distribution of body weight was fairly similar in the two populations, there was slightly less obesity in the Roma women of all age groups; however, the prevalence of smoking at least 20 cigarettes per day was two to five times higher among the Roma than among people in the general population. Furthermore, although no large differences were seen in the overall prevalence of moderate and heavy drinking between the two populations, a higher occurrence of abstinence was reported by the Roma men in all age groups than in all of the general population.

Environmental hazards in Hungary are also contributing to poor health. Approximately 48% of the population in Hungary resides in just 11.5% of the country. A major causal factor of respiratory disease is air pollution, primarily as a result of vehicle emissions. In addition, surface waters are polluted from geologically based arsenic (WHO, 2008).

 ## GENERAL HEALTH AND NUTRITIONAL INDICATORS SUMMARY

In 2006, the population of Hungary was approximately 10,058,000 with a median age of 39 years. The annual growth rate of the population between 1996 and 2006 was –0.3%. The fertility rate among Hungarian women in 2006 was 1.3. Between the years 2000 and 2006, 100% of births were attended by skilled personnel, with 23% of deliveries occurring by Caesarean section. During the period from 2000 to 2002, approximately 9% of newborns had a birth weight less than 2500 g (WHO, 2009).

In 2004, the neonatal mortality rate, or probability of death between the time of birth and 28 days of life, was 5/1000 births. In 2006, the infant mortality rate, or probability of death between birth and exactly 1 year of age, was 6/1000 births. In 2006, the under-5-years mortality rate, or probability of dying by the age of 5 years, was 7/1000 live births. Among children under the age of 5 years, neonatal deaths accounted for 56.9% of the mortality rate, whereas injuries and pneumonia accounted for 5.6 and 3.9%, respectively. Approximately one third of the deaths in this category were due to other causes; none were reported as being related to HIV/AIDS, measles, or malaria (WHO, 2009).

Observations from the Author (Mary Louise Kranyak)

My father is Hungarian and my mother is German. My mother learned German cooking from her mother and Hungarian cooking from her mother-in-law. Thus, her cooking expertise includes both German and Hungarian cuisine, both of which share many similarities. As I delved deeper into this project, many of the peculiarities I encountered with food and meals when I was growing up suddenly began to make sense. For example, Farkas (1998) indicated that Hungarians eat soup with spoons that are larger than the "soup spoons" that are included in a contemporary American flatware set. Actually, Hungarians eat soup with what might be termed a "serving spoon" in a contemporary flatware set. Whenever my mother served soup, she always gave my father a "serving spoon" to use, from which he slurped the soup. Actually, I am not sure if he slurped the soup because the spoon was too large to adequately fit in his mouth or if it was out of habit. When I asked my mother why she gave my father that size spoon, she indicated that this was how my grandmother had always set the table for a meal that included soup. Now I understand why my father was accustomed to eating soup with a "serving spoon."

Furthermore, this project provided me with additional insight regarding the communication style of Hungarians. Specifically, Hungarians are direct when conversing with others and tend to say exactly what is on their minds. In retrospect, I have observed this characteristic in many of the Hungarians I have met. As an example, one Hungarian I have known all my life was born and raised in Hungary. As a young adult, she moved to the United States where she later married a Hungarian. Remaining bilingual in Hungarian and English, she continues to associate within a small Hungarian community. She is a warmhearted and caring person who is always giving to others. Yet, her candidness and inquisitive manner can sometimes be perceived as offensive to those who do not realize that this is generally the way Hungarians communicate. Thus, when speaking with Hungarians, it is best to be aware of their communication traits so that conversations can be maintained in proper perspective.

In 2005, 99% of vaccines routinely administered to protect Hungarian children were financed by the national government. During 2005, 99% of 1-year-old children in Hungary received vaccines against tuberculosis, diphtheria, pertussis (whooping cough), tetanus, polio, measles, and influenza type B (UNICEF, 2007). During 2000–2006, the primary-school-enrollment ratio for males was 90% and for females was 88% (WHO, 2009).

The adult Hungarian mortality ratio, or the probability of dying between the ages of 15 and 60 years, was 177/1000 of the populace; however, this ratio was higher for males than for females at 249 and 104, respectively, per 1000 in the population. In 2006, the entire population of Hungary was reported to have access to improved sanitation and improved drinking-water sources (WHO, 2009).

COMMUNICATION AND COUNSELING TIPS

A sense of bonding and familiarity is important to Hungarians, and they prefer to do business with those whom they know and trust (OneWorld, 2007; PTG, 2008); therefore, taking time to build relationships is worthwhile (OneWorld, 2007). Hungarians prefer face-to-face interaction over other forms of communication (KCCS, n.d.). Punctuality, an important virtue for Hungarians, is deemed to be essential (eHow, 2008). Being on time or up to 5 minutes early for all social situations is traditional (TJC Global, 2007). In the case of a delay, an immediate telephone call with an explanation is in order. Canceling a meeting at the last minute is considered to be extremely rude (KCCS, n.d.).

For both men and women, the standard form of greeting is a handshake (PTG, 2008); however, a man should pause for a woman to extend her hand first (eHow, 2008). Visitors should stand when introduced to someone (PTG, 2008). Verbal greetings are particularly important (OneWorld, 2007). Hungarians introduce themselves by saying their full names, beginning with their family name or surname first, followed by their first name; however, as familiarity increases, they may ask to be addressed by their first name (Martire & Kelly, 2005). Asking "How are you?" is not considered to be a rhetorical question and requires an answer (OneWorld, 2007). Hungarians view eye contact during a conversation as being indicative of sincerity and believe that those who fail to do so are insincere and have something to hide (KCCS, n.d.; Martire & Kelly, 2005).

The intent for an initial meeting is to become acquainted with one another and evaluate the trustworthiness of the other person (KCCS, n.d.). The focus should be on small talk and developing familiarity with one another prior to discussing the business at hand. The Hungarian should be the one to lead the conversation into the business realm (KCCS, n.d.). Being fairly open and direct, Hungarians tend to say what they think and expect the same of others (KCCS, n.d.; Martire & Kelly, 2005). They dislike euphemisms and vague statements and are inclined to use stories, anecdotes, and jokes to prove their points (KCCS, n.d.).

Although Hungarians perhaps tend to use less personal space than others during conversations, it is not customary to physically touch others, such as giving a pat on the back or putting a hand on the shoulder. In essence, it is best to maintain a conservative approach with respect to body language and basic mannerisms (PTG, 2008). When conversing with others, Hungarians do not wave their hands about, gesture wildly, signal with their fingers, nod their heads, or dramatically roll their eyes (Martire & Kelly, 2005). Nonetheless, their candidness is evident in their conversation. Their inquiries, which can be quite personal, are merely a means of getting to know others, since they tend to become suspicious when others are reticent and guarded with their thoughts (eHow, 2008; KCCS, n.d.; Martire & Kelly, 2005).

Hungarians are very detail oriented and their preference is to understand everything before reaching an agreement (KCCS, n.d.). In business-related issues, it is best to be thorough in the discussion and record all the details in writing. Expectations need to be clarified to preclude any misinterpretations or misunderstandings of agreements (TJC Global, 2007). A meeting is typically concluded by shaking hands (OneWorld, 2007).

PRIMARY LANGUAGE OF FOOD NAMES WITH ENGLISH AND PHONETIC TRANSLATION

In general, the stress in Hungarian is on the first syllable of a word, with less stress on the first syllable of the second word of a phrase. For example, *csirke paprikás* (chicken paprikash) is pronounced CHEER-ke pah-pree-kahsh. Vowels have short or long sounds. Consonants are pronounced as in English, exclusive of the letters and combinations given in Table 15-1.

Table 15-2 lists some Hungarian food names with phonetic translation.

TABLE 15-1 Hungarian Consonants

Consonant	Pronunciation	Example
C	ts ("soft" c)	Floats
cs	tch	Porch
g	"hard" g	Garden
gy	dge	Fudge
j	y	Yard
s	sh	Sure
sz	s	Salami
Z	z	Zip
Zs	zh	Measure

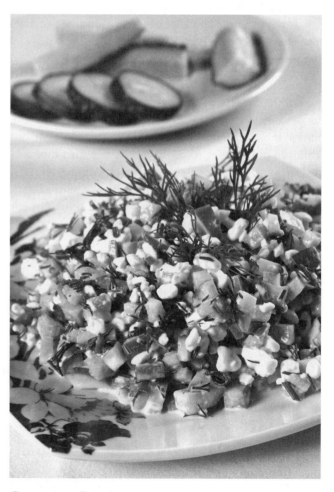

Cucumber Salad

TABLE 15-2   Hungarian Food Names with Phonetic Translation

Food (*ennivaló*; en-ni-vo-lā)	Hungarian Name	Phonetic Translation
Soup	*Levesek*	le-ve-shek
Goulash soup	*Gulyás leves*	gū-yahsh le-vesh
Fisherman's soup	*Halászlé*	ha-lahs-lay
Soft dumplings	*Galuska*	gah-lūsh-kah
Pinched noodles	*Csipetke*	chi-pet-ke
Egg barley	*Tarhonya*	tahr-hohn-yah
Cabbage dumplings	*Káposztás gombóc*	kah-poh-stahsh gom-bohts
Noodle dishes	*Laskák*	lahsh-kahk
Noodles with cabbage	*Káposztás kocka*	kah-poh-stahs kohts-kah
Palacsinta	*Palacsinták*	pah-lah-chin-tahk
Meat	*Hús*	Hūsh
Pork	*Sertés*	shayr-taysh
Pork paprika stew	*Sertés pörkölt*	shayr-taysh pur-kult
Pork sausage	*Disznóhúsból készült kolbász*	
Veal	*Borjú*	bawr-yū
Veal paprika stew	*Borjú pörkölt*	bawr-yū pur-kult
Beef	*Marha*	mahr-ha
Lamb	*Bárány*	bah rahny
Goulash	*Bogrács gulyás*	boh-grahch gū-yahsh
Fish	*Hal*	Hal
Poultry	*Szárnyas*	sahrn-yahsh
Chicken	*Csirke*	cheer-ke
Chicken paprikash	*Csirke paprikás*	cheer-ke pah-pree-kahsh
Turkey	*Pulyka*	pu-y-ko
Duck	*Kacsa*	kah-chah
Goose	*Liba*	lee-ba
Eggs	*Tojásos*	toi-ahsh-osh
Vegetables	*Zöldség*	zuld-shay gek
Cabbage	*Káposzta*	Kah-poh-sta
Stuffed cabbage	*Töltött káposzta*	tul-tot kah-poh-sta
Sauerkraut	*Savanyú káposzta*	shah-vahn-yū kah-poh-sta

(continues)

TABLE 15-2 Hungarian Food Names with Phonetic Translation (Cont.)

Food (*ennivaló*; en-ni-vo-lā)	Hungarian Name	Phonetic Translation
Cauliflower	*Karfiol*	kahr-fee-ohl
Green pepper and tomato stew	*Lecsó*	leh-choh
Stuffed green peppers	*Töltött paprika*	tul-tot pah-pree-ka
Kohlrabi	*Kalarábé*	ka-la-rah-bay
Potatoes	*Krumpli/burgonya*	krump-lee/bur-gon-ya
Cucumber salad	*Uborka sálata*	ū-bor-ka sha-lah-ta
Pickled beets	*Cekla salata*	tsayk-la sha-lah-ta
Fruit	*Gyümölcs*	dyew-meulch
Plum	*Szilvás*	sil-vahsh
Apple	*Alma*	ol-mo
Apricot	*Sárgabarack*	shaar-go-bo-rotsk
Walnuts	*Diós*	dee-ohsh
Noodle desserts	*Édes tészták*	ay-desh tay stahk
Stuffed palacsinta	*Töltött palacsinták*	tul-tot pah-lah-chin-tahk
Strudel	*Rétes*	ray-tesh
Poppy-seed roll	*Beigli*	bī-glee
Dobos torte	*Dobos torta*	doh-bosh tor-ta
Jam	*Dzsem*	Jem
Water	*Víz*	Veez
Mineral water	*Ásványviz*	aash-vaań-veez
Coffee	*Kávé*	kaa-vay
Tea	*Tea*	te-o
Wine	*Bor*	Bawr
Milk	*Tej*	te-y
Fat	*Kövér*	kea-vayr
Oil	*Olaj*	aw-lo-y
Bacon	*Szalonna*	so-lawn-nu
Butter	*Vaj*	vo-y
Cream	*Tej-szín*	te-y-seen
Sour cream	*Tejfol*	te-y-fuel

Compiled from Derecskey (1972) and Martire and Kelly (2005).

FEATURED RECIPES

Goulash
(Gulyás: gū-yahsh)

1½ lbs. boneless pot roast beef

3 cups prepared beef broth

4 slices bacon, diced

1 large onion, chopped

1 tbsp. paprika

¼ teaspoon freshly ground pepper

1 small green pepper, chopped

½ cup cold water*

¼ cup water*

1. Cut beef into 1½-inch pieces and set aside.
2. Place bacon into 3-qt. sauce pot; cook slowly, stirring frequently until bacon is lightly browned.
3. With a slotted spoon, remove bacon from sauce pot to a small bowl and set aside.
4. Add chopped onion to the bacon fat in the sauce pot and cook over medium heat until onion is transparent, stirring occasionally.
5. With a slotted spoon, remove onion from sauce pot and place in the bowl containing bacon; set aside.
6. Add meat to bacon fat; stir occasionally to slowly brown on all sides.
7. Sprinkle evenly over meat a mixture of the paprika and pepper. Stir in the bacon–onion mixture and the green pepper. Slowly pour in the beef broth and bring to a boil.
8. Reduce heat, cover sauce pot, and simmer for 2 hours, or until meat is tender when pierced with a fork.
9. Remove meat with slotted spoon to hot serving dish.

*If desired, thicken cooking liquid as follows: Put cold water into a 1-pt. container with a tight-fitting lid and sprinkle in flour; cover tightly and shake until mixture is well blended. Slowly pour half the mixture into the sauce pot, stirring constantly. Bring to a boil. Gradually add enough of the remaining flour–water mixture for the desired consistency. Bring to a boil after each addition. After the final addition, cook 3–5 minutes longer. Serve immediately.

Cucumber Salad
(*Uborka Sálata*: ū-bor-ka sha-lah-ta)

3 medium-sized cucumbers

1 tsp. salt

¼ cup white vinegar

½ cup water

1 tsp. sugar

Fresh or dried dill (optional)

Sour cream (optional)

1. Wash and peel cucumbers. Slice them ½ inch thick and place in a bowl. Mix lightly with salt and set cucumbers aside for 1 hour.
2. Mix vinegar, water, and sugar together, adjusting vinegar and sugar to taste, and set aside.
3. With clean hands, squeeze the liquid from cucumber slices, a few at a time, and put into a clean bowl; discard liquid.
4. Pour the vinegar mixture over the cucumbers and toss lightly together. If desired, sprinkle dill on top and mix in.
5. Chill for at least 1 hour. If desired, top each serving with a dollop of sour cream.

More recipes are available at http://nutrition.jbpub.com/foodculture/

REFERENCES

Advameg, Inc. (2007). *Food in Hungary forum.* Retrieved March 24, 2008, from http://www.foodbycountry.com/Germany-to-Japan/Hungary.html/

Animal Science Database (ASD). (2008). *Reproduction in the Hungarian mangalica pig.* Retrieved March 31, 2008, from http://www.animalscience.com/Reviews.asp?action=displayandopenMenu=relatedItemsandReviewID=871andSubjectID=/

Asturias, M.A., & Neruda, P. (1969). *Sentimental journey around the Hungarian cuisine.* Budapest, Hungary: Franklin Printing House.

Berkoff, N. (2002). Hungarian cuisine. *Vegetarian Journal, 21*(1), 9–12.

Biró, G. (2007). Public health nutrition in Hungary: Facts and hopes. *Hungarian Medical Journal, 1*(1), 7–12.

Budapest Hotels. (2008). *Religion in Hungary.* Retrieved March 31, 2008, from http://www.budapesthotels.com/tourist-guide/Religion.asp/

Cleveland Heritage Museum. (2007). *Christmas in Hungary.* Retrieved March 25, 2008, from http://www.jcu.edu/language/hunghemu/hunghe7g.htm/

de Proft, M., Albrecht, B., Bell, R., Buchanan, E., Clifford, K., Fulde, L., et al. (1955). *The Hungarian cookbook.* Chicago: Culinary Arts Institute.

Derecskey, S. (1972). *The Hungarian cookbook.* New York: Harper and Row Publishers.

eHow. (2008). *How to learn Hungarian etiquette.* Retrieved March 23, 2008, from http://www.ehow.com/how_2046424_learn-hungarian-etiquette.html/

Ember, M., & Ember C. (Eds.). (2001). *Countries and their cultures* (Vol. 2). *Denmark to Kyrgystan.* New York: Macmillan Reference.

Encyclopedia of Hungarian Food and Drink (EHFD)—Hungarian cuisine website. (2008). Retrieved March 25, 2008, from http://www.chew.hu/zoldseg.html/

Ender, B. (Ed.). (1986). *Hungarian cuisine.* Switzerland: Berlitz.

Farkas, E.T. (2005). *Hungarian cuisine and personal memories from the 1950s to present* (2nd ed.). Ithaca, NY: Author.

Freeman, J.B. (2004). *Lake Héviz—the biggest bath in Hungary.* Retrieved March 31, 2008, from http://www.hungarian-connections.com/Articles/Heviz/Heviz.htm/

Hungarian Food and Culture (HFC) website. (2008). Retrieved March 16, 2008, from http://www.food-links.com/countries/hungary/hungary.php/

Hungarians. (1998). In *Worldmark encyclopedia of cultures and daily life: Europe* (Vol. 4, pp. 186–189). Detroit, MI: Gale Group.

Hungary. (2001). In *Worldmark encyclopedia of the nations: Europe* (pp. 225–237). Detroit, MI: Gale Group

Kósa, Z., Vóko, Z., Széles, G., Kardos, L., Kósa, K., Fésüs, G., et al. (2007). A comparative health survey of the inhabitants of Roma settlements in Hungary. *American Journal of Public Health, 97*(5), 853–859.

Kwintessential Cross Cultural Solutions (KCCS). (n.d.). *Hungary—language, culture, customs and etiquette.* Retrieved March 30, 2008, from http://www.kwintessential.co.uk/resources/global-etiquette/hungary-country-profile.html/

Lang, G. (1994). *George Lang's cuisine of Hungary* (rev. ed.). New York: Atheneum.

Levinson, D. (1998). *Ethnic groups worldwide: A ready reference handbook.* Phoenix, AZ: Oryx Press.

Magyar, E. (1989). *The gourmet's cookbook* (2nd ed.; C. Bodóczky, Trans.). Budapest, Hungary: Kner Printing House, Békéscsaba.

Martire, J., & Kelly, P. (Eds.). (2005). *Hungarian phrasebook.* Victoria, Australia: Lonely Planet Publications.

Ministry of Foreign Affairs for the Republic of Hungary (MFA). (2007). *Fact sheets on Hungary.* Retrieved March 24, 2008, from http://www.mfa.gov.hu/kum/en/bal/hungary/about_hungary/

National Institute for Strategic Health Research (NISHR) (2005). *Health information, health data.* Retrieved March 24, 2008, from http://www.medinfo.hu/new3/adatok_en/adatok_en.php/

OneWorld. (2007). Retrieved March 22, 2008, from http://www.oneworld.com/ow/airports-and-destinations/city-guides/budapest-letter.pdf?

Professional Travel Guide (PTG). (2008). Retrieved March 23, 2008, from http://www.professionaltravelguide.com/etiquette/hungary/destinations-672809/

Rodler, I., & Zajkás, G. (2002). Hungarian cancer mortality and food availability data in the last four decades of the 20th century. *Annals of Nutrition and Metabolism, 46*(2), 49–56.

Rurik, I. (2006). Nutritional differences between elderly men and women. *Annals of Nutrition and Metabolism, 50,* 45–50.

Sasvari, J. (2005). Paprika: A spicy memoir from Hungary. Vancover, Canada: Canwest Books.

Skrabski, A., Kopp, M., Rózsa, S., Réthelyi, J., & Rahe, R.H. (2005). Life meaning: An important correlate of health in the Hungarian population. *International Journal of Behavioral Medicine, 12*(2), 78–85.

TJC Global. (2007). Hungarian translation. Retrieved March 22, 2008, from http:// http://www.tjc-global.co.uk/?pid=perlanguage&q=1&ln=44

UNICEF. (2007). *The state of the world's children 2007: Women and children, the double dividend of gender equality.* Retrieved April 14, 2009, from http://www.unicef.org/sowc07/statistics/tables.php

Venesz, J. (1982). *Hungarian cuisine* (rev. 4th ed.; G. Szabó, Trans.). Budapest, Hungary: Corvina.

Water and Fire. (n.d.). *Hungarian cuisine.* Retrieved March 24, 2008, from http://waterfire.fas.is/Hungary/hungariancuisine.php/

World Health Organization (WHO). (2008). *Hungary.* Retrieved March 31, 2008, from http://www.who.int/countries/hun/en/

World Health Organization (WHO). (2009). *World health statistics 2008.* Retrieved April 29, 2009, from http://www.who.int/whosis/whostat/EN_WHS08_Full.pdf/

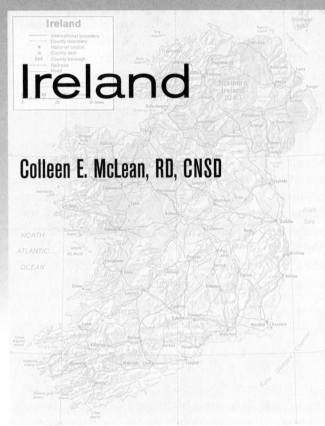

CHAPTER 16

Ireland

Colleen E. McLean, RD, CNSD

 CULTURE AND WORLD REGION

Today, Ireland is home to about 4.2 million people. The native Irish continue to hold the ethnic majority accounting for 87% of the population. The country is governed by a parliamentary democracy and twice elected a woman president. There is no official church, but 87% of the population is Roman Catholic according to the World Factbook (World Factbook, 2008). Blackwell and Hackney (2004) report that the Catholic Church still has a tremendous influence on the Irish government.

Ireland is known for fresh cooking ingredients but also for bland recipes of fried meats and overcooked vegetables. Immigration and travel to foreign countries for vacation helps bring a more worldly cuisine to Ireland. Also, the Irish are growing herbs to season foods and using the recipes of Darina Allen (1995). Wine can now be found throughout the country.

Similar to other industrial nations, Ireland is evaluating and addressing the rise in obesity. The Policy Challenges Report states that Irish children are over-consuming food from the "top shelf" (top of food pyramid), such as sweets, hamburgers, sodas, French fries, and potato chips (National Taskforce on Obesity, 2005). The SLÁN report showed similar findings for adults (Morgan et al., 2008).

Éire, Irish for Ireland, is an island located in Europe, west of Great Britain, that is slightly larger than West Virginia. The country is divided into 26 counties: Carlow, Cavan, Clare, Cork, Donegal, Dublin, Galway, Kerry, Kildare, Kilkenny, Laois, Leitrim, Limerick, Longford, Louth, Mayo, Meath, Monaghan, Offaly, Roscommon, Sligo, Tipperary, Waterford, Westmeath, Wexford, and Wicklow. The two largest cities are Dublin and Cork, respectively. Dublin, the capital, is located along the eastern coast and the Irish Sea at the mouth of the River Liffey in the Dublin region. It is home to more than a quarter of the country's population (Encyclopedia Britannica, 2008).

Ireland, fondly called the Emerald Isle for its abundance of verdant grasslands, has 1448 km of coastline and shares its only land border with the United Kingdom to the northeast. The interior is made up of mostly lowlands with many lakes, large bogs areas, and low ridges surrounded by low hills. The island's highest peak is Carrauntoohil at 1041 m. A small percentage of land is used for agriculture. On the west coast, there are sea cliffs. River Shannon was an important waterway in the 19th century. It is the longest river in Ireland flowing south and draining the central lowlands into an estuary below Limerick City.

The climate in Ireland is described as western maritime and influenced by the North Atlantic current. Winters are mild (39–45°F) and summers are cool (57–61°F). It is overcast half the time and consistently humid with rainfall averaging between 30 and 100 inches per year (Encyclopedia Britannica, 2008). Ireland's rainfall and climate are beneficial to the grasslands, which give the country its emerald appeal.

 LANGUAGE

In the 1500s, Irish Gaelic was the most spoken language in Ireland, but the use of the Irish language sharply declined due to restrictions on its use by the English and basic survival during hard times. Ireland introduced the language into schools in 1922 as part of an effort to revive the language and culture. Presently, there are a little over 1 million Irish Gaelic speakers; however, only about 20,000–30,000 speak the language on a daily basis (Hughs & Couglan, 2007).

Irish, the first official language of Ireland, is still taught in schools and is required for some civil service positions. It is spoken as a community language along the western seaboard in an area referred to as the Gaeltacht. English, the country's second official language, is most commonly spoken. All government documents are required to be published in both Irish and English (see Table 16-1 for a sampling of Irish Gaelic food names).

The Irish language originated from the Celtics with influences from the Vikings and Anglo-Normans. Irish Gaelic has greatly influenced the way the Irish speak and use the English language. You may notice that the Irish rarely answer a question with a direct yes or no. The Irish language does not contain these words. Also, the Irish may turn a negative adjective into a positive (e.g., "What an awfully nice day.")

Similar to other cultures, the Irish have their own set of colloquial words and phrases. You may hear the

TABLE 16-1 Irish Gaelic Food Names with Phonetic and English Translation

Irish Gaelic Name	Phonetic Translation	English Translation
Anraith	on-ra	Soup
Arán	a-rawn	Bread
Bainne	bahn-nyeh	Milk
Beoir	byohr	Beer
Cál	kawl	Cabbage
Cianneann	kyu-nun	Leek
Feoil	fee-oil	Meat
Glasraí	glos-ree	Vegetables
Iasc	ee-asc	Fish
Im	im	Butter
Mílseog	mil-shog	Dessert
Pióg	pee-ohg	Pie
Prátaí	praw-tee	Potato
Stobhach	sto-ukh	Stew
Subh	Soov	Jam
Torthaí	tor-hee	Fruit
Oraíste	or-awsh-te	Orange
Uisce	ish-ke	Water
Uisce beatha	ish-ke ba-ha	Whiskey
Úll	ool	Apple

Irish call food grub, nosh, scran, or tucker. Breakfast is called brekkie; main (evening) meal is tea or supper; appetizers are starters, desserts are afters; drink is alcohol; beverage is everything except alcohol; and they call the potato murphies, poppies, praities, purdies, shpuds, spuds, tatties, and totties.

 FOOD HISTORY WITHIN THE CULTURE

The earliest recorded inhabitants of Ireland, from 8000 to 7000 BCE, were hunter-gathers with tools of stone, wood, and bone. Between 4000 and 3000 BCE, domestic herding and farming was introduced and developed along with pottery making. Metal tools and cooking pots made during the Bronze Age were great assets to hunting, harvesting, and meal preparation.

The Celtic people, who were pagans, arrived in 350 BCE; however, little is known about them beyond the biased reports from Romans and Christians. The Celts could not write and did not record their history. They were violent people, but they brought social structure to Ireland by organizing clans and tribes governed by kings and chieftains. They were known for their metal art, using a distinctive interweaving and spiral design, and poetry. Along with metal, the Celtics valued cattle. They used their milk, butter, cheese, and eventually meat. During this period, Celtic and Christian beliefs became entwined.

Christianity and literacy came to the country during the 5th to 7th centuries. At that time, cereals and dairy were staples of the Irish diet. Invasion by the Vikings brought boat building, other trade skills, and construction of the first towns in Ireland. Dublin was founded by the Vikings in 840 CE. During the 12th and 13th centuries, more spices were used, agriculture increased, ovens were constructed, and trading between towns and overseas prospered.

Although Ireland was conquered and colonized by many peoples throughout the ages, including Celts, Norsemen, Normans, and Scots, it is the English who hold the pivotal role in Irish history. In 1536, Henry VIII signed the Act of Supremacy naming himself the head of the Church of England (Protestant). The Tudor and Stuart dynasties conquered Ireland in the 16th and 17th centuries, and famine and plague ensued. Pheasant, turkey, and potato were introduced. Ironically, the potato became a famine food. The Irish people saw a greater divide in food culture between the upper class and peasants. This gap widened during the 18th century with the peasants relying heavily on potato in their diet.

The Great Famine began in 1845 following the failure of one third of the potato crops infected with the fungus *Phytophthora infestans*. It struck again the following year with a blight of two thirds of the crops, as the previously year's failed crops were left to rot and the spores continued to infect the soil. In 1847, the crops survived, but not enough was planted. The third potato blight occurred in 1848. While many suffered greatly from malnutrition, it also left them vulnerable to disease, which spread quickly in the cramped living quarters of the peasants. Typhus, yellow fever, and cholera were common diseases during that time.

The Great Famine occurred during the heyday of laissez-faire economics where free markets were encouraged and government involvement discouraged. As a result, the British did little to aid the Irish during the famine. Death resulting from famine and plague struck the peasants. An estimated 1 million people died throughout the 5 years of famine (Blackwell & Hackney, 2004). Another 2 million people emigrated from Ireland during the famine (Allen, 1995). Anger directed at the English led to a rise in Irish nationalism.

Initially after the famine, people avoided traditional Irish dishes they associated with famine foods. There was a surge in Catholicism and movement into ecclesiastical vocations. In the late 19th century, Ireland experienced a rapid movement in commercialization. Processed goods, such as sugar, tea, and white bread, were now available in rural areas.

Ireland gained independence from the United Kingdom by way of treaty on December 6, 1921 (World Factbook, 2008), and was declared a free state in 1923. In 1925, Ireland joined the League of Nations (and later the United Nations). To avoid further conflict, the Irish agreed to form the Republic of Ireland by splitting from Northern Ireland, which remains under British rule. This resulted in conflict between Protestants and Catholics in Northern Ireland.

In the early 20th century, there was an increase in restaurants and people eating outside the home. Ireland experienced great economic prosperity during the 1960s. More Irish were going on vacation and traveling outside the country. In the 1980s and 1990s, more multicultural foods were available in supermarkets. It was during that time that Ireland earned the name "Celtic tiger" for its fierce economic recovery. There was also resurgence in traditional Irish products.

 MAJOR FOODS

 Protein Sources

The importance of pork in the Irish diet is evidenced by the many recipes calling for various parts of the pig. A traditional Irish breakfast may include three or more pork dishes: bacon, bangers (sausage), white pudding, and black pudding. White pudding is made from organs (liver, lung, and heart), trimmings, and meal. Black pudding is a combination of pig's blood, trimmings, lard, and meal. The renowned corned beef and cabbage is traditionally made with bacon, as beef was not affordable to the majority of Irish. Coddle is a mixture of bacon, sausage, potatoes, and onions. A testament to how little of the pig is wasted, crubeens, or boiled pig's feet, is another dish using offal.

Fish is a popular source of protein, as it is readily available to those living on the coast. Fish is also used extensively for Christian days of fasting and meat abstinence. Herring has always been popular because it can be preserved by pickling or salting and kept through winter. Once in abundance, herring was over-fished, resulting in a dramatic decrease in stock, and is now subject to government protection through quotas.

Cold-water fish thrive in the waters around Ireland and are included in the Irish diet. Some common cold-water fish are cod, haddock, mackerel, salmon, and trout. Fish and chips consists of cod or haddock coated in a flour-and-egg batter, deep fried, and served along with fried potatoes. Fresh fish is also served baked, boiled, or cooked into pies or fish cakes.

 Starch Sources

Potatoes were brought to Ireland from the New World in the 17th century. They are a mainstay in the diet. Some popular varieties are Home Guard, British Queens, Kerr's Pinks, Golden Wonders, Champions, and Records. The importance of the potato is emphasized by the names given to the different varieties, colloquial names the Irish call it (see *Language*), and the many dishes it adorns. Champ is a recipe of mashed boiled potato with milk, butter, and various other ingredients such as onions, scallions, parsley, chive, seaweed, peas, nettle, or leeks. Colcannon is a very traditional Irish casserole of potatoes, onions, and cabbage. It may also contain parsnips and curly kale. Boxty are a potato cake. This dish increased in popularity during the famine, as potatoes inappropriate for boiling could be used for this dish. French fries and potato chips are also consumed. Potatoes are also an ingredient in coddle.

Since Ireland became an agrarian society, oatmeal has been a staple in the diet. Oats are mixed with water, milk, buttermilk, or cream, and then seasoned with salt, butter, honey, or sugar to make porridge. Gruel is a simple dish of strained oatmeal and water. Soda bread is a daily staple of the traditional Irish diet. This simple-ingredient bread includes flour, salt, baking soda, and buttermilk. The buttermilk may be from the milk of a cow or goat.

 Fat Sources

Dairy products provide extensively to the fat in the Irish diet. The green grasslands provide well for the raising of dairy animals. Butter is used as a fat and a seasoning in Irish cooking and baking. Cheese making dates back to the 7th century and some people believe the Irish monks brought and helped shape cheese making in both France and Germany (Allen, 1995).

Lard is obtained from the fatty tissues of animals through a process called rendering. This fat is used in cooking and baking.

 Prominent Vegetables

Cabbage grows wild in Ireland but was not cultivated until the 17th century. It was used as an emergency food during the Great Famine. The Irish eat boiled or buttered cabbage and add it to popular dishes such as bacon and cabbage or colcannon.

Parsnips have existed in Ireland since early Christian times. It was not until the famine that the parsnips gained popularity in the Irish diet. Keeping with Irish cooking tradition, parsnips are boiled, mashed, and mixed with butter. Sometimes they are combined and mashed with boiled carrots.

Swede turnips (known as rutabagas in the United States) were initially introduced for cattle fodder and relatively unknown to the Irish until the famine. The seeds were distributed to people during the famine. The Irish substituted the Swede turnip into recipes that called for potatoes, boiling and mashing them with caramelized onion and parsley.

Sea kale grows wild along pebbly and sandy shores. It is native to the shores of Eurasia. This perennial cabbage-like plant has waxy and course-toothed green–blue leaves. It can be boiled and served alone or can accompany fish dishes.

Nettles, shrub plants with stinging hairs, are an abundant wildly grown food in Ireland. The eating of nettles is more common in rural areas. They are used in soups, broth, and in some champ recipes.

Wild, chanterelles, morels, deceivers, and hedgehog mushrooms are found throughout the Irish woods. The Irish may be suspicious of unusual mushroom varieties due to stories of poisonings during the famine. Mushrooms are typically stewed in milk or fried with butter.

 Prominent Fruits

Apple trees thrive in the temperate climate of Ireland. You will find many cakes, pies, soufflés, dumplings, tarts, jams, mincemeat, and wine made from apples. Strawberry, blackberry, gooseberry, and other berries are hardy plants that also grow well in the temperate climate. In season, these fruits are eaten ripe or used to make desserts of cakes, pies, and tarts. Fruits are commonly dried, preserved, or made into jams and jellies for use throughout the winter months.

 ### Spices and Seasonings

Honey was the only sweetener until the 12th century, and sugar was not widely introduced until the 16th century. Honey is used for cooking, basting, mead making, and as a condiment for meat, fish, and fowl.

 ### Beverages

Tea, pronounced tay, was brought to Ireland in the 19th century from India. Initially a drink of privilege, it was too expensive for most Irish. Now, it is enjoyed by the entire nation and consumption is about four cups a day on average (Blackwell & Hackney, 2004). The Irish drink more cups of tea, or "cuppa," per capita than any other nation. Tea time is traditionally at 4 PM and the pubs are legally required to provide it. The Irish prefer their tea with sugar and lots of milk.

Along with tea, Ireland is the largest consumer of beer. Stout, formerly known as porter, is a strong-flavored beer popular in Ireland. There are three well-known brewers of stout, but Guinness is most famous worldwide. Stout is made from barley, hops, and water, like other beers; however, the hops are roasted before brewing to give the beer its unique flavor and deep ruby

coloring (called black). It is used in beef and Guinness stew and porter cake.

 ### Desserts

Cakes, traditional desserts for all occasions, are made with seasonal and dried fruits. Barm brack is a fruited yeast bread or cake. The world "barm" comes from how these cakes were yeasted with fermented liquor before yeast was available. Other favorite desserts made with seasonal, preserved, and dried fruits are pies, soufflés, steamed puddings, and tarts.

 ## TYPICAL DAY'S MENU

The three meals of the day in order of appearance are breakfast, main meal, and light meal. Portions are said to be hefty in Ireland. The traditional Irish breakfast consists of fried eggs, black pudding, bangers (sausage), bacon, fried tomatoes with butter and chives, mushrooms, toast, jam, and tea. Today, these elaborate breakfasts are enjoyed mostly on weekends and holidays. An everyday breakfast is cereal or tea and toast, with an estimated 10% of Irish skipping breakfast (Morgan et al., 2008). Main meal is served midday and typically includes a meat, potato, and two vegetables. Light meal, the most frequent meal consumed outside the home, is eaten after work (Morgan et al., 2008).

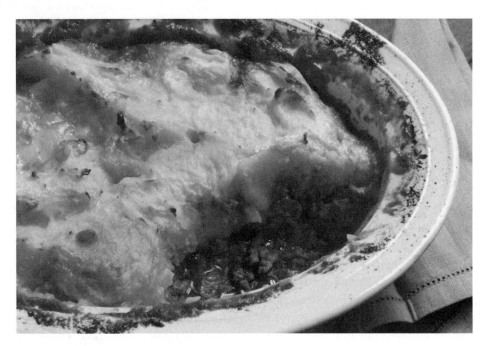

Shepherd's Pie

With almost 50% of people reporting snacking on biscuits and cakes, snacking habits play a significant role in the Irish diet.

HOLIDAY MENUS

The most festive holidays in Ireland are Christmas and Easter, as the majority of Irish are Catholic. Saint Patrick's Day, named after the patron saint of Ireland, was celebrated with a simple religious service and feast until the Irish adapted practices from the United States to benefit tourism. It is an Irish tradition to bake cakes for ceremonies and festivals. Bram brack, a fruit cake, is commonly made for Halloween.

While Christmas decorations are traditionally simple with a candle in the window and a wreath on the door, the menus are much more elaborate. Christmas is a time of family celebration around the meal table. A common holiday feast consists of roast turkey, thyme and onion stuffing, potato puree, smoked salmon on potato cakes, cranberry sauce, gravy, honey-glazed ham, roast potatoes, and brussels sprouts. Dry spiced beef with chutney is also a seasonal favorite. This holiday is not complete without Christmas cake made from dried raisins and currants, candied cherries, candied peel, almonds, apples, and whiskey. Sloe gin, a popular holiday drink, is a mixture of sloe berries, sugar, and gin. In the city of Cork, potato bread is served, as some traditions are regional.

GENERAL HEALTH AND NUTRITIONAL INDICATORS SUMMARY

Both public and private health care is available in Ireland. Cost for public health services depends on one's ability to pay, with some people receiving free comprehensive services. Affluent people usually obtain private insurance and health services; however, all are permitted to use the public system.

Much like the National Health and Nutrition Examination Survey (NHANES) in the United States, Ireland conducts a study called the Survey of Lifestyle, Attitudes, and Nutrition (2008), abbreviated SLÁN. Based on the third survey conducted in 2007, most Irish reported good health, visited with their general practitioner, and afforded enough food for their household. Excessive drinking (six or more drinks at least once a week) was reported by nearly a third of respondents. Current smoking was reported by 29% of respondents.

The fact that 39% of respondents were overweight and 82% had raised cholesterol is not surprising, as most consumed more than three servings from the top shelf of the food pyramid (foods high in fat, sugar, and salt), and 22% were physically inactive.

The European Union conducted studies on nutrition (Kafatos et al., 1999) and fitness health attitudes (Franz Zunft et al., 1999). They found that the Irish perceived smoking, food, stress, and physical activity, respectively, to be the most important factors on health. Food and fat were attributed to weight gain more often than inactivity and genetics. While the Irish were drawn to the health benefits and outdoor aspect of being physically active, work and study commitments were the most reported barrier to increasing physical activity. The less-educated respondents had a higher incidence of physical inactivity and were more likely to believe that exercise was not beneficial in the absence of weight loss.

Often, alternative and complementary medicine is not disclosed to the medical professional. A study of Irish children in a healthcare setting found that 57% of parents provided these therapies to their children, with less than half informing the general practitioner (Low, Murray, O'Mahony, & O'B Hourihane, 2008). Allen's (1995) cookbook provides a smattering of traditional Irish home remedies, including buttermilk to cure eczema and improve complexion, nettle stings to cure rheumatoid arthritis, and sorrel (clovers) to cleanse and heal ulcers, and improve jaundice.

UNICEF (2007) lists low birth weight, defined as weighing less than 2500 g at birth, affects 6% of newborns in Ireland. In addition, 100% of Ireland's urban population uses improved drinking-water sources.

COMMUNICATIONS AND COUNSELING TIPS

When speaking with or counseling someone from Ireland, it is important to be patient, avoid colloquial phrases, not overpraise, use conservative body language, and consider religious and health beliefs. Most people from Ireland speak English; however, they may have a brogue (heavy accent), making it difficult for you to understand them. Be patient and kindly ask them to speak slowly and repeat themselves when you do not understand. Colloquial phrases need to be avoided. They are unnecessary and may lead to misunderstandings. The Irish will deride themselves for enjoyment and out of modesty. They are not necessarily looking for praise and are suspicious of it (Hughs & Couglan, 2007). According to the Lonely Planet's *Irish Language and Culture* (2007), the Irish prefer keeping an arm's length away and limiting contact to a handshake with new acquaintances. Many Irish are Roman Catholic and this may influence religious and health beliefs. Fasting and abstinence is common during the Lenten period before Easter and for penance during other times of the year.

The sections *General Health and Nutritional Indicators Summary* and *Language* provide additional guidance for communication and counseling. As always, the best way to improve communication with a client is simply to ask questions and listen.

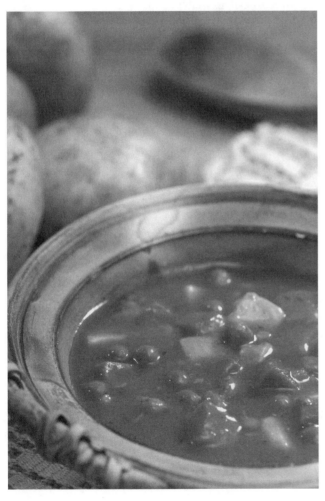

Irish Stew

FEATURED RECIPE

Irish Stew

2.2- to 3.3-lb. neck or shoulder of lamb

Bouquet of parsley, thyme, and bay leaf (tied together with twine)

3 large onions, finely chopped

Salt and freshly ground black pepper

3–4 carrots, chopped into bite-sized pieces

1 small turnip, chopped into bite-sized pieces

Some small new potatoes, peeled and quartered, or large potatoes, peeled and chopped

2.6–3.5 oz. cabbage, shredded

Finely chopped parsley and dash of Worcestershire sauce

1. Remove the meat from the bone, trim off all the fat, and cut into cubes.
2. Keep the bones, place the meat in a pot, and cover with cold salted water.
3. Bring to a boil, drain, and rinse the lamb.
4. In a fresh pot, put the meat, bones, bouquet of herbs, onions, seasoning, carrots, leeks, and turnip, and cover with water. Simmer gently for 1 hour. Skim off the foam as it rises. (This is very important for the final flavor and appearance of the stew.)
5. Add the potatoes and continue cooking for 25 minutes. For the last 5 minutes add the cabbage.
6. When the meat and vegetables are cooked, remove the bones and bouquet of herbs. Stir in the chopped parsley and a dash of Worcestershire sauce. Serve in deep bowls with soda bread.

Yields 4–6 servings

More recipes are available at http://nutrition.jbpub.com/foodculture/

REFERENCES

Allen, D. (1995). *The complete book of Irish country cooking: Traditional and wholesome recipes from Ireland.* New York: Penguin Group.

Blackwell, A.H., & Hackney, R. (2004). *The everything: Irish history and heritage book.* Boston: Adams Media.

Bord Bia. (2008). *Recipes home.* Retrieved October 30, 2008, from http://www.bordbia.ie/aboutfood/recipes/pages/recipehome.aspx/

Encyclopedia Britannica. (2008). *Ireland.* Retrieved October 26, 2008, from http://www.britannica.com/EBchecked/topic/293754/Ireland/

Franz Zunft, H.-J., Friebe, D., Seppelt, B., Widhalm, K., Remaut de Winter, A.-M., Vaz de Almeida, M.D., et al. (1999). *Public Health Nutrition, 2,* 153–160.

Hughs, M., & Couglan, G. (2007). *Irish language and culture.* Victoria, Australia: Lonely Planet Publications.

Kafatos, A., Manios, Y., Markatji, I., Giachetti, I., Vaz de Almeida, M.D., & Engstrom, L.M. (1999). Regional, demographic and national influences on attitudes and beliefs with regard to physical activity, body weight and health in a nationally representative sample in the European Union. *Public Health Nutrition, 2,* 87–95.

Low, E., Murray, D.M., O'Mahony, O., & O'B Hourihane, J. (2008). Complementary and alternative medicine use in Irish paediatric patients. *Irish Journal of Medical Science, 177,* 147–150.

Morgan, K., McGee, H., Watson, D., Perry, I., Berry, M., Shelley, E., et al. (2008). *SLAN 2007: Survey of lifestyle, attitudes and nutrition in Ireland. Main report.* Dublin, Ireland: Department of Health and Children.

National Taskforce on Obesity. (2005). *Obesity: The policy challenges.* Retrieved November 10, 2008, from http://www.dohc.ie/publications/pdf/report_taskforce_on_obesity.pdf?direct=1/

UNICEF. (2007). *The state of the world's children 2007: Women and children, the double dividend of gender equality.* Retrieved April 14, 2009, from http://www.unicef.org/sowc07/statistics/tables.php

World Factbook. (2008, October 23). *Ireland.* Retrieved October 29, 2008, from https://www.cia.gov/library/publications/the-world-factbook/geos/ei.html/

CHAPTER 17

Italy

JoAnna Siciliano, RD, LDN

WORLD REGION AND CULTURE

The Italian peninsula extends into the Mediterranean Sea between Spain and Greece in the distinct shape of a boot, with the two islands of Sicily and Sardinia to the west. The country is divided east and west by the Apennines Mountains, which historically interfered with the development of a unified culture, as the mountains isolated towns into creating their own unique cultures. The 20 regions of Italy are further subdivided into provinces and communes, which is significant because of the influence of traditional and local characteristics in shaping Italian culture (Capatti, 2000).

Italy's culture comprises food, wine, art, architecture, music, drama, and sports. Opera houses, particularly La Scala (Milan), are very popular, and the Roman Coliseum holds up to 50,000 spectators. Family is the most important aspect of Italian culture, as it provides their foundation in society. Small family businesses are led by sons or daughters of the founders and are the backbone of Italy's economy (Abbott, 2007). Italians are more loyal on a personal level than in the context of commitment to universal or state-instituted laws, because Italy as a country did not form officially until the 19th century. Even though Italy has a low birthrate (1.2 per family), family continues to be Italy's most solid bond (Shankland, 2005).

Italians are devoted to their local community. A piazza is a symbolic meeting place, usually in the center of town. In the evening, Italians take a *passeggiata* (evening walk) to meet up with well-dressed friends and families arm in arm, stopping by the local gelateria (ice cream bar) or for an *aperitivo*. The teenagers may spend time at a pizzeria. Watching the local soccer (*calcio*) team is common on Sunday, and the teams are owned by leading business and political figures (Shankland, 2005).Gatherings in public places are encouraged but not open to outsiders, a tradition that can be traced back to the Romans (Capatti, 2000). Most Italians live and work near where they were born, and they identify with their local culture, region, and city over the national level (Abbott, 2007).

Bella figura is a common expression used for the stylish dress of Italian people, as making the right impression is considered very important in Italian culture. Valentino, Versace, Armani, Gucci, wool, linen, and silk have been important parts of Italian identity. The silk trade started in Lake Como in the 10th century, and the art of shoe making began in Venice in the 12th century (Moramarco, 2000). Casual attire includes a t-shirt or polar-neck sweater with an expensive front-zip jacket with sunglasses and a tan. Men wear a tailored dark suit: a three-button navy-blue blazer with a shirt, tie, and classy shoes. Women also wear designer suits and shoes, with a matching handbag, gold earrings, bracelets, and pearl necklaces. Casual wear includes designer sweatshirts and jeans (Shankland, 2005).

Until the late 19th century, the regions of Italy were ruled by monarchs, foreigners, lords, or popes. Italy was the battleground of wars between the French, Spanish, English, and Austrians. The Italian people had no voice in their own destiny. The three leaders who emerged to bring all of Italy under one flag were King Vittorio Emanuel II of Piedmont, Count Camillo Cavour, his diplomat, and Guiseppe Garibaldi, a general.

RELIGION

Even though Italy has no official religion, Roman Catholicism is the main religion. Many feasts are church related, and most of the magnificent art, architecture, and sculptures are in the churches. Currently, about 87.8% of Italians are Roman Catholic, 36.8% consider themselves practicing Catholics, and 30.8% attend church every Sunday. In 1956, church attendance was 69%; it dropped to 48% in 1968, and to 35.5% in 1972, which can be related to the Second Vatican Council in which the church separated itself from the country because Italians did not agree with Vatican policy regarding, for example, birth control and divorce. The strong family ties, however, remained a dominant and cohesive force in Italian culture.

In 1978, the Catholic Church inaugurated its first non-Italian pope, John Paul II, in 450 years (Capatti, 2000). The public's relationship to religion remained unchanged, and the tradition of everyday Italian religious life continues to be structured around the celebrations of church holidays such as Easter, Christmas, and the days of patron saints.

Every town and village has its own patron saint; on that day there is a celebration and a day off from work, which includes processions, pilgrimages, and sacred rituals (Abbott, 2007). The Italian lifestyle is also partly influenced by the belief in, or opposition to, the Catholic hierarchy. Catholicism is autocratic hierarchy of authority starting with the pope, cardinals, archbishop, bishop, and local parish priest (Abbott, 2007). This is then reflected in society with the male being the head of the family or family business. Many celebrations in Italy are specific to the Catholic religion, but nonreligious persons also participate in the festivities (Parasecoli, 2004). Religious rituals that were considered a rite of passage remain a strong part of Italian customs that start with baptism, first Holy Communion, confirmation, marriage, and funeral mass (Horne & Kiselica, 1999). Today, 98% of Italians are baptized, and 80% are married in the church (Capatti, 2000). Presently, *Famiglia Cristiana* (*The Christian Family*) is the most widely read magazine in Italy (Abbott, 2007).

 ## LANGUAGE

Italian, a romance language, is the official language of Italy and is spoken by 90% of the people (Capatti, 2000). With the 20 different regions, there are 20 regional dialects, making communication between the regions somewhat difficult. For example, the Venetians speak Veneto, the Sicilians speak Sicilian, the Calabrians speak Calabrese, and the Tuscans speak Toscano. In the regions of Trento and Alto Adige, German is spoken. In the northwest region of Italy, Valle d'Aosta, French is spoken. In the northeast regions of Trieste and Gorzia, Solvene is spoken (Abbott, 2007).

 ## CULTURE HISTORY

The strong ties within the Italian community are a result of the oppression that Italians suffered from invading foreign nations, as well as from their own governments. As a result, the Italian people learned to rely on members of their extended family and community, and to distrust outsiders and have a general mistrust toward the government (Horne & Kiselica, 1999).

The Romans initially dominated Italy. The country was left in destruction and desolation after northern Italy was invaded by the barbarians from northern Europe (Killinger, 2005). In 1798, under Napoleonic rule, Italy was divided into three republics, which eliminated medieval traditions that included church privileges and title to much of its land. In the 1840s, the Italian revolution began in Sicily and Naples, and then spread to the rest of the peninsula. The Economic Miracle of the 1950s and 1960s raised the standard of living substantially and created significant prosperity.

As late as World War II, 50% of Italians worked in agriculture, 25% worked in industry, and 25% were service workers. In the 1990s, only 5% worked in agriculture and 50% were service workers. In the 21st century, four of five Italian businesses are family owned and employ fewer than 50 people. The largest private company for over 100 years is FIAT, owned by Gianni Agnelli (Capatti, 2000). Although family is important, large nuclear families of four to five children are not typical of Italian households, especially in urban areas. The gender roles of male dominance are not as rigid, and fathers are also nurturing. Large families are not viewed as financial assets that improve family earnings, but instead are viewed more as a financial strain. Due to the decrease in agriculture and industrial sectors, the stereotype of Italian women marrying early and bearing many children was shattered in the early 1980s (Capatti, 2000). There is greater individual expression and more time spent with friends, with less socializing around the family.

FOOD HISTORY WITHIN THE CULTURE

Food was traditionally and currently is the focus for family life in Italy. It identifies the specific regions in Italy with a positive image of Italians throughout the world. In northern Italy, Piedmont, at the base of the Alps, is the northwesternmost region and is characterized by high mountains, a hill at its center, and rolling plains in the south. The terrain is rugged and the climate is cold. Foods in this region include boiled meats, polenta, soups, and rich desserts, all of which characterize a diet for outdoor people.

The communities along the Po River grow rice, onions, celery, artichokes, peppers, and asparagus. The region is known for its cheese, fontina. In the region of Liguia/Genoa along the Italian Riviera, freshly caught seafood is abundant. Herbs, such as basil, which is used for, among other things, Pesto Genovese, are grown on hillsides. The Lombardy/Milan region, also known as dairy country, is notable for its butter and cheese, aperitif Campari, panettone, and balsamic vinegar. Milan is known for herbs, tomatoes, and wine. In Venice, the spice-trading center, rice, seafood, polenta, beans, and salt cod are prevalent. Emilia-Romagna and Parma are associated with milk, the vital ingredient for the third most important product of the region, parmesan cheese.

Fertile land on the Adriatic Sea produces cheeses, pork products, meat and pasta, seafood parmesan, and *prosciutto di Parma*. In Florence, beef from Tuscan cattle and Chianti (grapes) are grown in the mountains between Florence and Siena. Fresh pasta is more common in the north and central regions compared with the dried pasta in the south. The geographical difference of the mountainous south provides pasta made with durum wheat, which requires a less humid climate to dry more quickly and uniformly. In central Italy, the Marches region provides an ideal agricultural mild climate for wheat, fruit, corn, beets, tomatoes, pasta, polenta, and local berries for peasant cuisine. Sheep also graze in these lands.

Rome is the political, religious, and gastronomic capital of Italy; its cosmopolitan cuisine (influenced by northern, southern, and foreign cuisines) includes flat and tubular pasta, lard/bacon fat, olive oil, butter, and cheese pecorino, as well as mozzarella and ricotta cheeses. Highly seasoned pork and lamb dishes are a result of the Abruzzo farming, which is related to the mountainous region coastline on the Adriatic Sea, where goats and sheep graze on mountain slopes, cow's milk is drawn to make cheese, (scarmoza, provolone, caciocavallo), and pigs and lambs are raised for their meat. Other crops include wheat and eggplant, as well as sweet and hot peppers. Abruzzo has two distinct cuisines, the coastal one based on fish and the mainland cuisine based on pork and lamb.

Southern Italy, which was influenced by Greeks, Arabs, Normans, French, and Spaniards, is one of the poorest regions (Killinger, 2005). Naples is known for its pizza, mozzarella cheese, tomato-sauce spaghetti, macaroni pasta, and seafood. The Napoletans eat well and are known for their desserts. Basilicato Apulia is at the southernmost tip of Italy. In the mountains are locally raised goats, lambs, pigs, and small game, and foods enjoyed are sausages, artichokes, cabbage, hot peppers, provolone, and sweet pastries. In the region of Apulia, Bari borders the Adriatic Sea and is known for its pasta, bread, and seafood. In the region of Calabria/Catanzaro, mountainous terrain is surrounded by the sea on three sides, and food sources include pasta, vegetables, tuna, and swordfish. In the region of Calabria, the fish is grilled and accompanied with vegetable soups, pasta, and large loaves of bread.

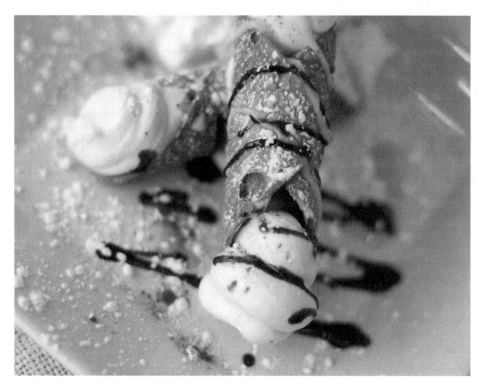

Cannoli, tubes of crisp, fried pastry dough filled with a sweet cream mixture, are a common dessert of Sicilian origin.

The island of Sicily is mountainous, with ancient cooking traditions, fertile land, and a sunny climate. Food grown on this island includes wheat, citrus fruit, figs, eggplant, peppers, tomatoes, broccoli, and squash, with little meat. Tuna, swordfish, mullet, sardines, and anchovies are staples of this region. Sicilians make their own bread and make tubular pastas that are topped with strongly seasoned sauces. Colorful sweet pastries made with cream, candied fruit, honey, and almonds are traditional desserts of this region (cassata: layered pound cake with ricotta cheese, chocolate, and orange-flavored liquor; cannoli: cylindrical pastries filled with ricotta cheese and sugar). Caponata, a marinated eggplant and tomato dish, serve as an accompaniment to swordfish, tuna, or sausage. In Sardinia, the cuisine includes sheep and goats, cheese, pork, wild boar, fowl, beef, pasta, and bread. Fresh meat is rare, but all types of salami are produced (capocollo, soppressata).

Women were in charge of transmitting their knowledge and experiences in all culinary matters to new generations. In the countryside, when women learned to read and write, recipes for traditional dishes were still communicated verbally. No quantities, weights, or measurements were given; everything was prepared according to the cook's eyes, nose, hands, and taste (Parasecoli, 2004). At the end of the 18th century, men wrote recipes as business. During the Fascist era, with world war and scarce supplies, magazines and recipe books insisted on dishes that would save money and resources. After World War II, families left their land of origin and moved to nearby cities or other regions for a better life.

In rural Italian communities, food existed as the vital form of economic and social exchange. Food was used as a form of payment for laborers. If the family's breadwinner passed away or a natural disaster or disease struck a village, starvation was the primary concern. Subsequently, in times of prosperity, people demonstrated their good fortune by utilizing food to pay their respects to God and the community. Food was dual purposed: firstly, as a form of payment for labor, and secondly, it brought the community together during their leisure time. Due to the difference in climate, growing season, proximity to water, and historic trade connections with other parts of the world, diets varied in the regions of Italy (Poe, 2001). The daily diet in the south included spaghetti made at home from rye and wheat flour, salt, and water. Common pasta toppings included sheep or goat cheese, tomatoes, beans, herbs, and vegetables. Because of their long growing season, vegetables incorporated were greens such as Savoy cabbage, escarole, lettuce, chicory, and turnip. Other common vegetables were eggplant (aubergine), peppers, onion, garlic, artichokes, asparagus, squash, broccoli, celery, and peas. Root vegetables, such as turnip roots, carrots, and beets, were considered fit only for animal feed.

Sicilians were noted for their abundant and creative use of seafood for holiday seasons because they lived close to the sea. Potatoes, rice, and cornmeal were used on occasion, but generally in the north. Fruits and vegetables were eaten raw or with minimal cooking for taste preference, but also due to the lack of wood in southern Italy that resulted in an insufficiency of cooking fuel. The simmering tomato sauces developed later in southern Italian life. Tomatoes, brought to Spain by Christopher Columbus in 1522, were initially thought to be poisonous (Barry, 2008). During the winter months, Italians ate the food they had dried, salted, or preserved in vinegar or rendered pork fat during the summer and fall. Cured meats, such as ham and sausage, were common, but fresh meat was rare, as southern Italy's hot climate meant that slaughtering was inadvisable except December through March. If a pig or cow was owned, the person kept the less valuable organ parts for him- or herself and sold the rest. Unless an animal died unex-

pectedly, families ate chicken or fish about once a week. Goats and sheep were more valued than cows, as dairy animals related to the open pastureland. The milk was used for cheese, because this method of preservation compensated for lack of refrigeration. Fresh milk and eggs were reserved primarily for babies or medicine. Pizza Margherita, named for Italy's Queen Margherita, came to Naples in 1889, and tricolored pizza, which represented the colors of the newly adopted Italian flag, was made especially for her.

The origins of Italian cooking can be traced back to the ancient Etruscans and Greeks (Dalrymple, 1985). Roman cooking influenced that of the whole empire, and during the Renaissance, Italiana cooking became the inspiration for most of the cuisines of western Europe. With 20 regions and 94 provinces, Italy was not united until 1870 under King Victor Emmanuel II (Dalrymple, 1985).

Geography also separates the regions. The Apennine Mountains form a crooked spine that runs the length of the country, dividing and subdividing it into valleys, plains, plateaus, and coastal strips. Pasta is served almost every meal, using fresh ingredients such

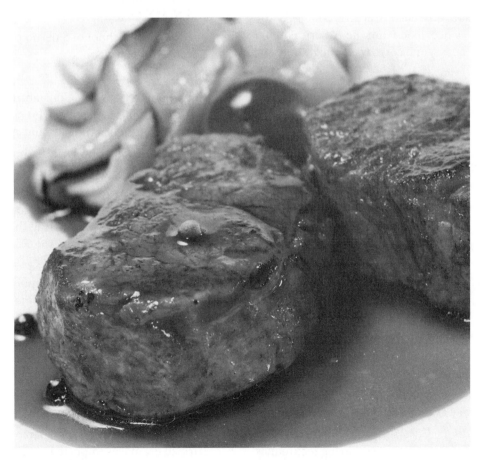

Roasted Veal

as cheeses, olive oils, wines, sausages, herbs, and garlic. Cooks in the prosperous industrial north, dairy country, use butter as well as olive oil and prefer fresh egg-based pastas (tagliatelli, lasagna, and ravioli). In the south, cooks use less luxurious ingredients; olive oil and dried tubular pastas (macaroni and spaghetti) made from flour and water. Northern Italy's upper class uses butter, cream, veal, and white truffles. In the south the land is more mountainous: olive oil, sheep, and goats rather than cattle and dairy products; and rice for special dishes, boiled and fried in small balls filled with different ingredients and powdered with bread crumbs (arancini).

In the Roman era, wild boar from Tuscany, bass from the Tiber River, radishes from the Alban Hills, onions and cabbage from Pompeii, asparagus from Ravenna, leeks from Ostia, semolina from Campania, and bread and wine from Piceno were the common fare. The Romans shared with the Greeks a diet based on bread, wine, and olive oil. A diet of beer, meat, and butter was incorporated from the Germanic culture after the invasion. Southern Italy was under Arabic influence, which led to the use of citrus fruits and cane sugar to replace the vinegar and honey, respectively, used under Roman influence (Capatti, 2000). At the end of the Renaissance, food from the Americas, such as tomato, green beans, and corn, was brought to Italy.

CHRONOLOGICAL CUISINE AND CULTURE LISTING

The following is a chronological listing of the culinary influences on Italy:

12th century BCE, the Italic people in Italy: introduction of rudimentary agriculture techniques.

11th century BCE, the Etruscans in Tuscany: probable arrival of olive trees and vines in Tuscany.

8th century BCE: foundation of Phoenician bases in Sardinia and Sicily, which become part of the food and product trade routes connecting the shores of the Mediterranean.

770 BCE: foundation of Petecus, the first Greek colony in Italy, and arrival of olive trees and vines in southern Italy.

575 BCE: Etruscan domination over Rome, who adopts culinary customs from its neighbors.

5th century BCE, Celts infiltrate northern Italy: introduction of salt-based meat-curing techniques and greater appreciation for pork.

237 BCE: Rome expands power to Sardinia, reinforcing its role in the Mediterranean and exposing itself to new influences including culinary ones.

210 BCE: Rome imposes the cultivation of wheat in Sicily.

188 BCE: Rome extends its power to Asia Minor (present-day Turkey) and begins to absorb the lavish and refined culinary customs of the East.

180 BCE: law limits number of guests invited for dinner.

171 BCE: foundation of the Guild of Bakers; formed by free slaves.

128 BCE: Rome forbids the populace beyond the Alps from planting olive trees and vines in an attempt to limit the cultivation of cash crops to Italy.

30 BCE: Rome conquers Egypt, a new major source of wheat.

552: Byzantine Emperor Justinian conquers Italy and reinvents traditional agricultural products that had disappeared under German influence.

902: Muslims conquer Sicily and introduce products and culinary techniques from the Middle East and North Africa.

1101: Medical School of Salerno produces the first European dietary book.

5th century: Italian cooks use olive oil.

1204: Fourth Crusade, Constantinople conquered on behalf of the Venetians, who take control of the trade of spices with the East and Asia.

1464: Master Martino writes a book on the art of cooking.

1492: Spanish monarchy conquers the Muslim Kingdom of Granada. Christopher Columbus lands in the Caribbean starting the Columbian exchange, which transforms the European diet in a few decades.

1570: Bartolommeo Scappi publishes his monumental *The Works*, about cuisine in papal Rome, which explains all methods and recipes for preparing each ingredient that was available in markets of Rome (local and imported).

1571: Venice, Spain, and the papal troops defeat the Turks. Coffee is introduced in Venice.

1606: chocolate becomes popular in Italy.

16th century: tomato and maize are introduced; Turkish grain was imported, and in Northern Italy polenta was utilized.

18th century: coffee drinks were first documented. Expedition of 1000 men, led by Giuseppe Garibaldi, topples the Bourbon Dynasty and delivers southern Italy to Vittorio Emmanuelle II, who becomes king of Italy. Northern soldiers are exposed to southern dishes such as pasta with tomato sauce.

1915: Italy enters World War I; victuals are granted to soldiers, such as coffee, dried pasta, and cheese, everyday food for the whole population.

1917: Olindo Guerrini publishes *The Art of Using Leftovers*.

1963: introduction of Regulation of Controlled Denomination of Origin for wines.

20th century, *macchina a vapore*: steam espresso machine was invented in Naples (Moramarco, 2000). Espresso refers to the manner in which the coffee is made; steaming hot water pressed through a small amount of finely ground, tightly pack coffee beans.

2004: first 4-year university program in gastronomy starts in Pollenzo (Piedmont).

MAJOR FOODS

Italians buy their food fresh in small, specialized neighborhood shops or in street markets.

Protein Sources

Pulses (legumes) traditionally constituted the main source of protein for most Italians, and meat was limited to festive and special occasions due to its high cost, although, over the past 50 years, the per capita consumption of meat has dramatically increased due to improved economic conditions. Recently, since the scare of mad cow disease, Italians are consuming less meat, especially beef (Parasecoli, 2004). Traditionally, pork and poultry were easily raised. Horse meat was sold in specialty shops; special breeds produced better meats in the regions of Veneto and Puglia. Small animals, such as rabbits, chickens, pigs, and pigeons, were easy to keep in the villages or on farms, with a small investment of money. All parts of the animals were used but mostly cured, seasoned, aged (salami, proscuitto, culatello), and pork buttock. Mutton and goat were common in central and southern Italy, because of the mountainous areas.

Italian cheese is enjoyed worldwide. The following is a list of cheeses traditionally produced in Italy:

Cow milk and cheese are produced in the north.

In the south, sheep and water buffalo cheese (*mozzarella di bufala*), made from the milk, are produced.

Gorgonzola, accompanied with grapes or walnuts as a pasta sauce, might serve as a first dish in any meal.

Provolone is packaged in long tubes and tied with ropes, and hangs from the ceilings of Italian delicatessens.

Ricotta is a soft, creamy cheese that is blended with fruits, salads, and desserts, such as cannoli, or pasta dishes, such as ravioli, manicotti, or lasagna.

Marscapone, a dessert cheese, is the main ingredient in tiramisu.

Other cheeses include tallegio, asiago, romano, pecorino, fontina, and scamorza.

Fish is sometimes marinated, mostly seasoned with herbs (e.g., oregano, dill, parsley, rosemary, sage, and basil), and baked in a crust of salt or broiled. The following is a list of popular fish in Italy:

Shellfish (mussels, clams, lobster, shrimp)

Other fish (octopus, squid, calamari)

Cod, flounder, whitefish, and swordfish

Common meats in Italy include:

Coppa/capocollo: pressed and dry-cured pork shoulder

Genoa salami: strong-flavored pork sausage with garlic and whole white peppercorns

Pancetta: Italian bacon, cured not smoked

Prosciutto: dry-cured unsmoked ham, dark pink and mild in flavor

Sausages: fresh pork and seasoned with fennel seed, garlic, and red pepper (hot)

Soppressata: large flat oval sausage of coarsely ground pork, highly seasoned

A common use of nuts in northern Italy is to mix them with raisins and apples and wrap them in sweet dough to make strudel. In Central Italy, whole hazelnuts are kneaded with flour, honey, pepper, and other ingredients to make *pan pepato* (pepper bread). Almonds are a main ingredient in many pastry traditions, such as amaretto cookies, *torrone* (a nougat candy with toasted almonds, honey, and sugar), and marzipan (almond paste), which are shaped and painted to look like peaches, apples, cherries, and so on.

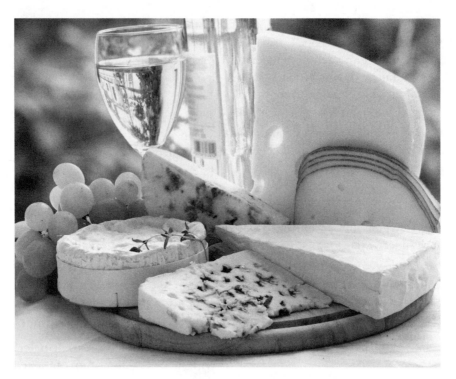

Italian cheeses, including gogonzola, provolone, ricotta, and marscapone are enjoyed around the world.

 ## Starch Sources

Pasta is a traditional staple food of the south made from flour, water, and eggs, and is kneaded, rolled, and cut into shapes such as farfalle (butterfly), penne (pen), spaghetti (string), or orecchiette (little ears) (Poe, 2001). Stuffed pasta, ravioli, tortellini, agnolotti, cappeleti, and manicotti are made of pasta dough wrapped around leftover meats, vegetables, and cheese from a previous meal (Anderson, 1994).

Polenta, a stiff cornmeal mush, is primarily a northern dish, served in place of pasta or risotto. In Apulia, polenta is served with shellfish or mussels; in Emilia-Romagna polenta is served with onions and pork. Venetians serve polenta with chicken livers. In Piedmont polenta is served with fontina cheese. The texture of polenta differs depending on the length of time cooked and amount of time before it is served. If served immediately, it is hot and creamy; if it sets, it becomes thick and solid and can be served in slices.

Other starch sources include rice, couscous, and potato. Risotto is a type of rice originated in Milan. This type of rice absorbs all the water, and is rich and creamy in texture; a common example is Risotto Milanese (seasoned with saffron). Couscous is used in Western Sicily as it was the only region influenced by Middle Eastern cuisine. Potato, a starchy vegetable, is used to make gnocchi, which is made of flour, water (or egg); and *frittata di patata* (potato omelet).

Many carbohydrate sources use refined semolina flour; examples include pane (bread), grissini (bread sticks), and focaccia. Bread is usually eaten with antipasti (Parasecoli, 2004). Bread in the south tends to be shaped in large, round loaves, densely textured, and usually torn apart by hand rather than sliced and passed around the table. In the north, the bread is lighter, longer, and crispier, and the loaves are long and thin and used for paninis. Pizza crust also varies between regions (Parasecoli, 2004), described as follows:

Sicilian pizza has a thick, bready crust.

Naples pizza has a paper-thin crust that is crisp and well-done on the bottom and soft and slightly undercooked on top. The dough is covered by the ingredients instead of sauce and includes toppings such as anchovies, mushrooms, cheese, sausage, prosciutto, zucchini, salmon, and rugola (Parasecoli, 2004). Pizza bianci (white pizza) may be filled with hazelnut spread or fresh figs, and folded.

Calzone is oven-cooked pizza folded in half, with ricotta cheese, diced mozzarella, diced salami or prosciutto, and egg (Parasecoli, 2004).

Fat Sources

Olive oil is the primary source of added fat in Italian dishes (Welland, 2008), whereas butter is reserved for pastry making (Poe, 2001). Olive oil is used in pasta sauces, salad dressings, as a base to coat and sauté vegetables, as part of a marinade for meat or fish, and to dip crusty Italian bread. Olive oil comes in a variety of styles and grades. Extra virgin olive oil is the premium grade; it is the oil made from the first cold pressing of the fruit.

Heavy cream is used in sauces and pastries, and pancetta (Italian bacon) is another source of fat.

 Prominent Vegetables

Prominent vegetables vary by season. An Italian vegetable garden is characterized by variety as well as abundance. Vegetables that are not consumed fresh are usually given to a neighbor or jarred with olive oil or pickled in vinegar for winter consumption (Moramarco, 2000). Vegetables can be cooked *al dente* (just tender enough to bite into), steamed briefly, or sautéed lightly in olive oil. Besides pulses and potatoes, vegetables are a main part of the Italian diet, due to the frequent lack of meat, which is expensive and difficult to find in rural areas.

Fresh salads became popular in the 16th century as a side dish. Onions, once a peasant food, are now the main ingredient for a cooking base in dishes and sauces. Raw or sautéed garlic, with its intense flavor, is not eaten raw but mashed with olive oil and cloves as a base for meat, fish, and vegetable dishes. Tomatoes are a central part of the Italian diet and are available all year. Several varieties of tomato are staggered, so crops continuously grow throughout the summer and early fall. Tomatoes typical of southern Italy can be sun-dried, puréed, boiled, and made into paste, peeled, crushed, or raw. Other seasonal vegetables include zucchini, red and green peppers, carrots, celery, peas, lettuce, onions, scallions, garlic, beans, cauliflower, asparagus, fennel, spinach, rugola (greens with a bitter aftertaste, mixed with other greens), broccoli rabe (long edible stems, narrow leaves), fennel (faint taste of licorice), radishes, wild chicory, Swiss chard, artichokes, and mushrooms. Sweet peppers can be served fresh, sliced, pickled, sautéed, fried, grilled, baked, or stuffed. Truffles are rare and expensive, and are found near Alba (Piedmont) and, in smaller quantities, in Tuscany. The Muslims introduced eggplant to Sicily. The most common dishes that include eggplant are eggplant parmesan, stuffed eggplant, and caponata (an eggplant appetizer).

 Prominent Fruits

Whole fruits are eaten every day, nearly with every meal (Welland, 2008). Some of the most common fruits include persimmons, grapes, and chestnuts in the fall; oranges, tangerines, pears, and apples in the winter; strawberries and cherries in the spring; and peaches, plums, apricots, figs, melons, and watermelons in the summer. In recent years, kiwi (originally from New Zealand), mango, papaya, and avocado have been commonly grown in Italy.

A bowl of fruit is usually found on the table all day for quick snacks in the home. Fruit is used as a dessert, but also as an appetizer (figs and melons with prosciutto). Dried fruit is used in the winter and includes plums, figs, and dates, and apricots are candied for pastry making.

 Spices, Seasonings, and Herbs

Spices are used in smaller quantities in Italy in order to not drown out the taste of the food (Wright, 2008). These spices include the following:

Coriander (*coriandolo*): used in lamb and pork dishes, crushed.

Nutmeg (*noce moscata*): used in sweet dishes. Nutmeg is a common ingredient in ravioli and dishes that contain spinach or cheese.

Pepper (*pepe*): black peppercorns are widely used, freshly ground. White pepper is also used.

Saffron (*zafferano*): most often used in risotto and in fish soups and stews. This spice is used sparingly, as it is very expensive.

Salt (*sale*): sea salt is used throughout Italy. Coarse sea salt is used at the table or in cooking.

Vanilla (*vaniglia*): vanilla is a popular flavor in sweet dishes; vanilla sugar sold in sachets is frequently used with regular sugar to give flavor to cakes and pastries. Vanilla beans, rather than extract, is used by most Italians.

Basil (*basilica*): sweet basil and bush basil are the most common forms of the numerous varieties of basil. It is mostly used in dishes that contain tomatoes, in salads, soups, and on pizzas. Fresh basil is most often used. If using dried basil, the sweet kind is more flavorful.

Bay leaf (*alloro*): used as a flavoring for casseroles, soups, and roasts.

Oregano (*origano*): also known as wild marjoram, oregano is used on pizzas as well as in sauces and casseroles; flavors differ from region to region.

Italian parsley (*prezzemolo*): Italian parsley is flat-leaved and more pungent than curly parsley.

Thyme (*timo*): not used except in Sardinia.

Fennel (*finocchio*): used in three ways: the bulb, *finocchio*, is used whole, sliced, or quartered as a vegetable, and either braised or baked or baked au gratin, or chopped raw in salads.

Wild fennel stems (*finocchiella*): used along with the leaf (bitter tang of aniseed) in cooking to flavor sauces (fish and pork dishes). Fennel seeds are used in sausages and cooked meats.

Balsamic vinegar was introduced about the same time as *nuova cucina* in Italy. The original vinegar can be found only in Modena and Reggio, two provinces in northern Italy (Anderson 1994). This vinegar is labor intensive and requires special processes that have been passed on from generation to generation in this region since the 15th century. It is made from the pulp of crushed grapes, which are heated, aged, and stored for long periods. The best balsamic vinegar is at least 12 years old.

Most Italians grow their own herbs or use fresh herbs from the market. If they grow their own herbs, any excess is shared among neighbors. In the winter months home-dried herbs are used. They can be grown easily in pots on the windowsill or in the garden. The herbs should be picked in the summer at the height of the growing season, stored in the freezer, or hung up to dry and then stored in airtight containers.

 Beverages

Bottled mineral water, carbonated or not, is served with all meals. Bottled water is assumed to be more pure than tap water (Parasecoli, 2004); however, *Guidelines for a Healthy Italian Diet* was published in 2003 with a chapter about water and common misconceptions.

Coffee is a typical after-meal beverage for Italians. Cappuccino, coffee with a thick layer of foamy milk, topped with a shake of cocoa, is served before 10:30 AM, usually with breakfast. Espresso is a small, strong black coffee. Caffé lungo is a small black coffee, weaker than espresso. Caffé corretto is black with a shot of grapa. Caffé macchiato is a black coffee with a dash of milk. Caffé latte is a large coffee with milk. Children may be served latte macchiato, warm milk with a shot of coffee; otherwise, they drink water, juice, or soda with their meals.

Red wine is typically served with meals, even during the work day, and if ordered at a bar, tap water must be served free. It is customary that the head of the household pour the first round of wine with a toast, usually *Salute!* (to good health). An aperitif (light drink), such as prosecco or verdicchio, is typically served before meals, or spumante (sparkling wine) (Abbott, 2007). The meal is followed by a digestive aid, such as *amaro* (a bitter drink, made from herbs and water, with a low sugar content), *sambuca*, *limoncello*, or *grappa* (a distillate made from the leftovers of wine production, mainly skins, but also seeds and stems; only the drink of poor people at one time).

Soda is served for special occasions; usually 1 L of soda is placed on the table to be shared among the guests. Wine is to complement the meat, and if not consumed by a guest, it is considered to be insulting to the host. Because of the regulations instituted in 1966, *Denominazione di Origine Controllata* (Denomination of Controlled Origin) was given to certain wines that met specific standards of taste, aroma, longevity, alcohol content, color, and acidity, and this gave rise to wine's renewed popularity. Italy, though mostly known for its wines, started producing beers (Moretti, Peroni) in the 19th century due to new techniques for refrigeration.

 Desserts

Desserts are reserved for special occasions, such as Sundays, holidays, or as celebration for when uncles, aunts, and cousins join the family table, but are not typical of daily meals (Welland, 2008). Desserts can be purchased at local pastry shops; typically, a boxful of assorted Italian pastries are served. A very common Italian dessert is cannoli (of Sicilian origin), which are tubes of crisp, fried pastry dough filled with a sweet cream mixture of ricotta cheese, sugar, spices, and cocoa, and may include chocolate chips, dried fruits, or nuts. Sfogliatelle are triangular-shaped pastries made of thin, layered flakes of pastry dough wrapped around a moist, creamy filling, usually almond flavor.

Pastries vary from region to region, described as follows:

Panforte is a strong bread of Siena, served as a fruitcake at Christmas tables.

Zeppole is a fried, sweetened puff of pastry dough for St. Joseph's Day throughout southern Italy.

Cassata is a rich, spongy Easter cake made in Sicily.

Panettone of Milan is made at Christmas and Easter.

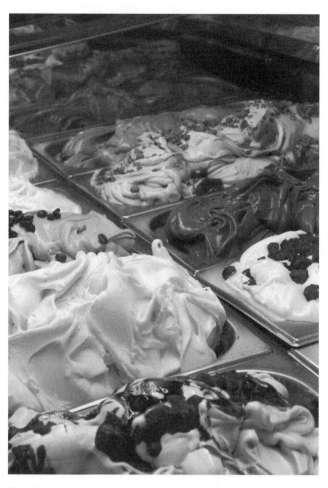

Gelato

Biscotti, which literally means "twice baked," are long, dry cookies for dipping into wine or coffee. Baked with almonds or other nuts, they are now coated with chocolate.

Gelato is a thick, sticky, creamy custard.

Granitas (Italian ices), made by hand, consist of a frozen mix of water, sugar, and flavor base of watermelon, lemon, orange, or espresso (Barry, 2008).

Pastarelle (éclairs), large and small, have fillings that can include chocolate, egg custard, zabaione, hazelnut, coffee cream, and plain or sweetened whipped cream.

Sfogliatelle-layered and crunchy dough filled with beam and boiled wheat grain. Many pastries are made of fried dough with different fillings.

Francesco Procopio dei Coltelli, a Sicilian aristocrat, established a chain of coffeehouses throughout Europe in the late 17th century. In 1675, he opened the Café Procope in Paris and developed a new frozen

dessert made with eggs and cream, called *spumone* or *spumoni*. *Spumone* was brought to Naples in three flavors, vanilla, strawberry, and pistachio, mirroring the colors of the Italian flag.

FOODS WITH CULTURAL SIGNIFICANCE

Easter (Pasqua)

The Easter basket contains an egg covered with cookie dough. The egg symbolizes fertility, resurrection, and rebirth. Lamb eaten on Easter Sunday is a symbol of Christ's sacrifice to the people, according to the Bible, a reference to the flight from Egypt where all Jews were required to butcher a lamb. Chocolate eggs are brightly wrapped and sold in pastry shops throughout Italy. Smaller eggs are for children and larger eggs contain a surprise inside such as a toy for a child or a small picture frame for an adult (Barry, 2008).

Christmas

Eating eel on Christmas Eve symbolizes renewal and new beginning in the coming year, because eels shed their skin and replace it with new skin (Barry, 2008). Panettone, a bread often given as gifts and consumed on Christmas Day with espresso or wine, is made with eggs, butter, candied fruit, and raisins, and is tall with a wide, round top that resembles the domed churches and cathedrals throughout Italy. Traditionally, each family member takes a bite of the first three slices of the cake, and by doing so Italians believe that they will have good luck until next Christmas (Bucciarelli, 2008).

New Year's Day

On New Year's Day, the amount of lentils eaten is believed to be directly proportional to the amount of money that will be earned in the coming year, because the lentils resemble coins (Bucciarelli, 2008).

Spring

Virtú is a traditional dish prepared at the beginning of spring in Abruzzo, with at least seven kinds of dried pulses, seven kinds of fresh vegetables, and seven kinds of pasta, cheese, lard, prosciutto, and pork rinds. In the local rural culture, whatever was left in the cupboard after the cold days of winter ended up in the boiling pot: the virtú symbolizes the passage to the new season (Capatti, 2000).

Epiphany

According to legend, on January 6, LaBefana leaves toys and gifts for good children, and bad children get lumps of garlic mixed with licorice that look like coal.

Feast Day of San Michele

On September 29, small round potato dumplings called *gnocchi* are cooked and said to bring good luck (Abbott, 2007). Now they are used for weddings and other special occasions. Confetti colors are traditional and symbolic; for example, white symbolizes purity, green signifies an engagement or hope, pink or blue announces the birth of a girl or boy, and silver and gold are associated with wedding anniversaries. The confetti are always packaged in odd numbers, which can be traced back to religious beliefs, and are considered to bring good fortune.

Saint Joseph's Day

Saint Joseph's Day is celebrated in the beginning of spring. The table is covered with all kinds of foods to feed the community. Many bean dishes are served on this day (fava beans and chick peas), and bread to look like a basket, boat, or fish. At the end of the meal, everyone takes home a loaf of bread from the bread altar, and the loaf stays in the house for a year. It is supposed to bring good luck.

Other Occasions

Garlic in foods originated in ancient times, because the herb has been prescribed medicinally since at least 1500 BC, when it was listed in an Egyptian document as a remedy for over 20 ailments, including headaches, insect bites, tumor, and heart problems (Moramarco, 2000).

 TYPICAL DAY'S MENU

Southern staple foods include pasta, dried beans, greens, and tomato sauce, whereas northern staple foods include risotto, meat, cheese, and white sauce. Breakfast is served about 8 AM and consists of cappuccino or espresso, sweet rolls, cookies, croissants, and toasted bread, either homemade or purchased that morning from a local bakery (Poe, 2001). Jams, preserves, honey, or a chocolate spread, such as Nutella, are used on the croissants or toast. Because of the media, American cold cereals are being introduced in Italian households. Children may drink Ovomaltina or Nesquick along with their breakfast.

For a midmorning snack, adults drink espresso or cappuccino with a pastry, croissant, or fruit left over from breakfast. For children, classes stop for a 15- to 20-minute recess and small paninos, pizza, cake, fruit, or more recently, a commercially produced snack, are served. Snack machines at the school mainly sell chocolate bars, chips, and soda (Low, 2008).

On weekends and vacation days, adults go to bars for an aperitivo (prosecco), a light sparkling wine, along with mixed nuts, crackers, potato chips, or olives, prior to lunch.

Lunch (pranzo) is traditionally the main meal of the day, about five courses, served around 1 or 2 PM and lasting up to 3 hours depending on the region and whether a person is at work (Abbott, 2007). Office workers tend to eat and leave faster. If a heavy lunch is eaten, the evening meal consists of a light snack. A typical lunch meal includes antipasto, "before the meal," because it is a custom in Italian homes never to keep people waiting for food. Antipasto is served before guests are seated; for example, bruschetta (crusty bread with chopped tomatoes, pesto, olives, cheese, and garlic) or an assortment of slices of meat (salami, prociutto, carpaccio), cheeses (provolone, scarmoza), marinated vegetables (eggplant, zucchini), and olives (or maybe cantaloupe wrapped in prosciutto or tomato with a basil leaf, extra virgin olive oil with light salt and pepper, and a side of breadsticks). An elegant "raw" antipasto is carpaccio, very thinly sliced, chilled raw meat or fish, lightly sprinkled with olive oil, various herbs, and shaved parmesan cheese (Anderson, 1994). Both the first and second courses are equal in portion size and smaller in portion than a main course. The first main dish includes pasta, risotto, soup (minestra, a vegetable broth soup), and tortellini in broth.

The second main course includes meat or fish seasoned according to the region, plus a cooked vegetable that is served separately as a side dish (*contorno*). *Contorni* (a plain salad that includes potatoes, zucchini, asparagus, broccoli rabe, and green beans) follows the second dish and is used to cleanse the palette rather than as an accompaniment to meat or fish (Shankland, 2005). Bread of the region is included in this meal, which may be used to clean the plate of sauce during informal dining. Pasta is never eaten as a meal in itself, except for lasagna or pizza (Shankland, 2005).

A regional wine, such as Chianti or Sangiovese, is often served after the first dish. The second dish is followed by a cheese-and-fruit platter in everyday dining. Dessert, which may include *torta*, *gelato*, or *biscotti* (cookies), and espresso, is served only when guests are present or on special occasions.

An afternoon snack might consist of a panini (tomato, mozzarella cheese, and salami), fruit, yogurt, cake, or cookies.

A typical Italian dinner may be eaten as late as 10 PM, but is usually consumed around 8 PM and includes pasta or meat/fish, salad/greens, fruit, bread, and wine. On Friday, fish is served as a meal (Poe, 2001). If the breadwinner is not home for lunch, dinner becomes the main meal (Abbott, 2007).

A late snack, especially during the summer or after a night out, may consist of plain bread, meats, cheeses, wine, or water (Abbott, 2007).

 ## HOLIDAY MENUS

The main Italian holidays are New Year's Day (January 1), Epiphany (January 6), Easter (March/April), Liberation Day (April 25), Labor Day (May 1), Republic Day (June 2), Ferragosto (Assumption Day, August 15), All Saints Day (November 1), Immaculate Conception (December 8), Christmas Day (December 25), and Santo Stefano (December 26). The birth of Christ is one of two major festivals of the Christian liturgical calendar and is celebrated at home.

Christmas Eve is called the Feast of the Seven Fishes, which began in the 7th century (Ruperto, 2008). Most Italians give up meat on the day before Christmas for religious reasons, and fast during the day. The meal consists of seven different fish dishes, representative of the sacraments 7 days of the week, or the seven hills around Rome (Ruperto, 2008). Fish is a symbol for Christianity in the Bible. Some of the fish dishes include squid, octopus, clams, eel, lobster, crab, shrimp, flounder, codfish (always served), salmon, and tuna. The fish can be fried, grilled, baked, served cold, tossed in salads, or stuffed in pasta, with olive oil or sauces. Also served are seasonal cheeses and nuts, chestnuts, candied fruit, sweets, and various breads (panetone, panforte). Dishes are served one at a time, and after dinner people go to church for midnight Mass.

Other holiday meals are as follows:

1. On Easter Sunday, melon and proscuitto, tossed salad, ravioli, marinated lamb, asparagus parme-

san, Easter bread, fruit, and lamb cake (southern Italy) are served.
2. On Pasquetta (Easter Monday), Italians travel to the countryside for a picnic or lunch to welcome the spring season. A picnic may include panini, wine, mineral water, fruit, cookies, and hard-boiled eggs from Easter Sunday.
3. Carnevale (*Martedi Grasso*) is celebrated 10 days before Ash Wednesday; this is when the Catholics enter a 6-week period of fasting and abstinence leading to Easter. The festivities include masked balls and gondola procession, medieval fairs, horseback sports and costumes, and they indulge in sensual pleasures and the feast of abundances including meats, breads, and sweets (fritters dusted with powdered sugar and filled with fruit and cream, fritole, and frappe). Carnevale is celebrated in many regions of Italy, although Venice is where the main celebration is held.
4. For birthday celebrations/Name's Day (*Animastico*), hors d'oeuvres, sandwiches, pizza, finger food, soft drinks, and birthday cake are served.

 ## HEALTH BELIEFS AND CONCERNS

Italians are sentimental and not afraid to express their feelings, and this extends into the healthcare environment (Hillman, 2008). Italians often discuss health-related issues, such as their blood pressure, visits to the doctor, and tests performed, even with newly met acquaintances (Abbott, 2007). This may be related to the belief that illness can be caused by suppression of emotions, and stress from fear, grief, and anxiety, because it is not healthy to keep emotions bottled up (Ragucci, 1981). Older Italians, especially women, are more likely to report pain experiences, express symptoms, and expect immediate treatment. Overall, Italians are one of the healthiest and longest-lived people; men live to an average age of 78 years and women live to an average age of 81 years (UNICEF, 2007). This is the highest life expectancy among Europeans, and many people believe it to be related to the Mediterranean diet, which includes red wine and olive oil. Olive oil is monounsaturated oil and does not affect the level of cholesterol in the blood, one of the reasons that the heart attack rate in Italy is low. Italian doctors and medical staff are among the best trained in the world, with the highest number of doctors per capita (1 doctor per 160 people) (Abbott, 2007); however, Italy also has the fewest dentists per capita, and the dentists they do have are expensive (Abbott, 2007).

Many Italians believe that bigger babies are healthier (Hillman, 2008). The amount of weight is perceived as a measure of successful maintenance of maternal and wifely responsibilities. Breastfeeding is expected by new mothers for health benefits to mother and baby. Strong religious influence among Italians, prayer and having faith in God and saints, are believed to improve illness (Hillman, 2008). Terminal illness and death is said to be God's will. Death is not discussed between the dying person and family members (Spector, 2004). The healthcare providers may need to help the client obtain the basic rites of Sacrament of the Sick, which includes Anointing, Communion, and a blessing by a priest. Many Italians may attribute the cause of illness to the "evil eye." The evil eye is a belief that someone (God or an evil person) can project harm by gazing or staring at a person or his or her property (Spector, 2004). Individuals can protect themselves from the evil eye by using symbols, such as amulets, cornicelli (little red horns), or with a gobo (man), which are believed to be good-luck charms or for health protection (Hillman, 2008). Another practice that is believed to remove the evil eye is to take an egg and olive oil and drip them into a pan of water, make the sign of the cross, and recite prayers. If the oil spreads over the water, the cause of the problem is the evil eye, and the illness will get better (Spector, 2004).

Some past health-protection beliefs include the use of garlic cloves and red ribbon or cloth on an infant or child (used to prevent colds and evil looks from other people, which could cause headaches and a pain or stiffness in the back or neck). Chicken soup was used for everything from preventing colds to encouraging delivery of a baby. Cooked oatmeal wrapped in a cloth (steaming hot) was applied to drain infections on the skin. Herbal tea (chamomile) was used for upset stomachs and honey was added for sore throats. If a person had a fever, he or she would be covered with blankets to sweat it out. Hot pepper was applied to the thumb to prevent a child from sucking his or her thumb. Live leeches were put on a person's skin, because they thought this would lower blood pressure. If the leech died, the person had to see a doctor, because it meant that something was wrong with the person's blood. For cold treatment, boiled wines or coffee with anisette was the cure. To prevent blemishes, hot flaxseed was applied. For a toothache, whiskey was applied topically. All members of the family would share in the responsibilities for a sick family member, as health care was often managed at home (Spector, 2004).

As the next generations become more educated, home-remedy treatment is decreasing. Physicians do not regard nutrition and diet as a high priority; they are only considered in cases of chronic illness and controlled diets in a hospital setting (Parasecoli, 2004). In addition, Italians, who believe in some superstitions, warn about the following: avoid spilling salt or oil; do not pour wine "backwards" (with your hand held under the bottle); do not leave a loaf of bread or bread roll upside down; and do not toast with water or bad luck will come to you (Shankland, 2005).

GENERAL HEALTH AND NUTRITIONAL INDICATORS SUMMARY

The Italian population, overall, exceeds the estimated nutritional requirements for a healthy diet. Food security has become a minor issue for the poor households; however, the poor groups may consume less healthy food as compared with the average household, given the heavier weight of their expenditure for food (Arcella & Conforti, 1998). The intake of traditionally rich foods was fairly equal between the average household and the poor groups according to Arcella and Conforti (1998).

Life expectancy of Italian males at birth is 78 years and for females 81 years. Italy ranks 182 out of 190 for the under-5-years mortality rate through the year 2005, which is a critical indicator of the well-being of children. For every 1000 live births, the probability of dying between birth and exactly 5 years of age is 4%, with the infant mortality rate (age under 1 year) at 4% out of a population of 58,093 in 2005. Infants with low birth weight (< 2500 g) equaled 6% of the live births between 1998 and 2005 (UNICEF, 2007).

Deficiencies in micronutrients, such as iron, iodine, vitamin A, and folate, are widespread throughout the world. In 1993, over 11% of Europe's population suffered from goiter. Since iodized salt became universally available, due to the mass-media campaign, medical education, and cooperation of industry, iodine deficiency is nearly nonexistent (Fraser, 2006). In Italy, iron deficiency was only 7% and noted as a cause of disability-adjusted life-year (DALY). The DALY is a summary that combines the impact of illness, disability, and mortality on population health. According to the World Health Organization (WHO, 2002), some of the leading risk factors include low fruit and vegetable intake; 3.9% of total DALYs that may contribute to cardiovascular disease and cancer. The WHO Europe

(2006) recommends an intake of more than 400 g of fruits and vegetables per person per day, and the average intake in Italy was 479 g in 1994–1995.

A higher prevalence of hypovitaminosis D was found in winter compared with summer in healthy and hospitalized patients living in Central Italy. The need to increase vitamin D intake in Italy, fortification of foods, and/or supplement use must be considered in order to prevent negative effects of vitamin D deficiency (Romagnoli, Caravella, Scarnecchia, Martinez, & Minisola, 1999).

COMMUNICATION AND COUNSELING TIPS

When communicating with Italians, it is important to remember that topics about family are typical conversation (Abbott, 2007; Horne & Kiselica, 1999). Willingness to share thoughts and feelings among family members is a prominent characteristic of Italians (Hillman, 2008). Immediate and extended family are important to the identity of Italians. Relatives typically live in close proximity to one another and visit on a regular basis to share the sorrows and joys of life (Horne & Kiselica, 1999). Sunday dinners are a symbol of the strong ties across generations, and family matters are discussed over meals (Horne & Kiselica, 1999).

Communication is often based on feelings and emotions, rather than on objective thoughts. Decisions are often made based on feelings, but also taking into consideration any other information presented. Details are considered and decided upon based on their merits. Whatever the rule, however, there is always an exception if a case is made for it (Abbott, 2007).

After conversation about the family, other topics of conversation include Italian culture, art, food, wine, and films. At social gatherings it is considered insulting to ask someone you have just met about his or her profession. The Italian male typically dominates the household, expecting the family to cater to his decisions, but in return he provides financial stability for his family. The mother is often dominating in household duties, with the responsibility of cook, counselor, interior decorator, fashion consultant, nurse, and manager of the family for emotional balance (Moramarco, 2000). Daughters have close ties with both parents, particularly as they age (Hillman, 2008). This family structure is changing in Italian households, with males becoming less dominant and the family sharing household responsibilities.

As researched by Horne and Kiselica (1999), several counseling techniques can be utilized when counseling Italians. As a counselor, present yourself as a friendly, genuine person welcoming the family. Upon initial greeting, male or female, young or old, the two parties may embrace and give the other a friendly kiss on each cheek. This exchange forms the basis of the communication that indicates friendliness, intimacy, and animation of the Italian people (Moramarco, 2000). First, establish rapport by using the family-system approach (making reference to immediate and extended family members). This can be accomplished by the counselor sharing some kind of food or drink with the family while revealing some general details about the counselor's own life, such as where he or she was born, the number of members in his or her own family, if he or she is married, and/or the number of children he or she may have. When family lifestyle is shared between family and counselor, a comfort level is established. The family may bring food, and acceptance of the food offered to the counselor creates a bond of acceptance with an Italian family. Not accepting food may insult the mother and prohibit therapeutic progress with the family. Traditional fathers view counseling as a sign of weakness and will be insulted if their authority is ignored. It is important to meet with the father before the first session to enlist his "help" in therapy. By stating how much the counselor "needs the father's strength and guidance" for the counselor to assist the family, the father's commitment is taken as a huge asset in counseling. Watch for hand gestures, as they may be a physical manifestation of emotions that cannot be expressed verbally. The gestures are a natural extension of the language and may provide insight into what the client is communicating. The mother is the source of the family's emotional, spiritual, and moral orientation, although the father is most often its final word.

PRIMARY LANGUAGE OF FOOD NAMES WITH ENGLISH AND PHONETIC TRANSLATION

Pesce (fish): pé-sce

> *Calamari* (squid): ca-la-mà-ri
>
> *Capitone* (eel): ca-pi-tó-ne
>
> *Baccala* (codfish): bac-ca-là
>
> *Acciuga* (anchovy): ac-ciù-ga

Gamberi (shrimp): gàm-be-ri

Arsella (clam/mussel): ar-sèl-la

Carpa (carp): càr-pa

Polpo (octopus): pól-po

Carni (meat): càr-ni

Prosciutto (ham): pro-sciù-to

Porchetta (roast pork): por-chét-ta

Agnello (lamb): a-gnèl-lo

Coniglio (rabbit): co-nì-glio

Bistecca (steak): bi-stéc-ca

Mortadella (ham): mor-ta-dèl-la

Pancetta (bacon): pan-cét-ta

Pollo (chicken): pól-lo

Salame (salami): sa-là-me

Salsiccia (sausage): sal-sìc-cia

Soppressata (cooked, pressed pork): sop-pres-sà-ta

Tacchino (turkey): tac-chì-no

Uovo (egg): uò-vo

Nocciola (nuts): noc-ciò-la

Mandorla (almond): màn-dor-la

Nocciola (hazelnut): noc-ciò-la

Pistacchio (pistachio): pi-stàc-chio

Pinolo (pine nuts): pi-nò-lo

Fagio'lo (beans): fa-g-o-lo

Fava: fà-va

Ceci (chick peas): cé-ci

Lupino (lupine): lu-pì-no

Spezie (spices): spè-zie

Alloro (bay leaf): al-lò-ro

Noce moscata (nutmeg): nó-ce mo-scà-ta

Origano (oregano): o-rì-ga-no

Cacao (cocoa): ca-cà-o

Zafferano (saffron): zaf-fe-rà-no

Pepe (pepper): pé-pe

Dolce (dessert): dól-ce

Panettone (fruitcake): pa-net-tó-ne

Biscotti (cookies): bi-scòt-to

Cannoli: can-nò-lo

Torrone (nougat candy): tor-ró-ne

Tiramisù: ti-ra-mi-sù

Gelato (ice cream): ge-là-to

Granita (Italian ice): gra-nì-ta

Amaretto: a-ma-rét-to

Torta (cake): tòr-ta

Panna cotta (cream pudding): pà-ne còt-ta

Colomba (Easter cake): co-lóm-ba

Pasta (pasta): pà-sta

Orecchietta (ear shaped): o-rec-chiét-ta

Orzo (rice shaped): òr-zo

Bucatini: bu-ca-tì-no

Fettucini: fet-tuc-cì-ni

Gnocchi (potato dumpling): gnòc-chi

Lasagna: la-sà-gna

Spaghetti: spa-ghét-ti

Risotto (rice): ri-sòt-to

Aranciono (rice ball): a-ran-cì-no

Raviolo (ravioli): ra-vi-ò-li

Rigatoni (tube pasta): ri-ga-tó-ni

Formaggio (cheese): for-màg-gio

Mozzarella: moz-za-rèl-la

Provolone: pro-vo-ló-ne

Parmigiano reggiano (parmesan cheese): par-mi-già-no reg-già-no

Ricotta: ri-còt-to

Mascarpone: ma-scar-pó-ne

Scamorza: sca-mòr-za

Taleggio: ta-lég-gio

Fontina: fon-tì-na

Pane (bread): pà-ne

Grissini (bread stick): gris-sì-ni

Focaccia (pizza bread): fo-càc-cia

Polenta (cornbread): po-lèn-ta

Panettone (fruitcake): pa-net-tó-ne

Bruschetta (bread with tomatoes): bru-shet-ta

Pizza: pìz-za

Frutta (fruit): frút-ta

Arancia (orange): a-ràn-cia

Cachi (Sharon fruit): cà-chi

Castagna (chestnut): ca-stà-gna

Ciliegia (cherry): ci-liè-gia

Fico (fig): fi-co

Fragola (strawberry): frà-go-la

Kiwi: kì-wi

Lampone (raspberry): lam-pó-ne

Limone (lemon): li-mó-ne

Tiglio (lime): tì-glio

Mela (apple): mé-la

Melone (melon): me-ló-ne

Pera (pear): pé-ra

Pesca (peach): pè-sca

Vegetale (vegetables): ve-ge-tà-le

Pomodoro (tomato): po-mo-dò-ro

Melanzana (eggplant): me-lan-zà-na

Cipolla (onion): ci-pól-la

Peperoncino (hot red pepper): pe-pe-ron-cì-no

Carciofi (artichoke): car-ciò-fi

Asparago (asparagus): a-spà-ra-go

Broccolo (broccoli): bròc-co-li

Patata (potato): pa-tà-ta

Porcino (mushroom): po-cì-no

Radicchio (chicory): ra-dìc-chio

Spinacio (spinach): spi-nà-cio

Bevande (beverages): be-vàn-de

Caffè (coffee): caf-fè

Espresso (strong coffee): e-sprès-so

Cappucino (coffee with steamed milk): cap-puc-cì-no

Cioccolata (chocolate drink): cioc-co-là-ta

Amaro (liquor): a-mà-ro

Vino rosso (red wine): vì-no rós-so

Vino bianco (white wine): vì-no biàn-co

Birra (beer): bìr-ra

Latte (milk): làt-te

Aranciata (orange drink): a-ran-cià-ta

Acqua minerale (mineral water): àc-qua min-ne-rà-le

Succo (juice): sùc-co

Tè (tea): tè

Other Items

Olio di oliva (olive oil): ò-lio di ò-lì-va

Burro (butter): bùr-ro

Panna (cream): pàn-na

Zucchero (sugar): zùc-che-ro

Besciamella (white sauce): be-scia-mèl-la

Frittata (omelette): frit-tà-ta

Avena (oats): a-vé-na

Farina (flour): fa-rì-na

Aceto balsamico (balsamic vinegar): a-cé-to bal-sà-mi-co

This list was compiled from *I Grandi Dizionari* (2006).

FEATURED RECIPE

Typically, carnevale lasagna is made only during the 3 days of Carnevale. It is eaten in the days before Ash Wednesday and Lent, because meat could not be eaten for 40 days.

Carnevale Lasagna

1 box of lasagna or homemade lasagna (flour, eggs, water, salt)

4 boiled eggs

5 fresh Italian sausage links

1 fresh sopressata

1 lb. ground beef

3 raw eggs

½ lb. dry, hard bread

Salt

Garlic

Black pepper

Parsley

Parmesan cheese

Mozzarella or caciacavallo cheese

Tomato sauce

1. For homemade pasta, make a well of flour in a bowl. Add 3 eggs and as much water as needed. Salt is optional. Add more flour if needed. Knead dough until smooth, but not too hard. Roll dough until thin and cut strips. (You might want to use a pasta machine to make it easier.) Let strips dry.
2. To make mini meatballs for the lasagna, in a bowl mix ground beef, 3 raw eggs, and hard bread (moistened). Add pressed garlic, salt, pepper, parmesan cheese, and chopped parsley to your liking. Form mini meatballs the size of marbles and fry until they are partially cooked, then put them aside.
3. Cut fresh sausage into thin round pieces and partially fry them. (You do not want the pieces to be overcooked and dry.) Put them aside.
4. Cut the sopressata (not too thin and not too thick) and put it aside.
5. Shred the mozzarella or caciacavallo in a bowl (as much as you need), then put it aside.
6. Heat the tomato sauce in a pan with some olive oil and garlic.
7. Peel boiled eggs and cut them into a bowl.
8. Only if using commercial pasta, boil water with a few drops of olive oil to partially cook it for 5–10 minutes. Then put pasta strip by strip on a piece of linen cloth.
9. Turn the oven on to 350°F. Using a 9×11-in. pan, add tomato sauce to cover the bottom and sprinkle parmesan cheese over it.
10. Put one layer of pasta strips on the bottom of the pan. Add tomato sauce over the pasta and sprinkle parmesan cheese. Sprinkle sausage, sopressata, boiled eggs, meatballs, and shredded cheese over the pasta. Add another layer of pasta over the filling. Spread tomato sauce over the pasta and sprinkle parmesan cheese. Sprinkle filling again over the pasta. Keep repeating layers. You should have three or four layers.
11. Cover the last layer of pasta with tomato sauce. Add some water to the sides of the pan so the lasagna will not burn. Cover and cook for 45–60 minutes.

(Courtesy of Enrica Cesario)

More recipes are available at http://nutrition.jbpub.com/foodculture/

ACKNOWLEDGMENTS

The author thanks Vanessa Low for providing useful information in the *Typical Day's Menu* section.

REFERENCES

Abbott, C. (2007). *A quick guide to customs and etiquette. Culture smart! Italy.* London: Bravo Ltd.

Anderson, B. (1994). *Treasures of the Italian table.* New York: William Morrow Publishers.

Arcella, D., & Conforti, P. (1998). Nutritional adequacy and relative poverty in Italy: A multidimensional fuzzy approach. *La Rivista di Scienza Dell'Alimentazione, 27,* 51–62.

Barry, L. (2008). *"Gelato and granita" Montreal foods.* Retrieved August 19, 2008, from http://www.montrealfood.com/granita.html/

Bucciarelli, P.D (2008). *Pour the wine, pass the baccala: Traditional Italian holiday foods.* Retrieved August 19, 2008, from http://www.accenti.ca/article_cover.php/

Capatti, A. (2000). L'osteria nuova. Bra, Italy: Slow Food Editore.

Dalrymple, M. (1985). *Great meals in minutes: Italian menus* (pp. 7–11). Chicago: Time–Life Books.

Fraser, D. (2006). Pediatric micronutrient deficiency, epidemiology, and prevention. Retrieved April 19, 2009, from www.bibalex.org/supercourse/supercoursePPT/1011-2001/1321.ppt

Hillman, S. (2008). *Transcultural healthcare: A culturally competent approach. People of Italian heritage.* Philadelphia: F.A. Davis Company.

Horne, A., & Kiselica, M.S. (1999). *Adolescent males: A pratictioners guide* (pp. 145–150). Thousand Oaks, CA: Sage Publications.

I Grandi Dizionari. (2006). *I grandi dizionari.* Garzanti nuova edizione 2006. Milano: Garzanti Linguistica.

INRAN. (2003). *Guidelines for a healthy Italian diet.* Italy: National Food and Nutrition Research Institute.

Killinger, C. (2005). *The culture and customs of Italy.* Westport, CT: Greenwood Press.

Low, V. Messina, Italy. Personal communication on August 30, 2008.

Moramarco, F. (2000). *Italian pride: 101 reasons to be proud you're Italian.* New York: Kensington Publishing.

Parasecoli, F. (2004). *Food culture in Italy.* Westport, CT: Greenwood Press.

Poe, T. (2001). The labour and leisure of food production as a mode of ethnic identity building among Italians in Chicago, 1890–1940. *Rethinking History, 5*(1), 131–148.

Ragucci, A.T. (1981). Italian Americans. In A. Harwood (Ed.), *Ethnicity and medical care.* Cambridge, MA: Harvard University Press.

Romagnoli, E., Caravella, P., Scarnecchia, L., Martinez, P., & Minisola, S. (1999). Hypovitaminosis D in an Italian population of healthy subjects and hospitalized patients. *British Journal of Nutrition, 81,* 133–137.

Ruperto, M. (2008). *The tale of the fishes.* Retrieved August 19, 2008, from http.www.pitt.edu/~dash/type0002.html

Shankland, H. (2005). *Customs and etiquette of Italy.* London: Kuperd.

Spector, R.E. (2004). *Cultural diversity in health and illness.* Upper Saddle River, NJ: Pearson Prentice-Hall.

UNICEF. (2007). *The state of the world's children 2007: Women and children, the double dividend of gender equality.* Retrieved April 15, 2009, from http://www.unicef.org/sowc07/statistics/tables.php

Welland, D. (2008). Return to roots: A Mediterranean makeover for "American" Italian Cuisine. *Todays Dietitian, 10*(6), 30–34.

WHO Europe. (2006). *Highlights on health in Italy 2004.* Retrieved April 19, 2009, from http://www.euro.who,http://data.euro.who.int/hfadb

World Health Organization (WHO) Regional Office for Europe. (2002). *Micronutrient deficiencies.* Retrieved April 19, 2009, from http://www.euro.who.int/nutrition/deficiency/20020731_1

Wright, J. (2008). Italian spice and herbs. In *Encyclopedia of Italian cooking.* Retrieved August 26, 2008, from http://www.calascio.com/spicesand.htm

INTERNET RESOURCES

www.cyborlink.com/besite/italy.htm/

http://www.corriere.it/Primo_Piano/Cronache/2006/01_Gennaio/17/cattolici.shtml/

http://www.who.int/countries/ita/en/

http://www.randomhistory.com/1-50/038italian.html/

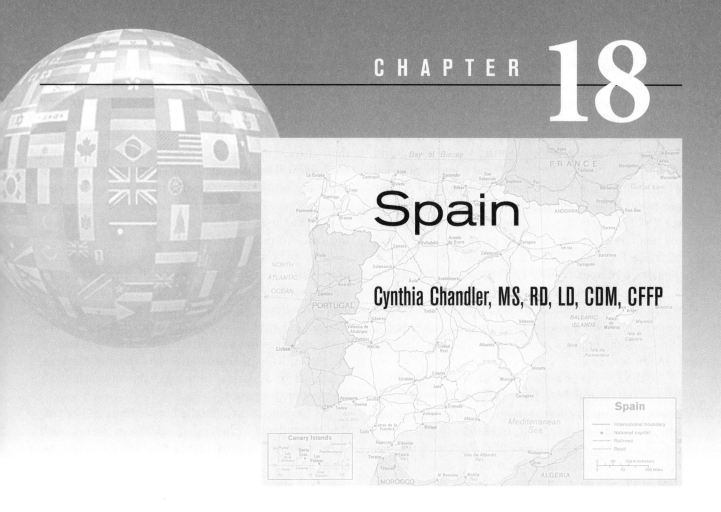

CHAPTER 18

Spain

Cynthia Chandler, MS, RD, LD, CDM, CFFP

 CULTURE AND WORLD REGION

Welcome to the land of flamenco, bullfighting, and soccer! The land rich in the artistic heritage of El Greco and Diego Velasquez and Francisco Goya! The land of diverse peoples that have come together under one flag! Spain is a land that comes to life in a variety of ways, depending on the region of the country you visit. Stretching from the Atlantic Ocean to the Mediterranean Sea, the Iberian Peninsula is home to the ancient country of Spain and neighboring Portugal.

Spain carries with it today the influences of its earliest inhabitants: the Phoenicians, the Greeks, and the Carthaginians. This prized land was fought over and cultivated by many peoples as they fought for land and power.

The Iberians settled into central Spain, perhaps as early as 3000 BC, and continued to live there for many centuries. It is from these settlers that the peninsula is named. "Iber" is a term that is similar to their word for "river." Iberian culture centered around Valencia on the Mediterranean coast.

In the early 200s BC, the Romans arrived and brought their government, wine making, and olive cultivation and pressing techniques. The Romans called the peninsula Hispania and made it part of the Roman Empire for approximately 500 years. The Visigoths crossed over the Pyrenees mountains and ruled Spain for a time.

The Greeks settled in the coastal areas of Spain by the 8th century BC and the Celts were occupying more of the interior regions. The area had already become a melting pot of civilizations such that each culture had brought their customs to the land.

The Moors traveled into Spain from North Africa by crossing the Strait of Gibraltar. They invaded in the 8th century and conquered many Spanish areas, establishing their culture in southern Spain. They introduced spices, fruits, vegetables, and agricultural techniques into the peninsula. They left a strong influence on the sweets of Spain today with the incorporation of such ingredients as orange and lemon zests, nutmeg, cinnamon, rice, and ground almond flours.

The two most important Spanish states from the 12th century until the 15th century were Aragon and Castile, joined when Ferdinand and Isabella married in 1469. They began the tremendous expansion of their newly joined and enlarged country. Columbus went in search of new worlds under their flag. Upon discovering new lands, the voyagers returned to Spain, bringing back new foods such as avocados, beans, corn, papayas, peppers, tomatoes, vanilla, and chocolate.

Present-day Spain has a parliament and operates with a democratic style of government. It is part of the European Union and uses the euro as its currency. It still has some political unrest, but remains a relatively tranquil country.

Although Spain remained neutral in both World War I and World War II, it suffered from internal chaos. The country lost many lives during the Spanish Civil War, which lasted from 1936 to 1939. The war ended with the establishment of a dictatorial regime, headed by Franco, who remained in power until he died in 1975. A new constitution under King Juan Carlos I in 1978 saw the return of democratic rule to the country, as well as a monarchial system. Spain entered the European Economic Community in 1986 and has continued to experience economic growth ever since. It is a country with diverse ethnic groups. The predominant religion is Roman Catholicism, although there is religious tolerance of all faiths today.

Spain is the third largest country in Europe and second only to Switzerland in its number of mountain ranges. It is a cultural crossroad stretching between the Atlantic Ocean and the Mediterranean Sea. Spain is divided into 17 regions, each having unique characteristics. The mountains in Spain formed natural boundaries within the country that separated the different tribes as they migrated and settled into the land. These barriers made transportation and communication difficult. The diversity of the land varies from snowcapped peaks of the Pyrenees Mountains on the northern border to the tropical Mediterranean region in the south and the east. To the north of Spain lies France, with the Pyrenees mountain range serving as a natural barrier between the two countries. The Pyrenees Mountains stretch almost 300 miles from the Mediterranean Sea to the Atlantic Ocean. To the south of Spain, less than 10 miles from its southern tip, lies Morocco, in Africa.

Spain also occupies the Balearic Islands and the Canary Islands, which are both near the mainland, in the Mediterranean Sea. The "garden of Spain" follows the southeast Mediterranean coast and includes the provinces of Murcia, Alicante, and Valencia. Together, these three provinces are known as El Levante. In this land you will find orange groves abounding. This area along the southeastern Mediterranean coast is where rice is grown. Pastries are in abundance in El Levante as well. The region is known for its factories that make the delicious nougat called *turron*.

The regions of Navarra and La Rioja are fertile grounds for fresh produce, especially the grapes that go into making Spanish wine. The Camino de Santiago, a medieval pilgrimage route, runs through both regions and attracts many tourists to view the monasteries and churches along the route. La Rioja is known mainly for its wine. Pamplona, the capital of Navarra, is famous for its annual running of the bulls, which attracts many tourists.

El Levante and Catalonia border France. The cuisine of Catalonia includes delicacies from the sea, such as baby octopus in garlic sauce or tallina, a clam stew. During the right season, using a rake at the water's edge will allow one to gather enough clams for a rich stew from the sea.

The Central Plains include the regions of Castile–Leon, La Mancha, and Extremadura. Known as the land of the conquistadors, Extremadura was long fought over by Christians and Moors. The land was the frontier for many centuries when there were wars waged against the Moors. The land, located to the west of Madrid along the Portuguese border, is a harsh mountainous land. La Mancha is the land where Don Quixote, the literary character created by Cervantes, had his adventures. It is located in the mesa of Spain, a dry, rural region. It is a land of cattle and sheep, vineyards, olive groves, and poppies. The capital of La Mancha, and its most known city, is Toledo.

The northern coast includes the Basque country, Asturias and Cantabria, and Galacia. This region of Spain is both green and humid. Galacia has a uniquely Celtic heritage and its people are fond of meat and fish pies, scallops, and veal. Galician cuisine is simple and based on an ample supply of food from the sea along with crops of potatoes, tomatoes, onions, and fruits. Asturias is famous for its legendary bean dish known as *fabada*. It is also known for its *queso Cabrales*, a strong blue cheese.

The Basque country serves a lot of fish dishes such as baby eel and squid. Catalonia, in the northeastern corner of Spain, is a region of creative cuisine as well as fine art and architecture. Barcelona, a very cosmopolitan city, is the capital and attracts many tourists. It is home to the stunning architectural designs of Antoni Gaudí.

The northeast interior includes Aragon, La Rioja, and Navarra. La Rioja is a land of high plains and dry valleys giving way to the mountain ranges of the Pyrenees.

Valencia is home to the famed Spanish dish paella.

Andalusia is located in southern Spain, an area that covers over 2 million acres. It is crisscrossed heavily by mountain ranges. Andalusia, with its Moorish palaces still in existence, was strongly influenced by the Moors, who had easy access to Spain by crossing through Gibraltar. (Morocco and Algeria lie just south of Spain.) It is one of the poorest regions of Spain. There is an abundance of fresh vegetables, fruit, and seafood available to Andalusian kitchens, keeping the cuisine simple, fresh, local, and delicious. It is not considered to be "gourmet" food due to its simplicity. Two internationally recognized products of Spain, gazpacho and flamenco, come from Andalusia.

Madrid, Spain's capital, located in the middle of the country, has no true distinct cooking style of its own, but it is a place where each region of the country can be experienced in various restaurants.

There are two sets of islands that are part of Spain: the Balearic Islands and the Canary Islands. The islands Mallorca, Menorca, and Ibiza are the Baleric Islands. The Canary Islands are closer to the Moroccan coast and a major tourist destination. Most of the income is derived from tourism. The volcanic soil is growth friendly to the tomatoes and potatoes that were brought back from the New World. The volcanic islands actually form an archipelago.

The population of Spain is over 40 million people. It is approximately the size of Texas. The official national language is Castilian. The climate varies with the region. The interior of the country has sultry summers and cold, cloudy winters. The coastline has a more moderate summer season with a cloudy and cool winter season.

FOOD HISTORY WITHIN THE CULTURE

There is no single word that describes the diversity of food in Spain. The cuisine varies extensively with the region. It is interwoven with the flavor of the Romans, Moors, French, Italians, and Aztecs. Spanish cuisine reflects the diversity of its background. Food is plentiful and hearty throughout the land.

Three predominant themes concerning food in Spain are freshness of ingredients, time spent on meals with friends and family, and an abundance of food for all to enjoy. The three ingredients that transcend the natural barriers in the country are olive oil, garlic, and bread. Garlic is used liberally everywhere in Spain. Traditionally, Spanish cuisine is uncomplicated and based on the freshness of ingredients from the earth and the sea.

Spanish cuisine most clearly resembles a Mediterranean diet combined with Moorish influences. The Moors introduced rice, saffron, nutmeg, cumin, and oranges into the culture, and they still hold a prominent place. Viticulture has flourished since the times the Phoenicians inhabited the land. Wine and sherry are served with or before a meal. Spanish cuisine is distinguished from Mexican cuisine by, among other things, its lack of hot chilies and sauces. Corn tortillas are not even used in Spain; thus, tacos, enchiladas, and chilaquilles are not on a Spanish menu. Spanish cooking is classically Mediterranean. The early spice routes to the east of Spain infused the flavors in Spanish cooking that are prevalent today. When Christopher Columbus returned from the New World, he brought with him potatoes, tomatoes, and peppers. These popular ingredients are harvested and integrated into the various stews served throughout Spain.

The influence of the Moors contributed to the cuisine in what is now Andalusia. The Arabs introduced olives, lemons, and oranges into the country. In October, in Extremadura, peppers are harvested for the prized paprika. Once the peppers are gathered, they are smoked for about 2 weeks and hand turned daily. As they age, they develop their deep coloring so characteristic of Spanish paprika. Their smell and taste also intensifies in the aging process. It is noteworthy that these peppers are not hot, as in Mexican cooking, but generally mild and sweet. Spanish cooking is not seasoned as a hot cuisine, but a flavorful cuisine.

Known as the land of the conquistadors, Extremadura (the area of Spain that borders Portugal) is known for its "peasant cuisine"; basic, nourishing food. Smoked paprika (*pimenton de la Vera*) is its best-known product.

Tapas

Food in Spain is denoted by a *Denominación de Origen* (DO), which describes where the food is grown. Andalusia, the primary producer of olive oil, is also the place where *tapas* probably began. *Tapas* are synonymous with Spanish cuisine. *Tapas* are not a certain type of food, but a way of eating small amounts of food. It is said that *tapas* originated in Andalusia, the land where sherry is made, in the 19th century. The custom arose of serving a morsel on top of the sherry glass, perhaps to keep out flies or to retard the absorption of the alcohol. *Tapas* started out with a simple piece of cheese laid across the rim of the sherry glass. It evolved into small plates of simple foods, such as marinated olives or almonds, being placed on top of the glass. (The word *tapa* means "cover" in Spanish.) *Tapas* do not cover sherry drinks any longer but are always offered to accompany sherry or any other drink. *Tapas* vary by region in Spain. The Basque country calls their tapas *pintxos*.

There are countless *tapas* bars scattered throughout the country that invite the passerby in for a leisurely drink and food. *Tapas* may be on display along the full length of the bar with people crowded around. *Tapas* are meant to be meal teasers, starters of sorts, to be consumed with your drink.

Some ideas for *tapas* include the following:

Anchovy-stuffed olives

Pickled mussels

A wedge of manchego cheese topped with a bit of quince preserves

Fried marcona almonds

Pan con tomato y anchoa (garlic, olive oil, and fresh tomato on toasted bread rounds)

Clams in garlic sauce on toast

Paella

Paella could be considered Spain's national dish. It hails from the Arab introduction of rice to the flatland area of Valencia. (Spain grows a medium- to short-grain round rice that easily swells and absorbs the flavors in which it is cooked.) Paella is cooked over an open flame with seafood, meat, and vegetables. The word *paella* actually describes the pan in which the dish is cooked, a style of pan introduced by the Romans. The original paella included rice, tomatoes, olive oil, paprika, saffron, and snails. Paella is seasoned with saffron, which gives the dish its characteristic light-orange color.

 MAJOR FOODS

Spanish cuisine rests comfortably on a tripod of wine, oil, and bread with an ample infusion of garlic. Ham is prized in Spain, with several museums devoted to

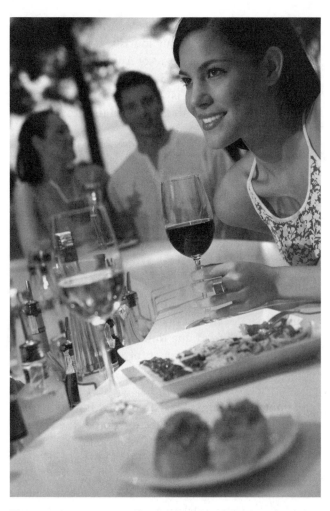

Tapas are not a certain type of food, but a way of eating small amounts of food.

the art of curing their Spanish hams. Like traditional Mediterranean cooking, there is extensive use of olive oil, fresh produce, rice, pasta, seafood, and bread. Potatoes and corn have been infused into Spanish cuisine from the early expeditions to the New World. Cuisine based on rice thrives in El Levante, a stretch of coastline along eastern Spain, including the provinces of Valencia.

 Protein Sources

Spain takes great pride in its sausages. Chorizo sausage is a national specialty. It is a pork sausage made with paprika. Lamb, veal, and pig are all protein sources favored in Spain, with baby lamb and suckling pigs being particularly popular.

Spain is a top producer of almonds, hazelnuts, and walnuts. Although not known for cheese, there is a manchego cheese that is made from sheep's milk

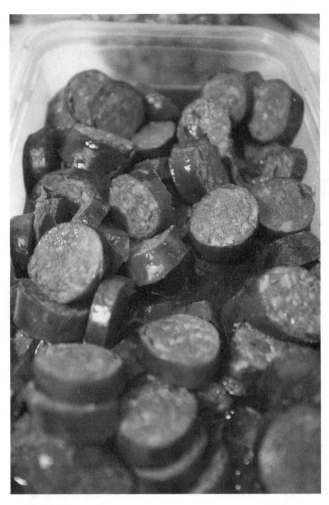

Chorizo is a type of pork sausage made with paprika.

in the La Mancha province. It is a hard cheese that is highly desired. It has its own *Denominación de Origen*. The Canary Islands produce a cheese made from goat's milk called *majorero* that is semicured. It is usually sold covered in paprika. In the Galician region, in the northwest corner of Spain, there is a soft cream cheese known as *tetilla* that is popular. Cheese is typically eaten plain in *tapas* or as part of a dessert. It is not used in traditional cooking.

Eggs are a staple of all Spanish diets, and fried eggs (fried in a generous amount of olive oil until the edges of the whites are crisp) are a part of most early meals. Eggs are used for making mayonnaise, a mainstay ingredient in Spanish cuisine.

Being surrounded by so much water, it is logical that seafood is a big part of Spanish cuisine. The Spanish particularly enjoy tuna, sardines, anchovies, and cod. Dry salted bacalao (cod) has been a part of their cuisine for centuries. There are plenty of fish markets

that offer fresh bass, tuna, cuttlefish, bonito, and many other varieties of fish. Merluza is on many menus. Merluza is a European hake that is eaten plain as well as incorporated into a variety of recipes. The southern region of Spain serves large rings of calamari.

Ham is a favorite meat among all Spanish provinces and has been since the days of the Spanish Inquisition. Ham was actually a food associated with being a good Christian. *Jamón iberico* (ham from the sierra) is prized in the country and people pay much money for it. It is made from the leanest part of the wild Red Iberian pig. It is salted and dried on the Spanish sierra and is similar to Italian prosciutto. Spanish ham has a high fat content and is a significant protein source, as opposed to the tender, thin prosciutto slices. You are likely to see hams hanging in bars, restaurants, and even homes. Hams are served thin sliced as *tapas* or in thicker pieces as part of stews. *Jamón serrano* is an everyday part of Spanish cuisine. It is from the domestic white pig. (Spanish hams are classified by the breed of pig.) Iberico hams are from black-skinned pigs indigenous to the Iberian Peninsula. *Jamón iberico* hams are made from pigs that have a diet based on acorns, which imparts a nutty flavor to the hams. This is considered the premier ham in the world. Serrano hams are from white-skinned pigs that came from northern Europe in the 1950s. Serrano ham is a bit more affordable than Iberico ham. Spaniards eat the ham plain in slices and also cook with it.

The Pyrenees valleys have long been the grazing ground for sheep and goats, and you will see these protein sources incorporated into dishes in this mountainous region. In addition to Manchego, which is processed either semicured (which makes it a mild cheese) or well cured (which makes it a sharp cheese), there is Idiazzagal, which is made there by Basque shepherds.

Spaniards use a lot of legumes in meals. Lentils and chickpeas are incorporated into many recipes. There is a dish called *Moros y Cristianos* ("Moors and Christians") that is a simple combination dish of rice and beans, which relates the food to the group that brought it to the region. Chickpea stew, a thick, hearty stew, is often served in Madrid.

 Starch Sources

Rice forms the base for the classically Spanish dish, paella. Valencia, Calasparra, and Catalonia each produce a short-grain rice that is used in many Spanish dishes. There is the special rice, *arroz bomba*, which requires special care but results in a grain that resists

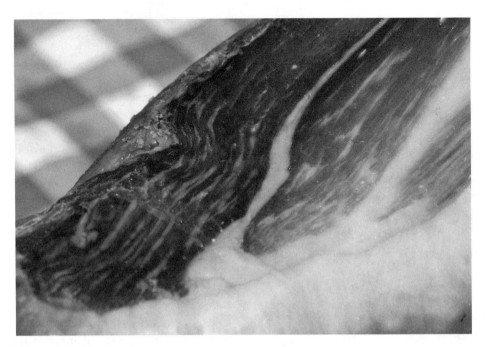

Jamon Serrano

overcooking. *Arroz bomba* requires more liquid in cooking than other short-grain rice and has a unique texture when done.

 Fat Sources

Olive trees grow abundantly in Spain, with over 262 varieties. It is from these olive trees that the oil that predominates in Spanish cooking is produced. Spain reigns supreme as the largest producer of olive oil. The time the fruit is harvested greatly affects the flavor. Early fall harvests yield a greener olive oil that is somewhat more on the bitter side. Later harvests yield a golden olive oil. Olives are picked and crushed into a thick paste called a "mash." The mash is pressed or centrifuged to extract the oil. If it is pressed, the oil is allowed to stand until it has floated to the top. If the mash is centrifuged, it goes through two spins to free it from impurities. The oil is allowed to age for 3–6 months. The aging process reduces some of the natural bitterness that is characteristic of olives.

Olive oils range from a deep green to a golden color. Earlier autumn harvests are greener and slightly more bitter. Later harvests yield more golden oil. Heat destroys the nuances of extra virgin oils, so those should be saved for salads and bread dips.

Olive oil is used in a variety of ways: to marinate, fry, sauté, and in desserts. It can be used as a frying agent if the heat is controlled. Extra virgin olive oil has a stronger taste than the lighter version, so a couple of varieties of this prized oil are usually found in kitchen pantries.

Types of olive oils are as follows:

Extra virgin olive oil (acidity level of no higher than 1%)

Average virgin olive oil (acidity level no higher than 3.3%)

Strong virgin olive oil (acidity level above 3.3%)

Refined olive oil (lacks the full taste of virgin olive oil)

Standard olive oil (a blend of virgin and refined olive oil)

Lard is traditionally used in Spain as well and imparts very flaky pastry dough to many pastries. It is high in saturated fat but does not have any trans fats, so a limited amount could certainly replace butter.

 Prominent Vegetables

Spain produces more fruits and vegetables than the rest of Europe. The Navarra region is known for its white asparagus, which is grown by covering the young shoots with dirt. This is to prevent them from turning green. The asparagus is considered best if canned or bottled. It forms the base for a simple salad with aioli. Navarra grows a pepper known as *pimento*

del piquillo with its own Denomination of Origin. It is wood roasted and stuffed with meat or fish. Onions are kept on hand to use in the famous Spanish omelets. Potatoes, brought from the New World, are a staple in Spanish stews and some side dishes, including *tapas*. *Tortilla española* is a potato omelet served throughout Spain for a simple supper. Tomatoes are used for soups, paellas, and sauces. The most basic tomato sauce that is used frequently in a variety of recipes is a Spanish *sofrita*. The most traditional Spanish dish that uses fresh vegetables fused with garlic is a cold tomato soup called *gazpacho*. Traditionally, it was ground in a special dish called a *dornillo*, but today a blender is used to pulverize the various vegetables. Gazpacho is very popular in the hot summer months in Andalusia. Chickpea stew is a staple in Madrid in cooler months, whereas gazpacho will be on the menu during hot summer days.

 ### Prominent Fruits

Spain has numerous *fruterias* (fruit shops). Fruit is often eaten as a last course in a meal. Seville oranges are famous worldwide, and Valencia is also known for its oranges. Chirimoyas, which are native to South America, are enjoyed throughout Spain. Their appearance is one of a green, heart-shaped fruit with bumps on the outside. They are usually eaten raw with seeds removed. Some enjoy chirimoyas for breakfast.

 ### Spices, Seasonings, and Nuts

The purple crocus flower, brought to Spain by the Moors and grown in Spain's central region, is prized for its stigmas. The autumn blooms are used to harvest the flowers from which the saffron will be extracted. This is the classic ingredient that makes a paella a true Spanish paella. The crocus stigmas, which produce saffron, are what yield this remarkable spice. Most crocuses are grown in the central region of La Mancha. It takes 75,000 flowers to yield 1 lb. of saffron. The spice is very expensive (about $20 in the United States for an ounce or two), mainly because the saffron must be harvested by hand. Saffron lends a deep color as well as a unique flavor to paellas and stews. It is always best to purchase saffron in strands rather than pulverized, and to look for a deep red color. Paprika is sold as sweet or spicy and can be smoked or not, depending on the flavor profile of a recipe. Garlic is the most commonly used spice in Spanish cookery. It is a staple in pantries and is best stored in a cool, dry place to avoid sprouting. La Mancha is known for its paprika, garlic, and saffron. Thyme, rosemary, and oregano are kept on

hand in most Spanish kitchens to round out the spice profile for various dishes.

When Columbus returned from his first trip to the New World, he brought back the *Capsicum annum* pepper (the chili pepper). This pepper is used in making the prized Spanish chorizo. It is called *pimenton* in Spain and paprika in the United States. *Pimenton* has an earthy, smoky aroma and flavor. It is from the ground, sweet red capsicum. Extremadura is known for its *pimenton de la Vera*, a delicious smoked paprika.

Hazelnuts are very popular mixed with chocolate. Grown in Catalonia, they are also used as an ingredient in romesco sauce. Marcona almonds, sweet yet delicate, are prized and used in many desserts or are roasted in olive oil as part of *tapas*.

 ### Beverages

Café con leche (coffee with milk) is a popular drink among Spaniards. *Jerez* (sherry) is a type of wine produced in Jerez, which is in southwest Spain. The production of sherry dates back to Phoenician days when their peoples introduced grape vines to the region. Jerez has the necessary sun, arid climate, and soil to produce the grapes needed for the sherry that bears the town's name. Cava is a Spanish sparkling wine that is served either very sweet or extra dry. Spanish wines, both red and white, are kept in most homes for cooking. The grapevines grow freely in the dry, arid climate of Spain's interior. La Rioja wines, from north–central Spain, are considered good for cooking with and drinking. Wine tends to be more of a beverage with *tapas*, rather than a drink consumed by itself. Spaniards are also associated with sangria, a wine that is mixed with fruit juices and soda, and perhaps some sugar syrup.

 ### Desserts

Dessert is typically reserved for special meals and holidays. The Moors brought almonds, sugar, eggs, and honey into Spanish territory as sweets ingredients, but sweets have been made in convents since the days that Moors and Jews were expelled from the country and Catholicism became the predominant influence. Nuns became known for their wonderful sweets, which have been sold in the countryside since 1500. Winemakers also utilized egg whites to clarify their wine. The egg yolks were donated to the convents to further the preparation of sweets by the nuns.

Turron, an almond-and-honey nougat, can be cooked to a crisp, hard stage (Alicante style) or bought soft and chewy (Gijona style), and *flan* is an internationally popular Spanish dessert that is based on a rich egg custard and usually served cold with a caramelized sauce.

 FOODS WITH CULTURAL
SIGNIFICANCE

Paella is a culturally significant food that is available and enjoyed throughout the country. Paella is a saffron-seasoned dish based on the rice that is grown in the homeland. The word "paella" actually refers to the style of pan that is used, which is a flat-bottomed pan that was used when the dish originated near Valencia where the freshest foods available were cooked together with a short-grain rice that was grown in the fields. Spain grows a medium- to short-grain round rice that easily swells and absorbs the flavors it is cooked in. The flat bottom allows the heat to disperse evenly across the contents and a handle is always on the pan to allow ease in handling. Many other foods, served either as main dishes or as *tapas*, carry particular significance in Spanish cuisine and culture. Additionally, *cocido*, or Spanish stew, made with chickpeas or vegetables and meat is also a characteristic meal found in the regions of Spain.

 TYPICAL DAY'S MENU

In Spain, meals are long, leisurely, and meant to be enjoyed with friends and family. A typical day's style of eating would begin with a very simple breakfast of coffee and bread with jam, or perhaps a simple breakfast pastry. There might be a simple snack about midmorning. From there, work would ensue and continue until midday when there is a large meal (the largest of the day). This meal might occur between 2 and 3 PM. Depending on the region, a siesta often follows the meal, and even stores close during the long hours of the afternoon. The evenings linger long and the final meal of the day is anywhere from 10 PM till midnight. This leaves time for *tapas* before dinner. You might find a very simple serving of *tapas* such as an olive pâté spread on a garlic toast slice or an open jar of olives. Alternatively, there are cookbooks devoted entirely to preparing *tapas* that are as varied in the ingredients as those used in Spanish cuisine. Bread is a part of every meal. Empanadas are quite popular and use bread to house layers of fillers ranging from chopped olives to sausages.

 HOLIDAY MENUS

Nochebena (the good night) of Christmas Eve is always heralded by a special dinner. Christmas in Catalonia and Valencia sees *turron*, a very sweet nougat that usually contains almonds and honey, on the dessert tables. Dozens of types of *turron* are available during the holiday season. The Christmas season continues until the *Dia de los Tres Reyes* (Feast of the Three Wise Men, or Epiphany) on January 6. There are parades held to welcome the three wise men, Balthasar, Gaspar, and Melchior, who will arrive bearing gifts for the children. There is a sweet bread called *Roscon de Ryes* that is baked with a small surprise inside. The person lucky enough to cut the piece of cake with the surprise can expect to enjoy an extremely good year. *Mantecados* are traditional crumble cakes that are served on special occasions. On New Year's Eve, Spaniards traditionally have 12 grapes to coincide with the 12 chimes ringing in the new year.

COMMON NAMES OF FOODS ITEMS

The following are common names of food items:

Ajo: garlic

Almendras: almonds

Arroz con pollo: rice with chicken

Avellanas: hazelnuts

Azafran: saffron

Café con leche: coffee with milk

Jerez: sherry

Jamone: cured ham

Cabrito: baby goat

Cazuelas: casseroles

Chilllindrones: sautéed peppers, tomatoes, and onion dish

Chorizo: a sausage made with pork and flavored with garlic and pimento

Cocido: chickpea stew

Pan: bread

Pimenton: paprika

Huevos: eggs

Puntillatas: squid

Pestinos: sweet fried potatoes

Garbanzos: chickpeas

Ternera: beef

Torrijas: French toast

USEFUL VOCABULARY

Bomboneria: candy shop

Buen provecho: good meal

Cena: supper; evening meal

Desayuno: breakfast

Comida: lunch; midday meal; main meal of day

Merienda: an early evening snack

Pasteleria: cake shop

Cazuela: earthenware casserole used for cooking and serving

Empanadilla: filled pastry pie

Helageria: ice cream shop

Panaderia: bread shop

Tascas: tapas bars

La cuenta: the bill

Cuanto cuesta?: How much does it cost?

 ## HEALTH BELIEFS AND CONCERNS

Spain is a land of fresh vegetables, fruit, hams, shellfish, fish, and wine. They grow their foods close to their homes and use the freshest ingredients. The Spanish diet rests on olive oil, garlic, and bread. Although it is high in fat and calories, the fat is a heart-friendly one. Walking and outdoor activities are part of Spanish culture, which contributes to their health. Sleep is not a priority for many people, but in many parts of the country it is a habit that comes from the traditional afternoon *siesta*. Late-night eating and lingering over a meal is the profile of many Spaniards. The history of the land has allowed a blending of various ancient cultures into a truly unique and culturally rich country that has its own flavors and identity.

 ## GENERAL HEALTH AND NUTRITIONAL INDICATORS SUMMARY

Spain has a reputation for being a healthy place to live, probably due to its climate and Mediterranean diet. Even with its almost ideal environment and healthy eating culture, the World Health Organization estimates the prevalence of overweight to be 70% for men and 60% for women. This is based on body mass index (kg/m^2) levels over 25 (Centers for Disease Control, 2009). Life expectancy in 2003 was 70 years for males and 75 years for females. Current life expectancy is 78 years for males and 84 years for females (Mataix et al., 2003).

Upon researching the dietary deficiencies in Spain, several publications report vitamin B deficiencies. Mezquita-Raya et al. (2001) noted deficiencies of vitamin B_1 in 6% of the general population and vitamin B_2 in 5% of the general population. Additionally, postmenopausal women were found to experience a prevalence of vitamin deficiencies, as is also common in the United States (Mezquita-Raya et al., 2001).

FEATURED RECIPE

Gazpacho

3½ lbs. vine-ripened tomatoes (peeled, seeded, and chopped)

1 cucumber (peeled, seeded, and chopped)

1 green bell pepper (roasted, peeled, seeded, membrane removed, and chopped)

3 garlic cloves (peeled, roasted till golden brown, chilled, and chopped)

1 serrano pepper (roasted, peeled, seeded, membrane removed, and chopped)

1 cup Spanish extra-virgin olive oil

1 tsp. white balsamic vinegar

To taste: gray sea salt, ground black pepper, hot sauce

Tomato juice (as needed to thin)

1 oz. golden tequila (optional)

1. Place all ingredients into an electric blender and puree until smooth.
2. Slowly pour oil and vinegar into activated blender. Add tomato juice and tequila until proper consistency. Season the mixture with salt, pepper, and hot sauce.
3. Chill and let flavors set for at least 2 hours.
4. Mix to re-emulsify the soup and then pour into chilled bowls.
5. Serve with bite-sized raw vegetables and wedges of hard-boiled egg on the side.

Yields 6 servings

(Courtesy of Chef Thomas Smith)

More recipes are available at http://nutrition.jbpub.com/foodculture/

REFERENCES

Caruso, J.C. (2004). *El Farol: Tapas and Spanish cuisine.* Layton, UT: Gibbs Smith Publishers.

Casas, P. (2005). *The food and wines of Spain.* New York: Alfred A. Knopf.

Centers for Diesease Control. (2009). Body mass index. Retrieved on November 30, 2009, from www.cdc.gov/healthy weight/assessing/bmi

Mataix J., Aranda P., Sanchez C., Montellano M.A., Planells E., & Llopis J. (2003). An assessment of thiamine and riboflavin status in an adult Mediterranean population. *British Journal of Nutrition, 90*(3), 661–666.

Medina, F.X. (2005). Food culture in Spain. In M. Williams (Ed.), *Food culture around the world.* Westport, CT: Greenwood Press.

Menden, J. (2006). *Cooking from the heart of Spain.* New York: William Morrow Publishers.

Mezquita-Raya P., Munoz-Torres M., De Dios Luna J., et al. (2001). Relation between vitamin D insufficiency, bone density, and bone metabolism in healthy postmenopausal women. *Journal of Bone Mineral Research, 16,* 1408–1415.

Norman, B. (1969). *The Spanish cookbook.* New York: Athenaeum Publishers.

Sterling, R., & Jones, A. (2000). *World food Spain.* Oakland, CA: Lonely Planet Publications.

von Bremzen, A. (2005). *The new Spanish table.* New York: Workman Publishing.

Walker, A. (1992). *A season in Spain.* New York: Simon & Schuster.

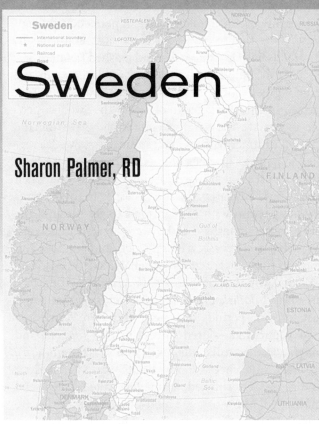

CHAPTER 19

Sweden

Sharon Palmer, RD

 CULTURE AND WORLD REGION

The country of Sweden is perched in northern Europe between Finland and Norway and is bordered by the Baltic Sea and gulfs of Bothnia, Kattegat, and Skagerrak. It is a beautiful land accented by patchwork farms, pristine birch and pine forests, and crystal lakes. Sweden has great diversity in climate, ranging from temperate weather and cold winters in the south to sub-Arctic conditions in the north. Because of its location, parts of Sweden experience extremely long summer days and equally long winter nights. Within this country, which is roughly the size of California, live about 9 million people. Although the first inhabitants probably arrived after the ice cap withdrew northward, it was not until about 1000 years ago that a central Swedish realm began to form in the country's fertile farmlands.

Today, Sweden's capitalist system, which includes social welfare programs, has been proven to be a successful economic model, contributing to a high standard of living for its population. Traditionally a homogeneous society, Sweden is now home to foreign-born and first-generation immigrants from Europe, South America, and the Middle East. In addition, the country has two minority groups of native inhabitants: the Finnish-speaking people of the northeast and the Sami (Lapp) population in the north. In Sweden, 87% of the people are Lutheran by faith. Swedish is the major language spoken and 99% of the population is literate. Sweden takes pride in doing their share to preserve the earth's natural resources, taking part in a number of international environmental agreements.

 FOOD HISTORY WITHIN THE CULTURE

Swedish food history and culture has forever been shaped by the land and climate. Cultivated farmland enables crops, such as wheat and potatoes, and livestock, including cattle and swine, to thrive throughout Sweden. Yet these farmlands are interspersed with forests and wetlands that nurture wild game, mushrooms, herbs, and berries such as lingonberries, blueberries, and cloudberries. Examples of such foods are woven together into Swedish food culture. A perfect example of this can be seen in one of Sweden's most iconic meals, meatballs with lingonberries and mashed potatoes.

Swedish food traditions are interlaced with the growing season and food-preservation skills that gained such importance in order for the Swedish people to survive the lengthy, cold winters. During the vibrant summer with its long, sunny days, Swedes reveled in nature's luscious bounty of fruits and produce, always with a watchful eye for the coming winter when food would be scarce. It was a necessity to fill the pantry to the brim with enough food to get through the dark winter months. Berries were cooked into jams, vegetables were preserved or pickled, and potatoes and root vegetables were stored in cellars. Rye breads were baked slowly into dark loaves (*kavring*) or dried into crispbread (*knäckebröd*) or rusks (*skorpor*) that could last for long periods of time. Milks were fermented into yogurt-like soured milks such as *filmjölk* and *långfil*, curdled milk (*filbunke*), sour cream (*gräddfil*), or made into cheese. Local meats, seafood, poultry, and game were smoked, fermented, salted, dried, and marinated. Many of these food-preservation styles are seen in some of the country's most beloved foods today, from *sill* (pickled herring) to *flädersaft* (concentrated elderberry beverage).

The motto of Swedish cooking was "you take what you have," which was penned by the 18th-century Swedish cookbook author, Cajsa Warg. This culinary philosophy persists today, as Sweden continues to make use of traditional and local foods found throughout the country. During the winter, dishes typically focus more on root vegetables, potatoes, and cabbage. But the summer months are celebrated with fresh local produce such as strawberries, a source of national pride highlighted in traditional desserts like *jordgubbs torta* (strawberry cake). It is common even today to mark a beautiful summer day by foraging for wild blueberries and mushrooms in a nearby forest or to fish in a quiet lake. With the exception of a few imports, Sweden is self-sufficient in agriculture, even though agriculture accounts for only 1% of its gross domestic product and 2% of employment. Farming takes place primarily in the south and central part of the country but extends even to the far north during the intense, short growing season. Most Swedish farms are still small and operated by individual families. Since entry into the European Union, more two-way trade of foodstuffs has occurred.

The Swedes have cultivated their own unique meal patterns, such as enjoying sandwiches at the breakfast meal and pancakes with strawberry jam for the dinner table. Nothing is more uniquely Swedish perhaps than *fika*, which means "to take a coffee break." Both used as a verb and a noun, *fika* goes far beyond a standard coffee break. In the workplace, it means a relaxing respite over steaming cups of strong coffee and a little sweet roll, such as a *kanelbulle* (cinnamon roll). On a weekend, it tends to translate into a leisurely social hour with friends or family on an enclosed patio with trays of traditional cookies and baked goods and coffee served in pretty cups and saucers. It is no surprise that Sweden has the highest coffee consumption per capita in the world.

Different regions within Sweden developed their own unique culinary traditions, which were often based upon climactic variations, urbanization, agriculture, economics, availability, and conservation. For example, the Samis lived largely on reindeer that was plentiful in the northern region. Salt was more available and thus used more heavily for preservation in southern Sweden. Bread was typically made of oats in the western region where rainfall was more plentiful, but in the north the grain of choice was barley, which could withstand colder temperatures. A variety of cheeses were developed throughout the country as a result of climactic conditions, preservation techniques, and economic situations, establishing a celebrated cheese culture that continues today. Many regional food preferences and traditions within Sweden's borders still thrive; some are even enjoying a revival among the modern Swedish population. For instance, in the Swedish Baltic island of Öland, a local food specialty is *kroppkaka*, a potato dumpling stuffed with chopped pork and fried onions served with mustard. This traditional food has become virtually a regional symbol that is sold in local hot dog stands and shops around the island. But *kroppkaka* has its roots in something less glamorous. A century ago, the dish was merely a frugal way of using up all the meat bits and leftovers from the week to fill up a dumpling.

Sweden's food traditions have also been shaped by modern issues such as immigration and assimilation. Ethnic foods from tacos to stir-fry are becoming increasingly popular, both at restaurants and at home. Supermarkets stock a growing variety of ethnic foodstuffs such as spices, tortillas, and Asian sauces. Some ethnic foods have undergone "Swedification," so that original ethnic flavors have been married with traditional Swedish elements to produce a new, popular dish. An example of this can be seen in the popular fast-food establishments (known as *gatu kök*, translated literally as "street kitchen") sprinkled across the country. In addition to the standard fare of burgers and hot dogs, a popular choice among Swedes at their neighborhood *gatu kök* is *tunn bröds rulle*, flat bread filled with mashed potatoes, sausage, and a choice of condiment such as curry sauce or shrimp salad. Chinese, Indian, Thai, pizza, and kebab restaurants are ubiquitous in Sweden.

Like other industrialized countries, Sweden's food culture is facing new challenges. Swedish dining habits are usually focused on family meals eaten together at the kitchen table or outside in the open air during the summer months. But as more women entered the workplace, families became busier and expendable income became more available for food purchases. Naturally, dining habits have steadily changed. An estimated 20% of Swedish meals are eaten outside of the home, a number that is expected to increase. Fast-food consumption has soared, fueled by expansion of chain outlets and an increasing number of gasoline stations that sell fast food. American restaurant chains abound in Sweden, from McDonald's and Burger King to TGI Friday's and Applebee's. Gourmet restaurant sales have also grown due to an interest in food culture and quality of food. Ready meals sold in supermarkets have also increased in popularity. Market researchers have identified a strong growth in Swedish demand for convenience foods, as well as foods that demonstrate health, environmental, and social awareness such as certified-organic and fair-trade-labeled products.

 ## MAJOR FOODS

 ### Protein Sources

Common protein sources include beef, pork, fish, shellfish, reindeer, game meat, poultry, smoked/salted pork, sandwich meats, cheese (typically full fat), sausage, liver pâté, fish (including salted, pickled, or smoked fish), caviar, dried beans and peas, nuts, eggs, and milk products.

 ### Starch Sources

Starch sources include bread (refined, rye, and whole grain), crispbread (refined and whole grain), potatoes (the most common staple food), turnips, rutabagas, rice, pasta, dried beans and peas, porridge (oat and rice), breakfast cereal, and crackers.

 ### Fat Sources

Fatty meats, full-fat cheeses, full-fat dairy products, margarine spreads, oil for cooking, butter and hard margarine for baking, salad dressings, cream for cooking, whipping cream for desserts, and nuts are common sources of fat.

 ### Prominent Vegetables

Prominent vegetables include potatoes, turnips, rutabagas, lettuce, tomatoes, bell pepper, onions, carrots, broccoli, cabbage, cucumbers, beets, and mushrooms.

 ### Prominent Fruits

Prominent fruits include berries, fruit juice, melon, apples, and pears.

 ### Spices and Seasonings

Common spices include black pepper, garlic, dill, chives, saffron, cardamom, cinnamon, and ginger.

 ### Beverages

Popular beverages include coffee, tea, milk products, juices, sodas, beer, snaps (strong alcohol-based drinks), and vodka.

 ### Desserts

Popular desserts include buns, pastries, rolls, cakes, tarts, cookies, ice cream, chocolate, and candy.

 ## FOODS WITH CULTURAL SIGNIFICANCE

Many Swedish dishes are laden with cultural significance. A good example might be *ärtsoppa*, pea soup made from dried yellow peas, which is served in restaurants and homes throughout Sweden on Thursdays. The tradition dates back to the pre-Reformation era when pea soup was eaten as preparation for the Friday fast. The typical recipe is a thick soup cooked with onions, marjoram, and thyme, and sometimes accompanied with smoked or salted pork pieces. The diner adds a stripe of Swedish mustard to suit his or her own taste. The meal is often accompanied with thin, crepe-like Swedish pancakes served with berry jam.

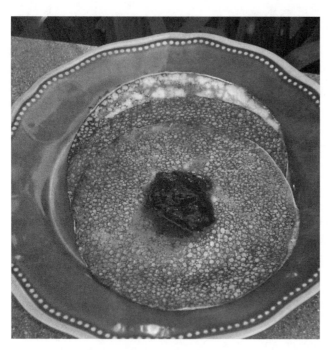

Swedish Pancakes with Jam

Lutfisk, an unusual dish made of stockfish (air-dried white fish) that is prepared using a long process involving soda lye, is a traditional food that is typically served with the Christmas meal. *Lutfisk* has its roots in Sweden's Catholic past before 1527, when people were permitted to eat fish during periods of fasting.

Janssons frestelse (Jansson's temptation) is a popular creamy potato and anchovy casserole said to be named after Pelle Janzon, a food aficionado and Swedish opera singer of the early 20th century. While Jansson's temptation has become a Christmas table classic, it is also a favorite side dish for many occasions and suits a number of meat dishes.

 TYPICAL DAY'S MENU

Breakfast

A typical breakfast may consist of porridge (oats or rice), muesli, cold cereal, boiled egg, open-faced sandwich with refined or whole-grain bread or crispbread

Observations from the Author (Sharon Palmer)

When visiting Sweden, I am always struck how tall and lean the people are. Yet the word "diet" does not seem to be part of their routine vocabulary as it is in the United States. Creams, butter, and sweets seem to be part of the daily diet of many people. A typical breakfast consists of full-fat cheeses and meats with white bread. Sauces are often made with cream. A great deal of red meat is consumed over fish and poultry, and a sweet or pastry is traditional with coffee breaks during the day. To top it off, fruits and vegetables (excluding potatoes) are not a huge part of the traditional diet. They are often enjoyed seasonally, which is typically limited to the short growing span during the summer.

I often ponder how Swedes stay so fit based on their unique eating pattern. Upon observing the Swedish lifestyle over the years, I find their secrets to be hidden in moderate eating patterns, plenty of meals eaten at home, and lots of physical activity. The traditional Swedish family eats most of their meals around the kitchen dining table. Portions are moderate, even when dining out. With Sweden's landscape of sky-high gasoline prices, emphasis on the environment and reduction of greenhouse gas emissions, wonderful public transportation, and difficult parking in major cities, people frequently rely on public transportation, bicycles, and walking—or a combination of these modes—to get to where they need to go. It is not unusual to see people even walk or ride their bikes to their nearby grocery store to bring home supplies for dinner. Walking and lots of fresh air is considered important for health, and even chilly weather does not keep people from taking to the neatly groomed walking paths that are found in many suburbs. There is less concern over violence and child abduction in Sweden; thus, children freely roam their neighborhoods and local forests on bike and foot. Lastly, the Swedes's positive attitude about food, which includes enjoying their favorite foods in moderation without guilt, instead of a culture of dieting interspersed with indulgence, is an important part of their healthy relationship with food that creates harmonious weight.

Unfortunately, lifestyle patterns are gradually changing in Sweden, resulting in increased concern over obesity. Like in the United States, Swedes are turning more often to fast-food meals, convenience foods, and soft drinks. Children are staying more often indoors to play video games and watch television instead of running and playing. In addition, more "diet" foods, including fat-free, low-fat, and sugar-free products, are available in Swedish supermarkets. It will be interesting to observe how Sweden's diet and health status evolve in the years to come.

with margarine spread, cheese, cured meats, liver pâté, or caviar; yogurt, milk, juice, coffee, or tea.

Lunch

A typical lunch may consist of an open-faced sandwich, sausage, hot dogs, meatballs and potatoes, *pyttipanna* (corned beef hash), baked potato with topping, potato pancakes, omelet, soup, cheese pie, pizza, or hamburger.

Dinner

A typical dinner may consist of ham, beef, pork, fish, fishballs, or chicken with potatoes; spaghetti Bolognese, curry or stir-fry and rice; pancakes, pea soup, meat-filled cabbage rolls, stroganoff, or tacos.

 ## HOLIDAY MENUS

Many holidays simply cannot be celebrated without traditional Swedish foods gracing the table. While modernization has made its impact on changing dietary patterns in Sweden, people are reluctant to break from these traditions during festive occasions. In addition to the traditional holiday foods that are required on the table, regional foods are often added. The *smörgåsbord*, literally translated "sandwich table," is often an important part of the festivities that mark special events and holidays, from weddings to Christmas. But you will find much more than sandwich fixings at an authentic Swedish *smörgåsbord*. The *smörgåsbord* is typically laden with many small dishes of traditional Swedish dishes including meatballs, ham, sausages, smoked salmon, herring, red cabbage, cheeses, potatoes, and fresh breads.

The Swedish *Jul* (Christmas) is the most highly anticipated holiday of the year. During the dark winter, Christmas is a season of joy and light, as homes blaze with candles in the windows, Christmas trees with twinkling lights, and holiday decorations. During the entire Christmas season, people enjoy social visits accompanied with treats of *glögg* (hot mulled wine) and *pepparkakor* (thin ginger cookies). The holiday meal is celebrated on Christmas Eve with a *smörgåsbord* of many requisite foods, starting with the Christmas ham that is specially prepared with a mustard and breadcrumb coating. Other traditional Swedish foods appear on the Christmas table including pickled herring, sausages, beet and herring potato salad, meatballs, brown beans, boiled potatoes, Jansson's temptation, *lutfisk*, saffron rolls, and *limpa* (rye bread with grated orange). Families often introduce their own regional specialties onto the Christmas menu, as well. The table is well stocked so that Christmas leftovers are enjoyed for days after the holiday repast. After dinner, one must leave room for *Julgröt* (Christmas rice porridge). With one almond hidden in the rice, legend predicts that the lucky finder will get married during the coming year. In addition, a bowl of porridge must be left for the house elf, who in return will behave and guard over the home in the new year.

Midsommar (Midsummer) is another hallowed holiday on the Swedish calendar. The longest day of the year, Midsummer has been celebrated in Sweden for thousands of years as a magical night when spirits roam the forests. For reasons of convenience, Midsummer is now celebrated in Sweden on the Friday and Saturday between June 20 and June 26, separated slightly from the authentic day of summer solstice on June 21. Cities empty en route for the country, where outdoor Midsummer festivities include singing and dancing around a Midsummer pole and open-air dining. The Midsummer menu features *sill* (pickled herring) in a variety of sauces such as dill sauce, mustard sauce, and cream sauce; hard-boiled eggs decorated with caviar, Swedish cheese, crispbread; summer potatoes served with sour cream and chives; and fresh strawberries. Each family usually adds a few favorite dishes as well, from cheese and vegetable pies to small sausages. As is the custom with many festive meals, ancient drinking songs are interspersed between bites of food with the resounding chant of "*skål!*" (cheers) and shots of aquavit and vodka.

The Swedish *Kräftskiva* (crayfish festival) is celebrated each year throughout the month of August. The crayfish party includes the consumption of enormous quantities of freshwater crayfish cooked with dill, washed down with liberal amounts of alcohol. The tradition began when freshwater crayfish was almost exclusively consumed by the ruling elite. But with the rise of the middle class at the end of the 19th century, the entire land celebrated crayfish parties, prompting legal regulation of crayfish catches in August.

 ## HEALTH BELIEFS AND CONCERNS

Sweden has a long history of public healthcare policy that includes national responsibility to provide health care to all and preventative health measures that underscore the country's commitment to equality and security. Sweden has a relatively low infant-mortality rate, 3 per 1000 live births, compared with a rate of 10 for Europe overall. Life expectancy in Sweden is 82.6 years for females and 77.6 years for males, compared with an overall rate for Europe of 78.2 and 70.1, respectively. Public health experts are concerned about Sweden's growing problems with obesity, mental health issues, and alcohol abuse; however, surveys do show that Swedes believe that physical activity, smoking, food choices, and body weight have an impact on health status.

GENERAL HEALTH AND NUTRITIONAL INDICATORS SUMMARY

Sweden is a modern European nation with a very high standard of living. The State of the World's Children 2007 Report issued by UNICEF (2007) offers insight into important health indicators of countries and territories across the world. The report lists the under-5-years mortality rate (U5MR), a critical indicator of the well-being of children in a particular country, listed by countries and territories in descending order. In the 2005 U5MR, Sweden ranks at 182 on the list along with the Czech Republic, Finland, Italy, Japan, Liechtenstein, Norway, and Slovenia. For purposes of comparison, the top rank in the 2005 U5MR is Sierra Leone. The United States ranks 156 on the list. On the 2005 U5MR list, Sweden's ranking of 182 is followed by countries with a ranking of 190 including Andorra, Iceland, San Marino, and Singapore.

The UNICEF report (UNICEF, 2007) includes other important basic indicators. Sweden's infant mortality rate (< 1 year) for 1990 was 6 per 1000 live births, with an improvement in 2005 of 3 per 1000 live births. The neonatal mortality rate in 2000 was 2 per 1000 live births. The total population of Sweden in 2005 was 9,041,000. The number of births in 2005 was 96,000. The number of under-5-years deaths in 2005 (in thousands) was 0. The 2005 gross national income (GNI) per capita in U.S. dollars was $41,060. The life expectancy at birth in 2005 was 80 years. The net primary school attendance and enrollment in 2000–2005 was 99%. The percentage share of household income during 1994–2004 was 23% (lowest) and 37% (highest). The percentage of infants with low body weight in 1998–2005 was 4%.

The UNICEF health indicators look at many aspects within a country. In Sweden, 100% of the population used improved drinking-water sources in urban and rural settings in 2004, and 100% of the population used adequate sanitation facilities in urban and rural settings in 2004. The estimated adult HIV prevalence rate (≥ 15 years) ending 2005 was 0.2. The estimated number of people (all ages) living with HIV in 2005 was 8000. The estimated number of women (≥ 15 years) living with HIV in 2005 was 2500.

The UNICEF education indicators in Sweden included 180 phones and 75 Internet users per 100 people in 2002–2004. The gross primary school enrollment ratio for both males and females in 2000–2005 was 99. The gross secondary school enrollment ratio in 2000–2005 was 101 for males and 105 for females.

Sweden's demographics, according to the UNICEF report, include a total population in 2005 of 1,943,000 under the age of 18 years and 488,000 under the age of 5 years. The population annual growth rate percentage during 1970–1990 was 0.3% and during 1990–2005 was 0.4%. The crude death rate was 10 in 1970, 11 in 1990, and 10 in 2005. The crude birth rate was 14 in 1970, 14 in 1990, and 11 in 2005. The life expectancy was 74 in 1970, 78 in 1990, and 80 in 2005. The total fertility rate in 2005 was 1.7. The percentage of population that was urbanized in 2005 was 83%. The average annual growth rate percentage of urban population in 1970–1990 was 0.4% and in 1990–2005 was 0.4%.

Economic indicators for Sweden include GDP per capita average annual growth rate percentage in 1970–1990 of 1.8% and in 1990–2005 of 2.1%. The average annual rate of inflation percentage in 1990–2005 was 2%. The percentage of central government expenses in 1994–2004 was allocated as 3% to health, 6% to education, and 5% to defense.

Indicators among Swedish women include life expectancy of females as a percentage of males in 2005 at 106%. Enrollment ratios of females as a percentage of males include primary school 2000–2005 (gross) of 100% and secondary school 2000–2005 (gross) of 104%. Maternal mortality ratio in 2000 was reported to be 5% and adjusted to 2%.

COMMUNICATION AND COUNSELING TIPS

According to the Swedish National Food Administration, the primary nutritional concerns for people in Sweden are that they typically eat the wrong kinds of fat, too much sugar and salt, and too little dietary fiber. The Swedish National Food Administration has developed a food circle to help guide people's food choices. The Swedish Nutrition Recommendations Objectified

(SNO) is a basis for general advice on food consumption for healthy adults with Swedish eating habits.

The SNO calls for improving the quality of the fats consumed rather than merely reducing the total fat intake. The typical Swedish diet is high in saturated fats through a dependence on full-fat cheeses, dairy products, and meats. Keeping the saturated fat level low without the total amount of fat becoming too low is difficult within this eating pattern. The SNO indicates that the choice of spread is critical for achieving recommended fat intake. Margarine, preferably low-fat margarine, and oil or liquid margarine are needed to offset the saturated fats that originate from milk, cheese, meat, and cured meat products.

Salt intake should be limited to 5 g/day. This recommendation is very difficult to achieve for Swedes, because the amount of salt in processed products, bread, cheese, and cured meat products is very high.

The consumption of fruits and vegetables is too low in the Swedish population. The Swedish National Food Administration has previously recommended 0.5 kg of fruit and vegetables per day, based on the minimum amount at which positive effects on cardiovascular disease and obesity have been observed in epidemiological studies. In the SNO, vegetables are divided into two groups depending on their fiber content. Half the vegetables come from the high-fiber group with over 2 g of dietary fiber per 100 g. Fiber can also be increased through whole-grain breads and cereal choices.

The typical Swede takes in too many "leeway" foods according to the SNO. These foods include savory snacks, buns, pastries, cakes, ice cream, desserts, sweets, jams, fizzy drinks, sugar, and alcohol.

PRIMARY LANGUAGE OF FOOD NAMES WITH ENGLISH TRANSLATION

The primary language of food names with English translation is as follows:

Ägg: egg

Äpple: apple

Banan: banana

Biff: steak

Björnbär: blackberry

Blåbär: blueberry

Blodpudding: black or blood pudding

Blomkål: cauliflower

Brysselkål: Brussels sprouts

Bröd: bread

Bulle: bun, roll

Champinjon: mushroom

Choklad: chocolate

Citron: lemon

Dryck: drink, beverage

Fet: fatty

Filbunke: processed sour whole milk

Filmjölk: processed sour milk

Fisk: fish

Flask: pork

Fläskkotlett: pork chop

Frukt: fruit

Gås: goose

Getost: goat's milk cheese

Glass: ice cream

Glögg: mulled, spiced wine

Godis: sweets, candy

Grädde: cream

Gräddfil: sour cream

Grapefrukt: grapefruit

Gräslök: chives

Gravlax: raw, spiced salmon

Grönpeppar: green pepper

Grönsak: vegetable

Grönsallad: green salad

Gröt: porridge

Gurka: cucumber

Hallon: raspberry

Hamburgare: hamburger

Hasselnöt: hazelnut

Havre: oats

Honung: honey

Jordgubbe: strawberry

Kaffe: coffee

Kaka: cake, pastry, cookie

Kål: cabbage

Kalkon: turkey

Kålrot: rutabaga

Kalv: veal

Kanel: cinnamon

Kardemumma: cardamom

Kaviar: caviar
Kavring: black rye bread
Keso: cottage cheese
Kex: cracker
Knäckebröd: crispbread
Körsbär: cherry
Korv: sausage
Kött: meat
Kräfta: crayfish
Krusbär: gooseberry
Kyckling: chicken
Lammkött: lamb
Leverpastej: liver pâté
Lök: onion
Majonnäs: mayonnaise
Majs: corn
Makaroner: macaroni
Mandel: almond
Margarin: margarine
Mat: food
Mjöl: flour
Mjölk: milk
Morot: carrot
Öl: beer
Olja: oil
Ost: cheese
Paj: pie
Pannkaka: pancake
Päron: pear
Peppar: pepper
Persika: peach
Persilja: parsley
Plommon: plum
Potatis: potato
Rabarber: reindeer meat
Råg: rye
Räka: shrimp
Ris: rice

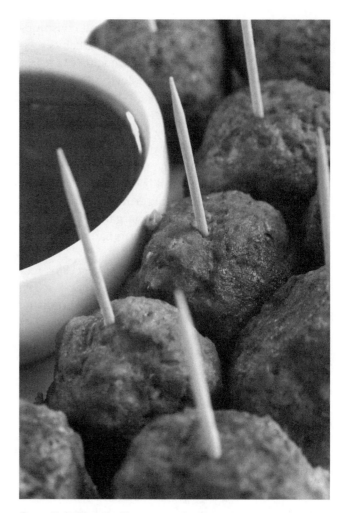

Swedish Meatballs

Rova: turnip
Saffran: saffron
Senap: mustard
Sill: herring
Smör: butter
Soppa: soup
Spenat: spinach
Sylt: jam
Te: tea
Tomat: tomato
Vanilj: vanilla
Vatten: water
Vitlök: garlic

FEATURED RECIPE

Köttbullar (Swedish Meatballs)

Meatballs:

- 1 lb. lean ground beef
- ½ cup fine breadcrumbs
- ⅓ cup milk
- 1 small onion, diced finely
- 1 egg
- ½ tsp. salt
- ½ tsp. black pepper
- Nonstick cooking spray

Sauce:

- 2 tbsp. margarine or butter
- 2 tbsp. flour
- 1 cup half and half
- 1 cup milk
- 1 cube beef bullion
- ½ tsp. salt
- ½ tsp. black pepper
- 1 tsp. soy sauce
- 1 tsp. blueberry jelly or lingonberry preserves
- Lingonberry preserves

1. In large mixing bowl, add ground beef, breadcrumbs, milk, diced onion, egg, salt, and pepper. Combine mixture well with wooden spoon.
2. Knead mixture an additional few minutes with hands to thoroughly mix ingredients. Shape into small meatballs (1–1½ inch in diameter).
3. Heat a large skillet over medium heat and spray with nonstick cooking spray. Place meatballs on skillet, covering the entire surface. Monitor the cooking process closely, turning the meatballs when one side is cooked and browned.
4. When the meatballs are cooked and browned evenly on all sides, remove to a serving pan and repeat the process to cook all meatballs.
5. To prepare sauce, in a clean skillet melt 2 tbsp. margarine or butter.
6. Stir in flour to make a roux. Gradually add the half and half and heat over medium-low heat.
7. Stir in milk and beef bouillon cube, stirring until beef bullion is dissolved. Mix in salt, pepper, soy sauce, and jelly. Stir with a whisk until all ingredients are dissolved and sauce is thick and bubbly.
8. Serve meatballs immediately with sauce and lingonberry preserves as desired.

Yields 6 servings

More recipes are available at http://nutrition.jbpub.com/foodculture/

REFERENCES

Barbieri, H. (2005). Rapport 20: Swedish nutrition recommendations objectified. Sweden: National Food Administration.

Euromonitor International. (2007, September). *Consumer food service in Sweden*. Retrieved November 30, 2009, from http://www.the-infoshop.com/study/eo50422-foodservice-sweden.html/

HRI Food Service Sector Report. (2001, November 7). Retrieved from http://stockholm.usembassy.gov/Agriculture/market.html/

UNICEF. (2007). *The state of the world's children 2007: Women and children, the double dividend of gender equality*. Retrieved April 14, 2009, from http://www.unicef.org/sowc07/statistics/tables.php

World Factbook (n.d.). *Sweden*. Retrieved March 12, 2008, from https://www.cia.gov/library/publications/the-world-factbook/print/sw.html/

Asia

Food, Cuisine, and Cultural Competency for Culinary, Hospitality, and Nutrition Professionals introduces the reader to nine prominent regions of Asia:

AFGHANISTAN

Afghanistan, a landlocked country, is located in South–Central Asia, north and west of Pakistan, and east of Iran. Afghanistan's economy is recovering from decades of conflict. Gross domestic product (GDP) growth exceeded 7% in 2008, but despite the progress of the past few years, Afghanistan is extremely poor and highly dependent on foreign aid, as well as agricultural trade with neighboring countries. Much of the population continues to suffer from shortages of housing, clean water, electricity, medical care, and employment. Afghanistan's standard of living is among the lowest in the world.

CAMBODIA

Cambodia is in Southeast Asia, bordering the Gulf of Thailand, between Thailand, Vietnam, and Laos. From 2004 to 2007, the economy grew about 10% per year, driven largely by expansion in the garment sector, construction, agriculture, and tourism. Growth dropped below 7% in 2008 as a result of the global economic slowdown. The major economic challenge for Cambodia over the next decade will be fashioning an economic environment in which the private sector can create enough jobs to handle Cambodia's demographic imbalance. (More than 50% of the population is less than 21 years old.) The population lacks education and productive skills, particularly in the poverty-stricken countryside.

FAR EAST

The "Far East" is a term used to describe East Asia, Southeast Asia, and the Pacific Rim. China is one of the countries located in eastern Asia. It borders the East China Sea, Korea Bay, Yellow Sea, and South China Sea, between North Korea and Vietnam. China's economy during the past 30 years has changed from a centrally planned system that was largely closed to international trade to a more market-oriented economy that has a rapidly growing private sector and is a major player in the global economy. Reforms started in the late 1970s with the phasing out of collectivized agriculture, and expanded to include the gradual liberalization of prices, fiscal decentralization, increased autonomy for state enterprises, the foundation of a diversified banking system, the development of stock markets, the rapid growth of the nonstate sector, and the opening to foreign trade and investment. China, in 2008, stood as the second-largest economy in the world after the United States, although in per-capita terms the country is still in the lower-to-middle-income category.

INDIA (SOUTHERN REGION)

India is in southern Asia, bordering the Arabian Sea and the Bay of Bengal, between Burma and Pakistan. India's diverse economy encompasses traditional village farming, modern agriculture, handicrafts, a wide range of modern industries, and a multitude of services. Services are the major source of economic growth, accounting for more than half of India's output with less than one third of its labor force. Slightly more than half of the work force is in agriculture, creating basic infrastructure to improve the lives of the rural poor and boost economic performance. The economy has posted an average growth rate of more than 7% in the decade since 1997, reducing poverty by about 10%. India is also capitalizing on its large number of well-educated people skilled in the English language, making the country a major exporter of software services and software workers.

NEPAL

Nepal is located in southern Asia, between China and India. Nepal is among the poorest and least-developed countries in the world, with almost one third of its population living below the poverty line. Agriculture is the mainstay of the economy, providing a livelihood for 75% of the population and accounting for about one third of the GDP. Industrial activity involves mainly the processing of agricultural products, including pulses, jute, sugarcane, tobacco, and grain. Bumper crops, better security, improved transportation, and increased tourism pushed growth past 5% in 2008.

JAPAN

Japan, an island chain between the North Pacific Ocean and the Sea of Japan, east of the Korean Peninsula, is in eastern Asia. In the years following World War II, due to government–industry cooperation, a strong work ethic, and mastery of high technology, Japan advanced at an extraordinary rate to the rank of second-most technologically powerful economy in the world after the United States. Today, measured on a purchasing-power-parity basis, Japan is the third-largest economy in the world after the United States and China. A tiny agricultural sector is highly subsidized and protected, with crop yields among the highest in the world. Usually self-sufficient in rice, Japan imports about 60% of its food on a caloric basis. Japan maintains one of the world's largest fishing fleets and accounts for nearly 15% of the global catch.

KOREA

Korea is located in eastern Asia by the Korean Peninsula bordering the Korea Bay, the Sea of Japan, and the Yellow Sea. North Korea, one of the world's most centrally directed and least-open economies, faces chronic economic problems. Severe flooding in summer 2007 aggravated chronic food shortages caused by ongoing systemic problems including a lack of arable land, collective farming practices, and persistent shortages of tractors and fuel. Large-scale international food-aid deliveries have allowed the people of North Korea to escape widespread starvation since famine threatened in 1995, but the population continues to suffer from prolonged malnutrition and poor living conditions. Since 2002, the government has allowed private "farmers' markets" to begin selling a wider range of goods. In contrast, South Korea has achieved an incredible record of growth and integration into the high-tech modern world economy. Four decades ago, the GDP per capita was comparable to levels in the poorer countries of Africa and Asia. In 2004, South Korea joined the trillion-dollar club of world economies.

RUSSIA

Russia is in northern Asia (the area west of the Urals is considered part of Europe), bordering the Arctic Ocean, between Europe and the North Pacific Ocean. Russia ended 2008 with GDP growth of 6%, following 10 straight years of growth averaging 7% annually since the financial crisis of 1998. Over the past 6 years, fixed capital investment growth and personal income growth have averaged above 10%, but both grew at slower rates in 2008. Growth in 2008 was driven largely by nontradable services and domestic manufacturing, rather than exports. During the past decade, poverty and unemployment have declined steadily and the middle class has continued to expand.

VIETNAM

Vietnam is in Southeast Asia, bordering the Gulf of Thailand, Gulf of Tonkin, and the South China Sea, alongside China, Laos, and Cambodia. Vietnam is a densely populated developing country that, in the past 30 years, has had to recover from the ravages of war and the loss of a financially supported economy. Agriculture's share of economic output has continued to shrink from about 25% in 2000 to less than 20% in 2008. Deep poverty has declined significantly and is now less than that of China, India, and the Philippines. Vietnam is working to create jobs to meet the challenge of a labor force that is growing by more than 1.5 million people every year.

CHAPTER 20

Afghanistan

Miho Sato, MA

CULTURE AND WORLD REGION

Afghanistan is a landlocked country, the size of Texas, bordered by Iran to the west, by Turkmenistan, Uzbekistan, and Tajikistan to the north and northeast, by China at the eastern-most corner, and by Pakistan to the east and south. Due to this specific location, Afghanistan was a crossroads on the Silk Route where merchants traveled from Europe to Asia, and vice versa. This strategic location within Central Asia has influenced the diversity that exists in ethic groups, religions, and languages among the people of Afghanistan. The main ethnic groups are Pashtun, Tajik, Hazara, Uzbek, Turkmen, Aimaq, Baluch, and Nuristani.

The majority of the population believes in Islam (80% Sunni; 18–19% Shi'a). A minority of 1–2% Hindu and Sikh also exist in the country. For the Afghan Muslims, Islam is the foundation of daily life. Major festivities coincide with the Islamic calendar of events (*Milad-Nabi*, the birthday of the Prophet Muhammad and the two *Eid*, for example).

According to UNICEF (2003), the average size of the Afghan household is seven, with children under 17 years accounting for four of every seven people in a household. The majority of Afghan families live with extended family of at least three generations. A typical Afghan family would consist of a couple and their children, the parents and grandparents of the husband, as well as siblings of the husband and their wives and children. Kinship is the basis of social life. As Dupree (1980) puts it, Afghan society can be categorized as patriarchal (authority in the hands of old men), partrilineal (inheritance through the male line), and patrilocal (bride moves to husband's place of residence upon marriage). Son preference is still prevalent in Afghanistan due to the fact that sons can help tend the field and cattle, and provide better protection for the parents, as opposed to the girls who will be married off to another family. Due to this social system, the official/public structure of Afghan society can be viewed as male dominant; however, informally, women, especially elderly women, have strong say and decision-making power within the household concerning, for example, all sales of homemade products, marriage negotiation, and decisions concerning reproductive health matters.

Hospitability is one of the major characteristics that describes Afghan people. Afghan's hospitality is best displayed when they receive a guest(s). Even when they come without advance notice, Afghan families receive them with a warm welcome. After the formality of a series of extended conversations about themselves, their health, the health and well-being of their family members, and so on, the host will take the guest to the guest room where he or she will be invited to sit down on the cushion (traditionally, Afghans sit on the floor) at the far end of the room away from the entrance door (the place designated for the guest/most respected person), which is *bala* (up). As soon as he or she sits down, the formal greetings repeat between each person in the room and then the host will ask if the guest wants black or green tea. If the guest is male, unless he is a close relative, female family members of the host do not come to greet the guest; they stay in the kitchen to prepare the tea and the food that will be offered followed by the tea. In such cases the host, the man of the house, serves the tea to the guest. This separation of men and women, often referred to as *purdah* (which literally means curtain and refers to the "seclusion of women"), is common practice particularly in rural Afghanistan. When the guest finishes the tea and is ready to leave, the host will insist that he or she take some food, which would be prepared by the women of the household. This is especially true if it is close to lunch or dinner time. Meals are sometimes served in another room. When the man of the house informs women that the guest will stay for a meal, they set up the dining room with *distarkhan* (a vinyl-coated mat on which dishes are placed to protect the carpets from crumbs) followed by *naan* (flat bread) and main dishes. When the guest is seated in the dining room with various dishes in front, usually a child in the family will come with a jug of warm water and a basin (*aftawa lagan*) and soap to wash hands, along with a towel, before eating, as the majority of Afghans eat with their right hand.

In the presence of a male guest who is not a family member/relative, women and children eat in a separate room observing *purdah*. The guest may be given a special serving while other family members share the food. For example, two or three people who sit together share one big plate with a heap of rice and stew. If it is *palao*, meat is hidden in the rice. One person breaks the chunk of soft meat skillfully into pieces to share by the right hand. In addition to the rice, usually there are accompanying dishes for the rice, such as stew, meatball (*kufta*) with tomato sauce (*korma*), sauce with vegetables, such as *banjan burani* (fried eggplant served with yogurt and mint), or cooked spinach (*sabzi*). If it is a special occasion, other meat dishes, such as kebabs, are also served. The representative dessert dish is *firni* (custard pudding spread with cardamom flavor with sprinkles of pistachio nuts) along with rice pudding and fresh fruits. When the guest finishes the meal and thanks the host, the host usually says something like, "You did not eat anything! Didn't you like the food in our house? Please have some more!" When the host is convinced that the guest is really full, he tells one of the children to bring the water jug (*aftawa lagan*) again to help the guest clean his or her hands. After the children take the dishes away from *distarkhan*, they promptly return with big plates full of seasonal fruits and desserts for the guest. After the fruits, tea is served to settle the food and conclude the feast. The host is pleased when he sees his guests leaving the house having enjoyed their food.

Mountain ranges form many parts of Afghanistan's terrain. Almost half of the total land area lies above 2000 m above sea level. The percentage of land types are arable land 12%, permanent pastures 46%, forests and woodland 3%, and other types 39%.

The major geographical characteristics can be represented by three regions. The central highlands are characterized as dry, with the average temperature in summer being 80°F, and very cold winters. The northern plains are known to have fertile land and spread to the Amu River. Lastly, the southern plateau is made up of high plateaus and sandy deserts.

Asian Development Bank (2007) estimates the total population of Afghanistan to be 24.1 million people; among them, 52% are 17 years of age or younger, 46% are female, and 44% are male (Ministry of Rural Rehabilitation and Development and the Central Statistics Office, 2007). Average life expectancy is 43 years and an Afghan woman would have 7.2 children by the end of her reproductive period (UNICEF, n.d.). Due to the mountainous terrain, access to health facilities, especially in the rural areas, is limited, which prevents people from having appropriate health care at the right time, and even more so among the most vulnerable population; women and children. Afghanistan's maternal mortality rate is 1600 per 100,000 live births.

The under-5-years mortality rate is estimated to be 257 and infant mortality (under 1 year) is 165 per 1000 live births, ranking as one of the highest in the world. In addition to geographical access, illiteracy prevents women from accessing relevant healthcare information (UNICEF, 2007). Twenty-eight percent of the total population 15 years or older are literate (males 43.1% and females 12.6%) (Anonymous, 2008).

LANGUAGE

Many Afghans are multilingual. Article 16 of the Constitution of the Islamic Republic of Afghanistan states that Pashto and Dari are the official languages of the state from among Pashto, Dari, Uzbeki, Turkmani, Baluchi, Pachaie, Nuristani, Pamiri, and other languages in the country. In areas where the majority of the people speak in any of the aforementioned languages, it shall be the third official language. It is estimated that 50% of the Afghan population speaks Dari and approximately 35% speaks Pashto. In the northern region, Turkic languages (Uzbeki and Turkmani) are widely spoken. There are more than 40 other languages and numerous dialects spoken by smaller groups throughout the country.

CULTURE HISTORY

Afghanistan was part of the Achaemenian Empire (559–330 BC), which extended from Macedonia and Libya in the west to the Hyphasis River in the east, and from the Caucasus Mountains and the Aral Sea in the north to the Persian Gulf and the Arabian Desert in the south. The Achaemenian Dynasty became extinct in 330 BC when the last king, Darius III, was defeated by Alexander the Great, who conquered most of the Afghan rulers by 327 BC. About 135 BC, five Central Asian nomadic tribes conquered what is the current territory of Afghanistan. One of those tribes, Kushan, reached its zenith in the 2nd century AD under King Kaniska (78–144 AD). His empire stretched from north–central India beyond what is now part of Afghanistan, Uzbekistan, and Tajikistan, as far as the frontiers of China. It was under the rule of the Kushans that the arts and religion prospered. Bactra (modern Mazar-e-sharif in Afghanistan) was a center of transportation on the Silk Route, carrying various goods, merchandise, and cultures between Italy, India, and China. Buddhism was introduced to China by Indian

pilgrims who were traveling the Silk Route during the early centuries AD. Under the Kushan Dynasty, Buddhist visual art in the style of Greco–Roman origin, called Gandhara art, flourished. One of the most famous figures represented in Gandhara art is Buddha, who was depicted in statues that were carved into a cliff at Bamyan in the central mountains of Afghanistan during the 4th to 5th centuries. The statues were destroyed by the Taliban in 2001.

In 1219, Genghis Khan invaded the eastern part of Afghanistan and soon after took control of the country. At the end of the 14th century, Timur conquered a large part of the country. Timur's fourth son, Shah Rukh, abandoned his father's capital of Samarkand for Herat. In 1504, Kabul became the capital and independent kingdom under the rule of Babur, who is a descendent of Genghis Khan and Timur. In 1526, he established the Mughal Empire, which lasted until 1707 and included all of eastern Afghanistan south of the Hindu Kush.

The Durrani Dynasty (1747–1842) established one of the greatest Muslim empires (second only to the Ottoman Empire) in the second half of the 18th century, and its control extended from Meshed to Kashmir and Delhi and from the Amu River to the Arabian Sea. Great Britain and Afghanistan had three conflicts (1839–1842, 1878–1880, and 1919) in which Great Britain sought to extend its control over neighboring Afghanistan and to oppose Russia, which was increasing its influence in the region. After winning the second war, the British took control of Afghanistan's foreign affairs until 1919, when Afghanistan regained independence. Afghanistan enjoyed stability from 1933 for the next 40 years under the rule of King Zahir Shah, until he was ousted by Mohammed Daoud Khan, brother-in-law and first cousin of the king, during a bloodless coup in 1973.

On December 24, 1979, the Soviets invaded Afghanistan. By early 1980, mujahideen (Muslim guerrilla fighters) had united to resist the Soviet invaders and the Soviet-backed Afghan army inside Afghanistan and across the border in Peshawar, Pakistan. Pakistan, along with the United States, China, Saudi Arabia, and several European countries provided small amounts of financial and military aid to the mujahideen. In May 1988, the Soviets began withdrawal of their troops and the last Soviet soldier left Afghanistan in February 1989.

The Taliban emerged in 1994, and by 2001 they had seized power over more than 90% of the country. The Northern Alliance, which was a coalition of mujahideen militias, maintained control of a small section of northern Afghanistan. Shortly after the terrorist attacks of September 11, 2001, the United States and Britain launched an intensive bombing campaign against the Taliban and provided significant logistical support to the Northern Alliance forces. On December 7, 2001, the Taliban surrendered Kandahar, their base and the last city under their control. The Loya Jirga held in June 2002 selected a transitional government to rule the country until national elections could be held and a new constitution drafted.

Afghanistan adopted its new constitution and declared itself as an Islamic Republic in January 2004. Hamid Karzai became the first democratically elected President of Afghanistan on December 7, 2004. According to the constitution, the Afghan government consists of a popularly elected president, two vice presidents, and a national assembly. Two houses constitute the national assembly: the House of People (*Wolesi Jirga*), lower house, with 249 seats, and the House of Elders (*Meshrano Jirga*), upper house, with 102 seats. The constitution stipulates that 25% of the seats in the lower house are reserved for women and half of the presidential nominees in the upper house have to be women. As a result of the parliamentary election, which took place in September 2005, 23 of the 100 members of the upper house and 68 of the 249 delegates in the lower house are women.

FOOD HISTORY WITHIN THE CULTURE

As mentioned previously, hospitality is an important part of Afghan culture. Food is an essential element of the hospitality offered to a guest. In welcoming special guests, an Afghan family is willing to slaughter chicken or sheep that they raise.

Although the basic diet of Afghans has not changed much, the origin of the food is different from what it was before the war. These days, many food items are imported from neighboring countries. For example, the majority of wheat flower and rice come from Pakistan. In the case of eggs, the price of those imported from Iran from factory-raised chickens was much cheaper than *watani* (local) eggs when the author lived in Afghanistan. Some of the contributing factors that force Afghan kitchens to rely on produce imported from neighboring countries are neglected land as a result of the Soviet invasion, mass exodus of Afghans followed by the mining and destruction of agricultural lands during the war, and many years of drought. As Afghans

in exile repatriate to their homeland, de-mining and restoration of once-damaged *karez* (irrigation system) are underway. It will take some time for Afghans to enjoy abundant *watani* produce again.

MAJOR FOODS

Protein Sources

Meat

If one can afford it, meat dishes are served for lunch or dinner a few times a week. Popular meat sources are lamb or goat, beef (various parts of sheep/lamb, goat, and cow, including the head, tongue, and feet), buffalo, mutton, and chicken. The traditional soup called *kalepache* includes lamb's head (including brain), tongues, and hooves. Afghanistan, being an Islamic country, has no presence of pork.

Fish

Fish from a variety of rivers, and also imported from Pakistan, is seen during the winter. Deep fried with a spicy batter is a common way of cooking fish. Most Afghans do not eat crustaceans.

Beans

Red kidney beans, mung beans, and lentils are common. Usually they are made into sauce (with or without meat) to accompany plain white rice (*chelao*).

Nuts

Almonds, walnuts, pistachio nuts, and pine nuts, as well as dried and roasted chickpeas are popular and served with tea. Sugar-coated roasted almonds and/or chickpeas are called *noql*.

Dairy

Afghanistan has a variety of dairy products made from the milk of cow, goat, sheep, and even camel. For nomadic people (Kuchis), cheeses, milk, and yogurt are not only important sources of protein but also income-generating products. In addition to milk, yogurt is offered to the guest as well as served in a meal (in the summer). Cheese, butter, and/or cream (*qaimaq*) are popular breakfast items with *naan* (bread). *Chaka* (drained and thus concentrated yogurt to garnish soup and other dishes) and *qrut* (dried and salted yogurt, in the shape of a ball, made from the milk of either sheep, goat, camel, or cow) are also common dairy products.

 Starch Sources

Rice (long and short grain) and bread made from wheat are key starch sources in the Afghan diet, followed by potatoes. *Naan* is a word for a flat bread as well as a general word for a meal or eating, as in the following sentences: *Naan tayor ast* (Food is ready); *Naan-khor-dan berim* (Let's go and eat); and *Naan khordid* (Did you eat?).

 Fat Sources

It is generally observed that oil is generously used in Afghan cooking. According to a qualitative study conducted by Save the Children Japan (unpublished data), expenditure on oil occupied about 20% of overall household expenditure in two destitute communities in rural Afghanistan. The most common oil in household use is Malaysian palm oil (a vegetable-solid ghee in a big can), which is also the cheapest oil available in Afghan markets. Animal fat is consumed directly as a form of kebab or used in cooking. Butter, and cream, as well as nuts are also common fat sources.

 Prominent Vegetables

Afghan people consume vegetables very well cooked in sauces or raw, accompanying main dishes. Major vegetables in cooked form include tomatoes, onions, garlic, eggplant, squashes, carrots, pumpkin, potatoes, okras, turnips, and leeks (mainly as filling), in addition to beans. The common vegetables that are served fresh are cucumbers, radishes, daikon radishes, lettuce, cilantro, mint, scallion, carrots, tomatoes, and onions. Those who want a piquant taste eat fresh *murch* (green hot peppers). Local mushrooms (*samaroq*) are found only in season. Some vegetables, such as tomatoes, eggplant, and onions, are also dried for consumption during winter months, because they are not readily available and therefore costly.

 Prominent Fruits

Afghanistan offers many varieties of fruits, which are one of the major export items of the country. Depending on the season, people enjoy apricots, cherries, mulberries, peaches, plums, melons, watermelons, grapes, pomegranates, pears, and apples of various kinds. Most of these fruits are dried and exported along with the nuts (almonds, pistachio, walnuts, and pine nuts,

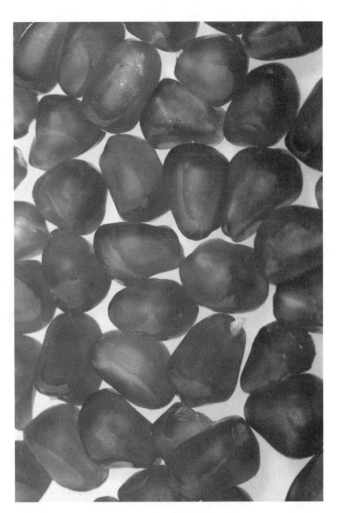

Pomegranate is a prominent fruit in Afghanistan.

jalghoza). Oranges, called *malta*, and sour oranges, called *narinj*, are grown in Nangarhar province, but those that are called *kino* (mandarin oranges) are imported from Pakistan along with bananas, mangoes, and pineapples.

 Spices and Seasonings

Afghan cuisine is not spicy hot and uses herbs and spices in a subtle way, which makes each dish tasteful. The herbs and spices commonly used in Afghan cuisine include anise, black pepper, cardamom, cilantro, cinnamon, clove, cumin, dill, fenugreek, ginger, mint, and turmeric.

 Beverages

Tea is the main beverage of Afghanistan. In destitute families, tea with sugar and bread can be a simple meal. There are two kinds of tea, black and green. Afghans put crushed cardamom seeds in the tea, which makes

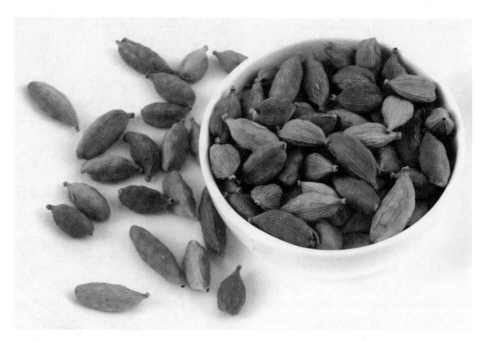

Afghans put crushed cardamom seeds in tea to add flavor.

the taste more flavorful. In the presence of guests, the host offers soft drinks to the guest with the meal. If it is summer, *dogh* (a salted yogurt drink with cucumber and mint leaves), a refreshing option that supposedly makes people sleepy after drinking it, offers a good reason for midday siestas.

 Desserts

Firni, custard pudding, or *sheer berenj* (rice pudding with cardamom and rose-water flavor with sprinkles of pistachio nuts) are very popular as dessert.

 FOODS WITH CULTURAL SIGNIFICANCE

The typical dish of Afghanistan is *qabli palao*, in which a lump of lamb tenderloin is buried in a heap of rice and decorated with glazed raisins and julienned carrots, along with peeled and sliced almonds and/or pistachio nuts.

For the Afghan New Year (*Naw Roz*, which literally means New Day; it is also the first day of spring), Afghan families begin the first day of the year by having a drink with soaked dried fruits and nuts called *haft-mewa* (which literally means "seven fruits"), which is prepared a couple of days in advance. Traditionally,

and still in remote areas of Afghanistan, only dried fruits are available in households during the winter. Seven kinds of dried fruits and nuts; namely, walnuts, almonds, pistachios, black and green raisins, dried apricots, and *sinjed* (the dried fruit of the oleaster tree), are soaked in water to give the water natural sweetness. People eat the fruits and drink the juice of *haft mewa* wishing good health and prosperity for the New Year. For the New Year lunch, Afghan mothers prepare a special pilaf called *sabzi palao*, which contains baby spinach that was germinated just before the *Naw Roz*. The young greens also symbolize the advent of spring.

 TYPICAL DAY'S MENU

The primary staple food in Afghanistan is wheat bread (*naan*). An Afghan family has *naan* three times a day.

Breakfast

Breakfast is called *chai sobh* (which literally means "morning tea"). Black or green tea with sugar or tea prepared with milk (*sheer chai*) is served with *naan* (bread) accompanied by *qaimaq* (cream), *maska* (butter), or *paner* (cheese) with honey or *murabaa* (fruit jam/preserve). Dried nuts, such as walnut (*chahr mags*,

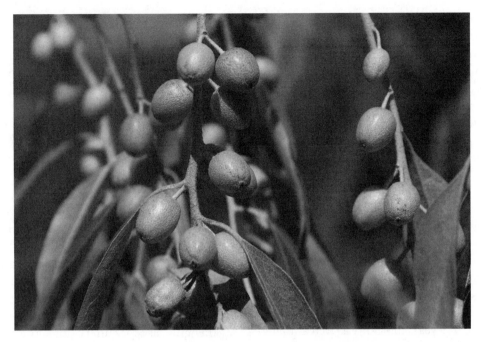

Sinjed, the dried fruit of the oleaster tree, are often soaked in water to add natural sweetness to the water.

which literally means "four brains") are also eaten. *Jelabi* (fried dough in a spiral shape soaked in honey/concentrated sugar), which is similar to funnel cake, is another popular breakfast item. Some people prefer *naan* with eggs fried with tomatoes. Afghan families do not eat rice for breakfast.

Lunch

Soup (*shurwaa*) and *naan* are popular for lunch, because rice is a luxury item for many families. Afghans break the *naan* into small pieces and soak them in the soup. More fortunate families might have rice (either *palao* or *chelao*) with sauce; for example, meatball sauce, and cooked vegetables with *naan*. Vegetable stew, yogurt, *torshi* (pickles), and/or fresh herbs and vegetables can be added as side dishes.

Dinner

Typically, women of the household decide the menu and a man/boy of the family goes to the bazaar to shop for the necessary ingredients to prepare dinner. If the family can afford it, meat is prepared for the main dish. Afghan people use pressure cookers so that the food item will be soft enough to be eaten by hand. Rice with meat and/or vegetable stew accompanied by salad/fresh assorted vegetables is a typical dinner menu.

 HOLIDAY MENUS

Afghans celebrate *Eid* twice a year. The first one is Eid ul-Fitr (after the end of the fasting month of Ramadan, also called Eid e-Ramadan) and Eid ul-Adha (Festival of Sacrifice, *qurban*, to commemorate the slaying of a sheep, instead of Isaac, as a sacrifice by his father Abraham, at the command of Allah). When Afghan families slaughter the sheep, they divide the meat into three: one third is used by the family, another third is distributed to relatives, and the rest is given to the poor who could not afford to buy the sheep. Both *Eid* dinners would have *qabli palao*, *mantu* (ravioli with lamb-meat filling decorated with yogurt sauce with lentils), and other accompanying meat dishes, such as kebab, *do-piyaza* (which literally means "two onions"; lamb cooked in onion sauce), *kofta* (meatballs), and *korma* (meat stew with vegetables). Prior to *Eid*, different kinds of cookies and pastries are purchased or prepared to serve to the guests who stop by to convey *Eid* greetings.

 HEALTH BELIEFS AND CONCERNS

As in other cultures, Afghan people classify food into hot and cold groups. For example, green tea would make you feel cold as opposed to black tea, which warms you.

People avoid drinking tea with certain fruits, such as melons, because they would cause indigestion, whereas drinking cola with a meal is considered to help digestion. People who have a sore throat would not consume *shirini*, because they believe that it would worsen the soreness. Traditional mothers-in-law advise their daughters-in-law who just had a baby not to consume such food items as yogurt, nightshade vegetables (tomatoes and eggplant), and citrus fruits.

 ## GENERAL HEALTH AND NUTRITIONAL INDICATORS SUMMARY

Afghanistan has one of the worst health indicators in the world. Its human development index, which is a composite measurement in education, longevity, and economic performance, ranked 174 out of 178 countries in 2007. Under-5-years mortality as well as maternal mortality rates are second worst in the world. Since the fall of the Taliban, once-collapsed health systems have been rebuilt. UNICEF (2007) shows a decline in the infant mortality rate from 165 per 1000 live births in 2001 to 135 per 1000 live births in 2006.

Afghanistan, being a landlocked country with hilly and mountainous terrain, makes people vulnerable to goiter due to lack of iodine. In addition to goiter, iodine deficiency causes mental retardation, which is otherwise preventable, and brain damage among fetuses and infants. Lack of iodine also increases the chance of infant mortality, miscarriage, and stillbirth. According to UNICEF (2003), 28% of households consumed iodized salt in 2007. Since 2003, local iodized salt plants have been producing iodized salt, called "Salt of Life," which has been made available at local stores for a minimal cost.

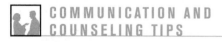 ## COMMUNICATION AND COUNSELING TIPS

When two men meet, they exchange greetings with a handshake, and if between close friends, with a firm embrace. If it is between male and female, greetings are verbal, because most Afghan women do not shake hands with men unless the man is her close relative. Afghan men do not openly talk about their wives, daughters, or sisters. While exchanging greetings, and if you want to know how a man's wife/female family members are, refer to them as "family" or "household" instead of using their names or asking about them directly. Pregnancy is also another taboo topic, especially in the presence of men.

When visiting someone's home, remove and leave your shoes outside the door, or ask where to do so. Then you will be guided to be seated on the floor. Never stretch the leg, especially the feet, in the direction of someone in the room, because it is considered disrespectful. Blowing one's nose with sound is also considered to be disrespectful. When the food is served, eat the food with the right hand and fingers. If it is too challenging, ask for cutlery (for a foreign guest, the Afghan host may have prepared cutlery already).

PRIMARY LANGUAGE OF FOOD NAMES

Table 20-1 gives the primary language of food names. More information on Afghanistan is available in Chapter 22.

TABLE 20-1 Primary Language of Food Names

English	Dari	Pashto
Bread	*Naan*	*Dodai*
Rice	*Berenj*	*Wreejay*
Milk	*Sheer*	*Sheeday*
Vegetable	*Tarkari*	*Sabah*
Fruit	*Mewa*	*Mewa*
Meat	*Gosht*	*Ghowashay*
Tea	*Chai*	*Chai*

REFERENCES

Anonymous. (2000). *Afghan meat dishes.* Retrieved March 14, 2008, from http://asiarecipe.com/afgmain.html/

Anonymous. (2008). Afghanistan. In *Encyclopedia Britannica.* Retrieved March 15, 2008, from http://www.britannica.com/eb/article-9106010/

Anonymous. (n.d.). *Afghan food.* Retrieved March 15, 2008, from http://www.embassyofafghanistan.org/brief.html/

Anonymous. (n.d.). *Afghanistan: Language, culture, customs, and etiquette.* Retrieved March 14, 2008, from http://www.kwintessential.co.uk/resources/global-etiquette/afghanistan.html/

Anonymous. (n.d.). *The constitution of Afghanistan.* Retrieved March 15, 2008, from http://www.president.gov.af/english/constitution.mspx/

Asian Development Bank. (2007). *ADB & Afghanistan 2007 fact sheet.* Retrieved March 23, 2008, from http://www.adb.org/Documents/Fact_Sheets/AFG.pdf/

Bonnier, J. (2007). *Dairy production and processing in Afghanistan.* Retrieved March 15, 2008, from http://www.ahdp.net/reports/Study%20on%20dairy%20production%20and%20processing%20in%20Afghanistan.pdf/

Dupree, L. (1980). *Afghanistan.* Princeton, NJ: Princeton University Press.

Dupree, L., & Dupree, N. (2008). Afghanistan. In *Encyclopedia Britannica.* Retrieved August 17, 2008, from http://www.britannica.com/EBchecked/topic/7798/Afghanistan/

Ministry of Rural Rehabilitation and Development and the Central Statistics Office. (2007). *The national risk and vulnerability assessment 2005: Afghanistan.* Retrieved March 23, 2008, from http://cso-af.net/nrva2005/main.php/

Najibullah, F. (2008, February 20). *Afghanistan: New party to focus on women's rights.* Retrieved March 16, 2008, from http://www.rferl.org/featuresarticle/2008/2/B39AFC45-C260-4A00-81DA-04FBB584049F.html/

Qazi, C. (2007). *Afghan cooking.* Retrieved March 14, 2008, from http://www.afghan-web.com/culture/cooking/

Raheel, Z. (2005). *Qabili pilau (chicken and rice)—Afghan.* Retrieved March 23, 2008, from http://www.myrecipefriends.com/recipe/4088.html?PHPSESSID=f084c0963419b03ef0c7b32f9bc8cd52/

Saberi, F. (2000). *Afghan food and cookery: Noshe djan.* New York: Hippocrene Books.

Saberi, F. (n.d.). *Afghan food and cookery.* Retrieved March 14, 2008, from http://www.inmamaskitchen.com/FOOD_IS_ART_II/food_history_and_facts/afganistan_cooking/afghan_cooking.html/

Sekandari, N. (2003). *Afghan cuisine: cooking for life.* Bloomington, IN: 1stBooks.

UNDP. (n.d.). *Human development report 2007/2008.* Retrieved March 16, 2008, from http://hdrstats.undp.org/countries/data_sheets/cty_ds_AFG.html/

UNICEF. (2003). *Moving beyond 2 decades of war: Progress of provinces multiple indicator cluster survey.* Afghanistan Central Statistics Office. Retrieved March 16, 2008, from http://www.childinfo.org/MICS2/newreports/afghanistan/AfghanistanMICS2003.pdf/

UNICEF. (2007). *The state of the world's children 2007: Women and children, the double dividend of gender equality.* Retrieved April 14, 2009, from http://www.unicef.org/sowc07/statistics/tables.php/

UNICEF. (n.d.). *Statistics.* Retrieved March 15, 2008, from http://www.unicef.org/infobycountry/afghanistan_statistics.html/

ACKNOWLEDGMENT

The author is grateful for the comments given by Ms. Gulbadan Habibi and Dr. Paul Ickx on previous drafts of this chapter.

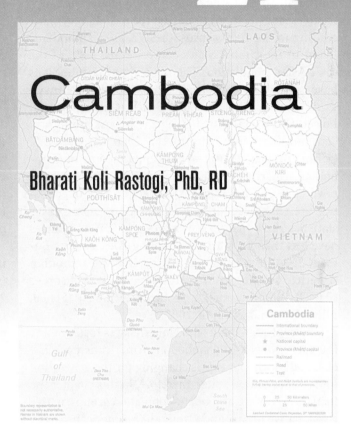

CHAPTER 21

Cambodia

Bharati Koli Rastogi, PhD, RD

 CULTURE AND WORLD REGION

Cambodia is a Southeast Asian country that borders the Gulf of Thailand to the south and is surrounded by Laos in the north, Thailand in the northwest, and Vietnam in the south. It is the smallest country in Southeast Asia. With an area of 181,040 sq. km (69,898 sq. miles), it is slightly smaller than Oklahoma. Cambodia is mostly low flatland with mountainous terrain in the north and southwest. Monsoons from May to November are followed by the dry season from December to April. The climate is hot and humid throughout the year (CIA World Fact Book 2007; New Encyclopedia Britannica Micropaeda Ready Reference, 2007).

The estimated Cambodian population of 14 million is 94% Khmer with minorities of 5% Vietnamese and 1% Chinese. The majority of the population speaks Khmer and practices Theravada Buddhism. Only a small minority, the Cham, who migrated to the northern part during the 3rd and 4th centuries, are Muslims. The official language of Cambodia is Khmer, but English is rapidly becoming the second language. Older educated Cambodians may speak French (CIA World Fact Book 2007; New Encyclopedia Britannica Micropaeda Ready Reference, 2007).

The Cambodian economy is primarily agrarian and involves nearly 80% of the population. Farmers, fishermen, and weavers live in rural areas, while the remaining 20% of the population lives in the cities and supports manufacturing and commerce (CIA World Fact Book 2007; New Encyclopedia Britannica Micropaeda Ready Reference, 2007).

The name *Cambodia* in English, or *Cambodge* in French, comes from the Khmer word *Kampuchea*, meaning *born of Kambu*, the eponymous prince sage. Cambodia has changed its official name five times in the past five decades, with regime changes indicative of the turmoil within the country. The historical name Kampuchea was used during the Pol Pot Regime (1975–1979) and the Vietnamese Sponsored Government

(1979–1989). The current official name is the Kingdom of Cambodia (Culture of Cambodia).

Cambodians are one of the most recent groups to immigrate to the United States, having left their country to escape persecution during the past 25 years. According to the 2000 census, the 172,000 Cambodians living in the United States comprise just 1.8% of the total Asian population. The majority of Cambodians have settled in California, Massachusetts, Pennsylvania, and Texas, with Long Beach (California) and Lowell (Massachusetts) having the largest immigrant communities. According to the 2000 census, (U.S. Census Bureau, 2000) the per capita income of Cambodian Americans is $17,693 and 25.4% live below the poverty level. The language barrier and lack of education are a handicap for Cambodian Americans. Census statistics show that 90% of males and 95% of females have less than 12 years of schooling (U.S. Census Bureau, 2000). Even after 20 years, 62% of Cambodian Americans suffer from posttraumatic stress disorder (PTSD) and other mental problems (Marshall, Schell, Elliot, Berthold, & Chun, 2005).

Even after being in the United States for 20 years, the eating habits of Cambodian Americans have not changed much, but this is changing for the generation born in the United States; therefore, in this chapter the focus is on three Cambodian population groups: native rural, native urban, and Cambodian American.

LANGUAGE

Khmer, or Cambodian, the official language of Cambodia, belongs to the Austro-Asian family of languages but is closer to Vietnamese, Mon, and other South-Asian languages. The Khmer writing system evolved from the Indian scripts. In the 3rd century, the upper strata followed Indian customs and adopted Indian names. Khmer borrowed many words from Sanskrit, such as for administration, politics, military, and literature. As Theravada Buddhism spread across the country, Pali was commonly studied and used by monks. Khmer also bears similarity to the Thai language. Khmer is a complex phonetic language with 66 consonants, 35 vowels, 35 superscripts, and 33 subscripts (Wetzel, 1995).

With the French occupation of Cambodia in 1863, French became the language of administration and the medium of education at the elite primary schools. Khmer, however, remained the vernacular of the poor

and uneducated. During the Pol Pot regime, education was completely halted. Now, the country is reviving the Khmer language and culture. In urban areas, English is more common than French. Ethnic groups, such as the Chinese, Vietnamese, and Cham, also freely use their own languages (Wetzel, 1995).

CULTURE HISTORY

The earliest evidence of human settlement in Cambodia dates back to 7000 BC. Evidence of rice cultivation dating back to 2000 BC was found near the Mekong delta region. This activity led to permanent settlements near the sea and other bodies of water. The trading center Oc-Eo on the South Vietnamese coast flourished between 200 BC to 200 AD (Chandler, 1991).

Around this time, the flourishing trading states near Phnom Penh and Tonle Sap were established. In Chinese annals, this region was called Funan (Forbes, 2004). This served as a seaport allowing the Indian, Chinese, and Arabian ships to enter Cambodia. This period is also marked by the early stages of Indianization, with the beginning of writing and implantation of Hindu religion, food, and culture. The Indian influence on the daily lives of the nobles, on food, poetry, writing, and other aspects of culture was noted by a Chinese visitor around 400 AD. Traders from other parts of the world, such as Persia, Europe, and China, also began to reach Cambodia (Chandler, 1991).

The civilization that flourished between northwest Cambodia and the northeast region of Thailand is known as Angkor. There are several hundred archeological sites and thousands of stone inscriptions left by the Angkor civilization. In all, 28 kings ruled Cambodia for over 600 years. During this period, vast irrigation systems were developed along the Mekong River. This was the golden age of Cambodia (Tully, 2005).

The Angkor Wat is the largest religious complex—visible from outer space—and has both Hindu and Buddhist monuments. Theravada Buddhism was established in Cambodia in the 6th and 7th centuries AD and was revived again in the 12th century. The Chinese scholar Chou Ta Kuan, who visited Cambodia during 1297–1298, described the lavish lifestyles of the king, nobles, and ordinary citizens of Angkor (Chandler, 1991).

Cambodia was invaded from the west by Thailand (Siam) and from the east by Vietnam. Both countries established their regimes in Cambodia. By the 16th century Portuguese and French traders had reached the shores of Cambodia (Chandler, 1991).

In 1863, Cambodia became a protectorate of France. With the establishment of French rule, Cambodia was exposed to European culture and cuisine. During World War II, the Japanese occupied Cambodia, but the day-to-day control remained in the hands of the French (Tully, 2005).

Cambodia gained independence in 1953. The Khmer Rouge revolutionary party, led by Pol Pot, took over Cambodia in 1975. Approximately 1.5 million people were either killed or died of starvation and disease. The events of that period still affect the psyche of the Cambodian people. The Khmer Rouge ruled for less than 5 years. The Communist Party of Vietnam ruled Cambodia until 1989. The country is moving forward with development and modernization. Hun Sen, a former Khmer Rouge member, is the present prime minister of Cambodia (Forbes, 2004).

 ## FOOD HISTORY WITHIN THE CULTURE

Archeological evidence indicates that in the 1st and 2nd centuries, the inhabitants of this region had already settled in small communities and were growing rice and rearing animals. As early as the 1st century, the communities along the Mekong River and the Tonle Sap (the Great Lake) areas were cultivating rice and harvesting the abundant seafood and fish from the sea, rivers, and lakes. Fish plays a pivotal role in this cuisine due to the 443 km of coastline (Cambodian Recipes Culinary History and Information, 2003).

Indians and Chinese immigrants in the 3rd and 4th centuries brought their own cultures and cuisines, which were gradually assimilated locally. Various spices from India were adapted to enhance the flavor in the dishes and continue to be used today. Cambodian cooking acquired the Thai influence after the 6th century, most notably in the use of coconut and chili peppers. Cambodian cooking can be described as a variant of Thai cooking, without the strong piquancy of chili peppers.

European contact with Cambodia started in the 16th century. The chili pepper spread throughout Southeast Asia through Portuguese traders, but as noted previously, the Cambodian cooking style did not adapt to it. Cambodia became a French protectorate in 1863. French cuisine has had an enduring impact since

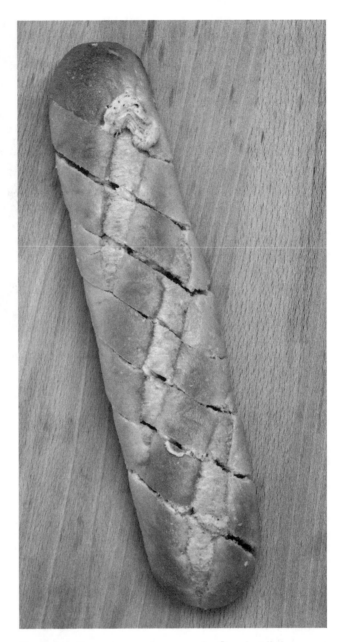

French influence can be seen in Cambodian cuisine in the prevalance of French baguettes and frog legs.

baguettes and frog legs were introduced. Even today, for Cambodians, eating bread is eating a baguette, and frog legs are still popular (Ray, Bewer, Burke, Hutiti, & Seng, 2007).

Vietnamese food influence escalated during the two centuries of Vietnamese rule, especially with the introduction of rice noodles. Over the centuries, Cambodian food has adopted some of the best qualities of Indian, Chinese, Thai, Vietnamese, and French cooking.

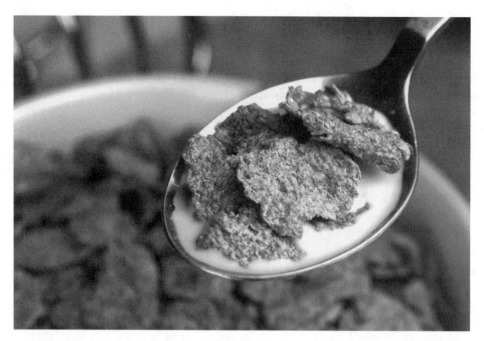

The western influence in urban populations appears in the use of cereal for breakfast.

Most Cambodians eat two to three meals a day. The rural population may eat just breakfast and dinner, but the urban population and the U.S. immigrants generally eat all three daily meals. Rice is eaten with all meals, and noodles are an alternative. Breakfast consists of rice porridge with dry salted fish and vegetables, rice with stir-fried fish, or some meat (beef, pork, or chicken) with vegetables. The western influence in urban populations appears in the use of cereal for breakfast. Meals generally have at least three dishes: soup, a stir-fry with vegetables, and rice. Soups and stir-fry always have some kind of protein in the form of fish, pork, chicken, beef, or tofu. All the dishes are served at the same time.

 MAJOR FOODS

 Protein Sources

Fish is the most important protein source in the diet, with chicken, pork, beef, and seafood eaten as well. Pork and beef are expensive, and their affordability is limited to the middle- and upper-class families in urban areas. Portion size for red meat servings depends on the economic condition of the family, but even among the rural population, the use of small quantities of finely chopped red meat for flavoring is common (Cambodian Recipes Culinary History and Information, 2003).

Unusual meats, such as wild chicken, bird, dove, and frog, are also part of the Cambodian diet. Organ meat, such as liver, kidney tongue, and feet, are consumed as well. Dried salted meats, fish, and seafood are consumed extensively. Eggs from chicken, duck, bird, or fish are a substantial source of protein in the Cambodian diet. Salted eggs provide variety, while fish eggs are eaten on special occasions or often combined with chicken eggs. Vegetable protein sources, such as beans, soybean, soy milk, tofu, or other soybean products, are eaten in small quantity. The baseline surveys conducted by UNICEF (2007) and the World Food Program (WFP) (2005) indicate high incidence of anemia in children and women (United Nations Food and Agriculture Organization, 1999). Proteins provide approximately 9.4% of the total calories in the Cambodian diet (United Nations Food and Agriculture Organization, 1999).

 Starch Sources

Rice and products made from rice flour are common in Cambodian cuisine. Rice is eaten at least three times per day with meals. It is also used as a snack between meals. White rice is eaten most often; brown rice has

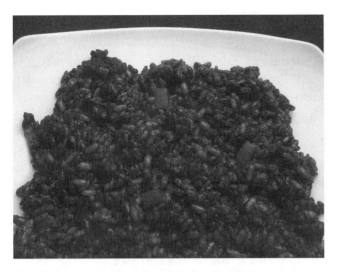

Black rice is used exclusively for desserts.

a strong association with the Pol Pot regime, because it was consumed during the revolution. Sweet white rice and black rice are used exclusively for desserts. The amount of rice consumed in rural areas is more than in urban areas or by Cambodian Americans. Starchy vegetables, such as potato, cassava, and sweet potato, are eaten often. Fresh corn is eaten in season, but corn flour is uncommon. Most of the desserts are made from rice or rice flour. All-purpose wheat flour is widely available in urban areas and used for making noodles and breads. On the other hand, whole-wheat flour is not very common.

Sugar is added in cooking to enhance flavor. White cane sugar is used in desserts and cane juice, which is served as a refreshment during the hot summer months. Brown sugar or partially refined sugar is also used in cooking. Condensed milk is used as coffee creamer because coffee creamer is not available in Cambodia. Palm sugar in used in rural Cambodia. Carbohydrates provide approximately 76.9% of the total calories in the Cambodian diet (United Nations Food and Agriculture Organization, 1999).

 Fat Sources

The rural population still uses fat from animal sources, such as pork or fish, as it is very inexpensive and easily available in villages. Fish fat is used in fried snacks. Fat pieces are skewered between meat pieces and vegetables to enhance the flavor. Vegetable oil is expensive but available and widely used for cooking in urban areas. Coconut milk is used in curries and all desserts.

Cambodian Americans generally use corn or vegetable oil, but the preference for olive oil in stir-frying is increasing due to health awareness. Most meats or chicken are cooked with fat or skin. Cambodian Americans, however, prefer fat-free or skinless meats or chicken, except for some special traditional dishes. Organ meats are eaten on special occasion. Fats provide approximately 13.6% of the total calories in the Cambodian diet (United Nations Food and Agriculture Organization, 1999).

 Prominent Vegetables

The Cambodian diet is high in leafy green vegetables. In rural regions, locally grown leafy vegetables are used in soups, stir-fries, and salads. Pickled vegetables are also traditionally used. A large variety of tropical vegetables is available and consumed throughout the year. These vegetables include cabbage, Chinese broccoli, watercress, pumpkin leaves, yard-long beans, tomatoes, potatoes, corn, eggplant, Thai okra, cucumber, various squashes (such as bitter melon, winter squash, summer squash, and luffa), and starchy vegetables such as taro, cassava, and sweet potato. Many unripe fruits, such as papaya, green banana, and mango, are used as vegetables (Thaitawat, 2000). The baseline surveys conducted by UNICEF (2007) and the WFP (2005) in rural Cambodia showed prevalence of night blindness in children as well as in pregnant and lactating women (United Nations Food and Agriculture Organization, 1999). In the United States, these vegetables are generally available in and near Asian neighborhoods and continue to be an important part of the Cambodian American diet. Due to the high price of these vegetables, consumption could be limited in older Cambodian Americans. During the summer, Cambodian American farmers bring their rich harvests of many of these vegetables to farmer's markets.

 Prominent Fruits

Cambodia has an abundant variety and supply of tropical fruits. Common Cambodian fruits are banana, durian, guava, jackfruit, longan, lychee, mango, mangosteen (often said to be the best fruit in the world), papaya, pineapple, tamarind, watermelon, and many other locally grown wild fruits. Banana and durian are the most popular fruits in Cambodia (Thaitawat, 2000). A larger variety is available in urban regions. Fruit shakes are very popular as desserts and snacks.

Shakes are generally made by blending fruit, coconut milk, ice, sugar, and raw egg for frothiness (Ray, 2007). Condensed milk, rather than sugar, is used with fruits. Durian is the preferred fruit in shakes. Cambodians eat plenty of fruit but consider vegetables as a more essential part of their diet.

 Spices and Seasonings

Indian traders introduced spices in Cambodia around the 2nd century. The Portuguese brought chili peppers in the 16th century. Spices are used with fresh local herbs to enhance the flavor of soups and meats. Herbs are always used fresh. The most common herbs are sweet basil, cilantro, Asian coriander, turmeric, garlic, ginger, galangal (a variety of ginger), kaffir lemon leaves, sdao (the bitter leaves of the margosa or neem trees), peppermint, lemongrass, chives, and scallions.

In each home, spices and herbs are freshly ground into a paste every day using a mortar and pestle. Chili peppers are used sparingly compared with Thai cuisine. The freshly ground herbal paste and sauces are added during cooking. Prahok, a fermented fish sauce, is the main ingredient that gives the distinct, unique flavor to Cambodian dishes (Thaitawat, 2000), although soy sauce and oyster sauce are also common.

 Beverages

Water is the beverage of choice in Cambodia. Potable water is not always readily available in rural areas. Water is boiled at home and consumed hot. Bottled water, soda, and sweetened fruit beverages are expensive but common in urban areas. Fruit shakes are becoming more popular with younger generations. Green tea (*te*) is consumed throughout the day. Coffee (*kafe*) is popular in urban areas and served usually with sweetened condensed milk, rather than black (Ray, 2007). In the countryside, locally brewed rice wine and fermented palm juice is very popular and inexpensive. It can be consumed as it is or with herbs, tree barks, or animal parts for medicinal purposes. This concoction is believed to give energy and vitality. Women consume these drinks after giving birth. Alcoholic beverages and hard liquor are available in urban areas but are expensive. Cambodian Americans drink sweetened beverages such as soda, juice, and coffee during the day. Alcoholic drinks, such as beer, wine, and hard liquor, are popular. Alcoholism is one of the biggest problems in Cambodian American communities.

 Desserts

Cambodian meals generally do not have formal desserts. Fruits are generally eaten as dessert. In urban areas, desserts are prepared and sold in specialty stores. Desserts are prepared mainly during holidays. Most desserts are made with rice, rice flour, tapioca, mung beans, and adzuki beans along with coconut milk. Cambodian Americans eat these desserts frequently and the younger generation has developed a preference for all American desserts.

 FOODS WITH CULTURAL SIGNIFICANCE

Cambodian cooking, though influenced by its neighbors, is distinct. Herbs and spices used in cooking often form a freshly ground paste with a unique flavor. *Prahok*, a fermented fish paste, gives a very distinct Cambodian flavor to soups and stir-fried food. Another fermented fish sauce, *Pahok*, common in eastern Cambodia, is prepared by marinating black and white sweet rice with salted fish for as long as 3 months. *Pahok* and *Prahok* are sold in both Asian and Cambodian stores.

Americans sometimes crave hamburgers when abroad for long periods. Similarly, Cambodians look for their staple dishes such as *Samlor Machu Khroeng* (Khmer lemongrass soup), *Samlor Kor Ko* (the Cambodian national dish, a flavorful soup made with eggplant, pumpkin, bitter melon, green banana, and other vegetables), *Samlor Krov Chhnang*, and *Tek Kroeung* (catfish with lemongrass).

 TYPICAL DAY'S MENU

In Cambodia, meals are freshly prepared three times a day (breakfast, lunch, and dinner). Due to lack of refrigeration, leftover foods are commonly discarded; however, in America, most families do the entire day's cooking in the morning, and the food is eaten throughout the day. Cooking once a day is still practiced by older Cambodian Americans. Traditional breakfast is preferred by most Cambodian Americans. Working Cambodians Americans may eat breakfast at fast-food restaurants and bring lunch from home. Younger Cambodians prefer Western foods. All the dishes are served at the same time.

Breakfast

A typical breakfast might consist of any of the following with warm or cold water:

> Rice porridge with dry salted fish
>
> Rice with dry salted fish and vegetables
>
> French baguette with condensed milk
>
> Rice or egg noodles with meat and leafy green vegetables

Lunch

A typical lunch might consist of the following:

> Rice
>
> Soup (made with fish, pork, chicken, or beef, and green leafy vegetables)
>
> Fried fish or any other meat
>
> Water
>
> Fruit as dessert

Dinner

A typical dinner might consist of the following:

> Rice
>
> Soup (made with fish, pork, chicken, or beef, and green leafy vegetables)
>
> Fried fish or another meat
>
> Water
>
> Fruit as dessert

 ## HOLIDAY MENUS

The Cambodian New Year, celebrated from April 13 to 15, is the most popular holiday. It marks the end of the harvest season as farmers enjoy the fruits of their labor before the next monsoons. *Moha Songkran* is the first-day celebration that signals the end of the old year and the beginning of the New Year. Prediction of arrival time, favorite foods, and items are announced on national television and radio. People select favorite fruits, foods, clothes, perfumes, and incense. Buddhist temples announce the arrival of the New Year time specified by astrologers by beating drums or ringing bells. In the afternoon, they visit the temple and offer foods to Buddhist monks. *Wannabat* is the second day of the New Year celebration. People contribute charity to less fortunate and homeless people as well as household servants. In the afternoon, people bring food for their deceased ancestors. Failure to do so will bring forth bad luck from them. *Thnei Loeung Sak* is the third and final day of the New Year. They begin by washing the statues of Buddha. Children bathe and perfume their parents on this last day and ask for forgiveness for all the sins committed by them, whether knowingly or unknowingly. In return, their parents forgive and bless them. By doing so, good fortune is bestowed upon the children. Food plays a big role in the celebrations. Specialty dishes are cooked in large quantities to be eaten during the 3-day festivities.

New Year's Menu

A New Year's menu might consist of the following:

> *Kari Sach Chrouk* with rice; pork with sweet potato, watercress, and green beans
>
> *Sach Chrouk Khor* with rice; pork, black pepper, and bamboo shoots
>
> *Misor* with rice; fried long noodles, pork, and Chinese leeks
>
> *Un-som slek jek* (sweet sticky rice, coconut wrapped in banana leaves)
>
> *Un-som chrouk* (sticky rice, pork with black pepper, mung beans wrapped in banana leaves)
>
> Watermelon for dessert
>
> Banana
>
> Custard-apple (fruit of the tree *Annona reticulata*)

 ## HEALTH BELIEFS AND CONCERNS

The traditional health belief is that ailments are caused by evil spells, by not performing rituals correctly, by mistakes made during life cycles, or by imbalance in natural forces (especially wind). Cambodians are generally comfortable with traditional as well as Western health practices. In illness, traditional medicine is usually tried first. They are aware that Western healthcare providers would view traditional treatment as ineffectual; therefore, they are reluctant to disclose such practices when they seek Western treatment.

The traditional treatment can be administered by family members or *kruu khmer*, the traditional healer who travels from village to village. The healers gather or grow the herbs necessary to produce medicine. These herbs are used singly or in combinations. Cupping, pinching, and coining are the most commonly used methods to cure many ailments. In cupping, a heated cup is used on the skin. In pinching, the healer pinches the skin. In coining, the skin is rubbed with a coin. Various dermal techniques are also used in illness. Usage of Chinese and Vietnamese herbs is common in rural areas. Families with Chinese ancestry may use the Chinese principle of hot and cold balance (Cambodian Health Beliefs and Practices, 2004).

Vegetables and roots of various plants are used in the treatment of diseases. Bitter vegetables, such as bitter melon and *sdao* (margosa leaves), are used to combat malaria and other fevers. Leftover rice is eaten for migraines. Durian, the favorite fruit of Cambodians, is supposed to give energy, but when eaten in large quantities it can make one feel very hot or even cause fever. Poisonous Egret's Drop (*Pis-Ach Kok*) is believed to be the most common ailment among young children. Those afflicted die due to severe malnutrition. The indigenous treatment is to slit the palm with a sharp instrument and squeeze the hand until fat from the adipose tissue is expelled.

There are many health beliefs and practices for pregnant and postpartum women. Pregnant women are discouraged from eating too much and taking prenatal vitamins, or from taking showers at night, because this is believed to make the baby too large and the labor difficult. Some foods, such as milk, are thought to change the baby's skin color. Drinking sugarcane juice can increase volume of amniotic fluid, and coconut juice decreases vernix caseosa in the baby. Certain meats and fish are forbidden foods during pregnancy and after delivery because they can make the mother sick. If sickness occurs, these forbidden meats or fish are charred and mixed with alcohol and consumed by afflicted women for recovery. Wine with roasted sesame seeds is supposed to ease delivery. Pregnant women are asked not to sit in front of a door or eat before others to avoid difficult labor. Rice is thought to be the only food that is needed for survival; fruits and vegetables are considered unnecessary. Although breastfeeding is prevalent, colostrum is discarded because it is believed to be unclean (Gill, Luttrell, & Conway, 2003).

The urban population and Cambodian Americans are more likely to be receptive to the Western health system; however, there remains a deep-rooted belief in the effectiveness of the traditional treatment.

 ## GENERAL HEALTH AND NUTRITIONAL INDICATORS SUMMARY

Health and Nutritional Status of Cambodia

Food insecurity and distribution are two major concerns in Cambodia. In 2004, one third of the population of 14 million lived below the poverty line. Ninety percent of this population living in rural Cambodia grows their own food, including staples such as rice. They grow vegetables, raise animals, fish in local rivers and streams, and gather food from forests. With the help from world organizations, Cambodian research institutes are gathering statistics on medical, nutritional, social, and economical status of the country. The Cambodian Demographic and Health Survey (CDHS) and Cambodian Socio Economic Survey (CSES) are conducted every 5 years. The CSES reports that with improving economic conditions, life expectancy has increased to 59 years for men and to 63 years for women (2008 estimate). In Cambodia, a third of the households are headed by women, who tend have lower income and spend nearly two thirds of their income on food.

Infant and Under-5-Years Mortality Rates

The nutritional status of the children has improved considerably during the rebuilding of Cambodia. Between the years 2000 and 2005, the infant mortality and the under-5-years mortality rates have declined. The CSES survey indicates a significant drop in the infant mortality rate from 96 to 66 deaths for every 1000 live births per year, although high infant-mortality rates of up to 120 deaths per 1000 live births have been reported in certain provinces. Under-5-years mortality rates have shown a 30% drop from 124 to 83 for every 1000 live births per year. Despite these improvements, 1 of 12 Cambodian children dies before the age of 5 years. Rural areas and certain provinces report a higher rate of infant mortality and under-5-years mortality than the national or urban figures. The UNICEF 2005 data reported that Cambodia ranked 25th among 190 countries for under-5-years mortality rate.

Nutritional Status of Children

Nutrition is important from the beginning of life. Breastmilk provides all the nutrients, disease-fighting antibodies, and emotional support to the infant. In Cambodia, due to traditional beliefs, colostrum is not fed to children. Only 11% of children are exclusively breastfed during the first hour of life. This deprives infants of a rich, natural source of antibodies at a time when they need it most. Other fluids, such as formula, water, and juice, are added at an earlier age than the World Health Organization (WHO, 2001) recommendation. Seventy percent of children under the age of 2 months are fed water. Introduction of solid foods is also done much earlier than the WHO recommendation.

Cambodia has the highest malnutrition rate among its Asian neighbors. Malnutrition is affecting the overall health of children. The economic progress achieved in the past 7–8 years has shown a dramatic drop in the number of children suffering from malnutrition. Between 2000 and 2005, the percentage of underweight children under 5 years decreased significantly from 45 to 35%. The number of children who are small in stature for their age has decreased from 45 to 37%, and wasting, based on body mass index (BMI), has decreased from 15% to half of this percentage.

In light of the recent economic downturn, the Cambodian government has announced that the progress made over the past years could be wiped out due to the high cost of food. Inflation reached 22% by July 2008 but dropped to 13.4% at year's end. In 2005, 8.4% of children under 5 years were malnourished, but the percentage rose to 8.9% last year.

Nutrient Deficiencies

Micronutrient deficiencies, such as iron-deficiency anemia, vitamin A, and iodine deficiency, have been reported in less diverse rural diets. Forty-one percent of the individuals reported inadequate food intake in the CSES 2005 survey. This was found also in higher-income families, indicating poor infant feeding practices and inadequate access to food. The CSES 2005 survey indicated rice as the main source of dietary energy providing 75% of calories. Less than 15% of calories came from fat and 10% from protein. Almost 25% of the protein was from fish.

Anemia

Inadequate intake of iron, folate, and vitamin B_{12}-rich foods leads to iron-deficiency anemia. Other causes of anemia are thalassemia, sickle cell disease, malaria, and intestinal worms. According to the CSES survey, 62% of children between the ages of 6 and 59 months are anemic. Children under 2 years were more likely to be anemic than older children, indicating improper feeding practices. Anemia has been reported in 57% of pregnant

women and in 47% of nonpregnant women. This could be a contributing factor in the slight increase in the maternal mortality rate (from 437 deaths per 100,000 live births in 2000 to 472 deaths per 100,000 in 2005).

Vitamin A Deficiency

Vitamin A deficiency in Cambodian children is due to low intake of foods rich in vitamin A and increased need due to infection. The CSES 2000 survey indicates that 22% of children had low serum–retinol levels. The vitamin A capsule distribution program is helping children and postpartum women in increasing vitamin A levels.

Iodine Deficiency Disorder

Iodine-deficiency disorder (IDD) was reported in 1997 by the First National Goiter Survey. It indicated that over 17% of children 8–12 years were low in iodine. In some provinces, prevalence of IDD was even higher. Distribution of iodized salt is slowly eradicating this problem. Close to 75% of the population is now consuming iodized salt.

Incidence of malnutrition and nutrient-deficiency diseases declines significantly with the mother's level of education. Research organizations and government authorities believe that educating women may eventually eliminate malnutrition or reduce the number of children suffering from these diseases, thus giving children a better start in life.

Effect of Economic Development

With economic development and modernization, Cambodia, in addition to its problem of malnutrition, is facing many of the same problems confronted in industrialized nations, such as overweight/obesity, diabetes mellitus, hypertension, and hyperlipidemia in urban and semi-urban areas. The CSES survey conducted in 2004 reported that about 2% of males and 4% of females have BMI over 30 and 18–20% are overweight (BMI = 25–29). The first diabetes survey conducted in 2005 estimated that 0.5–1% of 255,000 people under the age of 20 years had type-I diabetes. Data reported in 2009 indicated that 1 million Cambodians are diabetic (about 7% of the population). Sedentary lifestyle and excess food consumption by high-income families in urban and semi-urban areas have been implicated in the high prevalence of diabetes and other metabolic disorders.

Cambodia will need a two-pronged approach to combat the age-old problem of malnutrition and the modern problem of excessive food consumption and sedentary lifestyle.

COMMUNICATION AND COUNSELING TIPS

Cambodians are often slow to seek medical attention due to their traditional beliefs. Other barriers include denial of illness, high threshold for discomfort, scarcity of healthcare facilities, language, and the cost of health care. Immigrants who have lived in the United States for many years have been exposed to outreach activities conducted by healthcare agencies; therefore, they are familiar with medical terminologies, and signs and symptoms of common diseases. Recent immigrants, on the other hand, are not aware of the healthcare process.

Nutrition is a new concept to Cambodians. It is crucial that the relevance and benefits of nutritional counseling be explained at the individual and community levels. The rationale behind changes should be explained, and then those changes should be introduced gradually. Pamphlets and brochures should use simple language and graphics to circumvent the language barrier. Cambodians do not use recipes and are unfamiliar with measuring cups or spoons. The concept of portion size is also new to them. Food models should be used to show the correct portion size. Showing food packages can be an effective aid for shopping. Unfamiliar food products can be introduced through tasting.

Calories

Older Cambodian Americans are not aware that food has calories and that it is essential to eat a sufficient quantity to maintain healthy weight. Most Cambodians are fairly lean. Weight problems are seen in middle-aged women. Fuentes-Afflick, Hessol, & Pérez-Stable (1998) reported moderately low birth weight in Cambodians in California. Teenage boys, however, are becoming overweight, and even obese, as they eat more calorie-dense foods (e.g., potato chips, doughnuts, juice, soda, and other sweetened drinks). Stang, Kong, Story, Eisenberg, & Neumark-Sztainer, (2007) observed increased risk of obesity, body dissatisfaction, and unhealthy weight-control behavior among Cambodian adolescents compared with white adolescents. Food Security Statistics (United Nations Food and Agriculture Organization, 2003) indicated a dietary energy consumption of 2060 kcal/person per day in Cambodia in 2001–2003.

For counseling, the following is recommended:

- Encourage eating three meals per day, inclusion of all the food groups, and use of appropriate portion size.
- For teenagers, emphasize eating a more traditional fish, chicken, and vegetable-based diet, and fruits for dessert.
- Encourage nutrient-dense foods for infants and toddlers.

Protein

Protein in the traditional Cambodian diet provides 10–15% of the total calories. Protein intake has remained the same in older Cambodian Americans, who still prefer fish or chicken over red meat. The high cost of fish, however, limits consumption. In younger age groups, the intake of red meat and seafood has dramatically increased. Packaged meats, such as hot dogs, sausages, and lunch meats, are eaten frequently. Meats are boiled, steamed, grilled, or stir-fried. Food Security Statistics (United Nations Food and Agriculture Organization, 2003) indicated consumption of 51 g of protein per person per day in Cambodia in 2001–2003.

For counseling, the following is recommended:

- Consumption of lean meat and age-appropriate portion sizes for protein foods should be encouraged.
- Food handling and safety methods should be discussed. In Cambodia, due to lack of refrigeration, meat is often left at room temperature. The same practice is not uncommon in Cambodian American households.
- Eating undercooked meat should be discouraged.

Fat

Use of animal fat has decreased in Cambodian Americans. Vegetable oils, such as corn oil, are now used more often, so the percentage of calories from fat has increased over the years. Food Security Statistics (United Nations Food and Agriculture Organization, 2003) indicated consumption of 32 g of fat per person per day in Cambodia in 2001–2003.

For counseling, the following is recommended:

- Emphasize traditional cooking methods such as steaming, boiling, or grilling.

- Encourage stir-frying with small amounts of oil and to keep deep-frying to a minimum.
- Use pamphlets to show how to remove visible fat from meats, skin from chicken, and fat from soups.
- Discourage eating organ meats and consumption of coconut milk.

Carbohydrates

Rice, fruits, and starchy vegetables are the main carbohydrate sources in the Cambodian diet. A 2004 survey conducted in Lowell, Massachusetts, indicated that only 16.4% of Cambodians were consuming five fruits and vegetables per day, compared with 32.1% of Asians and 24.4% of the general population (Centers for Disease Control, 2004.)

For counseling, the following is recommended:

- Encourage use of whole-grain products. White rice is the staple food eaten with each meal. It provides energy, vitality, and comfort. Suggestions to change the amount and/or variety (e.g., use of brown rice instead of white rice) could cause anxiety, discomfort, and resistance due to historical associations (i.e., the use of brown rice during the Pol Pot regime). This should be considered in counseling.
- Cambodian Americans with diabetes should be made familiar with portion sizes for rice, noodles, starchy vegetables, and desserts.
- Discourage use of sugar in cooking for diabetics.
- Fruits are commonly eaten as dessert but not on a daily basis; thus, the USDA recommendation of five fruit and vegetable servings is not being fulfilled. Recommendations to increase fruit intake, with statements such as, "Fruits are an excellent source of vitamins, energy, and are vital for good health," will have greater impact.

Minerals

Dairy products are less common in the Cambodian diet. Southeast Asians are often lactose intolerant. Infants and children drink milk and eat cheese, because many are enrolled in the Women, Infants, and Children (WIC) program. Children over 5 years consume less milk. Most teenagers do not drink milk but eat cheese in sandwiches, and pizza is very popular. Low calcium intake is observed in pregnant teenagers. Older Cambodian Americans, even after living abroad for decades, do not drink milk or eat other dairy products.

For counseling, the following is recommended:

- The importance of calcium throughout the life cycle should be discussed with parents.
- Acceptable alternative calcium sources, such as tofu with calcium sulfate, calcium-fortified soy milk or fruit juices, sardines, and anchovies with bones, should be suggested.
- Instead of the traditional rice porridge for breakfast, WIC cereals should be suggested.

Salt

The Cambodian diet can be high in sodium. Dry salted fish, pickled eggs, vegetables, and salt-rich soy, as well as oyster and fish sauces are used extensively in cooking. Use of monosodium glutamate (MSG) is high.

Observations from the Author (Bharati Koli Rastogi)

My first encounter with Cambodian cuisine was in 1995 when I started working at Lowell Community Health Center (LCHC) in Massachusetts. Most of the Cambodian colleagues would bring their lunch from home. It was always rice with soup. The soups would have different varieties of Asian vegetables along with meat. Vegetables are cooked until they are soft but not mushy. Soups have two or three different meats, such as chicken, and pork can be added in the same soup, or beef and fish. Stir-fried meats and vegetables with rice indicate the influence of Chinese cuisine, and meats and vegetables served with noodles indicate Vietnamese influence.

I was exposed to Cambodian cuisine further at Metta Center, the Asian Health Center at LCHC. Around noon, the fragrance of jasmine rice begins to permeate the halls of the center. Almost magically, a big lunch table is set up within minutes with three to four hot dishes. Anyone who enters the lunch room is offered food. We have a joke in the clinic, that if someone at other sites has forgotten to bring lunch, they are always welcome at the Metta Center where no one leaves hungry during the lunch hour. Clients, as a sign of gratitude, bring food for the staff working in the clinic. In Cambodian culture, the rice cooker is always on! I am deeply touched by their generosity and warm hospitality.

For counseling, the following is recommended:

- Encourage use of herbs and spices.
- Introduce low-salt products.
- Discourage use of MSG.

Recommending food sources familiar to the client population increases compliance. Introduction of new food items, however nutritious and beneficial, requires willingness and acceptance on the part of the community; therefore, it is important in counseling ethnically diverse populations to know, and be sensitive to, their culture, beliefs, and food customs, as these play important roles in their lives.

FOOD NAMES IN ENGLISH WITH KHMER TRANSLATION

Table 21-1 gives food names in English with Khmer translation.

TABLE 21-1   Food Names in English with Khmer Translation

English	Khmer	English	Khmer	English	Khmer
Beverages		**Fats**		Chinese broccoli	*Khat Na*
Coffee	*Kafe*	Beef fat	*Klanh ko*	Chinese cabbage	*Spey Saw*
Fruit shakes	*Tirk Kroloc*	Chicken fat	*Klanh morn*	Eggplant	*Trop*
Juice	*Tirk Phle chheu*	Fish fat	*Klanh trey*	Luffa	*No Nong Proher*
Milk	*Tirk doh kow*	Oil	*Preng*	Potato	*Dam Long Barang*
Tea	*Tai*	Pork fat	*Klanh Chrouk*	Pumpkin	*Lpeou*
Water	*Teuk*	**Fruits**		Spinach	*P'ty or P'tee*
Wine	*S'ra*	Apple	*Phle Porm*	Sweet potato	*Dam Long Chvea*
Protein foods		Banana	*Chake*	Winter melon	*Tralach*
Beef	*Sach ko*	Durian	*Too rane*	Yard-long beans	*Sandek Veng*
Chicken	*Sach morn*	Gooseberry	*Kan Tourt*	**Spices**	
Duck	*Sach tia*	Guava	*Trabek*	Basil	*Slek Chee, Chi, Chy*
Egg	*Porng*	Jack fruit	*Phle Khnor*	Chili	*M'tase*
Fish	*Sach Trey*	Longan	*Mien*	Chinese parsley	*Che Vansuy*
Mung beans	*Sendek Bay*	Lychee	*Koulane*	Cilantro	*Che Vansuy*
Pork	*Sach Chrouk*	Mango	*S'vay*	Fish sauce	*Teuk trey*
Carbohydrate foods		Mangosteen	*Phle Mong khut*	Garlic	*K'tim Sar*
Bread	*Num Pang*	Orange	*Kroch*	Ginger	*Kh'nhey*
Flour	*M'sao*	Papaya	*L'hong*	Lemongrass	*S'lek K'rey*
Noodles	*Me (Kuy Teav)*	Rambutan	*Sao Mao*	Turmeric	*Ro Miet*
Rice	*Bay*	**Vegetables**			
Yellow noodles	*Me*	Bitter melon	*M'reas*		
		Bok choy	*Spey Bok Choy*		
		Cabbage	*Spey*		

FEATURED RECIPE

Cambodians do not use written recipes for preparing meals. The younger generation learns to cook by observing and assisting adults in food preparation. The following recipe was compiled by interviewing the staff at Lowell Community Health Center. The amounts of spices and herbs are approximate; they can be adjusted to suite taste.

Samlor Machu Kroeung Sach Chrouk (Lemongrass Pork Soup)

1½ lb. lean pork ribs

3 stalks lemongrass, finely chopped

2-inch piece galangal, finely chopped

1-inch piece turmeric, finely chopped, or ½ tsp. turmeric powder

4 kaffir lime leaves, finely chopped

4 cloves garlic, finely chopped

1 tbsp. tamarind paste

3–4 curry leaves

1 tsp. *prahok* (optional)

½ tsp. sugar

Salt to taste

½ tsp. fish sauce

Vegetables (a big bunch of watercress, Cambodian melon)

1–2 tbsp. corn oil

3 cups water

Hot pepper (according to taste)

1. Blend lemongrass, galangal, turmeric, and kaffir lime leaves with a little water to a fine paste (mortar and pestle can also be used), and set aside.
2. Chop watercress and Cambodian melon.
3. Remove visible fat from pork ribs and make 1- to 2-inch cubes.
4. Heat oil in a pot. Add chopped garlic and sauté for 1–2 minutes. Do not brown garlic.
5. Add cubed pork with tamarind paste and *prahok* (optional).
6. Cook for 3–4 minutes and then add blended or crushed herb paste. Let meat cook with all the herbs and spices for 2–3 minutes.
7. Add 3 cups of water, sugar, salt, and fish sauce. Let it boil for 1–2 minutes. Let it simmer for 10–15 minutes until the meat is soft and tender.
8. Add chopped vegetables. Cook for 2–3 minutes.
9. Roast curry leaves on a heated pan. Add crushed leaves to soup.
10. Serve with hot white rice.

Yields 4 servings

(Recipe courtesy of Sophie Greenwood, Connie Pen, and Sina Phou-Khoun)

More recipes are available at http://nutrition.jbpub.com/foodculture/

ACKNOWLEDGMENTS

I thank Dorcas Grigg-Saito, Director, Lowell Community Health Center (LCHC). Information about the Cambodian culture, customs, and food was gathered in my interactions with the Cambodian staff at LCHC. I thank them, especially Sonith Peou, Director, and Chan Touch, FNP, Metta Center, LCHC, for reviewing this chapter and their valuable suggestions during its preparation. I also thank S. Peou and S. Seang for assistance with the Khmer translations.

REFERENCES

Cambodian health beliefs and practices: A summary. (2004). Retrieved February 5, 2008, from http://www3.baylor.edu/ Charles_Kemp/cambodian_summary.html/

Cambodian Mirror. (2009). One million Cambodians have diabetes and hypertension. Retrieved April 15, 2009, from http://cambodiamirror.wordpress.com/2009/03/31/one-million-cambodians-have-diabetes-and-hypertension-tuesday-3132009/

Cambodian Recipes Culinary History and Information. (2003). Retrieved December 28, 2007, from http://www.recipes4us. co.uk/Cooking%20by%20Country/Cambodia%20Recipes% 20Culinary%20History%20and%20Information.htm/

Centers for Disease Control. (2004). *Health status of Cambodians and Vietnamese: Selected communities. United States. 2001–2002. Morbidity and mortality. Weekly Report, 53* 760–765. Retrieved February 2, 2008, from http://www. cdc.gov/mmwR/preview/mmwrhtml/mm5333a3.htm/

Chandler, D. (1991). *The land and people of Cambodia.* New York: HarperCollins.

China View. (2009) *Health, gov't survey finds health, nutrition problems of Cambodian children.* Retrieved April 18, 2009, from http://news.xinhuanet.com/english/2009-02/19/ content_10846417.htm/

CIA World Fact Book. (2007). Retrieved February 2, 2008, from http://www.cia.gov/library/publications/the-world-factbook/index.html/

Countries and Their Cultures. (2009). *Culture of Cambodia.* Retrieved December 21, 2007, from http://www.everyculture. com/Bo-Co/Cambodia.html/

Executive Brief. (2009). Cambodia Integrated Food Security and Humanitarian Phase Classification (IPC). Retrieved April 18, 2009, from http://www.ipcinfo.org/attachments/ Brief_IPC_Cambodia_24_May_2007.pdf/

Forbes, A. (2004). *Insight compact guide: Cambodia.* Singapore: APA Publications.

Fuentes-Afflick E., Hessol N.A., & Pérez-Stable E.J., (1998). Maternal birthplace, ethnicity, and low birth weight in California. Arch Pediatr Adolesc Med, Vol. 152 (*11*), pp. 1105–1112.

Gill, G., Luttrell, C., & Conway, T. (2003). *Food security in Cambodia.* Retrieved February 4, 2008, from http://www. odi.org.uk/publications/working_papers/wp231/wp231_ annex3_Cambodia.pdf/

Marshall, G.N., Schell, T.L., Elliot, M.N., Berthold, S.M., & Chun, C. (2005). Mental health of Cambodian refugees 2

decades after resettlement in the United States. *Journal of the American Medical Association, 294,* 571–579.

New Encyclopedia Britannica Micropaedia Ready Reference. (2007). *Cambodia.* (Vol. 2, pp. 757–758). Chicago: Encyclopedia Britannica.

Ray, N., Bewer, T., Burke, A., Hutiti, T., & Seng, S. (2007). *Vietnam, Cambodia, Laos & the Greater Mekong.* Victoria, Australia: Lonely Planet Publications.

Stang, J., Kong, A., Story, M., Eisenberg, M., & Neumark-Sztainer, D. (2007). Food and weight-related patterns and behavior of among adolescents. *Journal of the American Dietetic Association, 107,* 936–941.

Thaitawat, N. (2000). *The cuisine of Cambodia.* Bangkok, Thailand: Nusara & Friends Co.

Tully, J. (2005). A short history of Cambodia: From empire to survival. Melbourne, Australia: Allen & Unwin.

UNICEF (2005). Childhood under threat. Retrieved December 10, 2009, from http://www.unicef.org/sowc05/english/ index.html

UNICEF. (2007). *The state of the world's children 2007: Women and children, the double dividend of gender equality.* Retrieved April 14, 2009, from http://www.unicef.org/sowc07/ statistics/tables.php/

United Nations Food and Agriculture Organization. (1999). *Nutrition country profiles: Cambodia.* Retrieved February 2, 2008, from http://www.fao.org/ag/AGN/nutrition/ cmb-e.stm/

United Nations Food and Agriculture Organization. (2003). *Country profile and mapping information system—Cambodia.* Retrieved February 10, 2008, from http://www.fao.org/ countryProfiles/index.asp?lang=en&iso3=KHM&subj=4/

U.S. Census Bureau. (2000). We the people: Asians in the United States. Census 2000 special reports. Retrieved February 7, 2008, from http://www.census.gov/prod/2004pubs/censr-17.pdf/

Wetzel, L. (1995). *Cambodia.* Retrieved November 30, 2009, from http://ethnomed.org/culture/cambodian

World Food Program (WFP). (2005). *Children's nutrition status—Cambodia.* Retrieved April 18, 2009, from http:// www.foodsecurityatlas.org/khm/country/utilization/ childrens-nutritional-status/

World Health Organization (WHO). (2001). The World Health Organization's infant feeding recommendation. As stated in the Global Strategy on Infant and Young Child Feeding (WHA55 A55/15, paragraph 10). Retrieved December 1, 2009, from www.who.int/nutrition/topics/infantfeeding_ recommendation/en/index.html

CHAPTER 22

Far East
(Afghanistan, Pakistan, China, and Bangladesh)

Zaheer Ali Kirmani, PhD, RD

INTRODUCTION

As civilizations evolved and adequate supplies of food became available, humans started attributing certain characteristics to the foods they ate based on where they lived in the world. These associations of color, shape, size, mealtime, and so on underscore the cultural aspects of various foods. In this chapter, several countries of the Far East are explored with respect to their cuisine and culture. One important consideration is that, according to sociological studies of human populations, when cultures are influenced by religion a common thread emerges regardless of language or living environments. For example, in the East, one common thread is that adherents of Islam and Judaism, irrespective of where they live, seek foods that are free of pork or pork products.

AFGHANISTAN

 Culture and World Region

Afghanistan's culture can best be described as a mosaic of tribes with traditions spanning thousands of years that have never been truly intertwined. The reasons for the segregation among tribes may be poor means of communication and transportation. Ethnic diversity exists due to ancient trading and invading armies' routes to western and southwestern Asia from Central Asia and Europe. Over 40% of the people are Pashtun; others are Tajik, Hazara, and Uzbek. Islamic traditions and jurisprudence is practiced and is the uniting force in the country.

The entire country of The Islamic Republic of Afghanistan consists of 252,000 square miles, making it only slightly smaller than Texas. Its capital, Kabul, is populated with close to 2 million people. Inhabitants of Afghanistan are called Afghans. The majority of the population follows Islam (Muslims), with 1% of the population following Sikhism, Hinduism, Judaism, or Zoroastrianism.

Languages

Dari (Afghan Persian) and Pashto are the official languages.

Culture History

The Afghan people are an ethnically mixed population of peoples, reflecting the country's long history of being invaded. These invaders included Alexander the Great, the Scythians, the White Huns, and the Turks. Arabs were the last to invade (in 642 BCE), with the spreading of Islam. From ancient times to present, Afghanistan has been a tribal confederation country and a society where clan loyalty rules supreme. Mahmud of Ghazni (98–1030 CE) developed Afghanistan into a great empire with Ghazni as its capital. Ghazni eventually became a great bastion of culture. Genghis Khan's invasion in 1219 destroyed vast agricultural areas and large cities such as Ghazni, Herat, and Balkh. In the 14th century a man named Temurlane, one of Genghis Khan's descendents, incorporated Afghanistan into his vast Asian empire. In the 16th century, Babur, a descendent of Temurlane and the founder of India's Mughal Dynasty, created the Afghanistan principality with Kabul as its capital.

Afghanistan as we know it today was established by Ahmad Shah Durrani in 1747. His empire extended from Mashad in the west to Kashmir and Delhi in the east, and from the Amu Darya River in the north to the Arabian Sea in the south. All Afghan rulers since this time have been from Durrani's Pashtun tribal confederation including the present president, Hamid Karzai. The only exception is the short period of Marxist coup in 1978. During the reign of Amir Abdur Rahman (1880–1901), British and Russian officials reestablished boundaries of modern-day Afghanistan, but Britain retained the country's foreign affairs under their control until that authority was handed over to the Afghanistan government under the Rawalpindi Treaty in 1919. King Amanullah Khan (1919–1929) tried to shun isolation of the country and introduced several social and cultural reforms, especially for women in the society, but was not very successful and was forced to abdicate

the throne. Nadir Shah, another Pashtun, became king but was assassinated after 4 years. His 19-year-old son, Mohammad Zahir Shah, became king (1933–1973) and advanced several liberal constitutional reforms in the country by instituting central and provincial assemblies. During King Zahir Shah's regime there was some freedom to form political parties. As a result, the People's Democratic Party of Afghanistan was formed, which had ideological affiliation with the Soviet Union. King Zahir Shah appointed his cousin, Sardar Mohammad Daoud, as Prime Minister. Daoud instituted several social and cultural reforms, especially advancement of women in public life and dispensation with the traditional veil.

With the ethnic, class, economic, and ideological divisions in Afghan society, there was enormous dissatisfaction. Ex-Prime Minister Daoud took the opportunity and seized power in a military coup on July 17, 1973. Daoud declared Afghanistan a republic with himself as both the first president and the prime minister. The first constitution, promulgated in 1977, envisioned social and economic well-being for the country. Unfortunately, Daoud's efforts failed to curb the economic misery and political unrest that had prevailed for so long in Afghanistan.

Food History Within the Culture

Due to the political climate and isolative environment, the foods of this land have not evolved greatly over time. Much like its culture, in essence, Afghani food is a mosaic of Persian, Turkish, and Mongolian foods. Afghanistan is basically an agrarian culture; however, the agriculture is limited. Agriculturally, 12% of the total area is arable, but due to continued armed conflict, less than 6% is under cultivation. Irrigation techniques are primitive. There is hardly any use of chemical fertilizers, pesticides, or agricultural implements. Spring rainfall is erratic and water availability is dependent on the melting of the mountain snow in summer. Frozen products are rarely used because of lack of refrigeration in most households.

The majority of Afghan meals revolve around various *pilaos* derived from Persian influences, the most famous of which is *quabili pilao*. Other foods, such as *mantu* and *aash*, prepared with dumplings and noodles, most definitely stem from Afghanistan's Altaic neighbors in the north. Dill, mint, and yogurt remain some of the mandatory condiments at any Afghan dinner table.

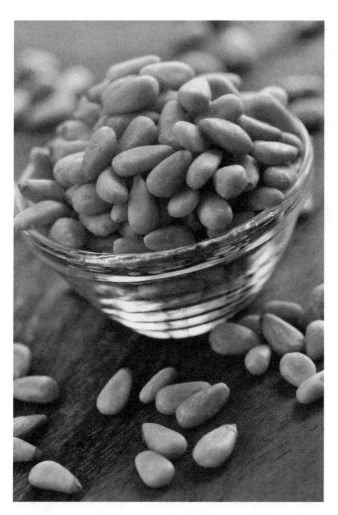

Pine nuts are served as a supplementary source of protein, and often are enjoyed while sipping a cup of green tea.

 Major Foods

 Protein Sources

The main protein source in Afghanistan is meat: lamb, sheep, goat, chicken, and beef. Mountain goats and deer are occasional meat sources depending upon hunting seasons. Various types of kabobs are extremely popular. Almonds, pistachios, and pine nuts also serve as a supplementary source of protein, often enjoyed while sipping green tea.

 Starch Sources

Wheat, rye, corn, barley, and rice are the main grains in the country and are grown by traditional means.

They are consumed in the form of rice, dumplings, and bread. *Tandoori naan*, a thick leavened bread cooked in an earthen oven, accompanies every meal.

 Prominent Vegetables

Vegetables grown are aubergines, carrots, chickpeas, cucumbers, leeks, onions, okra, potatoes, spinach, tomatoes, and zucchini.

 Prominent Fruits

A variety of fruits are grown in Afghanistan depending upon the topography of the land. Some of the prominent fruits include apples, grapes, melons, apricots, cherries, figs, mulberries, and pomegranates. Various types of raisins are also produced from grapes, and many of the fruits are utilized in Afghani cuisine, especially in the rice *palaus*.

 Beverages

Black or green tea is the most common beverage.

 Desserts

The most famous Afghani sweets include baklava and various types of *halva*.

 Typical Day's Menu

Afghan foods are usually a mixed affair and are spiced but not spicy. A breakfast can be as simple as a cup of boiled rice, a small amount of oil, and a spoonful of diluted yogurt all mixed together. A piece of *naan* and a cup of black tea are also common at breakfast. An egg omelet and *naan* is a breakfast presently reserved for the most fortunate people.

Afghans eat meats that conform to the Sharia, or Islamic laws, which ultimately means no pork. For the most part, lamb and goat meats are preferred. Lunch and dinners are usually interchangeable with staples such as lamb and goat kabobs and some form of rice or *naan*. When visiting an Afghan house, especially in rural areas, one must accept the offer of drinking a cup of black or green tea, called *kava*. It is the easiest way to make a good impression on your Afghan host or hostess.

 Holiday Menus

Palau is a food for special occasions and made with rice, meat (lamb, sheep, or chicken), carrots, raisins,

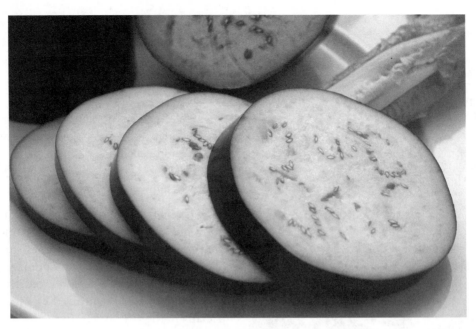

Eggplant is commonly grown in the Far East.

and pine nuts. Eggs, yogurt, pickled fruits and vegetables, and cheese are used quite often.

Afghanistan is discussed in greater detail in Chapter 20.

PAKISTAN

 ### Culture and World Region

Pakistani culture is largely dominated by Islam. Pakistan was once a part of the British colony of India before independence; therefore, Pakistan's culture is influenced by India and also by the British. Several important holidays are observed in Pakistan during the year, depending upon the Islamic calendar (lunar calendar). Ramadan, the 9th month of the calendar, is characterized by sunrise-to-sunset fasting for 29–30 days. Eid ul-Fitr is a celebration that follows at the end of Ramadan. In the second major festivity, which is Eid ul-Adha, an animal is sacrificed in remembrance of the actions of prophet Ibrahim (Abraham) and the meat is shared with friends, family, and the less fortunate. Both Eid festivals are public holidays. It gives people an opportunity to visit family and friends, and cook special meals, as well as make new clothes for the children and give presents and sweets to them. Muslims of Pakistan also celebrate Eid e-Milad-un-Nabi, the birthday of the prophet Muhammad, in the third month of the Islamic lunar calendar called *Rabi'al-Awal*. Muslims mark the

Day of Ashurah on the 9th and 10th days of the first month of the Islamic lunar calendar (Muharram) to commemorate the martyrdom of Husayn bin Ali (the grandson of Muhammad). These two days are national holidays and official and private businesses are closed, because people observe holidays with great reverence and respect. Food is distributed among the needy and mass prayers are held.

The Islamic Republic of Pakistan is a multiethnic, racially diverse country in South Asia. Its 540,403 square miles makes is slightly larger than Britain and France combined, and ranks it the 53rd country in population density in the world. It has 650 miles of Arabian Sea coastline in the south, Afghanistan and Iran as neighbors in the west, is bordered by India in the east, and China is located in the far northeast corner. Pakistan is divided into five administrative units called provinces; namely, Punjab, North West Frontier Province (NWFP), Baluchistan, Sindh, and Azad Kashmir (Pakistan Administered Kashmir Region).

 ### Language

Pakistan's national language is Urdu, but due to the British colonial legacy, the official language is English, which is also the language used in most of the schools and universities. In addition, the names of some of Pakistan dishes remain in Hindu, as the national language of Urdu was not proclaimed until 1950. Prior, both languages were commonly used.

Culture History

Pakistan became an independent state on August 14, 1947. Prior to this, it was part of the Indian subcontinent, and as a result, part of the British Empire. The area that became the country of Pakistan has been inhabited by ancient cultures including the Neolithic era Mehrgarh, and the Bronze era Indus Valley Civilization (2500–1500 BCE) at Harappa and Mohenjo-Daro. Imprints of successive migrations and conquests of Harappan, Indo-Aryan, Persian, Grecian, Saka, Parthian, Kushan, White Hun, Afghan, Arab, Turkics, and the Mughals can be traced back for several centuries. In present-day Pakistan, Punjabi and Sindhi populations show more of Indo-Islamic impressions, and the northwestern population shows cultural affiliation with Afghanistan and Iran. This area encompasses the historic trade routes to and from Afghanistan, Iran, and the Silk Route to China.

Arab General Muhammad bin Qasim conquered Sindh and Multan in southern Punjab in 712 CE. The Pakistan government's official chronology states that "its foundation was laid" as a result of this invasion: several Muslim empires followed including the Ghaznavid, the Ghorid Kingdom, the Delhi Sultanate, and the Mughal Empire. Islam spread through Sufi missionary work during Muslim empires among Hindus and Buddhist populations. Gradual decline of the Mughal Empire in the 18th century brought Afghan, Balochis, and Sikh control over large areas now called Pakistan until the East India Company gained power over all of South Asia.

Armed uprisings against British colonial power ensued in 1857 and were suppressed by the British Royal Crown for the next 90 years. Peaceful protests initiated the break in the chains of slavery for good under the banner of the Congress party and leadership of Ghandi. Hindus and Muslims struggled together for a number of decades for freedom.

British India's prominent poet and philosopher, Dr. Muhammad Iqbal, proposed in 1930 that an autonomous state be created for the Indian Muslims in the northwestern part of British India. Based on this idea, Muhammad Ali Jinnah, as the leader of the Muslim League and representing the Lahore Resolution of 1940, proposed the idea of two independent nations, which ultimately led to the formation of the independent state of Pakistan on August 14, 1947 (with Muslim-majority areas in the east and northwestern parts of the British Indian Empire), one province called East Pakistan separated by the Hindu-dominated independent state of India, and the other called West Pakistan comprising four provinces: Punjab, Sindh, Baluchistan, and the NWFP. Mass migration of people across the newly independent states of India and Pakistan followed.

An overview of Pakistan's history reveals a unique culture that is wrapped in rich ancestral traditions where religion plays a paramount role in every aspect of life but is learning Western-style democracy through traumatic experiences.

 Food History Within the Culture

Pakistan has been a part of the world where explorers' invaders' and conquerors' footprints can be seen everywhere. Food patterns show Afghani, Iranian, and Turkish influences with an overall impact made by the Islamic doctrine. There is zero tolerance of any porcine products or liquor in any recipes. Pakistan is basically an agrarian society as a whole, but international food franchises, such as McDonald's, Kentucky Fried Chicken (KFC), Pizza Hut, Burger King, and Subway, are common sites in large cities such as Islamabad, Karachi, and Lahore. The prices charged at these outlets are beyond the reach of common wage earners in Pakistan, but they all seem to be operating profitably. Local restaurants sell *pakoras* (fried vegetable in chickpea flour batter), *tikkas* (shish kabobs), and *chapli kabobs* (hamburgers with chopped onions and mild or hot spice) with *naan* (thick leavened bread) or *roti* (unleavened flat bread).

A variety of vegetables, especially potatoes, are eaten fried in the form of pakoras. Pakora is a generic term applied to any vegetable deep fried in chickpea batter. It can be *aloo* (potato) pakoras, *gobi* (cauliflower) pakoras, or *bengun* (eggplant) pakoras. Potatoes and spinach are quite often mixed to make pakoras. Pakoras are the favorite items on restaurant menus and at social affairs.

Pakistanis consume too much fat, trans fat, and saturated fat in their daily diet as a result of eating many fried foods. Incidence of coronary artery disease, diabetes, and stroke are on the rise, especially in the urban population, due to lack of exercise and excessive caloric intake. Dispensation of dietetic principles is almost nonexistent in Pakistani academic institutions and public health information systems.

Canning or freezing of fruits and vegetables is sparse; availability of such products is untested in Pakistani markets. Frozen products are rarely used because of nonavailability of refrigerators in most households.

Even though refrigerators and freezers are commodities that the upper middle class can afford, ever-menacing electrical brownouts make buying frozen products an unwise expense.

 Major Foods

 Protein Sources

Lamb, sheep, or beef is commonly consumed but not preferred over goat. Chicken is the most consumed meat in Pakistani meals due to its affordability and availability as compared with other meats.

 Starch Sources

Wheat flour is staple foodstuff in Pakistan; thin un-leavened tortilla-like bread, called *roti*, is made from wheat and accompanies every meal. Pakistanis consume an estimated 22 million tons of wheat every year. Rice is produced and consumed, but consumption is less as compared with wheat. A wide variety of beans (*dal*) are eaten on a daily basis. *Dal* is cooked with hot spices, garlic, and onion, and is eaten with *roti* just like tortilla and beans in Mexico. *Dal* and *roti* are the average Pakistani's mainstay, with occasional consumption of chicken or goat.

 Fat Sources

Vegetable oils, vegetable shortening that looks like ghee, or fat rendered from natural butter are the main cooking fats. Butter and ghee are liked very much but can be afforded only by the privileged few.

 Prominent Vegetables

A wide variety of vegetables are grown and consumed, but their availability is seasonal. Most common vegetables available in open farmers' markets are an assortment of beans, green peas, green chickpeas in pods, leeks, potatoes, artichokes, spinach, mustard greens, turnip greens, cauliflower, eggplant, turnips, beets, cucumber, squash, zucchini, and radishes.

 Prominent Fruits

A wide assortment of fruit is available depending upon the season. Mango is the preferred fruit; other fruits enjoyed are apples, apricots, grapes, bananas, oranges, grapefruit, pomegranates, guava, peaches, prunes, and an assortment of berries.

 Spices and Seasonings

Spices, such as hot chili, turmeric, coriander, cumin, black peppers, green and black cardamoms, cloves, and cinnamon, are frequently used in dishes. Generous use of cilantro is very common in various meat and vegetable dishes, either as an ingredient or a garnish.

 Beverages

Hot tea with milk and sugar is the staple beverage.

 Desserts

Desserts are most often served with dinner and can be *halva*, *kheer*, *firni*, or *methai*, which is a generic name for numerous types of sweets that are national and regional and made by an array of ingredients such as wheat flour, chickpea flour, sugar, milk, and other dairy products.

 Typical Day's Menu

Breakfast is the simple meal of the day. It usually consists of *roti* smeared with small amounts of butter, then stacked in a container with a lid. Those *rotis* are served with a cup of hot tea with milk and sugar. Quite often milk, water, tea, and sugar are boiled together for a few minutes and the contents strained in a cup while piping hot. This tea is said to keep one cool in the hot summers and warm in winters. Western-style bread has become popular in urban areas, especially for breakfast as a substitute for *roti*, due to the British influence of 200 years. Eggs are used commonly in breakfast in the form of fried, boiled, scrambled, or omelettes with onions as well as green and red peppers. Eggs are also made into a sweet dish called *halva*.

Lunch and dinner usually consist of an assortment of meat curries, vegetable *bhugias*, and/or *dal*. Most common dishes made from meat are named after the meat it contains, such as mutton *korma*, beef *korma*, and chicken *korma*. *Korma* is a term like curry in India. Indian curry has spice that is not used in korma in Pakistani dishes. The mixed dishes contain a meat (*gosht*) and vegetable combination; the most common example would be *aloo gosht* (potato and meat), *mutter gosht* (green peas and meat), and *phullian* and *gosht* (green beans and meat). *Bhugia* is a generic term for a Pakistani vegetable dish. It is usually served in conjunction with a meat dish or *dal*. Onions, whether fried or nonfried, make the base for most of the Pakistani dishes. Garlic, ginger, red chilies, red peppers, and green peppers are an essential part of Pakistani cooking depending upon the dish being prepared. As a whole, Pakistani cuisine is a greasy and chili-hot affair. Although ingredients vary from region to region and family to family, they tend to remain on the higher side of greasiness and spicy hot in Punjab and Sindh, but are a lot milder in terms of chilies in the NWFP and Baluchistan.

Holiday Menus

Rice dishes, such as *palao* and *biryani*, are two favorites for special occasions such as religious holidays and weddings. *Naan* and *korma* usually accompanies either *palao* or *biryani*.

Health Beliefs and Concerns

The meat used in most meals is goat or beef. Beef is preferred as a matter of taste and cultural tradition in most regions except the NWFP. The belief that beef has hot qualities for the body is commonly held by most Pakistanis in the Punjab region in particular, which is the reason for its low consumption.

General Health and Nutritional Indicators Summary

Low birth weight, defined as weighing less than 2500 g at birth, affects 19% of newborns in Pakistan (UNICEF, 2007). Sixteen percent of the nation's children are exclusively breastfed during the first 4 months of life. Thirty-one percent of infants 6–9 months are breastfed with complementary food, and 56% remain breastfed at 20–23 months of age.

Thirty-eight percent of the nation's children below the age of 5 years suffer from being moderately to severely underweight (UNICEF, 2007). Being severely underweight affects 13% of Pakistan's children. Moderate to severe wasting was found in 13% and stunting in 37% of this particular population. The nation has a 95% vitamin A supplementation coverage rate for individuals ages 6–59 months. Only 17% of all households in Pakistan consume adequately iodized salt.

Ninety-one percent of Pakistan's total population uses improved drinking-water sources (UNICEF, 2007). Specifically, 96% of the urban population and 89% of the rural population has access to improved drinking-water sources.

CHINA

Culture and World Region

The People's Republic of China, established by Mao Zedong on October 1, 1949, encompasses territories that are one of the most ancient civilizations on the planet. Fifty-six different cultures share this ancient land called China. A 5000-year history reveals that cultures developed independent of each other in different geographical regions. Each Chinese culture shuns the idea of learning from outsiders, whom they have always considered inferior. Of the many cultures, the predominant group is called Han. In spite of the cultural divide, the country as a whole has been under various rulers, three sovereigns and five emperors who belonged to various dynasties. During the Zhou Dynasty (1046–256 BCE), Chinese society was divided into a hierarchical system of socioeconomic classes known as the four occupations. The Chinese as a whole are proud to call themselves descendents of Huang Di, or Yellow Emperor, a tribal chief who lived in the Yellow River Valley more than four millenia ago. The socioeconomic distinctions and divisions became blurred during the Song Dynasty (960–1279 BCE) due to commercialization.

Chinese education has a long history; imperial examinations were administered to the national bureaucrats (Sui Dynasty 581–618 CE) and trades and crafts were taught by Sifu. Women's education was outlined by female scholars such as Ban Zhao during the Han Dynasty and those lessons were expanded by Zhu and Cheng Yi and other scholars. Chinese marriages are mixed influences of culture and Taoism.

China has over 1.6 billion people excluding the special territories of Hong Kong and Macao. At the end of 2000 China had 663 large cities of which 13 cities had a population of more than 2 million people, and 27 cities, between 1 and 2 million people. Beijing, the capital, has a population of about 12 million people.

Language

The official language of China is Chinese. Other languages spoken in the country include Mandarin, Cantonese, and Hakka.

Food History Within the Culture

Most of the cuisines in China originated in the emperors' kitchens of various dynasties. Over a period of time these cooking styles became commonplace. Still, most of the population living in rural China lives on a very simple diet of boiled rice and steamed vegetables with very little fat, and they are basically subsistence farmers, meaning they eat what they grow from the soil on which they live. It is a common misconception that all Chinese people eat rice as a staple food. A large number of Chinese living in the north, in arid China, grow wheat and subsist on it and eat rice only occasionally. The origin of wheat is traced back to 1500 BCE in China during the Han Dynasty. The way the wheat is consumed is quite different than in the West: it is consumed in the form of noodles, *mantou* (steamed bun), or a dumpling called *jiaozi*. Steamed wheat buns filled with pork, called *boazi*, are a common food in China. Some pan breads are also made. The demand for pan bread and processed foods is on the rise.

In China, the dominant part of cuisine is a starchy food: noodles or *mantou* in the northern areas, and rice in the southern regions. In the most formal cuisines no rice is served, and if served, it is fried at the end of the meal. Soup is served at the beginning and at the end of the meal in southern China. No dessert is served at the end of a formal Chinese meal; instead, delicately cut fruit or a sweet soup is served.

On the eighth day of the last month of the Chinese lunar calendar, people enjoy a multiple-grain porridge called *La Ba Zhou*, a tradition started by monks in ancient times but one that is still practiced by some country folk.

Coming home after a long period of being away signifies a special occasion for the Chinese in the northeast. They mark it by cooking noodles for the return (after having cooked dumplings for the departure).

China is rapidly changing from land subsistence to commercially driven agriculture. Coastal areas, such as Shanghai, Guangzhou, Shenzhen, Dalian, and Qingdao, are leading the way due to prosperity and fewer governmental restrictions. Foreign food operations, such as Pizza Hut, McDonald's, and Kentucky Fried Chicken (KFC) are cropping up. Still, about half of China's population live on farms and grow their own vegetables and grains, on which they subsist. According to China's Bureau of Statistics, rural Chinese still rely primarily on grains, whereas urbanites consume more red meat, fish, and shrimp.

 Major Foods

 Protein Sources

Red meat, fish, and shrimp are the main sources of protein consumed by the urbanites of China.

 Starch Sources

Rice, noodles, and *mantou* are the predominant sources of starch in Chinese diets.

 Fat Sources

Fatty fish, pork fat (lard), and butter comprise the Chinese fat sources.

 Prominent Vegetables

The Chinese eat various vegetables, mostly steamed, such as mushrooms, broccoli, cabbage, cauliflower, potatoes, and sweet potatoes.

 Prominent Fruits

Raw fruits that are commonly consumed in the Chinese diet include apples, bananas, pears, grapes, tomatoes, and various citrus fruits.

 Beverages

The most common beverages at a Chinese dinner table are hot green tea or hot water.

 Desserts

Very few desserts are eaten in China. In formal dinners there is no dessert other than thinly sliced fruit.

 Typical Day's Menu

Breakfast is not commonly deemed an important event in Chinese culture. It usually consists of rice porridge and soy-milk soup. At lunchtime one might find a hearty noodle soup or the traditional *dim sum*. For dinner one would find chicken, pork, fish, and shrimp dishes in various sauces served with noodles or rice. Many steamed vegetables are found alongside main dishes as well.

 Holiday Menus

Dragon Boat Festival is celebrated by most Chinese, although all of them cannot reach the river to watch the boat race but certainly enjoy a special meal called *zongzi*, a pyramid-shaped dumpling made with glutinous rice and wrapped in bamboo or reed leaves. The festival marks the patriotic poet Qu Yuan, who venerated scarcity of food (although foods are made in plenty of colors and styles today).

In Central China a baby's birth is celebrated by distributing boiled eggs with certain numbers of black pointed dots. An even number of dots, such as six or eight, with a point are marked for a boy, and an odd number, such as five or seven, and without a point, are for a girl.

Fish is considered a sign of prosperity and accumulation of wealth, and is a favorite in various dishes on Chinese New Year's Eve.

Chopsticks have historical significance in China. They spread from there to North Korea, South Korea, Japan, and Southeast Asia. Chopsticks are a simple but unique invention of Chinese people that can be used for eating, nipping, picking, ripping, and stirring the food. Chopsticks are given as a gift in marriage and other important ceremonies as a token of good luck.

 Health Beliefs and Concerns

It is believed by the Chinese that hot beverages, especially hot tea, aids in the digestion of food.

 General Health and Nutritional Indicators Summary

Low birth weight, defined as weighing less than 2500 g at birth, affects 4% of newborns in China (UNICEF, 2007). Fifty-one percent of the nation's children are exclusively breastfed during the first 6 months of life. Thirty-two percent of infants 6–9 months are breastfed with complementary food, and 15% remain breastfed at 20–23 months of age.

Eight percent of the nation's children below the age of 5 years suffer from being moderately to severely underweight (UNICEF, 2007). Moderate to severe stunting was found in 14% of this particular population. The great majority (93%) of all households in China consume adequately iodized salt.

Seventy-seven percent of China's total population uses improved drinking-water sources (UNICEF, 2007). Specifically, 93% of the population in the nation's urban areas and 67% of the rural population has access to improved drinking-water sources.

BANGLADESH

 Culture and World Region

The Democratic Republic of Bangladesh is a country that was carved out of the Bengal province of British India as the east wing of the newly formed country,

Pakistan, in 1947. Due to politico–cultural differences, armed civil unrest broke out against the federal government of Pakistan in the 1970s. Indian forces crossed the international boundary of East Pakistan in 1971, which resulted in the creation of the independent state of Bangladesh. Bangladesh has 159 million people within an area of 55,598 square miles. The country is surrounded by India, except in the south, where it borders the Bay of Bengal and Myanmar (formerly Burma). This is one of the most densely populated areas in the world. The majority of the population is Muslim. Dhaka is the capital of Bangladesh, with a population of 3.5 million people.

After the liberation war, with help from India and the Soviet Union, Bangladesh was born, but its development has since been marred by political turmoil, with 14 different heads of government and at least four military coups. Bangladesh is trying to adapt to a western style of democracy with a parliamentary system of government. Currently, there is a military rule in place with President Iajuddin Ahmed as head of state.

 Language

Bengali, the official language, boasts a rich heritage.

 Food History Within the Culture

Bangladesh has a beautiful deltaic landscape with three major rivers: the Ganges (local name *Padma* or *Pôdda*), the Brahmaputra (*Jamuna* or *Jomuna*), the Meghna, and their respective tributaries. The Ganges unites with the Jamuna (main channel of the Brahmaputra) and later joins the Meghna to eventually empty into the Bay of Bengal. The alluvial soil deposited by these rivers has created some of the most fertile plains in the world. Although the soil is fertile, there are relatively few hectares of land available for agriculture because of the deluge of water. Bangladesh has miles of marshy jungle called sundarbans, and it has the largest mangrove forest in the world. Mangrove forestations are good stabilizers of the environment. Agriculture is mostly cultivated by primitive methods. There is a constant decline of agricultural employment due to the lack of economic support, fertilizers, and low yield per acre due to primitive methods of cultivation. Bangladesh has not been able to find ways to use its own natural resources for domestic consumption; instead, much of the jute cultivated is exported to countries such as India. There is no significant industrialization of the country to justify allocation of national resources for land reform or manpower. Most of the foreign exchange comes to the country through remittances by the expatriates working overseas. Three fourths of the Bangladeshis are farmers, but the garment industry is flourishing due to foreign investment. Jute, rice, tobacco, tea, sugarcane, vegetables, potato, lentils, and beans are grown in the country. Jute is the principle export but has diminished due to the advent of polyester fiber. Mango, banana, pineapple, jackfruit, watermelon, green coconut, guava, and lichees are imported.

Bangladesh has a rich history of cuisine dating back to the Mughal Dynasty. Meat and vegetable dishes are relished. Kalia is a favorite meat dish. Most often rice dishes are favored, but wheat is also eaten in the form of *chapati*. Culinary cuisines are quite similar to Indian and Middle Eastern cuisines, with their own twist. Fish and rice are prominent in dishes that have a variety of spice.

 ## Major Foods

 ### Protein Sources

Fish is the main source of protein for the nation as a whole, although goat, sheep, and lamb are consumed by Muslims.

 ### Starch Sources

Rice is the main staple and largest source of starch in the country. Other sources include bread made of wheat called *chopattis*.

 ### Fat Sources

Mustard oil and other vegetable oils used in cooking are the main source of fat.

 ### Prominent Vegetables

Eggplant, cauliflower, okra, leafy vegetables, and small onions are most commonly used in Bangladesh.

 ### Prominent Fruits

Mango, banana, pineapple, jackfruit, watermelon, green coconut, and guava are the most common fruits.

 ### Beverages

Hot tea with milk and sugar added is the most popular beverage.

 ### Desserts

Bangladeshis make distinctive sweets from milk and rice, such as *rosghula*, *chomchom*, *sondesh*, and *kalojam*.

 ## Typical Day's Menu

Breakfast for the Bangladeshis usually consists of flour *naan* smeared with oil or butter and potatoes cooked in a curry sauce. Items made for lunch can also be eaten at dinner. Shukto, a bitter vegetable curry, can be served with rice, along with *dal* and something fried that is *bhajal* (vegetable, such as pumpkin or other seasonal vegetables). Fish is definitely at the lunch or dinner table, because it is part of the Bangladeshi staple diet.

 ## Holiday Menus

Eid ul-Fitr and Eid ul-Adha are two important festivals for the Muslim population. Other Muslim holidays are observed with religious fervor. Minorities, such as Christians, celebrate Christmas (*Borodin*), and Hindus celebrate Durga Puja and Saraswati Puja. Buddhists and Jews celebrate their holidays with complete religious freedom. Important secular festivals are Pohela Baishakh or Bengali New Year.

 ## General Health and Nutritional Indicators Summary

Low birth weight, defined as weighing less than 2500 g at birth, affects 36% of newborns in Bangladesh (UNICEF, 2007). Thirty-six percent of the nation's children are exclusively breastfed during the first 6 months of life. Sixty-nine percent of infants 6–9 months are breastfed with complementary food, and 90% remain breastfed at 20–23 months of age.

Forty-eight percent of the nation's children below the age of 5 years suffer from being moderately to severely underweight (UNICEF, 2007). Being severely underweight affects 13% of Bangladesh's children. Moderate to severe wasting was found in 13% and stunting in 43% of this particular population. The nation has an 83% vitamin A supplementation coverage rate for individuals ages 6–59 months. The majority (70%) of all households in Bangladesh consume adequately iodized salt.

Seventy-four percent of Bangladesh's total population uses improved drinking-water sources (UNICEF, 2007). Specifically, 82% of the population in the nation's urban areas and 72% of the rural population has access to improved drinking-water sources.

FEATURED RECIPE

Chinese Jiaozi (Chinese Dumplings)

Dough:

¼ tsp. salt

3 cups all-purpose flour

1¼ cups cold water

Filling:

1 tbsp. Chinese rice wine or dry sherry

1 tbsp. soy sauce

1 clove garlic, peeled and finely minced

1 tsp. salt

¼ tsp. freshly ground white pepper (or to taste)

3 tbsp. sesame oil

½ green onion, finely minced

1 cup ground pork or beef

1½ cups finely shredded napa cabbage

4 tbsp. shredded bamboo shoots

2 slices fresh ginger, finely minced

1. To prepare the dough, mix the salt into the flour. Slowly add the cold water, forming a smooth dough. Knead the dough into a smooth ball. Cover and let it rest for at least 30 minutes.

2. To prepare the filling, add the soy sauce, salt, rice wine, and white pepper to the meat, stirring in only one direction. Add the remaining ingredients, stirring in the same direction, and mix well.

3. To prepare the dumplings, divide the dough into roughly 55–60 smooth balls. Roll each ball out into a circle about 3 inches in diameter. Place a small amount of filling into the middle of each 3-inch-diameter dough wrap. Wet the edges of the dumpling with water. Fold the dough over the filling into a half-moon shape and pinch the edges to seal it. Repeat until all the dumplings are filled.

4. In a large pot bring water to a boil. Add the dumplings, stirring gently so that they do not stick to one another, then bring the water to a boil again. Add ½ cup of cold water to the pot; cover and bring water to a boil for a third time. Drain and remove.

More recipes are available at http://nutrition.jbpub.com/foodculture/

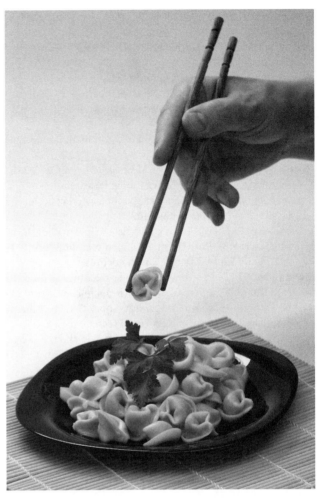

Chinese Dumplings

REFERENCES

Adamec, L.W. (1991). *Historical dictionary of Afghanistan.* Metuchen, NJ: Scarecrow Press.

Akand, M.K. (2005). Folk culture and urban adaptation. *Asian Folklore Studies, 64*(1), 39(14).

Balagopal, P. (2000). *Indian and Pakistani food practices.* Chicago: American Dietetic Association & American Diabetes Association.

Banerji, C. (2006). *Feeding the Gods: Memories of food and culture in Bengal.* Calcutta, India: Seagull.

Bangladesh: A policy analysis of their success or failure. (2008). *PA Times, 31,* 6(2).

Chan, A.L. (2001). *Mao's crusade: Politics and policy implementation in China's great leap forward.* Oxford, UK: Oxford University Press.

Chi-Tim, L. (1980–2002). Daoism in China today. *The China Quarterly, 174.*

Economic Overview. (2008). *Bangladesh Country Review, 79*(25).

Edmonds, R.L. (2002). China and Europe since 1978: An introduction. *The China Quarterly, 169.*

Environmental Overview. (2008). *Bangladesh Country Review, 147*(37).

Export Target Out of Reach. (2008). *Asia Monitor: South Asia Monitor, 14*(3), 6(0).

The Fishing Fields. (2004). *Economist, 372,* 76.

Gerth, K. (2003). *China made: Consumer culture and the creation of the nation.* Cambridge, MA, and London: Harvard University Press.

Gladney, D.C. (2003). Islam in China: Accommodation or separatism? *The China Quarterly, 174.*

Hobbs, F. (1987). *Afghanistan: A demographic profile.* Washington, DC: Center for International Research.

Kilara A., & Iya K.K. (1992). Food and dietary practices of the Hindu. *Food Technology,* 94–102.

Lindenbaum, S. (1987). Loaves and fishes in Bangladesh. In M. Harris & E. Ross (Eds.), *Food and evolution* (pp. 427–443). Philadelphia: Temple Unversity Press.

Moreno, M. (1992). Pancamirtam: God's washings as food. In R.S. Khare (Ed), *Eternal food: Gastronomic ideas and experiences of Hindus and Buddhists* (pp. 147–178). Albany, NY: State University of New York Press.

Nair, K.N. (1987). Animal protein consumption and the sacred cow complex in India. In M. Harris & E. Ross (Eds.), *Food and evolution.* Philadelphia: Temple Unversity Press

Parkinson, R. (1998). *Decadent desserts.* Retrieved April 2, 2008, from http://www.chinesefood.about.com/library/weekly/aa092499.html/

Political Overview. (2008). *Bangladesh Country Review, 7*(71).

Regional Indicators. (2008). *Asia Monitor: South Asia Monitor, 14*(3), 1(0).

Riyaja, A. (2003). "God willing": The politics and ideology of Islamism in Bangladesh. *Comparative Studies of South Asia, Africa and the Middle East, 23*(1)(2), 301–320.

Rizvi, N. (1986). Food categories in Bangladesh and its relationship to food beliefs and the practices of vulnerable groups. In S. Khare & M. Rao (Eds.), *Food, society and culture.* Durham, NC: Carolina Academic Press.

Roberts, J.A.G. (2002). *China to Chinatown: Chinese food in the west.* London: Reaktion Books.

Roger, D. (2000). The Middle East and South Asia. In K.F. Kiple & K.C. Ornelas (Eds.), *The Cambridge world history of food* (pp. 1140–1151). Cambridge: Cambridge University Press.

Sarker, A., et al. (2006). Entrepreneurships barriers of pond fish culture in Bangladesh: A case study from Mymensingh district. *Journal of Social Sciences, 2*(3), 68(6).

Sleeboom-Faulkner, M. (2006). How to define a population: Cultural politics and population genetics in the People's Republic of China and the Republic of China. *BioSocieties, 1*(04), 399–419.

Social Overview. (2008). *Bangladesh Country Review, 119*(27).

UNICEF. (2007). *The state of the world's children 2007: Women and children, the double dividend of gender equality.* Retrieved April 14, 2009, from http://www.unicef.org/sowc07/statistics/tables.php/

White, D. (1992). You are what you eat: The anomalous status of dog-cookers in Hindu mythology. In R.S. Khare (Ed.), *Eternal food: Gastronomic ideas and experiences of Hindus and Buddhists* (pp. 53–93). Albany, NY: State University of New York Press.

CHAPTER 23

India
(Southern Region)

Sudha Raj, PhD, RD

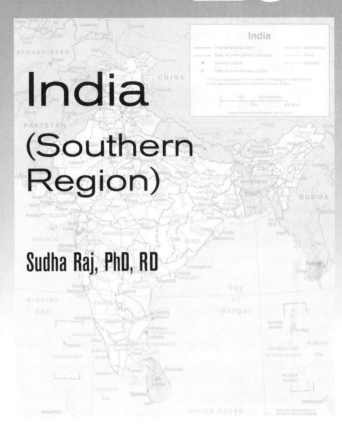

 ## CULTURE AND WORLD REGION

The triangular peninsular plateau in the South Asian subcontinent of India is known as the Deccan Plateau or *dakshin*, which means south in Sanskrit. This chapter focuses on the southern states of Tamil Nadu, Kerala, Karnataka, Andhra Pradesh, Goa, and the union territories of Lakshadweep, Pondicherry, Andaman Islands, and Nicobar Islands. In addition to geographic and religious diversity, each region is characterized by its own language, culture, customs, architecture, regional cuisine, and interregional culinary specialties. Despite the diversity, certain common elements define South Indian culture and cuisine, differentiating it from North India. The topography as well as the warm and moist climate of the peninsular plateau allow for the agricultural production of two or three rice crops annually along with a variety of tropical and subtropical food products that impact the regional cuisines.

The Deccan plateau is a kaleidoscope of geographic diversity bordered by the Vindhya mountain ranges in the north, the Arabian Sea in the west, the Bay of Bengal in the east, and the Indian Ocean at the southern tip. The western and eastern ends of the plateau culminate at the mountain ranges known as the Western and Eastern Ghats. The ghats begin as highlands and mountainous terrain in the north, gradually wind south parallel to the coastlines, and terminate as foothills along the waters of the Arabian Sea to the west and the Bay of Bengal to the east. At higher elevations, the Western Ghats are water fed by the southwest monsoon winds from June through August. Rivers that originate in the Western Ghats flow west through Goa and empty into the Arabian Sea. This region is home to lush, evergreen, and deciduous forests that support a diverse vegetation, flora, fauna, marine life, and animal habitat. Timber, sandalwood, and bamboo are well-known commercial forest products of this region. Plantations of coffee, tea, and spices abound in the relatively cool and adequately moist climate. Between the Western Ghats and the Arabian Sea lie the wide coastal strips of Konkan and Malabar, which are well known for natural harbors, sandy beaches, backwaters, lagoons, rice paddy fields, sugarcane, coconut, and palm groves, rubber and cashew plantations, and a vast array of seafood (Singh, 1976).

In direct contrast are the lower elevations of the Eastern Ghats, which consist of plateaus and flat terrain. This region is water fed by the retreating northeast monsoon winds from November through January and the rivers that flow through the ghats that create the narrow Coromandel coastal plain on the southeastern coast. The soil conditions and limited precipitation in this region are conducive to the farming of legumes, pulses, oilseeds, grains (such as sorghum, ragi, and millets), tobacco, groundnuts, and red chilies (Singh, 1976). The major rivers of the Deccan Peninsula, namely, the Krishna, Cauvery, and Godavari, rise in the Western Ghats and, together with smaller rivers, tributaries, and estuaries, cut through the Eastern Ghats into the Bay of Bengal, creating fertile deltas and rice granaries on the southeastern coast.

South India enjoys a tropical climate with three seasons: summer, winter, and monsoon. Summer extends from March through June; April and May are the hottest months with inland temperatures soaring to 40°C (Singh, 1976). The coastal plains experience considerable humidity during the summer with some respite offered by the cool night sea breeze. The intense heat of the south, complemented by the low pressure in North India, causes the southwesterly jet stream from the Arabian Sea to rise above the towering Western Ghats. This provides the needed precipitation and relief from the hot, humid weather from June through August to the states of Kerala, Karnataka, parts of Andhra Pradesh, and the coastal plains adjoining the Ghats. Following the monsoon, the plateau enjoys cool weather through November; however, the retreating northeast monsoon winds provide precipitation from November through January. The rain-shadowed Tamil Nadu and coastal Andhra Pradesh do not benefit from the southwestern monsoon winds.

 LANGUAGE

The official South Indian regional languages spoken are Tamil in Tamil Nadu, Malayalam in Kerala, Kannada in Karnataka, and Telugu in Andhra Pradesh. Marathi, Tulu, and Konkani are the regional languages of Goa;

residents of Pondicherry speak the southern regional languages of Tamil, Telugu, Malayalam, and French influenced by earlier colonial settlements. Malayalam is also the official language of the Lakshadweep Islands along with Mahl, an Arabic derivative (Maps of India, 2008), and other regional languages of the island's migrants. English is the official unifying language of communication throughout South India. Several academic institutions use English as the primary medium of oral and written instruction along with the secondary regional language specific to the state. Hindi is also an official language of India; however, it is spoken by only a small percentage of the southern population.

 CULTURE HISTORY

The South was generally insulated from the political struggles that shaped the history of North India. A limited but significant number of influences from the North included (1) the introduction of the Sanskrit language that had tremendous literary impact on the southern regional languages, and (2) the spread of Buddhism and Jainism by the powerful Mauryan Empire from the North (Shastri, 1955). Chandragupta Maurya and his successors, including Emperor Ashoka, were disillusioned by the perils of warfare and embraced Jainism and Buddhism. The Mauryan emperors are credited for spreading these religions to Karnataka and Andhra Pradesh during their sojourn to the South.

Archaelogical findings and Tamil literature draw attention to the existence of southern dynasties and the frequent internal political struggles between several smaller kingdoms after the 6th century. The Chalukyas of Badami in the Western Deccan, the Pallavas of Kanchi, the powerful Chola kingdom of the Coramandel coast, and smaller kingdoms, such as the Pandyas of Madurai and the Cheras of the Malabar Coast, were instrumental in shaping the region's history (Basham, 1959). Each dynasty and kingdom made significant cultural contributions in the realms of art, music, dance, architecture, literature, and trade.

Other historical developments of cultural consequence include the Muslim invasion in the 13th century; the subsequent rise of the sultanates in Karnataka, north Kerala, and the Nizam of Hyderabad; and the rise and fall of the Vijayanagar Empire, which prospered and fostered the arrival of the Europeans. Specifically, the Portugese were the first to arrive on the western coast. They introduced Christianity to the Malabar and Konkan coast. The Dutch and the French followed to expand seafaring operations and spice trade with Southeast Asia. Finally, the British arrived in the 1600s and established the East India Company in Madras, Tamil Nadu. The British eventually controlled trade in the entire Deccan with the long-term interest of monopolizing the entire country. All of these developments left an indelible impression on the cultural, religious, and social ethos of the land.

Religion

Hinduism

Hinduism is practiced by over 80% of the population in South India. Hindus believe in the Supreme Being, *Brahman* (Swami Tejomayananda, 1993), who creates as Brahma, preserves as Vishnu, and destroys evil as Shiva. A multitude of gods and goddesses are worshipped (Mitchell, 1982). Examples include Ganesh, the elephant-headed God; Lakshmi, the goddess of wealth and prosperity; Saraswati, the giver of knowledge; and Shakti, the mother goddess or provider of strength. Hindus believe in becoming one with the Supreme Being by transforming into a state of divine consciousness that occurs over several rebirths (reincarnation). Hindus follow the religious tenets of purity, self-control, detachment, renunciation, truth, nonviolence, and *bhakti* (emotional surrender to the Supreme Being).

Hinduism emphasizes the value of righteousness or acting according to *dharma* or the religious code. Religious scriptures, such as the Vedas, Upanishads, and Bhagavat Purana, encompass the religious teachings, codified rules, and observances. South Indian Hindu temples, the places of worship for Hindus, are architectural marvels built centuries ago based on astrological and religious laws. The South Indian temple has a central sanctum known as the *Garbagriha* that houses the deity and a superstructure known as the *vimana* that rises above the shrine. Temples have a colorful pyramidal tower or *gopuram* adorned with beautiful carvings of gods, goddesses, and other figures. Rituals are led by temple priests who belong to the Brahmin caste.

Islam

About 10% of South Indians follow Islam, with a greater concentration of Muslims in Andhra Pradesh (Hyderabad Muslims), Kerala (Mapillas), and Karnataka. Islam was introduced to South India in 636 (Shastri, 1955) by Muslim traders settling on the southwestern Malabar coast. Followers of Islam believe in the surrender to the will of Allah as codified in the religious scripture, the *Quran*. All Muslims follow the Five Pillars of Islam: *shahadah* (the declaration of their faith), *sala* (prayer five times a day), *zakat* (charitable donations or service for goodwill), *sawm* (fasting during Ramadan), and *haj* (pilgrimage to Mecca) (Kittler & Sucher, 2007).

Christianity

Less than 3% of the South Indian population is Christian. Historical accounts ascribe the introduction of Christianity to the Malabar region by St. Thomas in 52 AD; however, its presence strengthened after the arrival of the Portuguese and other Europeans (Shastri, 1955). The predominant Christian communities include the Syrian Christians of the Malabar coast; the Goan Christian community, which consists of the descendents of the Dominicans, Franciscans, and Jesuits in the former Portuguese colony in Goa; and the Protestant community, which was introduced by the Dutch and the British.

Other Religions

Religions with a smaller following include Jainism, founded by Mahavira in the 6th century, which follows the tenet of *ahimsa* (nonviolence toward all sentient beings); Buddhism, founded by Gautama Buddha in the 5th century and brought to South India by the Mauryan kings; Sikhism, founded in the 15th century by Guru Nanak; and Judaism, followed in the Malabar region of Cochin, which houses the oldest synagogue (Singh et al., 2007). Several tribal religions are also practiced in rural South India.

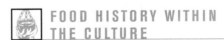

FOOD HISTORY WITHIN THE CULTURE

Food is often a limitless symbol of a culture's worldview. For example, all cultures have their own selective ways of defining "food," "meals and meal patterns," and identifying foods that are acceptable and prohibited for human consumption. Tastes, the ability to satisfy nutritional needs, selective use of particular foods, and food combinations for festivities, celebrations, and rituals are different ways that cultures symbolize foods. Hindu religious scriptures; namely, the Upanishads and the Bhagavat Gita, state, "From food do all creatures come into being" (Achaya, 1994). Food in the Indian cultures is not only a means of sustenance but a way of life. Over the centuries, a host of implicit but complex traditions, rules, and customs have developed in the realms of food production, processing, distribution, and consumption. Many of these traditions continue to be followed. This, coupled with regional varieties in agricultural products, have contributed to a rich diversity in food patterns and cuisines throughout India.

Feasts

Each religion has celebrations and festivals throughout the year during which food plays an important role. Celebrations are an expression of happiness related to the harvest, life events (e.g., births, an adoration of nature, birth of prophets), and other occasions. Rituals performed on special occasions, such as during pregnancy, and festivals are accompanied by feasts. Generous amounts of traditional foods and sweets are prepared and offered to the gods before distribution for human consumption (Patil, 1994). Festive meals include preparations that consist of ghee, rice, lentils (such as urad dal and chana dal), turmeric, native vegetables, jaggery, spices, coconut, and fruit such as bananas, desserts, betel leaf, and arecanut.

Fasts are common among followers of all religions. For instance, Muslims fast during the month of Ramadan from dawn to dusk, and orthodox Hindus fast on festival days and certain days in the lunar months, particularly the 11th day of the lunar fortnight (Achaya, 1994). The frequency and duration of a fast is variable and dependent on the individual. Fasts involve eating after moonrise, and abstinence from a particular food or food category either for the entire day or part of the day. Foods eaten during a fast include fruits only, fruits and milk, or preparations using cereals such as broken or puffed rice, or tapioca. Ghee and rock salt are permitted during certain fasts; others may eat sweets such as *ladoos* and *kesari bhath* during a fast.

 MAJOR FOODS

South India boasts a vast array of cereal grains, lentils, tropical fruits, vegetables, spices, and seafood.

 Protein Sources

Pulses (lentils, beans, and peas) form the basis for traditional dishes such as *dal, sambar, rasam,* and *kootu.* Red, green, and white lentils are commonly used in South Indian cuisine. The lentils are boiled and mixed with vegetables, spices, and/or coconut. Lentils are also combined with rice or other cereals in dishes such as

pongal, idlis, and *dosas,* and provide complementary proteins. Although the cuisine is largely plant based and vegetarian, fish is an important protein staple in the coastal regions. Chicken, eggs, lamb, and mutton are protein sources for nonvegetarians. Pork and beef dishes are popular among the Christian populations. Other protein sources include dairy products such as milk, yogurt, buttermilk, and ghee.

 Starch Sources

Rice and parboiled rice are the staple grains in all the southern states. Different forms of rice, such as puffed rice, beaten rice, rice sticks, rice flour, and cream of rice, are used in a variety of preparations. Other regional-based grains include barley, ragi, tapioca, jowar, millet, maize, and wheat products such as wheat flour, semolina, and vermicelli. Potatoes, sweet potatoes, green plantains, different varieties of yams, and colocasia provide starch in the diets.

 Fat Sources

The oils from coconut, sesame, peanut, gingelly, sunflower, and canola are used. Ghee or clarified butter is added to rice in everyday meals and also used in the preparation of dishes for special occasions. Hydrogenated vegetable shortening, vegetable oil, and peanut/gingelly oil are used for shallow and deep frying. Nuts, such as almonds, cashews, peanuts, gingelly seeds, and sesame seeds, are used in desserts and main-meal preparations.

 Prominent Vegetables

The tropical weather and fertile soil in South India are conducive to the cultivation of a variety of tropical vegetables and fruits. Local markets carry produce that is picked fresh daily. It is not uncommon to see vendors peddling their produce-laden carts in the early morning hours. Produce is purchased fresh daily, prepared, and eaten immediately. A variety of greens, such as green and red amaranth leaves, fenugreek leaves, drumstick and drumstick leaves, colocasia leaves, and agathi leaves, as well as gourds, such as ridge gourd, bottle gourd, and snake gourd, and cucumbers, okra, green beans, and yams, are commonly used in the South India.

 Prominent Fruits

Tropical fruits, such as mango, papaya, jackfruit, custard apple, sapota, guava, pomegranate, and banana, are grown and eaten along with temperate fruits such as grapes, apples, and oranges. It is not uncommon to see mango, banana, jackfruit, and coconut trees growing in the backyards of homes. Coconut palms grow in the coastal regions and the coconut fruit provides several products including coir from the husk, coconut water, and coconut milk, and the desiccated flesh is used in cooking, eaten fresh, or dried and used as copra. Betel nut palm is used in paan as a mouth freshener, and the palmyra palm is used for sugar and toddy production.

 ### Spices, Seasonings, and Herbs

South Indian cuisine employs a complex blend of spices and herbs with intraregional variations. Spices are used for their antiseptic, anti-inflammatory, and digestive properties (Patel & Srinivasan, 2004; Shobana & Naidu, 2000). Spices include coriander, cumin, fenugreek seeds, asafeotida, ginger, peppercorns, red chilies, mustard seeds, turmeric, garlic, cardamom, cloves, saffron, nutmeg, anise seeds, and mace. Fresh herbs, such as cilantro, are used for garnishing and preparing chutneys, and dill and mint are used in cooked dishes and chutneys. Herbs are used either in the fresh or dried form. Different combinations of whole spices and/or dried herb seeds are dry roasted until they release their aroma, then cooled and ground into a fine powder using a mortar and pestle or electric grinder. Dry spice powders can be stored for later use but are often made fresh as needed.

Spice powders (*podis*) are used for seasoning and enhancing flavors in dishes but are also mixed with plain cooked rice and ghee. Whole spices are sautéed in oil and then ground to a paste, with or without coconut and herbs such as cilantro and mint, for chutneys, or are added to vegetable or gravy dishes. Mustard seeds, cumin, asafeotida, red chilies, curry leaves, and black gram dal are tempered in a small quantity of oil added as a garnish to gravy-based dishes as well as rice preparations.

 ### Beverages

Coconut water, filter coffee, or drip coffee with added sugar and milk are popular beverages. Filter coffee is prepared by roasting the arabica seeds with chicory for aroma and grinding the roasted coffee to a very fine powder that is placed in a coffee filter to which boiling water is added. The resulting brew is heated with milk and sugar. Unspiced tea with milk and sugar is also popular. Other beverages include lemon juice, sugarcane juice, and toddy (alcoholic) made from the sap of the palm tree.

 ### Desserts

Sugar and jaggery are sweeteners used in a variety of desserts. Dessert preparations use liberal amounts of ghee. Common desserts include *appams*, *adirasams*, *payasams*, *chakare pongals*, *kesari bhaths*, *halwas*, *burfis*, and *ladoos*.

 ## TYPICAL DAY'S MENU

Regardless of the geographic region, a typical South Indian daily menu is an interesting blend of colors, textures, and flavors, and has certain common elements. The repertoire consists of breakfast, lunch, and dinner, with an afternoon *tiffin* (snack). Office goers enjoy sumptuous hot homemade meals provided by food carriers or *daba-wallas*. Regional variations in food patterns include the terminology for dishes, ingredients, and foods (see Table 23-1), the kinds of flesh foods, the extent of coconut use, the combination of spices, and the degree of spiciness in dishes.

All traditional meals are served on a stainless steel *thali* or on a banana leaf; the latter is used in some homes, restaurants, weddings, on festive occasions, and in religious ceremonies. Water is sprinkled on the leaf (a symbol of purification) and washed off before the food is served. Rice is served first with a few drops of ghee. Different food items are placed and served in a specific position and order. Regional variations exist in the arrangement of foods on the banana leaf. Food is eaten with the right hand and the use of fingers is preferred to silverware.

Breakfast in South India is cereal or cereal–legume based and includes a range of steamed, boiled, fermented, and shallow-fried delicacies. Typical breakfast dishes include steamed preparations such as *idlis* and *iddiappams*, and shallow-fried *dosas*, *oothapams*, *adais*, *pessarat*, and *pongal*. *Upumas* are also popular breakfast dishes and are made from cream of wheat, vermicelli, or beaten rice. Accompaniments include coconut chutney and *sambar*. Coffee sweetened with sugar and milk is the choice beverage, although non-spiced tea may also be consumed.

A South Indian meal is nutritionally well-balanced and consists of three courses. The first course is rice served with a few drops of ghee and *sambar*, followed by rice with *rasam*; the third course consists of rice and yogurt. Stir-fried vegetables (*poriyals*, *upperis*, *palyas*) and/or gravy vegetable dishes (*aviyals* and *kootus*), salads or *pachadis*, pickles, poppadums (fried or roasted),

TABLE 23-1 South Indian Regional Variations in Terminology Used to Describe Foods and Ingredients

English	Tamil	Telugu	Malayalam	Kannada
Rice (raw)	*Arasi*	*Beeyam*	*Ari*	*Akki*
Rice (cooked)	*Saadum*	*Annam*	*Choru*	*Anna*
Beaten rice	*Aval*	*Attukulu*	*Aval*	*Avalakki*
Rice flour	*Arasi-mavu*	*Beeyampindi*	*Aripodi*	*Akkihittu*
Corn	*Makka-jolum*	*Makkajannulu*	*Makka-cholam*	*Jolla*
Red gram dal	*Thovaram-paruppu*	*Kandhi-pappu*	*Thomara-pappu*	*Togri-belley*
Black gram dal	*Ulutham = paruppu*	*Minna-pappu*	*Ulundhu-pappu*	*Uddin-belley*
Bengal gram dal	*Kadala-paruppu*	*Sannaga-pappu*	*Kadala-paruppu*	*Kadale-belley*
Green gram dal	*Paitham-paruppu*	*Pessara-pappu*	*Cherupayyar*	*Hesre-belley*
Tamarind	*Puli*	*Chintapandu*	*Puli*	*Hunsey-hannu*
Sugar	*Chakarai*	*Panchadara/ chakara*	*Panjasara*	*Sakare*
Jaggery	*Vellam*	*Bellum*	*Shakara*	*Bella*
Salt	*Upu*	*Upu*	*Upu*	*Upu*
Milk	*Pal*	*Palu*	*Palae*	*Halu*
Ghee	*Neyye*	*Neyye*	*Neyye*	*Thupa*
Dry vegetable curry	*Karamdhu/karameedu*	*Koora*	*Uppekerri/ Meruzhukuvaratti*	*Palya*
Sambar	*Sambar/koluzmbhu*	*Sambar/paruppu pulusu*	*Sambar*	*Hilzhi*
Rasam	*Rasam*	*Charu*	*Rasam*	*Saru*
Yogurt	*Thayir*	*Perrugu*	*Thayir*	*Mosaru*
Vegetable with gravy	*Kootu*	*Kalagala-pappu*	*Malyalan/Thoran*	*Kootu*
Lemon rice	*Eluzhumbuchambalam saddum*	*Nimmakai-pulihora*	—	*Chitra-anna*
Yogurt rice	*Thayir-sadam*	*Perrugu-annam/ Dadhojanam*	—	*Mosar-anna/ Bagzhala-bhath*
Eggplant	*Kartharikai*	*Vamkaya*	*Vazhidannanga*	*Badanakai*
Potato	*Urulakalangzha*	*Bangaledumpa*	*Urulakalangzha*	*Alugede*
Okra	*Vendakkai*	*Bendakayya*	*Vendekka*	*Bendakaya*
Cucumber	*Vellarikai*	*Dosakaya*	*Vellarikai*	*Southekaya*
Green leafy vegetables	*Keerrai*	*Akukuralu*	*Keerrai*	*Soppu*

TABLE 23-1   South Indian Regional Variations in Terminology Used to Describe Foods and Ingredients (Continued)

English	Tamil	Telugu	Malayalam	Kannada
Pumpkin	Pushanikai	Gumadikayya	Matthanga	Gumblikayya
Cilantro	Kothumalli	Kothimira	Kothamalliyella	Kothumari-soppu
Curry leaves	Karavepalle	Karvepakku	Karvepalle	Kariven-soppu
Fenugreek seeds	Menthiyam	Menthulu	Uluva or Vengayam	Menthiya
Coriander seeds	Kothamalivarai	Dhaniyalu	Kothambalari	Kothamaribija
Turmeric	Manjal	Pasupu	Manjal	Arshana
Asafetida	Perungayam	Inguva	Kayam	Ingu
Cumin	Jeeragam	Jeelakara	Jeeragam	Jeeragai
Mustard	Kadagu	Aavalu	Kadagu	Sasve
Green chilli	Pachai-molaga	Pachi-mirapakaya	Pachai-molagu	Hasi-mensinkai
Red chilli	Vatha-molaga	Endu-mirapakaya	Chomana-mulaga	Vanna-mensinkai
Cardamom	Elaka	Elakaya	Elaka	Yalaki
Poppy seeds	Ghasa-ghasa	Ghasa-Ghasulu	Ghasa-ghasa	Ghasa-ghasa
Cloves	Lavangum	Lavangalu	Lavangam	Lavanga
Sesame seeds	Yellu	Nuvulu	Yellu	Yelzhu

and wafers are served on the side (Padmanabhan, 1994). *Sambar* powder is a dry-spice combination of roasted lentils, coriander seeds, fenugreek seeds, asafetida, curry leaves, and red chilies. Regional variations in sambar powder include the addition of mustard seeds, cumin, cinnamon, nutmeg, and dried coconut. *Sambar* powder can be prepared ahead or fresh at home, or purchased in Indian stores or Asian markets. *Sambar* is also an accompaniment to South Indian *tiffin* foods such as *vadais*, *dosas*, and *idlis*.

In contrast to the spicy *sambar*, the second course consists of rice served with a watery, cooked red gram dal-based soup known as *rasam*. It is made with tamarind, tomatoes, and/or citrus fruits such as lime. *Rasam* is eaten with rice and ghee or consumed as plain soup. *Vadais* can be soaked in *rasam* (*Rasa vade*) and enjoyed as a popular snack. *Sambar* and *rasam* powders share similar ingredients with the exception of cumin and black pepper, which distinguish the two powders. Tomatoes are used to prepare *rasam* and ginger *rasam* is popular as a digestive. Cumin seed, pepper *rasam*, and garlic *rasam* are used as an antidote for respiratory

ailments. Spicier versions, such as Mysore *rasam* from the state of Karnataka, have coconut in addition to the other ingredients and are eaten in lieu of *sambar*.

The meal ends with the curd or yogurt rice popularly known as *thaiyar sadam*. Homemade yogurt with a pinch of salt is eaten with rice or the yogurt rice is tempered with green chilies, ginger, mustard seeds, asafeotida, curry leaves, black gram dal, and cumin, and is garnished with cilantro and/or grated coconut; the latter is served on special occasions or preferred as travel food.

Meal Accompaniments

Poriyals, upkaris, thorans, and *kootus* are the vegetable accompaniments. *Poriyals* are prepared by dicing or shredding the vegetables, stir-frying with oil tempered with mustard seeds, cumin, black gram dal, asafoetida, green/red chillies, and curry leaves, and are garnished with cilantro. *Kootu* is semisolid in consistency, often substituted for *sambar*, and eaten with rice. Vegetable is the main ingredient; a ground paste that consists of black gram dal, pepper, cumin, and green chilies; coconut is added during preparation. Culinary *kootu* variations include *puli kootus* with tamarind and red gram dal, *poricha kootu* (tempered *kootu*), and *more kootu* (with buttermilk). *Aviyal, erisherri, pulisherri, rasavangis,* and *thoves* are regional versions of *kootus.*

South Indian salads consist of raw, chopped vegetables, seasoned lightly with or without green gram dal or mung bean (*kosumalli, kosumbari*) or mixed with yogurt (*pachadis*). Mung beans are washed, soaked in water for an hour, drained, and added to the vegetables. Popular vegetables for *kosumallis* include carrots, cucumber, tomatoes, raw onions, and sweet peppers.

Pickles (*urugas*) are aromatic, hot, and spicy, and an accompaniment to South Indian meals. Limes, lemons, mangoes, and gooseberries are commonly used to make pickles. They are cut into small pieces and marinated with turmeric and chili powder, and set aside for a couple of days. Pickles are seasoned with generous amounts of hot oil, mustard seeds, fenugreek seeds, asafoetida, and salt, and are left to marinate at least for a week before use. Mangoes are grated and cooked in oil with all the spices in the preparation of *thokkus* (a variation of pickles). Pickles and *thokkus* have a shelf life of more than a year. Chutneys, fresh or cooked (*thuvaiyals*), are popular accompaniments for snacks and appetizers. *Thuvaiyals* can be eaten with rice instead of *sambar* and *rasam* by mixing with ghee and are easily digestible.

Poppadums and *appalams* are deep-fried and served as crispy accompaniments in addition to plain or spiced deep-fried chips made from plantains, yams, or potatoes.

South Indian snacks (called *tiffins*) offer a large variety of flavors and textures. Snacks can be steamed such as *idlis*, shallow-fried such as *dosas, adais,* and *oothapams*, deep-fried such as *pakodas, bondas, chaklis/ murrukus, bhajjis,* and *vadas,* or lightly seasoned savory dishes such as *sundals* and *upumas*. Many snacks are breakfast treats or popular appetizers either with afternoon coffee and tea or before dinner. Nonvegetarian snacks, such as *kebabs*, may be baked, broiled, or grilled.

Desserts and sweets are the finale to a sumptuous meal served on special occasions or as a snack. *Payasams, halwas, burfis, appams,* and *adirasam* are popular desserts.

Spiced betel leaves, *paan*, and fennel seeds are used as mouth fresheners after a meal.

Selected Regional Cuisines

Goa

Goan cuisine (Indialine Expeditions, 2008) is a medley of Hindu, Muslim, and Portugese influences. Fish, curry, and rice are prepared in a spicy manner using ingredients such as red chilies, coconut, tamarind, and palm vinegar. Seafood preparations, such as curries, fries, pickles, and soups containing prawns, lobster, crab, clams, pomfret, mussels, and oyster, are common.

Karnataka

The culinary traditions of Karnataka are influenced by the bordering states of Maharashtra in the north, the Konkan coast in the west, Kerala in the southwest, Andhra Pradesh in the east, and Tamil Nadu in the south. Grains, such as ragi, jowar, and millet, are common in the north. Seafood and coconut-based dishes abound in the coastal regions. Mangalorean cuisine utilizes fresh or dried coconut with a special variety of red chili called *Gaati Mensu* or kumta chilies in most masala-based vegetarian and nonvegetarian preparations; rice preparations abound and fresh fruits, such as mango and jackfruit, are used in a wide array of dishes (Hegde, 1988).

Andhra Pradesh

The cuisine of Andhra Pradesh is the spiciest of all South Indian cuisines. The regional cuisines of Andhra share similarities with the cuisines of Tamil Nadu and Karnataka, whereas the Hyderabadi cuisine has a distinct Mughal influence. *Biryanis, bagara baingan,* and *kheema* are some popular Hyderabadi dishes. A variety of spiced powders, known as *podis*, are popular in this region, often eaten with hot rice and ghee.

Kerala

Kerala cuisine is a medley of vegetarian and nonvegetarian dishes popular among the Hindus, Muslims, and Christians in the region. Parboiled rice is the staple, eaten with dry curries (*upperis*) and other dishes such as *sambar, aviyal, kaalan, thoran, pulicherri,* and *kappa*. Vegetarian and nonvegetarian stews, fish moli, and biryanis are popular. Coconut products, including oil, are widely used in this cuisine. *Sadhya*, the traditional festival meal, is served on a banana leaf with rice in three courses, with vegetables, accompaniments, and *payasam*.

Chettinad

Chettinad cuisine, a regional specialty of Tamil Nadu, utilizes large amounts of pepper and savored meats with marinades and broths. Other popular spices used include saffron, mace, cashew nuts, and rose petals.

SELECTED LIST OF FESTIVALS AND HOLIDAYS CELEBRATED IN SOUTH INDIA

Table 23-2 gives a selected list of festivals and holidays celebrated in South India.

TABLE 23-2 Selected List of Festivals and Holidays Celebrated in South India

December to January	Pongal Harvest Festival (Hindu)
February to March	Shivaratri (worship of Lord Shiva) (Hindu)
	Muharram (Muslim)
March to April	Mahavir Jayanti (Jain)
	Ramanavami Birth of Lord Rama (Hindu)
	Easter (Christian observance)
	Eid-Milad-un-Nabi (Muslim)
April to May	Buddha Jayanti (Buddhist)
May to July	Regional Festivals
July to August	Naag Panchami; Narial Purnima (Hindu)
August to September	Ganesh Chaturthi (Hindu)
	Janmashtami (Hindu)
	Shravan Purnima (Hindu)
	Ramadan (Muslim)
September to October	Navaratri; Dussehra (Hindu)
	Eid-ul-Fitr (Muslim)
October to November	Diwali (Hindu)
November to December	Christmas (Christian)

 ## HEALTH BELIEFS AND CONCERNS

The scriptures advocate moderation by specifying that solid food should fill half the stomach, liquid one fourth, and the remainder should be left empty to facilitate proper digestion. All Hindus consider the cow as sacred (Kittler & Sucher, 2007), leading to the prohibition of beef consumption, although meats such as lamb, mutton, chicken, and poultry are permitted. Vegetarianism became popular in India following the introduction of Jainism and Buddhism, which emphasize *ahimsa* (nonviolence). The widespread availability of grains, legumes, fruits, and vegetables contributed to the spread of vegetarianism. The Brahmin caste in South India strictly follow lacto-vegetarian practices, with regional differences; for example, Brahmins in the coastal regions eat fish. Vegetarianism may be practiced by nonvegetarians on festive and/or religious occasions.

Ayurveda (which literally means "knowledge of life" in Sanskrit), the science of longevity and the classical system of Indian medicine, views the universe and everything in it, including the food, environment, and humans, as interconnected by the invisible energy pathways known as *prana* (Svoboda, 1992). Optimal health and well-being are achieved when all the aspects are in harmony. *Ayurveda* attributes improper diet and digestive action as the basis for all diseases and ill health. Treatment therefore employs a holistic approach involving nutrition, herbal therapies, massage, yoga, and meditation. The science further elaborates on the idea that the five elements in the universe; that is, fire (*tejas*), water (*ap*), earth (*prithvi*), wind (*vayu*), and ether or space (*akasha*), combine in the body to create three *doshas*: phlegm (*kapha*), wind (*vata/vayu*), and bile (*pitta*).

Doshas are believed to control the body's physiological, mental, and spiritual abilities. As a result, all human beings have one or more *doshas* that determine their constitution (*prakurti*) and state of health (*vikruti*). A further extension of this view, detailed in the scriptures, is the concept that food is capable of enhancing or evoking physiological and emotional responses by becoming part of the human body. This has led to the categorization of food on the basis of its effects on the body. *Sattvic* foods, such as milk, ghee, cereals, lentils, and vegetables, are believed to contribute to serenity, health, and longevity; *Rajasic* foods, such as meats, spices, and eggs, exert an aggressive disposition; and *Tamasic* foods, such as garlic, alcohol, and drugs, make an individual confused, sluggish, and dull. In

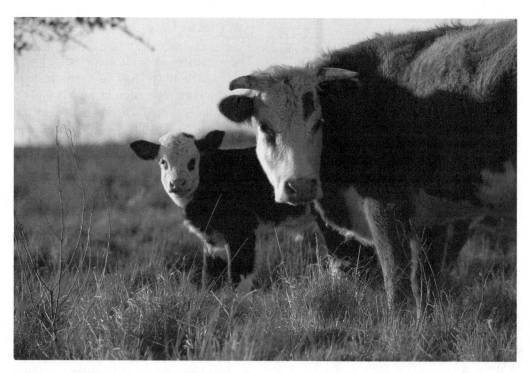

Hindus consider cows to be sacred.

light of this, *Ayurveda* emphasizes the importance of following the proper diet and lifestyle suited for one's *dosha*.

Disturbing the *dosha* or humoral basis of the body either due to environmental or dietary influences is thought to result in ill health and disharmony (Airey, 2002). The humoral counterparts of the universal elements in the human body are phlegm (*kapha*), wind (*vata/vayu*), bile (*pitta*), hot (*ushna*), and cold (*seeta*). *Kapha* foods, such as refined white sugar, millet, and buttermilk, are mucus producing and therefore avoided during respiratory illness; *vayu,* or gas-producing foods, such as beans and lentils, provoke flatulence; *pitta* foods (fried foods) are avoided during indigestion. The hot–cold food concept, originally developed by the Greeks and brought to Asia by Alexander the Great, was also integrated into the humoral balance theory over the centuries (Achaya, 1994). This continues to be a basis for food selection in India. Hot (*ushna*) foods, such as mung bean, spices, papaya, mango, chicken, and garlic, are believed to promote digestion, whereas cold (*seeta*) foods, such as cereals, legumes, fruits, and vegetables, are valued for their strength and nourishment. The hot–cold nature of foods is highly subjective; its use is variable and flexible. For example, cooking or the addition of spices can alter the hot or cold status of a food; food availability and usage based on regional variations can also alter the status. For example, rice, a staple grain in South India, is considered a "cold" food, whereas wheat, used less often, is considered a "hot" food. The hot–cold concept is followed very strictly when seasonal variations are extreme. For instance, cold foods, such as yogurt, buttermilk, and green mango, are popular summer foods, whereas hot foods, such as dried coconut, dried fruits, nuts, and fatty foods, are eaten during the monsoon season. This concept is also extended to health-related conditions (e.g., pregnancy) and diseases and is a "hot" condition, whereas arthritis is a "cold" disease.

Ancient food classification systems permitted the use of certain foods while prohibiting others for ritualistic purposes. Many of these beliefs are still followed. For instance, foods fried in ghee, clarified butter, or cooked in milk are *pucca* or ritualistically pure foods, whereas foods cooked in water, such as rice and lentils, are *kaccha* foods. Milk, turmeric, coconut, bananas, betel leaves, arecanut, and ghee are popular ceremonial foods. Furthermore, the authenticity of such foods is dependent on the observance of the concepts of purity and pollution. Foods, ingredients, equipment, preparation methods, and persons who are responsible for food preparation and serving are all subject to this classification. For example, foods served in brassware, raw foods, milk, and ghee are also pure or *pucca* foods, whereas alcohol and meat, foods prepared by lower castes, and leftovers are considered as *jhuta* (polluted) foods.

Food taboos for pregnancy, lactation, infants, and young children are also widely practiced. Hot foods, such as spices, mangoes, and papayas, may be avoided during pregnancy; vegetables that cause flatulence, and cold foods, are restricted for the lactating mother. Lactation foods, which include several herbal preparations, foods prepared with ghee (such as *ladoos*), and foods made with nuts and oilseeds (e.g., almonds for revitalization, ginger, and fenugreek) are considered as galactalogues. Therapeutic foods in use today include coconut water, lime and honey with warm water for digestive disorders; lightly seasoned boiled rice and mung lentils or green gram dal for a convalescing diet; honey, ghee, or the use of turmeric or saffron in warm milk as throat soothers; turmeric as an antiseptic; "hot" foods such as mangoes, eaten with a cold food such as milk; and buttermilk and fenugreek seeds, which are used as antidotes for diarrhea.

 ## GENERAL HEALTH AND NUTRITIONAL INDICATORS SUMMARY

It is difficult to describe an overall national dietary profile for a country such as India because of the existence of diverse dietary patterns that are influenced by geography, religion, and cultural differences. On the one hand, rural areas continue to suffer from the ravages of food insecurity, poor sanitation, high rates of infection, and resultant undernutrition. On the other hand, there is evidence that with economic development and higher purchasing power, a steady increase in noncommunicable diseases, particularly in urban areas, is becoming a problem. For instance, urban hypertension is twofold higher than in rural areas (World Health Organization, 2000). Similar trends are observed with the increasing rates of obesity, diabetes, and cardiovascular diseases (Shetty, 2002). A shift in dietary patterns to emulate Western diets rich in saturated fats, refined foods, and sugar, as well as diets low in fiber, with a concomitant disparity in physical activity patterns, has been blamed for what is described as "nutrition transition" (Griffiths & Bentley, 2001). A recent study in Karnataka (Griffiths & Bentley, 2005), using data from the National Family Health Survey, analyzed the differences in body mass index, diet, and

lifestyle among 4374 urban and rural women. The study showed that undernutrition was prevalent among rural women with limited resources and availability of healthy foods; urban women with more resources had a higher prevalence of being overweight. A number of barriers to healthy eating and physical activity were identified among urban and rural dwellers. The study underscored the urgent need for health and nutrition campaigns for urban women in order to prevent future increases in noncommunicable diseases such as obesity. In the long run, rural women will also likely benefit from such campaigns, which focus on changing the environments in which people live to prevent obesity, because poor physical activity patterns and the tendency to purchase unhealthy foods appear to be closely linked to economic development.

 ## COMMUNICATION AND COUNSELING TIPS

The following are communication and counseling tips:

1. English is spoken, written, and understood by the majority of South Indians. Use of regional languages is preferred among South Indians from the same region. For instance, people from Karnataka prefer to speak in Kannada with others from Karnataka. Many South Indians also understand other regional languages; however, relatively few South Indians speak Hindi.

2. South Indians, like others from the subcontinent, prefer a leisurely, personal style of communication. Loudness is considered rude. Self-control in demeanor and expression are followed; confrontation and a direct negative response may be avoided in the interests of maintaining harmony. Some people may indicate agreement by head wobbling (Kittler & Sucher, 2007). Emotional feelings, cultural values, and religious beliefs are all part of the decision-making process. Expectation of privileges, such as getting immediate appointments or service, may not be unusual.

3. Maintaining close family ties, adherence to family norms, and fostering interdependence are characteristic of South Asians, including those from South India. The elderly are respected for their wisdom and deferred to when making decisions.

4. Women are the primary gatekeepers of food and are responsible for food handling.

PRIMARY LANGUAGE OF FOOD NAMES WITH PHONETIC PRONUNCIATION

The primary language of food names with phonetic pronunciation is as follows:

Adai (a-dai): a shallow-fried thick pancake. Rice with two or three types of lentils is soaked, ground to a paste, and then shallow-fried to a golden-brown color. Onions, cilantro, ginger, and green chilies are added for a crunchier taste.

Adirasam (adhi-rasam): a deep-fried sweet pancake made from rice flour and jaggery.

Annam (a-nam): rice.

Appalam (app-alam): wafers made from rice and lentil flour either broiled or deep-fried.

Appam (a-pam): rice/wheat-based preparation steamed or made in the form of crepes in either salt or sweet varieties.

Aviyal (avi-yal): a gravy dish with 7–10 vegetables to which a paste made from coconut, cumin, green chilies, buttermilk, and coconut oil is added and boiled.

Bajji (ba-jji): vegetable fritters dipped in gram-flour paste and deep-fried.

Balchao (bal-chao): a Goan dish made with a ground paste consisting of coconut, red chilies, peppercorns, onions, tomatoes, and to which kokum (a red-colored sour fruit) can be added.

Bebinca (bebin-ca): a Goan layered pudding popular during Christian festivities.

Bisibele huli anna (bi-si-bele-huli-anna): a popular Karnataka specialty translated as a rice–lentil–vegetable dish cooked in tamarind juice and spiced with cinnamon, nutmeg, star anise seeds, and lots of ghee.

Bonda (bon-da): cooked vegetables (especially potatoes) shaped into balls, dipped in gram-flour paste, and deep-fried to a golden-brown color.

Burfi (bur-fi): a dessert made by cooking nuts, gram flour, coconut, or milk to a thick consistency, then transferred to a greased plate and cut into desired shapes.

Chakarai pongal (chak-a-rai pon-gal): rice and mung dal sweet dish, cooked with jaggery and milk, topped with ghee, nutmeg, cinnamon, raisins, and cashews.

Chakli/murruku (chak-li/mu-rru-ku): a deep-fried savory snack made from rice flour and lentil flour to which salt and chili powder are added, made into a stiff dough, and dropped into hot oil by pressing through a chakli maker to get the desired circular shape.

Chitranna (chitra-anna): the name given to lemon/tamarind-flavored spiced rice in Karnataka.

Chutneys (chut-neys): puréed condiments made with coconut, cilantro or mint, onions and tomatoes, vegetable peels, eggplants, or mango. Tamarind, fenugreek seeds, green chilies, dal, and peanuts are ingredients used to prepare chutneys.

Dhonos (dho-nos): a Goan pudding made from rice flour, jackfruit, coconut, and jaggery.

Dosa (do-sa): a shallow-fried crisp crepe made from rice and dal, soaked, ground to a paste, and left to ferment. Semolina and/or wheat flour may also be used for dosa. Dosa is eaten plain with chutney or stuffed with potato curry filling and eaten as masala dosa.

Huli (hu-li): a tamarind-based *sambar* in Karnataka.

Iddiappam (iddi-appam): a Kerala dish similar to the *idli*. *Iddiappam* can be made from rice sticks also known as *Noolputtuappa*.

Idli (id-li): a steamed dish made from fermented cereal–lentil batter. The batter is poured into a greased idli plate (tray) that resembles an egg-poaching dish with three or four circular compartments. Several of these circular trays are arranged on a stand (idli tree). The idli tree is placed in a steaming dish and allowed to cook for 10–13 minutes.

Kadala (ka-dala): a Kerala curry made from black chickpeas.

Kalan (ka-lan): a buttermilk-based gravy dish containing coconut and vegetables such as plantains or yams.

Kanji (kan-ji): a popular rice porridge in Kerala and Tamil Nadu.

Kappa (ka-ppa): the Malayalam name for tapioca.

Kootu (koo-tu): a vegetable–lentil combination gravy dish, with or without coconut, lightly spiced, served as an accompaniment or eaten with rice.

Kozhambu (ko-zham-bu): a tamarind-based vegetable stew with coriander, fenugreek, red chilies, asafoetida, and curry leaves, eaten with hot rice.

Laddu/ladoo (la-doo): a ball-shaped sweet made using, for example, semolina, wheat flour, gram flour, sesame seeds, gingelly seeds, peanuts, and so on. A syrup made from sugar or jaggery is mixed in, and then the mixture is shaped into balls.

Majjigehuli (ma-jji-ge-huli-anna): the name given to spiced yogurt rice in Karnataka.

More kozhambu (koz-ham-bu): buttermilk- and-tamarind-based stew similar to *kozhambu*.

Oothappam (oo-tha-ppam): a thick pancake made from dosa or idli batter, topped with sliced onion, tomatoes, and cilantro.

Pakoda (pa-ko-da): fritters made from onions, cashew nuts, or other nuts dipped in gram-flour paste and deep-fried.

Pal-appa (pal-appa): a Kerala specialty that consists of a pancake made from rice flour fermented with toddy or wine and served with vegetarian or nonvegetarian stew.

Payasam (pa-ya-sam): a thickened milk dessert made from cereals, nuts, sugar, and topped with cardamom and raisins.

Pessarat (pes-sar-at): a medium-thick pancake made from rice and green gram dal, ground into a paste to which onions and cilantro can be added.

Pongal (pon-gal): a rice and green lentil combination dish with salt, pepper, cumin, and freshly grated ginger.

Poppadam/pappadam (poppa-dam): see *Appalam*.

Poriyal (pori-yal): a dry vegetable dish sautéed in oil and lightly to moderately spiced according to taste and served as an accompaniment.

Pulisherri (pul-ish-heri): a Kerala version of *sambar*.

Puttu (put-tu): a Kerala breakfast dish made from rice powder and grated coconut in a cylindrical form.

Rasam (ras-am): made from cooked dal to which tomatoes and tamarind are added along with *rasam* powder, tempered with ghee, mustard seeds, and garnished with cilantro. Different varieties of *rasam* are prepared using citrus fruits, cumin, pepper, drumstick, buttermilk, ginger, and garlic.

Sambar (sam-bar): a thick, spicy lentil-based gravy dish with tamarind and vegetables to which spiced powder is added. The dish is tempered with oil, fenugreek seeds, mustard seeds, asafoetida, red chilies, and curry leaves.

Sar (sar): the Karnataka name for *rasam*.

Sorpote (sor-pote): a spicy pork and liver Goan curry.

Sundal (sun-dal): a lightly spiced dry dish made from chickpeas or lentils that are soaked and cooked.

Thayir sadam (thay-ir sa-dam): spiced yogurt rice in Tamil Nadu.

Thokku (thok-ku): fruits, vegetables, or herbs that are puréed or grated and cooked in oil with spices until the mixture thickens.

Thoran (thor-an): a Kerala dry curry.

Thuvaiyal (thu-va-yil): cooked chutney in which the main ingredient (vegetable) is sautéed before spices are added.

Upuma/uppitu (u-puma/u-pitu): a semolina-, vermicelli-, or beaten-rice-based dish with cooked vegetables and seasoned with fat and spices.

Vadai (va-dai): a deep-fried doughnut-shaped dish made from black lentils. Vegetables, such as cabbage and onion, can be added. *Vadais* can be eaten plain (*medhu vadai*), with chutney and *sambar*, soaked in *rasam* (*rasa vade*), or soaked in spiced coconut–yogurt mixtures (*thayir vadai*).

Vadams (va-dams): wafers made from cereal/dal that is dehydrated and deep-fried.

Vindaloo (vin-da-loo): a Goan stew (with pork, chicken, mutton, or prawn) seasoned with wine vinegar and garlic, local spices, and palm-sap vinegar.

Xacuti (sha-cu-ti): a Portugese, pungent spiced preparation made from tamarind, lemon juice, and nutmeg.

ACKNOWLEDGMENTS

Names of foods and ingredients were provided by Anita Rajan (Malayalam), Sailaja Sishtala (Telugu), Pramila Suryanarayana (Kannada), and Sudha Raj (Tamil).

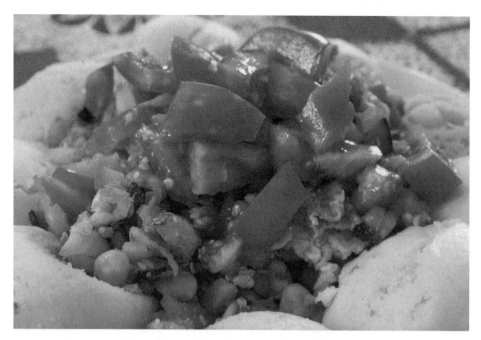

Idli is a steamed dish made from fermented cereal–lentil batter.

FEATURED RECIPE

Idli

2 cups raw rice

1 cup black gram dal (lentil)

4 cups water

Salt to taste

1. Soak the rice and dal for 4–5 hours.
2. Drain the water. Place dal in a blender and blend to a fine batter adding small quantities of water, then blend rice to a coarse batter.
3. Mix both batters together and add salt to taste.
4. Set aside to ferment for at least 8 hours.
5. Fill greased idli trays with portions of the batter, then place the idli stand in a steamer for 15 minutes.
6. Cool and remove from tray and serve with coconut chutney.

More recipes are available at http://nutrition.jbpub.com/foodculture/

Coconut Chutney

1 cup (8 oz.) grated fresh/grated frozen coconut

2 tbsp. roasted fried gram dal (lentil)

2 green chilies

1 small bunch cilantro leaves

Salt to taste

For Tempering:

2 tbsp. oil

1 tsp. mustard seeds

1 tsp. black gram dal (lentil)

1 red chili

Few curry leaves

A pinch of asafoetida

1. Place the coconut, dal, green chilies, cilantro, and salt to taste in a blender, adding small quantities of water to make a fine paste.
2. Heat oil in a frying pan. Add tempering ingredients. When the mustard seeds splutter, add this mixture to the ground paste. Serve with idlis, dosa, and vadai.

REFERENCES

Achaya, K.T. (1994). *Indian food: A historical companion.* New Delhi, India: Oxford University Press.

Airey, R. (2002). *Healing with Ayurveda.* London: Southwater.

Basham, A.L. (1959). *The wonder that was India.* New York: Grove Press.

Griffiths, P., & Bentley, M. (2005). Women of higher socioeconomic status are more likely to be overweight in Karnataka, India. *European Journal of Clinical Nutrition, 59,* 1217–1220.

Griffiths, P.L., & Bentley, M.E. (2001). The nutrition transition is underway in India. *Journal of Nutrition, 131,* 2692–2700.

Hegde, S.S. (1988). *Mangalorean cuisine.* Mumbai India: India Book House.

Indialine Expeditions. (2008). *Goa cuisine.* Retrieved March 25, 2008, from http://www.indialine.com/travel/goa/cuisine.html/

Kittler, P.G., & Sucher, K.P. (2007). *Food and culture* (4th ed.). Belmont, CA: Thomson.

Maps of India. (2008). *Languages in Lakshadweep.* Retrieved March 25, 2008, from http://www.mapsofindia.com/Lakshadweep/languages/index.html

Mitchell, A.G. (1982). *Hindu gods and goddesses.* Printed in England for Her Majesty's Stationery Office.

Padmanabhan C. (1994). *Dakshin: Vegetarian cuisine from South India.* San Francisco: Thorsons.

Patel, K., & Srinivasan, K. (2004). Digestive stimulant action of spices: A myth or a reality *Indian Journal of Medical Research, 119,* 167–179.

Patil, V. (1994). *Celebrations–festival days of India.* Mumbai, India: India Book House.

Shastri, K.A.N. (1955). *A history of South India.* New Delhi, India: Oxford University Press.

Shetty, P.S. (2002) Nutrition transition in India. *Public Health & Nutrition 5*(1A), 175–182.

Shobana, S., & Naidu, K.A. (2000). Antioxidant activity of selected Indian spices. *Prostaglandins, Leukotrienes and Essential Fatty Acids 62*(2), 107–110.

Singh, G. (1976). *A geography of India* (2nd ed.). New Delhi, India: Atma Ram and Sons.

Singh, S., Butler, S., Jealous, V., Karafin, A., Richmond, S., & Wlodarski, R. (2007). *Lonely Planet South India* (4th ed.). Victoria, Australia: Lonely Planet.

Svoboda, R.E. (1992). *Ayurveda: Life, health and longevity.* New York: Arkana Penguin Books.

Swami Tejomayananda. (1993). *Hindu culture: An introduction.* Mumbai, India: Central Chinmaya Trust.

World Health Organization. (2000). Global strategy for the prevention and control of non-communicable diseases. Geneva, Switzerland: World Health Organization.

OFFICIAL WEBSITES FOR THE UNION TERRITORIES AND STATES IN SOUTH INDIA

Andaman and Nicobar Islands: http://www.and.nic.in/

Andhra Pradesh: http://www.aponline.gov.in/apportal/index.asp

Goa: http://goagovt.nic.in/

Karnataka: http://www.karnataka.gov.in/

Kerala: http://www.kerala.gov.in/

Pondicherry: http://www.pondicherry.nic.in/

Tamil Nadu: http://www.tamilnadutourism.org/

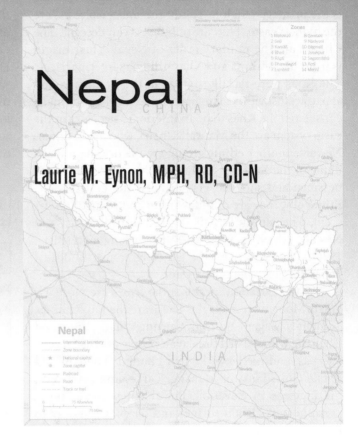

CHAPTER 24

Nepal

Laurie M. Eynon, MPH, RD, CD-N

 CULTURE AND WORLD REGION

Nepal is home to many groups of people. The country's cultural regions correspond to the three physical regions. The Tarai, an extension of the Indian plains, is the lowest area and is predominantly Hindu. The hill region is a mixture of Hindus and Buddhists, and people of Ido-Aryan origin. In the north and the mountainous area are the people of Tibetan origin who practice Tibetan Buddhism. There are also Muslims who live in the hills and the plains. Each ethnic group has some unique practices, but the primary influence on their culture is religion. The economy of Nepal is primarily subsistence agriculture and tourism, which has been negatively impacted by the political unrest of recent years.

Nepal is a landlocked country located between India and Tibet. "From an ethnic, cultural and socio-psychological standpoint, the midland and northern regions of Nepal represent an intermediate zone between South Asia on the one hand and East and Central Asia on the other" (Shaha, 1975).

 LANGUAGE

Nepali is the official language of Nepal, but over 26 different languages are spoken. English is also spoken in the schools. It is not uncommon for Nepalese to be multilingual.

 CULTURE HISTORY

Nepal is an ancient country. The Mahabharat and Purnas as well as Buddhist and Jain religious texts mention Nepal. The first Nepali texts, the Vamshawalis or chronicles, refer to King Sthiti Malla (1382–1395) and are the only record of Nepali history of the earliest time (Shaha, 1975).

Nepal's culture is greatly influenced by the two main religions: Hinduism and Buddhism. (The birthplace of the Buddha, Lumbini, is located in the Tarai.) The caste system still exists in Nepal, where Hinduism is the primary religion. The Brahmans, or priests, are the highest caste. They are of Indo-Aryan descent. The Chetris are the military order of Nepal. Their origin is from the Brahma and Khas hill-tribe intermarriage. The Khas were racially similar to the Brahmans and spoke a Sanskrit-like language; however, the Brahmans considered the Khas to be an inferior caste. Next in the caste system are the Matwali-Chetri, who drink liquor. Newars, another ethnic group, are the original inhabitants of the Kathmandu valley. They tend to be businessmen and shopkeepers, farmers, and craftspeople. Ethnically, they are of Indo-Aryan and Mongolian descent. They speak Nepali, derived from Sanskrit and Newari, which is a Tibeto-Burman language (Bista, 1976). The Newari can be either Hindu or Buddhist depending on where they reside.

As the elevation increases the tribes are more Tibetan/Mongolian in origin. These are the Rai, Limbus, Tamangs, Magars, Sunwar, Gurung, Pnachgunle, and Chepang tribes. The Himalayan people are the famous Sherpas, and the lesser known Lhoomi, Thudam and Topke Gola, Lopa of Manang, Larke, and Siar. With the increase in elevation, Buddhism becomes more prominent as Hindu shrines and temples give way to Buddhist stupas and prayer flags. It is not uncommon to see pictures of the Dalai Lama in homes and shops.

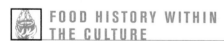 FOOD HISTORY WITHIN THE CULTURE

Food is influenced by religion and region. In the lower altitudes, where Hinduism is predominant, rice, *dal* (lentils), and curry are the mainstays of the diet. In the middle hill region, rice is supplemented with corn. In the west, potatoes are a staple of the diet. As the elevation increases, millet and buckwheat become the foundation of the diet. Hindus are mostly vegetarian and do not eat beef at all. The cow is considered an incarnation of the Goddess of Wealth, Laxmi. Some Hindus eat chicken, fish, male goat and lamb, and pigeon. Newars, Magars, and Tamangs eat water buffalo. The untouchables are the caste that handles cowhide, or sarkis, and will eat beef when a cow has died a natural death. Some groups eat pork or wild boar meat. Determining what meat is eaten involves a combination of caste, degree of religious adherence, and financial availability. Bud-

dhists might be vegetarian or they might be omnivores and eat all of the aforementioned meats, including yak. Only male animals can be sacrificed for Hindu religious ceremonies, and meat must be slaughtered by either cutting the throat as a saw would or by chopping off the head in one stroke.

The kitchen is a private part of the house, and a Hindu kitchen normally faces south. This is the most sacred part of the whole house, and persons belonging to a caste lower than that of the house owner are not allowed to enter it (Majupuria, 1980). The kitchen is also used for worship. Most Hindu homes have an altar at the top of a corner in their kitchen.

 MAJOR FOODS

 Protein Sources

Protein sources are water buffalo, yak or cow's milk, lentils, chicken, fish, eggs, pork, goat, lamb, and yak.

 Starch Sources

Starch sources are rice, corn, millet, buckwheat, wheat or white bread, or unleavened bread called *chapattis* or *roti*.

 Fat Sources

The Nepali diet is low in fat. The main fat source in the hill country is mustard seed oil, and in other areas it is clarified butter known as ghee. Sesame seed oil is also used. Meat is usually eaten only during festival days in the hill region.

 Prominent Vegetables

Prominent vegetables are potatoes, cherry tomatoes, cucumber, cauliflower, bitter gourd, cabbage, fiddle ferns, mustard greens, spinach, onion, okra, pumpkin, radish, turnips, carrots, eggplant, peas, string beans, taro-elephant ear tubers, coriander, and yams.

 Prominent Fruits

Prominent fruits are tangerine, mango, fig, guava, papaya, banana, apple, pineapple, and Asian pear.

 Spices and Seasonings

Turmeric, garlic, ginger, onion, and chili peppers form the spice base. Other widely used spices are cumin,

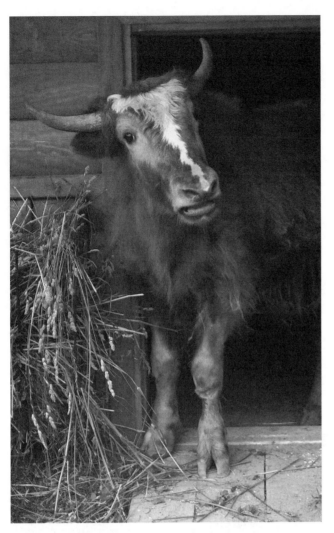

Yak is commonly consumed in India and is a good source of protein.

coriander (both the dried seed and the leaf), mustard seed, allspice, cinnamon, clove, coconut, nutmeg, pepper, salt, cardamom (white and black), saffron, and sesame seed.

 Beverages

Common beverages are spiced tea water, *lassi* (yogurt smoothie), *chung* (homemade beer), *raksi* (rice liquor), and orange or lemon squash (-ade).

 Desserts

Desserts are eaten only on special occasions. *Jilebi* or *jeri*, a deep-fried batter, is made by putting the batter in a coil and then submerging the coil into hot oil. It is served with sugar syrup, rice pudding, and cream or milk balls.

 FOODS WITH CULTURAL SIGNIFICANCE

Rice has a religious role as well as being a staple in the diet. Brahmans eat only rice that is cooked by a Brahman; otherwise, to them, it is ritually impure. They do not eat rice cooked by anyone of a lower caste. People of other castes eat rice cooked by any caste member who is higher in status than they are. Beaten rice (*chiura*) is eaten regardless of the caste group that prepared it. Rice is also offered to Hindu gods as a part of *puja* (worship). Rice is not eaten on certain Hindu holidays such as *Ekadasi* (the 11th day of the fortnight) and on the day of *Amavasya* or *Aunsi* (the dark-moon day). Nepalese fast as part of religious festivals such as the birthday of Lord Krishna, or Shivratri (the marriage anniversary of Shiva and Parvati) (Majupuria, 1980). A typical greeting is "Did you eat?" which translates as "*Bhat kanne?*" in Nepali. *Bhat* is the Nepali word for rice. This underscores the importance of rice in the Nepalese diet.

Water is considered to be ritually pure in Hinduism and is used to purify anything that has become religiously unclean. Nepal does not have safe drinking water or sanitation systems. It has been challenging to educate the Nepalese about the importance of safe water. Unclean water is the leading cause of infant and child mortality in Nepal.

Food is divided into three classes based on the qualities each food group has according to Hindu mythology. According to Majupuria (1980) these groups are:

1. Tamas—the quality that begets anger, envy, dullness, or inertia. Root vegetables are an example because they grow underground in complete darkness.
2. Rajas—the quality that evokes sexual passion and excitement of mind and body. Hot chili peppers are believed to do this.
3. Sattva—the quality that promotes harmony and elevation of the spirit for enlightenment. Vegetables and fruits that grow above ground are examples of this group (Majupuria, 1980).

It is believed that the food one eats affects one's temperament. Sattvic food is prescribed by the Hindu holy scriptures, because they are believed to increase energy, health, and cheerfulness. Salty, bitter, or sour foods are thought to cause pain, grief, and disease. Tamasic food is tasteless or rotten and is thought to cause extreme dullness (Majupuria, 1980).

Because most Nepalese are subsistence farmers who do not have money to buy food, the end of the growing season can be very limited in quantity and variety of fresh vegetables. *Gunduk* is a dried and cured green leafy vegetable like mustard leaf. This has been promoted as a way to prevent vitamin A deficiency, which is endemic in Nepal and the leading cause of blindness.

TYPICAL DAY'S MENU

Most Nepalese in the hill region eat two big meals and one to two snacks daily. They rise early to tend to their animals and fields. The people may have some popped corn and/or roasted soybeans for a snack. Around 9:00 or 9:30 AM they eat *dalbhat*, which is rice, *dal* or lentils, curried vegetables, and chutney or relish. Large quantities of boiled rice, coarsely ground corn, or millet are eaten. (Corn and millet are considered poor people's food, even though millet is nutritionally superior to rice or corn.) Millet is eaten by people in higher elevations in the hill country.

In the afternoon there is a snack of tea (served with milk and sugar), roasted soybeans, popped corn, biscuits (which are more like cookies), or perhaps some bread and curried vegetables.

At sunset a large meal of rice, lentils, vegetables, and chutney is eaten again. The menu differs depending on what can be grown in any given area with regard to rainfall and elevation. The farther east one goes, where the tribes are of Tibeto-Mongolian descent, more buckwheat and noodles are eaten. Farther west, potatoes are as important as rice. Women eat last and eat the least of the side dishes of vegetables and meat. Men, boys, and small children, regardless of gender, are fed first. This is not a beneficial practice for healthy pregnancy and lactation.

HOLIDAY MENUS

Most holidays are a religious festival in which a male goat or sheep is killed and offered to the gods in the temple before it is eaten. These festival days break up the monotony of hard labor and are an opportunity to eat meat. Most people cannot afford to eat meat daily, and when they do, it is a small portion of one or two ounces. *Pulao* is cooked on some holidays. This is a rich dish in which presoaked and drained rice is cooked in butter and vegetables, and spices, such as cardamom and cumin, cloves, and black pepper, are added. Sometimes meat is added as well. Fried puffed bread, called *puri,* may be made and served with chutney for some festivals.

Observations from the Author (Laurie M. Eynon)

I served for 2 years as a math and science teacher in the U.S. Peace Corps from September 1977 through December 1979, in the Village of Khudi Beni in the Lamjung province of Nepal. I lived with a local family and ate as they did. Kitchens in Nepal are dark; windows are small because there is no central heat. There is no electricity, so dinner is lit by small vegetable-oil, wick-burning lamps. Everyone eats with their right hand.

I developed an appreciation for eating a variety of foods year round, because with subsistence farming food was scarce right before the monsoons came and new vegetables could be planted.

The Nepalese are for the most part vegetarian; however, when they do eat meat, they eat barely 2 ounces and waste nothing. A man in our village had two large white domestic pigs. The day came for one to be butchered. My family asked me if I wanted a share, and I said that I would pay for my share if they would cook it. The pig was butchered in the open air, and each part was meticulously cut into thumb-sized chunks and doled out according to the number of buyers, so everyone got a piece of rump, shoulder, loin, and so on. The women in my family were very happy because my share was cooked with the family's share, and because women eat after everyone else (I ate with the men since I was American and a paying guest/teacher), that night they got the same portion as everyone else.

One Sunday the teachers at my school decided to have a picnic. We went to the creek to swim, and we cooked curried chicken and *pulao* (seasoned rice). I was served the whole chicken head from the neck up. I could not bring myself to eat it, so I discreetly (I thought) tucked it between a layer of newspaper that served as a plate. Later, while singing "Call and Response," in which the Nepalese love to create their own lyrics to fit the occasion, I heard, "She couldn't eat the chicken's head." It was a playful way to let me know they had noticed. At another time (I do not remember where I was) I was chewing on something, and not being able to chew it completely, I finally looked at it and saw that it was a chicken's foot—with all the toes intact!

HEALTH BELIEFS AND CONCERNS

Access to Western medicine is limited. Nepalese may self-medicate with herbs or visit a shaman or traditional healer. The shaman may use herbs, rituals, or a combination to rid the ill person of evil spirits. Babies wear a necklace and strings around their waist to protect them from evil spirits. Infant boy's ears are pierced to trick the evil spirits into thinking they are girls (and hence less valuable). Infants often wear kohl around their eyes to protect them from evil spirits. As in Ayurvedic medicine, which is also popular, foods and illnesses are labeled as hot (i.e., a hot illness is not fed a food believed to be hot). Diarrhea is a leading cause of mortality among Nepali infants and children. Food and water are withheld in the belief that such action will cure the illness, but it often compounds the dehydration problem. When someone has a cold, milk is withheld in the belief that it produces more mucus secretions.

 GENERAL HEALTH AND NUTRITIONAL INDICATORS SUMMARY

Because Nepal is a poor country, the health and nutritional status of the population is also poor. The average life expectancy at birth as of 2004 is 61 years (World Health Organization, 2007). Eighty-eight percent of the population had access to improved drinking-water sources in 2000; however, only 28% of the population was using adequate sanitation (UNICEF, 2004). Diarrhea is still a leading cause of death in children under 5 years. Between 1994 and 2002 the oral rehydration rate (in which they received increased fluids and continued feeding during the episode) in the 2 weeks prior to the survey was 11%; however, between 1990 and 2000 there was a 37% reduction in the under-5-years child mortality rate (UNICEF, 2004).

Eighty-eight percent of infants under 2 months are exclusively breastfed, and 63% of infants 6–7 months are breastfed and receive appropriate complimentary feeding. Of children 6–59 months, 87.5% received one dose of vitamin A in the previous 6 months (as vitamin A deficiency is endemic there) (World Health Organization, 2007).

Due to limited access to food in a subsistence agricultural society, 49.3% of all children under 5 years are stunted (low height for age), 12.6% of children under 5 years are wasting (low weight for height), and 38.6% of children under 5 years are underweight (weight for age) (World Health Organization, 2007). In addition, the prevalence of anemia among children 6–59 months was 48.4% (hemoglobin less than 11 g/dl). Thirty-six percent of women 15–49 are anemic (hemoglobin less than 12 g/dl) (World Health Organization, 2007).

 COMMUNICATION AND COUNSELING TIPS

Nepalese people are very seldom called by their first name. They are addressed according to their relationship to the speaker. For example, a woman older than the speaker might be called big sister, aunt, or grandmother depending on her appearance. A younger woman might be called little sister or daughter.

One should use a soft tone of voice and speak respectfully, especially to people older than oneself.

Traditional Nepalese are modest in dress; a woman does not show her ankles or wear pants. It is important to assess literacy skills. Nepal has a high illiteracy rate, especially for females except in the Newari caste where it is customary to educate girls. Nepalese are very family/friend oriented. They do not like to do anything alone, so communicating any health information will most likely be better received with family or friend(s) present. In social situations men and women usually stay in separate groups and eat in separate groups (outside the family). The head is sacred and should be treated very respectfully, which means not to touch it or point one's feet in its direction. Feet are considered dirty and ritually unclean. One never passes one's foot over or near another's head. In addition, it is considered disrespectful if one's legs are extended, either sitting in a chair or on the floor. Also, items are given or taken with the right hand, and it is considered more polite to use both hands to receive something, especially if the giver is from a high caste. Personal body space is less than that required by Westerners, especially if it is between two people of the same gender.

Gender of the health care provider is a consideration. It may not be proper for an unmarried woman to be with a man, or for a married woman to be examined by a man. Women are expected to be modest.

The Nepalese are friendly and hospitable people, and since they are often multilingual (e.g., they might speak their tribal language, Nepali, and English), they expect other people to be likewise.

TABLE 24-1 Common Food Names in English with Nepali and Phonetic Translation

English	Nepali	Phonetic Translation	English	Nepali	Phonetic Translation
Allspice	Battis masala	Baa-tee-ss ma-sa-la	Milk	Dudh	Dude
			Millet	Junelo	Ju-nei-lō
Almond	Badam	Ba-dam	Mustard	Rayo	Ray-ō
Apple	Syau	Ci-owe	Mustard greens	Rayo sag	Ray-ō-saag
Apricot	Khur pani	Cur-pa-nee	Mustard oil	Thoriko tel	To-ri-kō tell
Baking soda	Khanne soda	Connie soda	Nutmeg	Jaiphal	Jai(long i)-fal
Banana	Kera	Cara	Oil	Tel	Tell
Beans	Simi	Cimi	Onion	Pyaj	Pi(long i)-aj
Beaten rice	Chiura	Chi-u-ra	Orange	Desi suntala	Day-ci sun-ta-la
Bread	Roti	Row-tee			
Cabbage	Bandakobi	Bunda-kō-bi	Pea flour	Besan	Bay-san
Cardamon (white)	Sukumel	Sue-coo-mel	Peanuts	Badam	Ba-dom
			Pears	Naspati	Na-spa-tea
Carrot	Gajar	Ga-jar	Peas	Kerau	Kay-rau
Cauliflower	Kauli	Cow-li	Pepper (black, peppercorns)	Marich	Ma-reech
Chicken	Kukhura	Coo-ku-ra	Pepper (hot)	Khurseni	Coor-sani
Cinnamon	Dulchini	Dull-chin-ee	Puffed rice	Murai	Mu-rai
Cloves	Lwang	Lwang	Pumpkin	Pharsi	Far-cee
Coriander	Daniya	Dan-i-ya	Radish	Mula	Moo-la
Corn	Makai	Ma-kai	Rice	Bhat	Baa-t
Cumin seed	Jeera	Jee-ra	Salt	Nun	Noon
Egg	Phul	Fool	Sesame oil	Tilko tel	Teal-kō tell
Eggplant	Bhanta, brinjal	Bhan-ta, brin-jal	Sesame seed	Til	Teal
Fish	Macha	Ma-cha	Shortening	Ghiu	Gee-u(long u)
Fruit	Phalphul	Fal-fool	Spices	Masala	Ma-sa-la
Garlic	Lasun	La-soon	Spinach	Palung	Pa-lung(hard g)
Greens	Sag	Saag			
Lentils	Dal	Doll	Sugar	Chini	Chin-ee
Mango	Aanp	Aanp	Sweet potato	Sakarkhanda	Sa-car-con-da
Meat	Masu	Ma-soo	Tangerine	Suntala	Sun-ta-la

TABLE 24-1   Common Food Names in English with Nepali and Phonetic Translation (Continued)

English	Nepali	Phonetic Translation	English	Nepali	Phonetic Translation
Tea	Chiya	Chee-ya	Wheat	Gahu	Gow
Tomato	Golbeda	Gōl-bay-da	Wheat flour	Gahuko pitho	Gow-kō-pee-tō
Turmeric (powder)	Besar	Bay-sar	Whole-wheat flour	Ata	Ah-ta
Turmeric (root)	Haledo	Ha-lay-dō	Yam	Tarul	Ta-rul
Vegetables	Takari	Ta-car-ee	Yellow mustard	Sarseum	Sar-se-um
Vinegar	Sirka, amilo	Sir-ka, a-me-low	Yogurt	Dahi	Da-hee
Water	Pani	Pa-ni			

Compiled from Oppedal (1971).

FEATURED RECIPE

Whole Moong Dal

1½ cups whole moong dal

½ tsp. crushed red chilies

1 tsp. salt

½ tsp. turmeric

½ tsp. ground ginger

7 cups water

2 tbsp. ghee or butter

1 small onion, finely chopped

1 large tomato

½ tsp. cayenne pepper or paprika

1. Pick over the dal and wash thoroughly.
2. Put the dal into a crock pot or heavy saucepan with the chilies, salt, turmeric, ginger, and water.
3. Cook for 7–8 hours in the Crock-Pot. If you are cooking the dal on the stove, bring it to a boil, reduce the heat to medium, and cook for an hour or so. The dal should split when it is tender, but the liquid will still be separate from the beans.
4. Reduce the heat to medium-low and cook for another 45–60 minutes or until the dal has become creamy.

For the baghar:

1. Heat the butter or ghee and sauté the onions until they are golden brown.
2. Add the tomato, cover the pan, and cook for 2–3 minutes.
3. Uncover and stir constantly until the tomato is cooked and the ghee starts to separate.
4. Add the paprika or cayenne pepper. Gently stir the baghar into the dal.

From: Jain (2003)

More recipes are available at http://nutrition.jbpub.com/foodculture/

REFERENCES

Bista, D.B. (1976). *The people of Nepal* (3rd ed.). Kathmandu, Nepal: Ratna Pustak Bhandar.

Jain, S. (2003). *Vegetarian nirvana: A passage to North Indian cuisine.* Bloomington, IN: First Books.

Lispon, J.G., & Dibble, S.L. (Eds.). (2007). *Culture & clinical care.* San Francisco: University of California San Francisco Nursing Press.

Majupuria, I. (1980). *Joys of Nepalese cooking.* Gwalior-1, India: Summit S. Devi.

Oon, S.-F. (2004). The difficulties of western medicine in Nepal. *Trinity Student Medical Journal Essay,* 91–93.

Oppedal, D.L. (Ed.). (1971). *Himalyan gourmet* (2nd ed.). Kathamandu, Nepal: American Peace Corps.

Shaha, R. (1975). *An introduction to Nepal.* Kathmandu, Nepal: Ratna Pustak Bhandar.

UNICEF. (2007). *The state of the world's children 2007: Women and children, the double dividend of gender equality.* Retrieved April 14, 2009, from http://www.unicef.org/sowc07/statistics/tables.php

UNICEF. (2004). *State of the world's children 2004.* Tables 3, 10. Retrieved December 10, 2009, from http://www.unicef.org/media/media_15444.html

World Health Organization/South East Asian Region Organization. (2007). *Nepal DHS 2006 demographic and health indicators.*

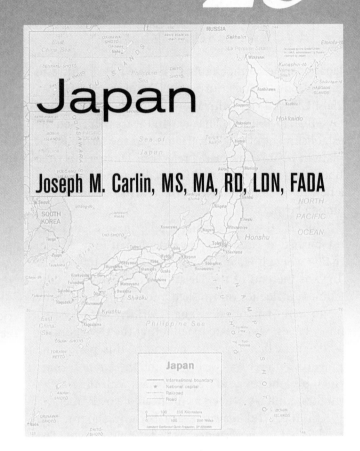

CHAPTER 25

Japan

Joseph M. Carlin, MS, MA, RD, LDN, FADA

"... an understanding and appreciation of Japanese cuisine implies a certain understanding and appreciation of the Japanese themselves."

—*Ka'ichi Tsuji* (Hosking, 2000)

 CULTURE AND WORLD REGION

Japan, called *Nippon* by the Japanese, literally means "the sun's origin" and is often translated as the *Land of the Rising Sun.* Located off the coast of the Asian continent in the Pacific Ocean, Japan's culture was heavily influenced by China and Korea. Most people observe both Shinto and Buddhist practices (84%), and about 1% identify themselves as Christians. The majority of Christians live in the west, where missionary activities were most intense during the 16th century.

Japan consists of four main islands (Honshu, Hokkaido, Kyushu, and Shikoku) and about 3000 smaller islands. The Japanese archipelago runs roughly north to southwest separated from the eastern coast of Asia by the Sea of Japan. Japan is about the size of California; if it were superimposed on North America, it would stretch from Montreal, Canada, to Tampa, Florida. About three fourths of the country is mountainous and two thirds is covered by forests and woodlands; only 11% percent is arable. Japan is politically structured into 8 regions and 47 prefectures. The population is just over 127 million people of whom 99% are ethnically Japanese.

 LANGUAGE

The language is Japanese but English is widely spoken and understood. Street signs in the urban areas, and a high percentage of store signs, advertisements, and food packaging, as well as menus, are printed in both Japanese and English.

CULTURE HISTORY

Japan's earliest inhabitants introduced agriculture to the volcanic islands during the Jōmon period (1000–250 BCE) and rice cultivation during the Yayoi period (300 BCE to 300 CE). The next 400 years witnessed the establishment of a political center in the fertile Kinai plain in what is now Nara prefecture. During this time Buddhism was introduced from China and Korea and a new tax system resulted in the redistribution of land among farmers.

In 710, the first permanent Japanese capital was established at Nara but moved to Heian (now Kyoto) in 794 where it would remain for the next 1000 years. Toward the end of the Heian period (710–1185 CE), Chinese influence diminished and ideas from outside Japan were "Japanized." Kana, a writing system based on syllables, was created facilitating the development of Japanese literature. At the end of this period the Emperor's power was weakened and the *samurai* (warriors) became the leading social class with the *shōgun* (highest military officer) as the head of government.

In 1603, Tokugawa Ieyasu became shōgun and established his government in Edo (now Tokyo). The Tokugawa shōguns ruled Japan in peace for the next 250 years. During the 1630s the shōgun forbade traveling abroad, banned all foreign books, and limited trade to China and the Netherlands. Japan entered a period of almost total isolation from the rest of the world.

In 1853, Japan was forcefully opened to the outside world by the American commodore Matthew Perry when he sailed into Tokyo harbor and pressured the Tokugawa government to open the country to international trade. In 1868, the modern period began with the restoration of the emperor when he moved from seclusion in Kyoto to Edo (now Tokyo), and took the name of Meiji.

FOOD HISTORY WITHIN THE CULTURE

Japan's earliest inhabitants are credited with introducing agriculture to the archipelago. Called the Jōmon period, these early people grew millet and root crops and supplemented their diet by hunting, fishing, and gathering. Rice cultivation was introduced from China and Korea during the Yayoi period. In fact, the early indigenous name for Japan was *mizu ho no kuni* (the land of the water stalk plant or rice).

Japanese food culture was influenced by delegations returning from China, who brought back Tang Dynasty (618–904 CE) high culture including chopsticks and scroll painting. One of these early scrolls depicts foods and dishes served at aristocratic feasts (Hosking, 2000). Throughout history the majority of the population led a poor and desperate existence in the rural areas toiling in the rice patties or as subsistence farmers. A small group of artisans, craftsman, and merchants catered to the needs of the aristocratic class.

During Japan's early history the majority of the population subsisted on millet, tubers, and rice. A high percentage of harvested rice was used for paying taxes (Ashkenazi & Jacob, 2003). By 700 CE rice became firmly established as the staple food and has remained so. During the 19th century annual consumption of rice per person was about 330 lbs. but has dropped to about 110 lbs. today. The Japanese prefer to grow their own short-grain Japonica variety (*Oryza sativa japonica*), as opposed to long-grain varieties (*jawa* and *indica*) found in Southeast Asia. When cooked, Japanese rice becomes slightly sticky, enabling it to be picked up in mouthfuls with a pair of chopsticks. It is appreciated for its rich, slightly sweet flavor.

Historically one-pot cooking on an open *irori* (hearth), a pot suspended from an adjustable trammel over a charcoal fire in a sand pit, was the traditional method of cooking. Whatever was on hand went into the pot: vegetables and seafood or just vegetables. With prosperity, particularly in the late Tokugawa and Meiji periods, the pattern of the ordinary meal (*ichijū issai*) evolved. This meal consisted of a bowl of soup, a pickled vegetable of some kind, and a bowl of rice (Hosking, 2000). This meal was first consumed by the samurai class and copied by the richer merchants. By the Meiji period, even townspeople and laborers were following the new meal pattern (Hanley, 1997).

As Japan's economy grew, farmers began to eat more rice (not only more rice, but more highly milled and polished rice). Those people who could afford the so-called highest-quality rice often developed a vitamin B deficiency. Because many low-paid workers tended to live in the cities, beriberi (a nervous system ailment caused by a deficiency of thiamin, vitamin B₁) became known as "Edo affliction" (Hanley, 1997). One measure of well-being and wealth of a people is the publica-

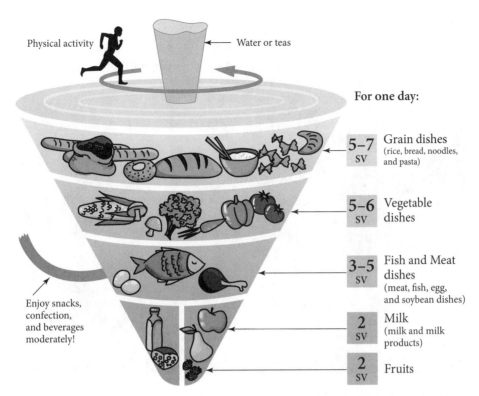

Physical activity

Water or teas

For one day:

5–7 SV   Grain dishes (rice, bread, noodles, and pasta)

5–6 SV   Vegetable dishes

3–5 SV   Fish and Meat dishes (meat, fish, egg, and soybean dishes)

2 SV   Milk (milk and milk products)

2 SV   Fruits

Enjoy snacks, confection, and beverages moderately!

SV is an abbreviation of "Serving", which is a simple, countable number describing the approximate amount of each dish or food served to one person

Japanese Food Guide Spinning Top

Source: Reprinted with permission from the Japan Ministry of Health, Labour and Welfare and Ministry of Agriculture, Forestry and Fisheries; Tohoku Regional Agricultural Administration Office.

tion of cookbooks. As people are exposed to new foods and dishes, they look to cookbooks as how-to manuals to help duplicate the experience. Japan's first cookbook was *Ryōri monogatari* (*The Story of Cooking*) published in 1643. Over 100 cookbooks had been published by the late Tokugawa period (Hanley, 1997).

MAJOR FOODS

Protein Sources

Products made from soybean, fish, and shellfish are the principle protein sources in the Japanese diet. Historically, meat made up a very small part of the Japanese diet. A 1918 study found that the yearly per-person consumption of beef was only 1.5 lbs. and milk consumption was less than 1 qt. per year (Morimoto, 1918). In 1873, Emperor Meiji encouraged the Japanese to eat meat to improve their physique. Today Japan produces

some of the most expensive beef in the world. Wagyu beef (also known as "Kobe beef") is appreciated for the "marbling," which refers to the fine white streaks of fat that run through the meat enhancing its flavor and tenderness. Kobe rib-eye steak can sell for as much as $300/lb. (2008 figures). Pork is also popular and horse meat has its devotees (Hosking, 2000).

Animal meat was never a major protein source in Japan until the country ended its isolation in the second half of the 19th century. The Western preference for meat slowly spread to the general population following its adoption as a protein source by the army during the Sino-Japanese War and the Russo-Japanese War. The army introduced beef calling it Japanese stew (*yamato-ni*). An instant market for imported meat was created by newly discharged soldiers.

The principle animal protein is fish. One of the most popular fast foods is sushi, which originated in the 19th century. Sushi can be made with many ingredients, but its most popular form is a thumb-size

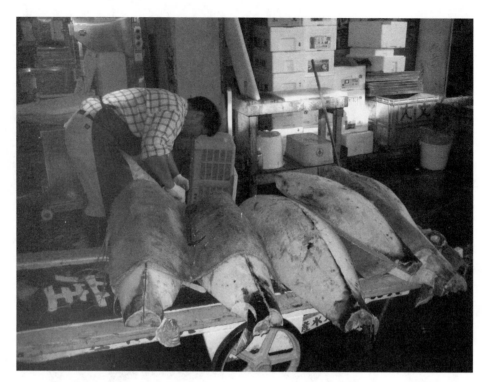

The Tsukiji Fish Market of Tokyo is the largest fish market in the world.
Courtesy of the author

mound of sticky rice with a slice of raw fish on top (*nigari-sushi*). *Maki-sushi* is rice wrapped in seaweed and stuffed with a filling such as vegetables or fish.

Soybean, a legume high in protein, is the raw ingredient for miso, *shōyu* (soy sauce), tōfu, and soy milk (*tonyū*). Buddhists, who avoided meat of any kind, very early promoted this legume in place of meat. Soybean foods, small bony fish, and seaweed are also important calcium sources (Kittler & Sucher, 2000).

Miso, a soybean paste fermented with *kōji* (mold spores), is ubiquitous in the Japanese diet. It is the principle ingredient in *misoshiru* (miso soup), a major protein source that is served at almost every meal.

 ## Starch Sources

The Japanese prefer short-grain rice, which possesses a high level of amylopectin, a highly branched starch that makes rice tender and lets it cling together. Rice (*kome*) is the element around which the meal is structured. The Japanese feel that a meal without rice is incomplete. Other cereals important to the Japanese diet are millet (*awa*), barley, sorghum (*kibi*), and buckwheat.

Wheat flour was introduced to the Japanese diet in a significant way following the Tokyo earthquake of 1923 and again after World War II, when the United States sent wheat as food relief. With no tradition of making Western-style bread, the Japanese made batter-based dishes or crepe-like dishes such as *issen-yoshoku* or "one-penny Western food." The first self-contained bread-making machine came on the market in Japan in 1986.

Wheat and buckwheat are consumed in the form of noodles, ramen, sōmen, and udon. Buckwheat noodles (*soba*) are appreciated for their aroma and subtle taste. Buckwheat cultivation originated in mountainous areas inhospitable to other crops and was a backup in case the rice harvest failed. Wheat flour is frequently mixed with buckwheat to prevent the noodles from breaking apart; however, 100% buckwheat noodles are available for those who know their soba from their udon.

Sōmen are very thin, white noodles made of wheat flour. The difference between sōmen and udon is that sōmen is stretched and udon are cut. Japanese mostly associate eating sōmen during the summer as it is served cold with a dipping broth.

Ramen are wheat-based noodles served in a broth and topped with sliced pork, green onions, mung beans, or seaweed. Every region of Japan has its own distinct way of serving ramen. In 1958 Momofuku Ando, founder of Nissin Foods, invented instant ramen noodles and they have become a Japanese cultural icon.

Fat Sources

The Japanese favor foods that are fresh and have a clean taste rather than the taste and oral feel of deep-fried or greasy food. Historically, very little food was deep-fat fried in Japan until the Portuguese introduced deep-fried foods such as tempura (fritters). Until that time (1500–1640 CE) the Japanese used sesame oil for deep-fried foods. This was replaced with rapeseed oil (canola oil). More recently, *furai* (fried foods), such as seafood coated in egg and breadcrumbs and deep-fried, are becoming more popular.

 Prominent Vegetables

Before World War II, the Japanese diet was largely vegetarian. Vegetarianism was promoted by the Buddhist belief that it is wrong to harm any sentient being (i.e., any animal capable of feelings). The practice of abstaining from animal flesh, including fowl and fish on Buddhist holy days, was adopted by the upper classes and led to the development of *shojin ryori*, meatless Japanese cuisine (Bergen, 1994). *Shojin* means the pursuit of a perfect state of mind. Ingredients for *shojin ryori*, also called "temple food," follow the seasons; new sprouts and shoots in spring, green leaves in sum-

mer, fruits and nuts in autumn, and roots in winter. The monks who developed this cuisine used a lot of soybeans, vegetables, and fat from walnuts, peanuts, and sesame seeds. Seaweed and mushrooms supplied calcium, phosphorous, and iron. Because they are believed to arouse desires, onions, garlic, and scallions are not used in *shojin* cooking.

Many vegetables are preserved by drying or pickling. Pickles (*tsukemono*) are served as a condiment at most meals and are an important accompaniment with sake (an alcoholic beverage) and beer. Besides salt and vinegar, which dominate Western pickling, the Japanese incorporate miso and *nuka* (rice bran paste). Regional pickled specialties are found throughout the country. Pickled vegetables are a Kyoto favorite. Western-style vegetable salads are frequently eaten for breakfast.

Many meals are accompanied by a dish called *sunomono* (*su* means vinegared and *mono* means things), which is made from a small Japanese cucumber sliced thin with turnips, bamboo shoots, and lotus root, and is marinated in sweetened vinegar. Vegetables, such as sweet peppers, asparagus, okra, pumpkin, and sweet potato, are eaten braised, cooked in *dashi* (Japanese soup stock), or dipped in tempura batter and fried.

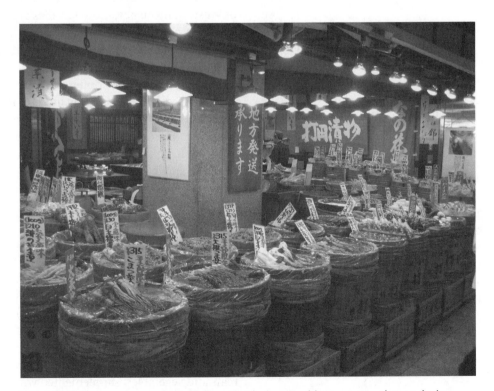

This pickle processor and retail outlet is located in a covered arcade in Koyto.

Courtesy of the author

The yam (*yama-imo*) grows in the mountains and is grated into soup or sliced and deep-fried in fat. Sweet potatoes (*satsuma-imo*) are a favorite snack food roasted over a charcoal stove mounted on open-backed trucks. Japan's climate makes it the ideal place for the cultivation of mushrooms and fungus. The shiitake, matsutake, shimeji, mai-take, and enoki-dake are the best known.

Young soybean pods (*eda-mame*) are Japan's most visible green vegetable to most foreigners. Bamboo shoots (*take-no-ko*) and spring onions (*negi*) are widely used as soup ingredients. The Japanese love eggplant (*nasu*), which come in a wide range of shapes—roundish, elongated, and egg shaped (*kuro-nasu*)—and varieties. They are prepared in a variety of ways including pickled, used in tempura, or grilled with tōfu.

Prominent Fruits

Four fruits stand out in importance; namely, plums, mandarin oranges, pears, and persimmons. Plums are dried and pickled (*umeboshi*) and used as an appetizer; pickled *umeboshi* is mostly eaten with rice and also used as filling in *onigiri* (rice balls) in the summer for its saltiness and its natural preservation qualities. Depending on the season, peaches, apples, grapes, figs, cherries, and other fruits are harvested in Japan or imported.

The Japanese have a particular fondness for strawberries. They were introduced into Japan from Holland during the first half of the 19th century. They are considered a winter fruit since they are grown in hot houses set up on empty rice fields. They are served with either condensed milk or cream.

Spices and Seasonings

Many restaurants put a spice mixture on the table called *shichimi togarashi* (*shichi* means seven, *mi* means flavors), which consists of *sansho* pepper (prickly ash seed pod; related to Szechuan pepper from China), chili pepper, sesame seeds, mustard, hemp, poppy seeds, dried citrus peel, and sometimes powdered seaweed (*nori*). It is sprinkled on *yakitori* and on bowls of noodles or soup. Thinly sliced peach-colored pickled ginger and green wasabi garnish many meals as a condiment. A bottle of soy sauce is always within reach.

Beverages

Sake is the national drink of Japan. Beer is the beverage of choice for toasting and social events. At home, sake is consumed daily at the evening meal by adults. Because sake is made from rice, it is not consumed when rice is eaten. There are 1500 sake brewers throughout Japan, each producing between 10 and 30 kinds of sake. The spectrum of up to 30,000 different sakes to choose from include champagne-like effervescent sake to 35-year-old Kurumazaka, which is said to have an intense layering of flavors reminiscent of aged balsamic vinegar (Sando, 2008).

Shochu is a beverage with a high alcoholic content that is growing in popularity. It can be made from a number of ingredients including barley, rice, and sweet potato. Besides yeast, the microbe koji (*Aspergillus* mold) is used in the fermentation. The final step is to age it in wooden barrels. *Shochu* is used at the beginning of the meal as an aperitif, or as an ingredient in cocktails (Benes, 2007).

The Japanese drink green tea after eating rice or at the conclusion of a meal. Tea is served in ceramic cups or bowls, whereas coffee is consumed from cups with handles. Sake is drunk from small ceramic or pottery cups, whereas milk, soda, and beer are served in glasses.

Desserts

Traditionally, sweets were consumed with tea. Because of Western influence, more families are adding dessert to meals consumed at home. French patisseries and Western-style pastry shops dot the streets in urban areas and at train stations.

One type of confectionery unique to Japan is *wagashi*, also called *chagashi* or literally tea sweets. *Wagashi* is a paste made from sugar and red azuki beans, white beans, sweet potatoes, and chestnuts or snow peas. From this basic paste (*an*) the confection is colored and made in various shapes.

FOODS WITH CULTURAL SIGNIFICANCE

The single most important food in Japan is rice. In the Japanese language, *gohan* means "cooked rice," and also "meal." Breakfast (*asa-gohan*) literally means "morning rice." The evening meal, the one meal that might bring the family together, is *ban-gohan*. For most of Japan's history the diet consisted chiefly of cereals and vegetables, supplemented with a little poultry and dried fish.

The perfect meal follows the ancient Chinese model containing five colors (purple, white, red, yellow, and green) using a variety of preparation methods (raw, grilling, steaming, boiling, braising, and deep-fat frying) and is composed of six tastes (sweet, bitter, salty, sour, peppery, and umami). Umami is a savory taste imparted by glutamate and ribonucleotides found in many foods including meat, fish, vegetables, and dairy products. It tends to expand and round out flavors and makes food taste better. Umami is associated with dried bonito flakes, kelp, and shiitake mushrooms in Japanese food (Ashburne & Abe, 2002). In 1908, Professor Ikeda Kiknae at Tokyo University isolated monosodium glutamate (MSG), the chemical that gives the umami taste to food.

The Japanese believe that food should be enjoyed as close as possible in its natural state and at the proper season. One expression of this philosophy is *sashimi* (raw fish). Next to raw fish would be grilled fish, followed by fish that has been simmered or lightly steamed, and then fried fish.

Japanese food is characterized by its cleanliness and aesthetics. Travelers to Japan in 1869 noted that "extreme cleanliness characterizes not only their dwellings, but their food, manner of cooking, serving it, etc." At a dinner they attended they observed that "everything was served on the most beautiful lacquer ware, no one set appearing twice throughout the evening" (Jephson & Elmhirst, 1869).

For the Japanese a good meal is more than just tasty food. The atmosphere, table setting, room, dishes, and artistic arrangement of food on the plate contribute to the visual appeal of the meal. Ka'ichi Tsuji, a tea-ceremony master said, "There is nothing more important in Japanese food than arranging it well, with special regard to the colors, or plates chosen to suit the food" (Hosking, 2000).

Under the influence of Zen Buddhism people ate from boxes and bowls set on small personal tables about 8 inches high. Tables were arranged on the floor in a hierarchy—children, the elderly, women, and men, in that order, based on distance from the kitchen. This arrangement was replaced by a low table (*chabudai*), about 12 inches high, at which the entire family sat around, women with their legs tucked under and men cross-legged. As the Japanese economy improved, Western tables and chairs were adopted.

At the beginning of the meal each person says *itadakimasu*, "I am about to take up," and at the end of the meal everyone will say *gochisosama*, "I have enjoyed my dinner very much."

The Japanese use *hashi*, chopsticks, just as most other cultures in Asia, but the Japanese chopsticks are traditionally made of lacquered wood and tapered to a point. They come in two sizes, long for men and shorter ones for women and children. Western-style utensils are also widely available.

Japanese food etiquette requires that food never be transferred from one's own chopsticks to someone else's chopsticks, because this is similar to a Japanese funeral rite whereby family members use chopsticks to transfer bones into an urn. They should never be stuck into the rice as this creates the image of burning incense at a Japanese funeral. Chopsticks should never be crossed because this symbolizes death. The Japanese never share chopsticks because they believe that if they touch another's mouth it could transmit a spiritual contamination. It is acceptable to hold a bowl of rice or soup with noodles close to the mouth when eating.

 ## TYPICAL DAY'S MENU

The Japanese generally eat three meals a day supplemented with an *oyatsu* (snack). The traditional breakfast, which includes *umeboshi* (salty sour plums), grilled fish, rice topped with nori, miso soup, and pickled vegetables, has not disappeared but is increasingly more confined to the weekends. Western-style breakfasts are the norm today. Children have cold cereal with milk and adults enjoy toast with butter, eggs (fried, scrambled, or as omelets), and pancakes.

A traditional lunch could be as simple as a bowl of rice topped with the previous night's leftovers or a bowl of noodles with added meat, fish, or vegetables. Increasingly more people are turning to pizza, Western-style hamburgers, and the Japanese-style hamburger made with teriyaki chicken provided by Mos Burger at its 1200 stores. Another form of fast food is *onigiri* (rice balls). *Onigiri* literally means "taking hold of (something) with your hands." It is made from cooked rice, pressed into a triangular shape, and often filled with grilled salmon, cod roe, *kombu* (kelp), or a pickled plum. It may be dusted with sesame seeds or wrapped in a sheet of *nori* (seaweed).

Eating outside the home is very common in Japan. Many restaurants specialize in just one type of food. The popular Edo-style finger-formed sushi (*nigiri-zushi*) originated in Tokyo early in the 19th century. Originally, cooked rice was packed around fresh fish fillets to prevent them from spoiling when transported into the countryside. At first the rice was thrown away, but then it was discovered that raw fish on top of vinegared rice tasted pretty good. The *sushi-ya* serves sushi either

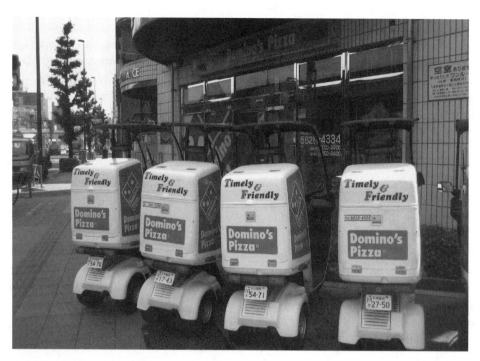

Domino's Pizza outlet in Tokyo. Four motor scooters lined up to dash across the city.
Courtesy of the author

at the table or at the sushi bar, directly in front of the sushi chef. Sushi restaurants that present their offerings on a conveyor belt are called *kaiten-zushi* restaurants. Sitting at the oval counter the customer picks the dish of choice off the moving belt and is charged according to the number of empty plates.

Yakitori-ya restaurants specialize in chicken grilled on skewers. Skewered items might also include

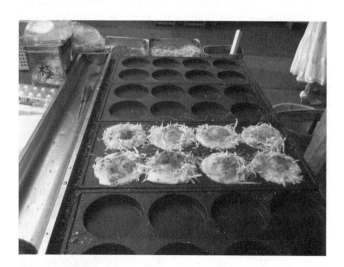

Street Food in Tokyo
Courtesy of the author

beef, vegetables, and even quail eggs. These places are very popular. Other specialized restaurants serve curry rice (*kare-ya*), freshwater eel (*unagi-ya*), and tempura dishes (*tempura-ya*). Tempura can be fish or vegetables dipped in a light batter and fried in vegetable and sesame seed oil. It was introduced by the Portuguese in the 16th century.

Some restaurants specialize in puffer fish (*fugu*), which is highly prized, very expensive, and potentially dangerous because it contains tetrodotoxin, a deadly poison that requires a well-trained cook to prepare it safely. These restaurants advertise by hanging a dried puffer fish outside the entrance.

The *izakaya* is the place where the Japanese go to after work to socialize over sake and small dishes of their favorite foods. The "I" in *izakaya* means to "stay" or "linger." The atmosphere in these neighborhood eateries is similar to that of an Irish pub, a café in France, a beer hall in Germany, or a neighborhood tavern in the United States. An *izakaya* is a relaxed and inviting place that many Japanese call their second home. *Izakaya* are known for their seasonal dishes priced relatively inexpensively.

You cannot walk the streets of Japan and not be aware of the great number of vending machines (*jidō-hanbaiki*) that dispense everything imaginable from fresh to prepared food. It is estimated that there are over 6 million machines that provide such things as yogurt drinks, fresh eggs, instant ramen, soba/udon, 10-kg (about 22 lbs.) bags of rice, and a wide selection of beer and liquor. Vending machines became popular during the Tokyo Olympics in 1964 when it was necessary to supply large numbers of people with goods and services quickly.

Japan's 40,000 convenience stores (*konbini*) are a daily destination for most Japanese because they are open 24 hours a day. Almost one third of the population visits a convenience store two or three times a week, and 17% go daily. Food products in demand at these stores include prepackaged microwavable meals, sushi, boxed lunches, curries, instant noodle products, bottled teas, snacks, and sweets such as rice balls and rice crackers. Cold dishes can also be heated up in the store for students and single men/women. Convenience stores also sell beer, sake, *shochu* (liquor), and wines.

Traveling by train or subway is a way of life for the Japanese. Since ancient times the Japanese have carried convenient packs of food while traveling. Today, these lunchboxes are called *bento*, a word that can be translated as "usefulness" and "eating quickly." In the 1800s,

bento boxes were created for people traveling by train. Today, eki bento (*ekiben, eki* meaning station) is a delicious custom still available to the traveler. The typical *ekiben* contains rice, egg omelets, grilled fish, a piece of teriyaki chicken, a vegetable, and pickles that reflect regional and/or seasonal specialties.

Despite having one of the most traditional and unique food customs in the world, Japan was no match for the global onslaught of fast food. McDonald's came to Japan in 1971, followed by Kentucky Fried Chicken, Mr. Donut, Wendy's, and Pizza Hut. Western fast foods have a strong hold on Japan, pizza being one of the most popular; however, toppings are quite different from those in the United States and Europe, including baby corn, fish, shrimp, squid, and tuna.

Foods prepared quickly are not new to the Japanese. Those wanting a quick lunch or dinner dine on noodles, rice with toppings (*gyūdon*), and street foods.

Yoshinoya and Sukiya are two home-grown fast-food chains that specialize in *gyūdon* (beef bowl). *Gyū* means "beef" and *don* is short for *donburi*, meaning bowl. It is a dish that consists of a bowl of rice topped with beef and onions simmered in a broth flavored with soy sauce. The dish is topped with pickled ginger

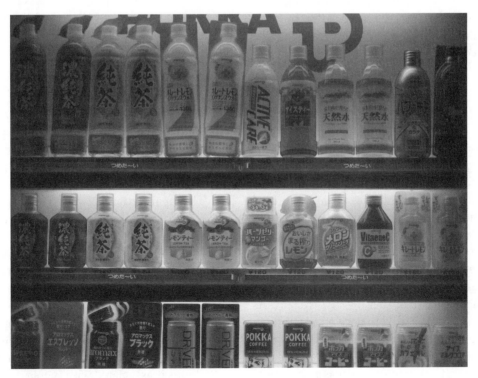

Vending Machine in Tokyo
Courtesy of the author

(*beni shoga*). In 2006, *gyūdon* chains stopped selling the dish due to fear of mad cow disease from imported American beef. American beef was banned and some *gyūdon* chains imported beef from Australia, whereas others switched to pork and/or chicken.

One of the most popular street foods in Osaka, Japan's second largest city (8 million people), is *takoyaki*, boiled octopus formed into balls and fried. Osaka's streets are dotted with *takoyaki* stalls. Many people own a special grill with hemispherical pockets for making this national food at home.

 ## HOLIDAY MENUS

Mochi is a rice cake made from steamed rice and pounded in a large wooden mortar with a wooden mallet until it takes on dough-like consistency. It is traditionally made as part of a New Year's celebration. Because of its dense consistency, *mochi* can be a choking hazard for the elderly.

The calendar is filled with festivals associated with harvesting or geared to celebrations centered on Buddhist temples or Shinto shrines. In homes and Buddhist temples an offertory presentation is made from two rice cakes, the largest on the bottom and topped off with a tangerine or mandarin. The large rice cake represents the older generations, the small cake represents the younger generation, and the orange symbolizes the generations to come.

 ## HEALTH BELIEFS AND CONCERNS

Lactose intolerance was very common in Japan, because after weaning, children rarely had access to milk; however, milk consumption has continued to increase in Japan and lactose intolerance has abated. Demand for milk products, such as yogurts, milk-fermented drinks, and cheese, is now close to Western levels. Yogurt beverages with live *bacilli* are popular and sold in vending machines.

The Japanese tend to have high rates of stomach cancer and other diseases of the digestive system. As early as the 1930s, Japan started to develop a lactic acid probiotic beverage called *yakult*. Japan is recognized as a leader in the development and marketing of prebiotic and probiotic food to promote good gastrointestinal health. Prebiotics, nondigestible food ingredients such as soluble fiber, are known to stimulate the growth

Observations from the Author (Joseph M. Carlin)

Japan has the reputation of being one of the most expensive countries in the world to eat in, particularly the city of Tokyo. Yes, it can be very expensive if you eat in hotel restaurants that cater to a Western clientele; however, Japan can be one of the most economical culinary destinations for the adventurous tourist or the budget-conscious student. A quick continental-style breakfast can be had at any convenience store. These stores sell single servings of instant coffee, and hotel rooms come equipped with an electric kettle for heating water for tea, coffee, or for making a bowl of noodles.

Because the Japanese eat out a lot, the streets, particularly around train and subway stations and markets, abound with noodle shops, and restaurants that sell "set" meals that are organized like a TV dinner on a single tray. Many restaurants display realistic plastic models of their dishes outside their shops. All you have to do is point to the meal you want.

A visit to Japan would not be complete without a bento box for at least one meal. These inexpensive meals are attractively packaged and always a joy to open. Street food and pastry shops are always nearby for a quick snack and there is always a vending machine nearby for a beer and a bowl of ramen noodles.

and activity of healthy bacteria in the colon. Probiotics are "friendly" bacteria introduced into foods such as yogurt and fermented milk to address gastrointestinal health issues. Prebiotic and probiotic products represent a $3.6 billion (2005 figures) industry in Japan (Bailey, 2008).

The Japanese have always had a high consumption of sodium chloride in their diet. A study conducted in 1918 found the per capita annual intake of salt to be almost 40 lbs. while the yearly intake of sugar was only 14 lbs. Salt intake is proportional to the consumption of pickled vegetables, miso, soybean products, and dried fish and shellfish. As the diet became westernized after World War II, salt consumption gradually decreased (Kimura, Yokomukai, & Komai, 1987). Epidemiologic studies indicate that consumption of salt or salty foods is associated with increased risk of stomach cancer. Despite this obvious health risk, the Japanese live longer than any other people.

GENERAL HEALTH AND NUTRITIONAL INDICATORS SUMMARY

According to UNICEF (2007), 8.6% of Japanese infants were in low-birth-weight categories from 1998 to 2005. This was parallel to the United States, which had an 8% rate during the same time period. The life expectancy of a Japanese person is 73 years as of 2007. Japan also boosts high child-immunization rates, low infant mortality rates, and an HIV rate of 0.1%, consistent with most industrialized countries. Malnutrition, for children under 5 years in the weight-for-age category, is 3.7%, and 5.6% in the height-for-age category (UNICEF, 2007).

FEATURED RECIPE

Miso pastes vary enormously in sodium content. Generally speaking, lighter color pastes are more mildly salted and somewhat sweeter; the darker the color, the saltier the paste. In this recipe, a medium-salty one, with about 735 mg sodium/tbsp. was used.

Salmon Marinated with Miso Paste

2 tbsp. miso paste
2 tbsp. mirin (sweet cooking sake)
2 tbsp. sake (rice wine, preferably dry)
12 oz. salmon fillet

For garnish:

4 stalks broccoli rabe
1 cup water
1 tsp. soy sauce
½ tsp. sesame oil
1 sheet of nori (dry seawed), thinly sliced using scissors

1. Place miso paste, mirin, and sake together in a shallow container, large enough to hold the salmon fillet, and mix well with a folk.
2. Rinse salmon with cold tap water and dry with paper towel. Cut the fillet into four pieces. Place the pieces in the marinade, coating both sides well. Marinate overnight, or for at least 4 to 5 hours.
3. Rinse the broccoli rabe. Boil water in a small saucepan, place the broccoli in the pan, cover, and parboil until tender, about 3 to 4 minutes. Remove from heat, drain, and immediately cool in cold tap water. Lightly squeeze out extra water. Cut into pieces 1 to 2 inches long.
4. Pour soy sauce and sesame oil in a mixing bowl, add broccoli rabe and nori, and mix together; divide into four portions.
5. Set oven to broil, 500°F, placing shelf in the middle position. Cover a baking sheet with foil for protection from grease, and spray canola oil on foil.
6. With fingers, remove any extra miso paste from surface of the fillet and place it on the foil, skin side up. Broil about 10 minutes, or until surface becomes slightly browned, then turn and grill other side not more than 5 minutes, until golden brown. Timing depends on thickness of the filet. While piping hot, serve with the prepared broccoli rabe.

Note: Nori and mirin are available in Asian outlets and some regular grocery stores. Nori comes in a flat packet, usually marked for sushi rolls. If you do not have nori, it can be replaced with roasted sesame seeds. Sake can be found in a liquor store. This recipe uses dry sake. Parboiled spinach or broccoli may be substituted for broccoli rabe. Also, ½ tsp. Dijon mustard can be used instead of sesame oil.

Courtesy of Setsuko Sasaki

More recipes are available at http://nutrition.jbpub.com/foodculture/

REFERENCES

Ashburne, J., & Abe, Y. (2002). *World food Japan.* London: Lonely Planet Publications.

Ashkenazi, M., & Jacob, J. (2003). *Food culture in Japan: Food culture around the world.* Westport, CT: Greenwood Press.

Bailey, R. (2008). Prebiotics and probiotics in Japan. *Nutraceuticals World, 11*(3), 26–27.

Benes, R.J. (2007). Shochu (show-chew). *Chef Magazine, 51*(10), 14.

Bergen, T. (1994). *Vegetarian Asia: A travel guide.* San Francisco: Noble Poodle Press.

Booth, S. (2002). *Food of Japan.* New York: Interlink Books.

Hanley, S.B. (1997). *Everyday things in premodern Japan.* Berkeley, CA: University Press.

Hosking, R. (2000). *At the Japanese table.* New York: Oxford University Press.

Jephson, R.M., & Elmhirst, E.P. (1869). *Our life in Japan.* London: Chapman and Hall.

Kimura S., Yokomukai, Y., & Komai, M. (1987). Salt consumption and nutritional state especially dietary protein level. *American Journal of Clinical Nutrition, 45,* 1271–1276.

Kittler, P.G., & Sucher, K.P. (2000). *Cultural foods: Traditions and trends.* Belmont, CA: Wadsworth/Thomson Learning.

Morimoto, K. (1918). *The standard of living in Japan.* Dissertation. Baltimore: Johns Hopkins Press.

Ota, K. (2008). Rediscovering Tokyo's Izakaya. *Kateigaho International Edition, 19* (Spring), 128–141.

Richie, D. (1985). *A taste of Japan.* New York: Kodansha International Ltd.

Sando, A. (2008). Savoring the golden age of sake. *Kateigaho International Edition, 19* (Spring), 144–149.

UNICEF. (2007). *The state of the world's children 2007: Women and children, the double dividend of gender equality.* Retrieved April 14, 2009, from http://www.unicef.org/sowc07/statistics/tables.php

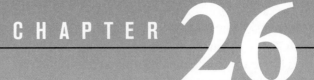

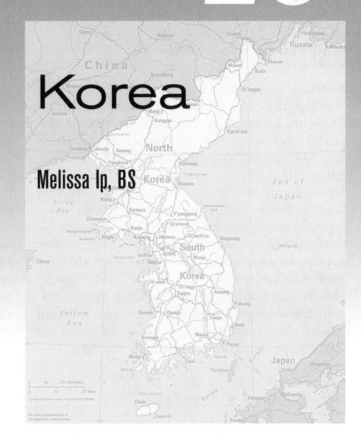

CHAPTER 26

Korea

Melissa Ip, BS

 CULTURE AND WORLD REGION

Korea is one of the oldest continuous civilizations in the world. Koreans are believed to be descendents of Mongol tribes that migrated to the Korean peninsula from Central Asia. While remaining a unified and independent nation for many millennia, in the past 50 years Korea has existed as two nations: the Democratic People's Republic of Korea (more commonly known as North Korea) and the Republic of Korea (South Korea). Despite its ethnic and cultural homogeneity, a variety of religions are practiced, including Christianity, Confucianism, Buddhism, and shamanism. Modern Korean values and social structure are largely based on Confucian values, which emphasize education, frugality, hard work, and strong family values. Koreans are well educated, with high literacy rates in both urban and rural areas. Confucian values enforce hierarchies by gender, age, and class. Seniors are highly respected, and children are expected to care for their parents in old age. As a patriarchal society, the oldest male serves as the authority figure not only in the home but in the workplace; however, in recent years a greater number of women have entered the workforce and have come to occupy leadership positions in many fields. Another change has been the significant migration both in and out of Korea. Koreans have migrated to the United States since the early 20th century, with the largest influx occurring after World War II. Today, there are over a million Korean immigrants in the United States, residing mainly in the western and northeastern states. The majority of immigrants arrive from South Korea.

North and South Korea are located in East Asia, which includes China, Taiwan, and Japan. The two countries are situated on a mountainous peninsula surrounded by the Yellow Sea to its west and the Sea of Japan (or the East Sea) to its right. Its neighboring countries are China and Russia across its northern border, and Japan across the Korea Strait. The total size of the peninsula, 218,600 km^2 (Central Intelligence

Agency [CIA], 2008a, 2008b), is about the size of Utah. North Korea is home to 23 million residents, and South Korea is populated by almost 49 million residents (CIA, 2008a, 2008b).

LANGUAGE

Korean is spoken mainly by residents of North and South Korea and by Korean immigrants living in China, the United States, Japan, Russia, and Australia, among other countries. Korean has some regional dialectal differences; however, compared with other languages, the Korean language is considered relatively homogeneous. Written Korean is known as *Hangul* in South Korea. In Korean, surnames are written before given names. When Romanized, some given names are written as one word, and some names are written as two with a space in between them. (Note: Although multiple systems for writing Korean in the Roman alphabet exist, in this chapter the 2000 Revised Romanization system is used. The exception is the word *gimchi*, which is more popularly known as *kimchi* and is written as such in this chapter.)

CULTURE HISTORY

The peninsula known today as North and South Korea has developed from centuries of rule by ancient dynasties. The earliest dynasty, Old Choson, existed from approximately 2333 to 562 BC. The Three Kingdoms period, between 37 BC and 935 AD, saw the separation of the peninsula into three warring tribal states, the Goguryo in the north, and the Baekje and Silla in the south. The state of Silla eventually took over and unified the three kingdoms. During this time, the religions of Buddhism and Confucianism were introduced from China.

During the successive Goryeo Dynasty (918 to 1392) the country became known as "Corea." Buddhism became the state religion, particularly that of the court and aristocracy. This period was not without its conflicts with its neighbors, and the dynasty fell after the Mongol invasion in 1388. The last dynasty, Choson, followed, lasting from 1392 to 1910. During this time Koreans were encouraged to adopt Confucian principles over Buddhism. Many cultural and scientific achievements were made during this dynasty, including the development of the written form of Korean, *Hangul.*

In the early 19th century, Japan colonized Korea in the aftermath of wars between Japan, China, and Russia. Japan occupied Korea until World War II, when it gained independence from Japan but was split into North and South Korea. Conflicts ensued between the two states, culminating in the Korean War from 1950 to 1953. Tension still remains, although there have been recent efforts made at creating peaceful relations.

FOOD HISTORY WITHIN THE CULTURE

Cereals, such as millet and sorghum, have been cultivated in Korea since 2000 BC. Millet is likely to be the only grain native to the country; however, rice, introduced from China, is considered the staple grain in the Korean diet. Barley was also introduced in Korea and is consumed widely as barley tea and in mixed-grain dishes. During the Three Kingdoms era, land-reform policies increased rice production as well as the cultivation of soybeans, red beans, mung beans, and buckwheat.

Many different fruits, vegetables, and nuts have been part of the Korean diet since ancient times, including radishes, turnips, lotus roots, taro, yams, leeks, lettuce, green onions, garlic, cucumbers, eggplant, pears, peaches, chestnuts, pine nuts, and hazel nuts. Wild plants eaten include bamboo shoots, ferns, mushrooms, ginseng, and bellflower. Foods from the Americas introduced into Korea include chili peppers, pumpkins, sweet potatoes, white potatoes, maize, and tomatoes. Potatoes, which grew well in the northern parts of Korea, became particularly popular, as did chili peppers, which are responsible for the characteristic spiciness of Korean cuisine.

There is a Korean saying that Korean cooking takes "ages to prepare, seconds to consume" because of how time-intensive the recipes are. With less time devoted to cooking, convenience foods (including instant noodles and Western fast food) are gradually finding their way into the daily diet of Koreans. With the economic prosperity South Korea has experienced in the past 50 years, Koreans have changed the way they eat, including eating more animal and milk products and fewer cereals and starchy foods. While rice remains the most important starch, breads and baked goods are becoming more popular.

Some Koreans have resisted changes to their traditional culture by embracing the concept of *sinto buri.* Rooted in a Buddhist philosophy, *sinto buri* literally means "body and soil are not separate." Touted by antitrade activists and farmers' associations, the slogan is used to promote the idea that food from Korean soil is best for Korean bodies. A continued interest in, and consumption of, wild plants in Korea is another example of steadfast preference for locally grown foods. Wild foods include green leafy vegetables, pine needles, flowers, herbs, and ferns. These foods are used to make *banchan* (side dishes), among other Korean dishes.

 MAJOR FOODS

 Protein Sources

Seafood, chicken, tofu, and eggs are eaten regularly. Koreans have a stronger preference for beef than is seen in other parts of Asia. Pork is less common but is used to prepare dishes such as *kimchi jjigae*, a *kimchi* stew. Because red meat is more expensive, small portions of meat are usually prepared mixed with vegetables. Living on a peninsula, Koreans have access to an abundant variety of seafood, including fish, shellfish, octopus, and squid. A popular snack is *ojing-eo*, dried squid jerky that is widely available in grocery and convenience stores. *Soon dubu* is a spicy stew prepared with soft tofu, clams, squid, shrimp, and scallions in a beef stock, and seasoned with plenty of red pepper flakes, garlic, salt, and sesame oil.

 Starch Sources

The Korean diet is largely carbohydrate based and low in fat. Short-grain white rice (*bap*) is the main staple of the Korean diet, although it is common to find beans, chestnut, barley, millet, or other grains mixed in for added nutritional value or taste. The predominance of rice in the diet has contributed to keeping fat intake among Koreans relatively low, even though the economic development that Korea has experienced is usually associated with increased fat intake (Kim, Moon, & Popkin, 2000).

Rice can be boiled to make *juk*, a thick porridge. *Juk* is eaten for breakfast, as a snack, or during sickness. Nuts and beans, such as pine nuts and red beans, can also be ground or mashed and added to the porridge. Meats, vegetables, or fish can also be added. *Tteok* (rice cakes) are another important part of Korean cuisine and can be prepared as a sweet or salty snack or as a component of soups and other dishes. Unlike the puffed rice cakes that are a popular snack in the United States,

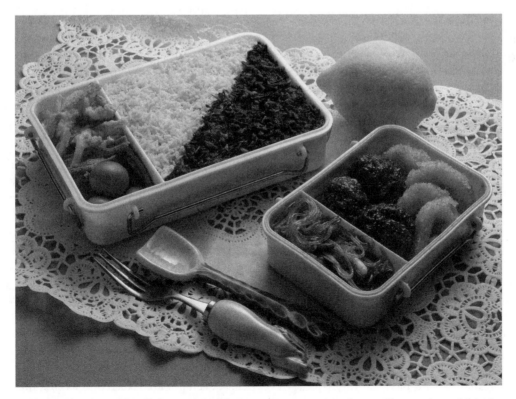

Japchae is a noodle dish made with sweet potato starch noodles, strips of fried egg, beef, mushrooms, and vegetables.

Korean rice cakes are made from rice flour and shaped into balls, coins, or cylinders. They can be steamed to a soft and chewy consistency or pan-fried.

There are a variety of noodles (*guksu*) eaten in Korean cuisine. They are made of wheat, buckwheat, potato starch, mung beans, or arrowroot, and can be eaten either hot or cold in broth or dry with meats and vegetables. Buckwheat noodles, which are thin, chewy, brown noodles, are very common in cold noodle dishes such as *mul naengmyeon*, a delicious dish of buckwheat noodles in a chilled beef broth with vegetables and boiled eggs often enjoyed during the summer. *Jap-chae* is another noodle dish made with sweet potato starch noodles, strips of fried egg, beef, mushrooms, and vegetables.

 ## Fat Sources

Sesame oil is a fragrant oil commonly used in Korean cooking for frying, flavoring, and as a component of sauces such as *doenjang*, a seasoned soybean paste made of fermented soybean paste, minced garlic, green onions, and sesame oil. Vegetable oils are also used in cooking. A study done by Gordon, Kang, Cho, and Sucher. (2000) found that Korean-Americans in the San Francisco Bay Area, California, often use corn oil in addition to sesame oil. Butter, margarine, and mayonnaise are rarely used in Korean cooking (Gordon et al., 2000).

 ## Prominent Vegetables

Seasoned vegetables (*namul*) are served at every meal, often in the form of colorful and tasty side dishes (*ban-chan*). *Namul* are fresh or lightly cooked vegetables such as bean sprouts, carrots, cabbage, white radish, green onions, potato, seaweed, and cucumbers. They are usually parboiled or stir-fried in sesame oil and seasoned with garlic, soy sauce, and sesame seeds. The fermented, spicy vegetable side dish, *kimchi*, is the most notable vegetable eaten. Other vegetables eaten include soybean sprouts, mushrooms, Korean zucchini, eggplant, bellflower root, leafy vegetables (including spinach, burdock, mugwort) lotus root, sweet potato, leeks, and pumpkin.

Vegetables are also added to rice, noodles, meat dishes, flatcakes (*jun*), and pancakes (*buchingae*). Pumpkins or winter squash will sometimes be boiled and blended with *juk*, (rice porridge). *Bibimbap* is a popular Korean dish with a base of white rice, covered in a variety of seasoned, cooked vegetables such as spinach, mushrooms, soybean sprouts, fern bracken,

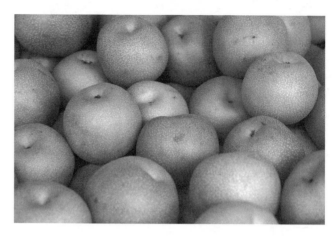

Asian Pears

Korean zucchini, and carrots. *Bulgogi*, or barbecued beef, and eggs can be served with it as well. This dish is usually eaten mixed up with a liberal serving of *gochu-jang*, a red chili paste.

 ## Prominent Fruits

Fresh fruits are often enjoyed at the end of the meal. Fruits that are commonly eaten fresh or used in dishes include apples, Asian pears, peaches, strawberries, cherries, dates (*jujubes*), grapes, melons, tangerines, persimmons, and plums. With modern growing practices, Koreans have been able to grow fruit not normally grown in its temperate climate, including oranges, kiwi, and bananas.

 ## Spices, Seasonings, and Condiments

Korean cuisine is characterized by its spicy dishes. A Korean proverb states that "spice is the power of the Korean." Preserved and fermented foods provide a spectrum of flavors in Korean cuisine. Koreans have traditionally relied on pickling, fermenting, salting, and drying foods to keep over the winter. Three types of sauces (*jang*) are most commonly used in Korean cooking: soy sauce (*ganjang*), chili paste (*gochujang*), and fermented soybean paste (*doenjang*). Other condiments commonly used to season dishes are salt, garlic, black pepper, vinegar, red chili pepper, ginger, and sesame seeds.

 ## Beverages

Hot beverages are referred to as *cha*, literally meaning tea. *Bori cha*, a roasted barley tea, is the most popular Korean beverage, drunken like water in Korea. Citron

tea (*yujacha*) is a hot, sweet drink made from citron, a fragrant citrus fruit. Other popular hot beverages include ginseng teas, green tea, rice tea, and ginger tea. Cold beverages are often made from fruit or grains. *Hwachae*, a fruit drink sweetened with honey, is a popular summer beverage. Citrons, pears, strawberries, mandarins, cherries, watermelon, and peaches are some fruits that are used to make *hwachae*. *Sikhye* is a cold, sweet beverage made from rice and lightly fermented with dried barley sprouts. It is widely available canned. *Songhwa hwachae* is a drink made of pine-blossom pollen mixed with honey.

Soju is distilled liquor traditionally made from rice and can be compared to vodka. Drinking *soju* with elders requires following strict etiquette, such as holding the glass with both hands when being served by an older person, and drinking slowly with your head turned slightly away. Other traditional alcoholic beverages include *makgeolli* ("quick brew"), a milky-white, sour wine made from fermented rice; *cheongju*, a rice wine comparable to the Japanese *sake;* and *imsamju*, ginseng wine often given as a gift.

Desserts

Desserts are rarely eaten after a Korean meal; rather, fresh fruit and tea are usually served. There is, however, an abundant variety of sweets in Korean cuisine, usually consumed with tea as a snack or during special occasions. *Hangwa* are traditional sweets and cookies that are eaten particularly during special occasions. There are a wide variety of *hangwa* made from rice flour, honey, fruit, flowers, and edible roots.

In addition to fruit, seeds, and rice, red beans (also known as adzuki beans) are a common ingredient in many Korean sweets. It is made into *pat*, a sweet red-bean paste, which in turn is used in desserts. For example, it is used as a filling in rice cakes or as an addition to *patbingsu*, a shaved ice dessert with fruit cocktail, condensed milk, fruit syrup, and jelly. *Patjuk*, hot red-bean porridge, is commonly eaten during the winter solstice.

FOODS WITH CULTURAL SIGNIFICANCE

Rice is more than just the basis of sustenance for Koreans. Rice has historical significance for having served traditionally as the center of Korean economy. Recently, rice has been at the center of a heated controversy over South Korea's transition into a free-market economy. Rice serves many roles: as the primary starch in the diet, as an offering to ancestors, as the commodity that farmers for centuries have relied on for their livelihood, and as a symbol of national heritage. The significance of rice is demonstrated in its usage in everyday speech: the word *bap* means both rice and food, and the question literally meaning "Have you eaten rice/food yet?" is asked to mean "How are you?"

Kimchi has been part of the Korean diet since ancient times. The spicy, red *kimchi* that is ubiquitous in Korean meals has been part of the diet since the 17th century, when chili peppers were introduced to Korea by Portuguese traders. There are over 200 varieties of *kimchi*. The most popular varieties are made with Chinese cabbage, daikon radish, cucumber, leeks, eggplant, sesame leaves, or scallions. Pickled fish is sometimes added as well. *Kimchi* was traditionally made and stored in large earthenware pots. The chili pepper, ginger, garlic, and salt added act to preserve the *kimchi*, which was a good source of vitamins during harsh Korean winters. The type of *kimchi* varies depending on the region in Korea where it is prepared. In general, *kimchi* from the south tends to be sweeter with a stronger flavor, whereas *kimchi* prepared in the north is milder and less salty. Individual households also have unique methods for preparing *kimchi*. It is said that the new wife of a Korean man must learn to prepare *kimchi* his family's way.

TYPICAL DAY'S MENU

There are few differences between breakfast, lunch, and dinner in traditional Korean cuisine. Rice and *kimchi* are eaten at every meal. Beverages are rarely served, but rather soup or *dongchimi*, a watery white radish *kimchi*, is provided. The most common soups include *kimchi jigae*, *kimchi* stew, and bean-paste soup. *Oi naengook* is a chilled watery soup with shredded cucumbers enjoyed in summer months. To accompany the rice, a series of side dishes (*banchan*), are served. Koreans traditionally use metal chopsticks to eat and spoons to mix and stir food and drink soup.

Korea is a historically agrarian country; meals usually featured local and seasonal ingredients. At the Korean table, all the dishes are served at one time. Traditional meals often include five colors: green, white, red, black, and yellow. These colors represent the five elements of wood, metal, fire, water, and earth, based on the Chinese yin yang philosophy. Contrast is

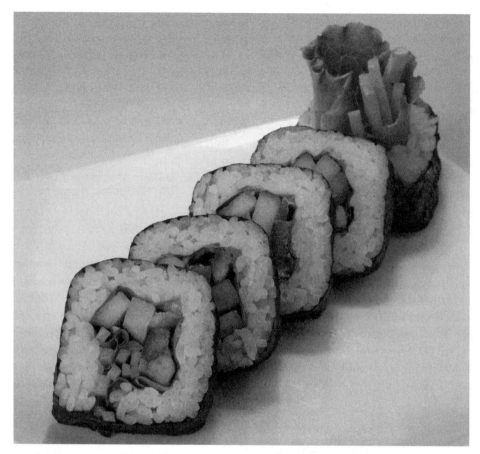

Gimbap, rice and vegetables wrapped in seaweed, is a popular snack.

important; for example, serving a spicy dish with bland rice, or serving cold noodles with hot soup.

Snacks are an important part of the daily menu. *Gimbap* (rice and vegetables wrapped in seaweed) is a popular snack. Flatcakes and pancakes that contain meat and vegetables are a common snack and party food. *Kimchi buchimgae* are flatcakes made with flour, eggs, *kimchi*, scallions, and chili pepper, and is served with a spicy dipping sauce. *Nokdu bindaetteok* are fried pancakes made of mashed mung beans, sticky-rice powder, minced pork, finely sliced onion, cabbage, and scallions. *Tteokbokki* are rice "sticks" (cylindrical rice cakes) that can be prepared in a variety of ways. One popular method is to sauté the rice sticks with sesame oil, soy sauce, chili paste, sugar, and sliced vegetables. *Tteokbokki* are so popular in Korea that in South Korea's capital, Seoul, there is a street lined entirely with *tteokbokki* stands.

Depending on the degree of acculturation, Koreans in the United States will consume a combination of American and Korean foods on a daily basis. Ac-

cording to a study by Lee, Sobal, and Frongillo (1999), Korean-Americans are more likely to consume American foods at breakfast and lunch, and consume Korean foods at dinner. Regularly consumed American foods include breakfast foods such as bagels and bread, whereas regularly consumed Korean foods include rice, stew, or soup, and *kimchi* (Lee et al., 1999).

 ## HOLIDAY MENUS

The lunar New Year is celebrated in Korea, and one of the most important New Year foods is *tteok guk* (rice-cake soup). It is made of sliced rice cakes boiled in a savory beef broth with scallions, shredded beef, toasted seaweed, and egg. *Tteok guk* is prepared and offered to the ancestors before it is eaten. *Soojong gwa* is a chilled, sweet ginger–cinnamon tea served with dried persimmons after the New Year's meal.

Chuseok is Korea's harvest moon festival celebrated in the fall. People often return to their hometown to spend the holiday with family, visit graves of ancestors, and make offerings. Special foods made during this holiday are *song pyon* (rice cakes in a half-moon shape) and *jun* (pan-fried flatcakes). These foods are offered first to ancestors, and then are eaten by the family, a ritual that symbolically connects family members with their ancestors.

The 100th day, 1st birthday, and 60th birthday are the most significant birthdays in Korean culture and are celebrated accordingly. Birthday foods usually include a variety of rice cakes and *miyeok guk* (seaweed soup). *Miyeok guk* is also often eaten by mothers to gain strength after giving birth. It is made with dried seaweed, sliced beef, and beef stock, and is seasoned with black pepper, soy sauce, and sesame oil.

 ## HEALTH BELIEFS AND CONCERNS

Today, Koreans in both Korea and the United States follow a combination of Western medical practices and *hanbang*, traditional Korean medicine that is based on principles of traditional Chinese medicine. These principles include the belief in maintaining balance between humans and the universe, yin and yang, and hot and cold. "Hot" conditions include hyperactivity, hyperthermia, dehydration, fever, tension, and seizures. "Cold" conditions include depression, hypothermia, colds, and indigestion.

The most common traditional treatments used by Koreans include acupuncture, moxibustion, and herbal medicines. Acupuncture is a preventative and healing treatment involving the insertion of special needles into designated points on the skin. Moxibustion involves heating pulverized leaves of mugwort (also known as moxa) and applying it over specific points on the skin. Herbal medicines are known as *hanyak*, medicines that derive from roots, wild flowers, leaves, vines, and animals. Koreans consult licensed practitioners of traditional Korean medicine, *hanui*, to prescribe the appropriate *hanyak* for their condition.

A Korean proverb says that "the mouth is the executioner and the doctor of the body." Koreans believe that nutrition plays an important role in maintaining the health of the body. Good appetite is a sign of good health. To boost stamina, ginseng is consumed in a variety of forms such as teas and soups. *Samgyetang* is a chicken ginseng soup with rice, garlic, and red dates consumed during illness to promote strength.

 ## GENERAL HEALTH AND NUTRITIONAL INDICATORS SUMMARY

According to UNICEF (2007), 7% of Korean infants were in low-birth-weight categories from 1998 to 2005. This was parallel to the United States, which had an 8% rate during the same time period. Sixty-five percent of infants are exclusively breastfed for the first 6 months of life in Korea. The life expectancy of a Korean is 67 years, a drop of 5 years since 1993. Forty percent of the population consumes iodized salt, which is low, but 95% of children receive vitamin A supplementation. Underweight, for children under 5 years in the moderate to severe category, is 37% (UNICEF, 2007).

 ## COMMUNICATION AND COUNSELING TIPS

How one communicates to another in Korean society is often dependent on age, gender, and status. Upon asking Korean acquaintances about social etiquette, they all reiterated that respect for seniors was a crucial aspect of Korean culture. Korean friends noticeably always refer to friends even slightly older than themselves as "older sister" or "older brother" more often than using their given names. At the table, seniors call for the start of the meal; eating before the most senior member at the table has started is inappropriate. Koreans further convey respect for elders by showing agreement and not questioning authority. This may also apply when Korean patients communicate with physicians or other health professionals.

Koreans have been described as stoic in their facial expressions; however, this need not be interpreted as disinterest. Many Koreans do not necessarily communicate feelings in their facial expressions. Koreans often greet one another by bowing; however, a handshake is also an appropriate greeting for most age groups. Adults should be addressed formally by their surname unless they are on friendly terms.

PRIMARY LANGUAGE OF FOOD NAMES WITH ENGLISH AND PHONETIC TRANSLATION

The primary language of food names with English and phonetic translation is given in Table 26-1.

TABLE 26-1   Primary Language of Food Names with English and Phonetic Translation

Korean Transliteration	English Translation
Gogi	Meat
Dubu	Tofu
Bap	Rice
Tteok	Rice cakes
Juk	Porridge
Myeon	Noodles
Namul	Seasoned vegetable
Banchan	Side dish
Gimchi	Fermented cabbage (or other vegetable)
Guk	Soup
Bori cha	Barley tea
Ganjang	Soy sauce
Doenjang	Soybean paste
Gochujang	Red chili paste
Bulgogi	Barbecued beef
Galbi	Beef short ribs
Japchae	Mixed noodles with vegetables
Bibimbap	Mixed vegetables on rice
Gimbap	Seaweed roll of rice and vegetables
Tteokbokki	Seasoned rice sticks
Mandu	Dumpling
Samgyetang	Ginseng chicken soup
Miyeokguk	Seaweed soup

FEATURED RECIPE

Kimchi jjigae is traditionally prepared with pork; however, it can also be made with beef or shrimp, or prepared with *kimchi* and tofu alone.

Kimchi Stew (*Kimchi Jjigae*)

2 cups *kimchi*
2 tbsp. sesame oil
1 tsp. garlic, minced
½ lb. pork, sliced thin
1 cup *kimchi* juice (the liquid in ripe *kimchi*)
3 cups water
8 oz. tofu, cut into cubes
2 stalks green onion, chopped

1. Cut *kimchi* into 1-inch squares.
2. In a pan over medium heat, stir the sesame oil, garlic, and pork until the pork is nearly cooked through. Transfer to a pot.
3. Add the *kimchi*, *kimchi* juice, and 3 cups of water, and bring to a boil.
4. Add the tofu and scallions and bring to a boil again.
5. Serve with rice.

Yield: 4 servings

More recipes are available at http://nutrition.jbpub.com/foodculture/

REFERENCES

Bak, S. (1997). McDonald's in Seoul: Food choices, identity, and nationalism. In J. Watson (Ed.), *Golden arches east: McDonald's in East Asia* (pp. 136–160). Stanford, CA: Stanford University Press.

Central Intelligence Agency. (2008a). *South Korea*. Retrieved May 31, 2008, from https://www.cia.gov/library/publications/the-world-factbook/geos/ks.html/

Central Intelligence Agency. (2008b). *North Korea*. Retrieved May 31, 2008, from https://www.cia.gov/library/publications/the-world-factbook/geos/kn.html/

Choe, J.S., & Moriyama, Y. (2003). *Korean cooking for everyone.* Tokyo: Japan Publications Trading.

Chun, H.J., Lee, H.G., & Han, Y.S. (2001). *Traditional Korean food.* Seoul, Korea: Korea Tourism Association.

Chung, O., & Monroe, J. (2003). *Cooking the Korean way.* Minneapolis, MN: Lerner Publications Co.

Chung, S.Y. (2002). *Korean home cooking.* Boston: Periplus Editions.

Clark, D. (2000). *Culture and customs of Korea.* Westport, CT: Greenwood Press.

Gordon, B.J., Kang, M.S.Y., Cho, P., & Sucher, K.P. (2000). Dietary habits and health beliefs of Korean-Americans in the San Francisco Bay Area. *Journal of the American Dietetic Association, 100*(10), 1198–1201.

Hoare, J. (2005). *Korea: A quick guide to customs and etiquette.* Portland, OR: Graphic Arts Center Publishing.

Kim, B.L., & Ryu, E. (2005). Korean families. In M. McGoldrick, J. Giordano, & N. Garcia-Preto (Eds.), *Ethnicity and family therapy* (3rd ed., pp. 349–373). New York: Guilford Press.

Kim, S., Moon, S., & Popkin, B. (2000). Nutritional status, dietary intake, and body composition: The nutrition transition in South Korea. *American Journal of Clinical Nutrition, 71*, 44–53.

Kittler, P., & Sucher, K. (2004). *Food and culture* (4th ed.). Belmont, CA: Wadsworth Thomson.

Kwak, J. (1998). *Dok Suni: Recipes from my mother's Korean kitchen.* New York: St. Martin's Press.

Lassiter, S. (1995). *Multicultural clients: A professional handbook for health care providers and social workers.* Westport, CT: Greenwood Press.

Lee, C. (2005). *Eating Korean.* Hoboken, NJ: John Wiley & Sons, Inc.

Lee, M. (2004). Korea. In C. Kemp & L. Rasbridge (Eds.), *Refugee and immigrant health: A handbook for health professionals* (pp. 221–227). Cambridge, UK: Cambridge University Press.

Lee, S.Y., Sobal, J., & Frongillo, E.A. (1999). Acculturation and dietary practices among Korean Americans. *Journal of the American Dietetic Association, 99*(9), 1084–1089.

Magner, L. (2000). Korea. In K.F. Kiple & K.C. Ornelas (Eds.), *The Cambridge world history of food* (pp. 1183–1191). Cambridge, UK: Cambridge University Press.

Pang, K.Y. (2000). *Virtuous transcendence: Holistic self-cultivation and self-healing in elderly Korean immigrants.* New York: Haworth Press.

Pemberton, R. (2001). Wild-gathered foods as countercurrents to dietary globalisation in South Korea. In K. Cwiertka & B. Walraven (Eds.), *Asian food: The global and the local* (pp. 76–94). Honolulu, HI: University of Hawai'i Press.

Purnell, L., & Kim, S. (2003). People of Korean heritage. In L. Purnell & B. Paulanka (Eds.), *Transcultural health care: A culturally competent approach* (2nd ed., pp. 249–263). Philadelphia: F.A. Davis.

Reinschmidt, M. (2007). Estimating rice, agriculture, global trade and national food culture in South Korea. In S. Cheung & C.B. Tan (Eds.), *Food and foodways in Asia: Resource, tradition and cooking* (pp. 96–111). New York: Routledge.

Son, C.H. (Ed.) (1997). *Korean cultural heritage* (Vol. 4): *Traditional lifestyles.* Seoul, Korea: Korea Foundation.

Song, J.J. (2005). *The Korean language: Structure, use and context.* New York: Routledge.

Stux, G., Berman, B., & Pomeranz, B. (2003). *Basics of acupuncture* (5th ed.). Berlin, New York: Springer.

Trang, C. (2003). *Essentials of Asian cuisine: Fundamentals and favorite recipes.* New York: Simon & Schuster.

UNICEF. (2007). *The state of the world's children 2007: Women and children, the double dividend of gender equality.* Retrieved April 14, 2009, from http://www.unicef.org/sowc07/statistics/tables.php

CHAPTER 27

Russia

Susan Levine Krantz, MA, RD

 ## CULTURE AND WORLD REGION

In December 1991, the original 1922 treaty that established the Union of Soviet Socialist Republics (USSR) was dissolved. Russia officially became the Russian Federation and a part of the Commonwealth of Independent States (CIS), also called the newly independent states (NIS), a group of 15 countries previously part of the USSR. The population of the Russian Federation was estimated at 144.2 million people in 2004 (World Health Organization [WHO], 2006), with about 75% living in cities, where two- or three-room apartments are common, and the remainder living in rural areas. Many city dwellers also have a *dacha*, a country house, where they have gardens to grow fruits and vegetables (Mack & Surina, 2005).

In terms of land mass, Russia, at 6,592,741 square miles, is the largest country in the world, and 1.8 times the size of the United States. Russia spreads over the European and Asian continents and borders China, Fin-

land, North Korea, Mongolia, Norway, and Japan, as well as most of the republics of the NIS. It is located at a latitude similar to that of Canada. It snows a great deal in the winter and the northern part of the country is especially cold, with short sunlit days and permafrost-laden tundra, ground so frozen that it cannot grow anything. South of the tundra is land covered with trees, constituting the largest forest of coniferous trees in the world. Most Russians will say that their favorite tree is the magnificent birch, with its characteristic white trunk speckled with black. Logging is a popular industry in Russia, although Russians have made efforts to preserve their forests. Farther south, the open prairie provides fertile ground for planting crops. Although most of the country is flat, Russia includes several mountain ranges, such as the Urals, which separate Europe from Asia, and the Caucasus, which lie between the Black and Caspian seas. Russia is also a land of lakes and rivers. The Volga, Europe's longest river, flows through the west. The Caspian Sea, a salt-water lake, is the largest inland body of water in the world. Russia has ports on the Black and Baltic seas that provide access to the Mediterranean and the Atlantic (Schultze, 2000).

Russian culture has been shaped by its history of governmental changes, economic class disparity, internal instability, pogroms, and famines. The republics of the former Soviet Union that became the NIS include Russia; the Baltic republics of Estonia, Latvia, and Lithuania; the Slavic republics of Ukraine and Belarus; landlocked Moldova; the southern states of Armenia, Georgia, and Azerbaijan; and the central Asian countries of Uzbekistan, Tajikistan, Kyrgyzstan, Kazakhstan, and Turkmenistan. Since 1991, about 5 million people have immigrated to Russia, including those from the NIS, especially from Armenia, Azerbaijan, and Tajikistan. Chinese and Koreans also have settled in Russia. These new immigrants influence Russian culture and cuisine (Goldstein, 1999; Mack & Surina, 2005; Schultze, 2000).

Most Russians are ethnically Russian (about 116 million people, or about 81.5%), while others are Tartar (3.8%), Ukrainian (3%), Chuvash (1.2%), Bashkir (0.9%), and Belarussian (0.8%). Much smaller numbers of Yakuts, Chechens, Mari, Moldovans, Jews, Germans, and Udmert also live in Russia. Eighty percent of Russians are Orthodox Christians and 18 million are Muslim (Mack & Surina, 2005; Schultze, 2000).

Due to migration and assimilation, it is hard to say what being "Russian" means. Russians have two words to define themselves: *russkiy*, meaning someone ethnically Russian who speaks the Russian language, and *rossiyskiy*, for all other Russian citizens (Mack & Surina, 2005).

The Slavs are the ancestors of today's Russians and by the mid-800s they had built many small towns, including Kiev, which was the first capital of Russia. Today's Russians are also descendents from the Tartars, or Mongols. They came west from central Asia in 1237 and destroyed many Russian towns, eventually taking control of Russia. Mongol-Tartars ruled Russia for about 350 years (Schultze, 2000).

LANGUAGE

The Russian language is part of the Slavic group of the Indo-European language family, which includes English, French, German, and Hindi, among others. As the native language of 145 million people, Russian is the most widely spoken of the Slavic languages (Stakhnevich, 2007).

In the 17th century, Russian became the country's national language and today it is the official language of the Russian Federation. The Russian language has many words of Slavic origin, but words from many other languages, such as English, French, Greek, and Latin, have been incorporated into Russian as well (Stakhnevich, 2007).

Russian uses the Cyrillic alphabet, which is based, in part, on Greek. Cyrillic may be named after St. Cyril, who along with St. Methodius tried to create a new alphabet in the 9th century. Their ultimate goal was to encourage the spread of Christianity among the Slavic population (Schultze, 2000; Stakhnevich, 2007).

FOOD HISTORY WITHIN THE CULTURE

Foreign trade as early as the 12th century brought spices, fruits, and nuts, such as walnuts and almonds, to Russia. Before the Mongol invasion in the 13th century, cabbage and turnips were the most common Russian vegetables. The poor ate porridge made from coarse millet, barley, and oats. By the 15th century, buckwheat groats were cultivated. Today, they are called kasha and are closely identified with Russian foods (Mack & Surina, 2005).

As in other areas of medieval Europe, famine and disease were common. During times when food was scarce, a typical dish was *tyurya*, made of stale breadcrumbs mixed with *kvas* (a fermented drink similar to beer) or water. Sometimes garlic or hemp oil was added. Russians have become accustomed to deprivation during lean times and feasts during good times (Mack & Surina, 2005).

By the mid-18th century, wealthy Russians began to imitate the French by entertaining on a grand scale. They imported chefs from France, Germany, and Switzerland. In France, food was served smorgasbord style, with all the dishes, from appetizers and entrees to the desserts, laid out on a banquet table. In Russia, food was served in courses, with each course served and removed before the next course began. This custom has persisted in Russia and has been adopted by most Western countries, including France (Mack & Surina, 2005; Schultze, 2000).

Russian meals begin with *zakuski* (appetizers). This tradition probably arose because people traveled great distances and arrived at any time of the day or night. The *zakuski* table was always set and the appetizers kept the guests satisfied until dinner was served.

Zakuski include caviar, fish roe, or eggs, and usually comes from expensive sturgeon or less-costly salmon. Caviar is served with bread and butter, on top of deviled eggs, or wrapped in *bliny*, very thin pancakes made from buckwheat or wheat flour. *Zakuski* also can include fish, such as pickled herring served with oil and vinegar, sour cream, or mustard sauce. Nonfish appetizers include sliced meat, marinated vegetables, and sauerkraut. By the late 19th century, most dishes on the *zakuski* table were topped by very elegant vegetable garnishes (Schultze, 2000).

Zakuski are followed by soup, including *borscht*, made from beets, and *shchi*, made from cabbage. Both *borscht* and *shchi* are often served with sour cream. Other soups include *Ukha*, made from one or more varieties of fish, and *rassolnik*, made from kidney meat and pickles. Mushroom barley soup is also popular. Usually accompanying the soup are *pirozhki*—baked or fried dough with various meat, cheese, or vegetable fillings—or slices of *kulebiaka*, a large pie filled with salmon or cabbage (Mack & Surina, 2005; Schultze, 2000).

The main entree consists of meat, chicken, lamb, pork, or fish. A popular choice is *pelmeni*, dumplings filled with beef and served with sour cream, vinegar, or mustard. *Shashlyk* (shish kebab) is an entree of marinated meat or poultry skewered and cooked over charcoal. Side dishes include boiled potatoes served with mushrooms, sour cream, and onions. Kasha is a Russian staple that may be served as a main or side dish with butter and milk, or onions and mushrooms. Dessert usually consists of vanilla ice cream served with jam, cookies, cakes, and pastries (Mack & Surina, 2005; Schultze, 2000).

Russians also have adopted the cuisines of their neighbors. Russians love the cuisine of the Baltic republics of Estonia, Latvia, and Lithuania, known for their dishes with butter, eggs, and cream. In addition, many Russian dishes, such as *borscht* and stuffed cabbage, originated in Ukraine (Goldstein, 1999).

Georgia borders Russia along the Caucasus mountain range and its proximity has affected Russian food as well. There are many Georgian restaurants in Russia that serve Georgian specialties, such as *khachapuri*, a Georgian cheese pie, and *tabaka*, chicken covered in a garlic sauce. Additionally, Georgia is known for its selection of fine wines, especially *kindzmarauli*, a red wine that supposedly was favored by Stalin, and *teliani*, which was preferred by the poets of the Communist era. In Russia, there is also rice pilaf from Uzbekistan, and *samsa*, fried meat pie similar to *pirozhki*, from Kazakhstan and Kyrgyzstan (Goldstein, 1999).

There are about 500,000 Koreans in the NIS, so Korean salads are found in the markets of Moscow and other cities. They are made with pickled vegetables and fish. Russians are very fond of the Korean carrot salad in particular. Markets also sell prepackaged Korean spice mixtures (Mack & Surina, 2005).

Historically, the basic recipes of Russian cooking were created in a slow-bake oven that also provided heat to the house. Placing food in different places in the oven allowed for it to be cooked at different temperatures. The oven also was used to dry berries, herbs, and mushrooms, and to accelerate the fermentation of dough and *kvas*. Bread baked in the oven was crusty and hearty. Peasants and serfs lived in villages and most of their staples came from small farm plots. They also foraged wild greens from the woods and fished from lakes and rivers (Mack & Surina, 2005).

Social stratification has been a big factor in Russian diet choices throughout the country's history, and continues to be today. The lives of the extremely wealthy have differed from the poor, both in culture and cuisine. Today, there are Russian billionaires who have profited from the privatization of industries at the end of the Communist era. Wealthy "New Russians," who flock to pricier new restaurants, nightclubs, and casinos, make up as much as 10% of the population. They also travel extensively, especially to Turkey, Spain, and Cyprus. The Russian middle class, estimated at 20–30% of the population, is attracted to new fast-food restaurants and supermarkets that provide both domestic and imported choices (Mack & Surina, 2005); however, about 70% of Russians live at or below the poverty line and cannot take advantage of the luxuries provided by Russia's strong economic growth (Mack & Surina, 2005). Many peasants cannot afford to own *dachas* and instead rent them for the summer. They cook with simple ingredients, using recipes that are similar to those of their ancestors (Goldstein, 1999).

 MAJOR FOODS

 Protein Sources

Sources of protein include beef, pork, poultry, and mutton. *Zharkoe* is a traditional slow-cooking stew of meat, potatoes, and vegetables. *Kotlety* is fried ground-beef patties made with breadcrumbs and diced onions. *Zalivnoe* is meat and vegetables covered with gel made from fish, meat, or poultry. *Kholodets* are boiled pigs'

knuckles served with gel. Both *zalivnoe* and *kholodets* are served as appetizers with mustard or horseradish (Mack & Surina, 2005).

Russia is known for its sausage, *kolbasa*, made from pork and beef. The high-fat *Moscovskaya* sausage is very popular. Russians prepare cured ham and *salo*, cured pork back fat, often spread on black bread (Mack & Surina, 2005).

Chicken usually is imported and is used in soups, salads, and other dishes. *Kotleta po-kievski*, chicken kiev, is chicken breast that is pounded, wrapped around herbed butter, breaded, and fried (Mack & Surina, 2005).

Fish, when served as an appetizer, is salted or smoked. Boiled, fried, or breaded fish is often served as a main dish during fasting days when meat, milk products, and eggs are prohibited. In addition to salmon, available fish include carp, perch, cod, flounder, northern pike, and catfish. Other available seafood include mussels and oysters. Boiled crayfish is used in salads or served whole. Anchovies from the Black Sea are canned in tomato sauce or oil (Mack & Surina, 2005).

Protein also is available from dairy products such as milk and cheese. The most popular cheese is *plaveny syr*, a processed cheese similar to American cheese. *Rossiyskiy*, a Russian semisoft cheese similar to Dan-ish havarti, is also popular. *Brynza*, originally from Switzerland, is a salted cheese made from sheep's milk and similar in texture and taste to feta cheese (Mack & Surina, 2005).

Fermented dairy products include *smetana* (sour cream); yogurt; kefir, a yogurt-like beverage; and *ryazhenka*, a breakfast drink made by baking sour milk until it is golden brown. *Prostokvasha* is a beverage that tastes like a combination of buttermilk and yogurt. When *prostokvasha* is gently heated, it produces *tvorog*, a cheese similar to, but thicker than, cottage cheese (Mack & Surina, 2005).

Starch Sources

In Russia, the word for hospitality is *khlebosolstvo*, derived from the words *khleb* (bread) and *sol* (salt). *Khleb* and *sol* were offered to guests who cut the bread and dipped the first slice in salt. Bread is served at every meal and can be sweet or salty. The traditional black bread is typified by *borodinskiy*, rye bread with coriander seeds. *Sushka*, which is sweet and looks like a small bagel, is often served with tea and sometimes given to teething babies. Larger *sushki*, softer and studded with poppy seeds, are called *bublik*. *Krendel* is like a large soft pretzel often baked with raisins or nuts. Many

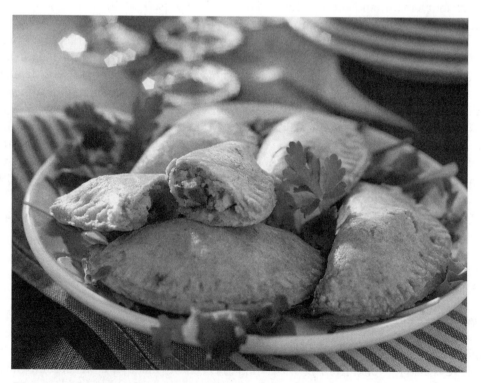

Pirogi, pies with various fillings including meat, fish, or berries, are usually served on special occasions.

Russian bakeries have signs in front of them that look like a *krendel* (Mack & Surina, 2005).

Russia is the largest producer and consumer of kasha in the world. Kasha is boiled with raisins and milk or water and served at breakfast. At other meals it may be mixed with eggs, fruit, cheese, pork, liver, onions, or mushrooms. *Pirogi* are 9- to 10-inch pies with various fillings, including meat, fish, or berries, that are usually served on special occasions. *Pirozhki*—smaller, similar pies of baked or fried dough—are served as snacks, appetizers, or accompaniments to soup (Mack & Surina, 2005).

Russians eat rice pilaf and pasta. *Makarony* are long tubes that are sometimes as long as 1 meter. *Makarony flotski* are boiled macaroni fried with ground beef. *Pelmeni* and *vareniki* are boiled dumplings that can be filled with sweet fruits, meat, or vegetables and served with butter or sour cream (Mack & Surina, 2005).

 ## Fat Sources

Russian cooking typically uses a large quantity of butter that is often clarified, melted, and stored as ghee. Bacon or pork fat is used to flavor soups, stews, and fried vegetables. Sunflower oil, the only fat permitted during Lent, is often used for salads and frying. Russia initiated commercial production of it in the 19th century and subsequently became a leading world producer (Mack & Surina, 2005).

 ## Prominent Vegetables

Cabbage, the most prominent Russian vegetable, is used in soups and salads. It may be served in both main and side dishes. *Kvashenaya kapusta*, homemade sauerkraut, is sour cabbage pickled in brine without vinegar. *Golubtsy* are cabbage leaves stuffed with ground meat and rice and cooked in tomato sauce, usually topped with sour cream. Cucumbers, pickled in brine, are added to many dishes. Mushrooms are used in fillings, stuffing, soups, and vegetable dishes. Collecting wild mushrooms is a sport-like pastime for Russians (Mack & Surina, 2005).

Potatoes often are peeled, boiled, and covered in dill, butter, and sour cream. Potatoes can be puréed or mashed and may be fried with mushrooms and bacon. They are also included in salads such as *salad Olivye*, named after Olivier, the French chef who owned Moscow's Hermitage restaurant in the 1860s. The salad is made with boiled and diced potatoes, carrots, onions, peas, pickles, and chicken, and mixed with mayonnaise.

Vinegret is a typical salad that combines potatoes, pickled cabbage, cucumbers, beets, and onions with an oil-and-vinegar dressing (Mack & Surina, 2005).

Turnips, rutabaga, red beets, and sugar beets are also typical Russian fare. Turnips are puréed or cooked as part of meat dishes. Red beets are part of salads and *borscht*, and sugar beets are used as a source of refined sugar. Russians grow other vegetables, including tomatoes, eggplant, squash, zucchini, peppers, peas, and string beans, in their gardens (Mack & Surina, 2005).

 ## Prominent Fruits

Fruits grown in the north include apples, pears, raspberries, gooseberries, cranberries, currants, and strawberries. Berries are made into jams, jellies, and preserves, but they are also eaten raw. The southern regions grow peaches, cherries, plums, and melons. Moreover, some fruits are imported from southern Asia, including watermelon, grapes, dried apricots, and raisins. Citrus fruits are imported from Morocco, Egypt, and Turkey. Today's world marketplace has made it possible for major cities to have fruits from all parts of the globe (Mack & Surina, 2005).

 ## Spices and Seasonings

The Black and Azov seas are harvested for salt, a vital source of revenue to the Russian economy as early as the 16th century (Mack & Surina, 2005). Parsley and dill are used as spices and garnishes. Bay leaves and sweet paprika are used in soups and stews. Allspice, anise, cinnamon, cloves, and nutmeg are used in baking. Citric acid, which comes from acidic fruits, is used in *borscht*, jams, and beverages (Mack & Surina, 2005).

Russian mustard is very spicy and used for roasts, pork dishes, and cold cuts. Horseradish is grated and mixed with vinegar to make the white variety and with beet juice to make the red variety. Horseradish is served with fish and meat or mixed with a cream sauce for entrees such as roast beef or poached sturgeon (Mack & Surina, 2005).

 ## Beverages

Alcoholic beverages have been common throughout Russian history. Mead is a fermented beverage of honey, water, and spices. Other beverages include *kumiss*, fermented mare's milk, and *kvas*, fermented from rye or barley and similar to beer. Homemade wine typically has been made from all kinds of fruit. Additionally, since 1991, drinking beer has become a trend for young adults, because it is less expensive and has less alcohol than vodka (Mack & Surina, 2005).

Alcoholic beverages are never served as cocktails or without food. Guests at Russian homes are encouraged to drink repeated toasts made to health, to the hosts, to accomplishments, and to other celebratory topics. Ice-cold vodka, usually plain and made from rye, also comes in many flavors such as orange, cinnamon, and coffee. Vodka and other alcoholic beverages are gulped down in a single swallow followed by a bite of appetizer after each toast (Mack & Surina, 2005; Schultze, 2000).

Although many people consider vodka the national beverage, *chai* (tea), a gift from a Chinese ruler, was used by Russian Tsars as early as the 17th century. Tea is served almost everywhere, both at meals and in between them. (Mack & Surina, 2005). Some people argue over whether the *samovar*, a large brass urn that was used not to brew but to boil water for tea, originated in Russia, was adapted from a pot used to make soup in Mongolia, or if Peter the Great brought it back from Holland (Mack & Surina, 2005). Russians usually drink strong black tea with lemon, and while holding a sugar cube in the mouth or between the front teeth. For the most part, wood-burning samovars have been replaced by electric ones, and many modern families use electric teapots (Mack & Surina, 2005; Schultze, 2000), but many poorer Russians simply boil water in pots on the stovetop.

 Desserts

Tea is usually accompanied by sweets such as chocolate, jam, candy, or cookies. Desserts include *pryanik* (spice cookies), tortes (European-style layer cakes), *khvorost* (deep-fried pastry strips), and Russian ice cream. *Blinchiki* are thin pancakes without fillings that are served as dessert or with tea. Traditional Russian beverages, part of the dessert course, include *kompot*, fresh or dried fruit boiled in water and sugar, and *kisel*, a thick beverage of pureed fruit mixed with sugar and pectin (Mack & Surina, 2005; Schultze, 2000).

 FOODS WITH CULTURAL SIGNIFICANCE

Russian cultural identity has been entwined with religion. Even though the USSR was officially atheist, the strong power and common language of Orthodox

Christianity has held the Russian people together since the 10th century (Mack & Surina, 2005). The Russian Orthodox calendar contains at least 220 fasting days. Fasting restricts the intake of animal protein such as meat, eggs, and dairy, so during fasting most Russians eat vegetarian and fish dishes including fruits, vegetables, and grains (Mack & Surina, 2005).

Maslenitsa is a week of celebration before the fast of Lent, which culminates with Easter. During the 10 days before *Maslenitsa*, Russians bake and eat rolls shaped like larks with eyes of raisins. During *Maslenitsa*, Russians make *bliny*, served with butter or sour cream and topped with jam, caviar, or smoked fish (Schultze, 2000).

 TYPICAL DAY'S MENU

Most Russians eat three meals a day. They drink tea, served with sugar and lemon, jam, or cookies, at meals and between meals. Breakfast often includes kasha, or other hot cereals, and a source of protein, such as eggs or meat. Nutritious whole-grain bread is served at breakfast, lunch, and dinner (D. Goldstein, personal communication, March 25, 2008).

Lunch is hearty and starts with *zakuski*, which may include dill pickles, cheese, smoked fish, or other appetizers. Next comes soup (cabbage or *borscht*) and *pirozhki* stuffed with vegetables. The main course can be *zharkoe*, beef stew, and a *vinegret* salad (Mack & Surina, 2005).

Dinner is a lighter meal and usually soup is not served. *Zakuski*, including pickled herring or sauerkraut, are followed by a grain such as kasha, served with mushrooms or onions. Dessert, such as ice cream, cake, or cookies, is served with tea (Mack & Surina, 2005; Schultze, 2000).

 HOLIDAY MENUS

The Russian Orthodox Easter is the most important religious holiday of the year. The meal begins with *zakuski* and vodka, followed by platters of salad, cooked leg of lamb, ham, turkey, and other dishes. The center of interest is the *kulich*, a sponge cake, shaped like a cylinder. It is about 12 in. tall and flavored with spices such as saffron, with raisins or candied fruit. The *kulish* has "XB"—the Russian abbreviation for Jesus Christ—on the top and it is ringed by Easter eggs. A tall candle decorates the top, sometimes with a paper flower as well. On Easter the *kulish* is brought to church for the midnight service, when it is blessed before it is eaten. Easter also showcases *paskha*, a cheesecake made of cottage cheese molded in the shape of a pyramid with "XB" and a cross on the sides, and topped with raisins, almonds, and candied fruit (Mack & Surina, 2005; Schultze, 2000).

On Christmas Eve, *kutia* may be served with almond milk. Originally made from wheatberries, honey, and poppy seeds, today's *kutia* is usually made from rice, raisins, and almonds. It is served in a bowl on a bed of hay to represent the Nativity. *Uzvar*, a soup made from dried fruit, is also popular (Mack & Surina, 2005; Schultze, 2000).

On Christmas Day a feast of 12 dishes, representing the 12 apostles, may be served. Christmas carolers go from house to house and are rewarded with cookies (Mack & Surina, 2005; Schultze, 2000).

 ### HEALTH BELIEFS AND CONCERNS

The average life expectancy for a Russian born in 2003 was 65 years (72 years for women and 58 years for men) (WHO, 2006); however, the "expected length of life spent in good health" was only 58.4–64.1 years for women and 58.4 years for men (WHO, 2006). In 2002, the top two health problems for men were heart disease and unintentional injuries, including motor vehicle accidents and poisoning. The highest risk factors were the use of alcohol and tobacco (WHO, 2006). For women, the two biggest health problems were heart disease, with risk factors of hypertension and hypercholesterolemia, and neuropsychiatric conditions, including depression, anxiety, migraine, and senile dementia. Although the neuropsychiatric conditions are not life threatening, they can negatively affect quality of life (WHO, 2003, 2006).

Darra Goldstein, a professor of Russian at Williams College and the founding editor of *Gastronomica: The Journal of Food and Culture*, noted that most Russians who grew up under Communism do not put much faith in physicians. "They often relied more on homeopathy remedies, which were actually very good (different herbal teas for stomach complaints, mustard plasters instead of medicine for coughs, etc.)" (D. Goldstein, personal communication, March 25, 2008).

Kasha is believed to have healing properties and it is given to children and the sick. Honey is considered to have healing powers as well, and it is often mixed with milk, mineral water, or lemon juice to treat colds and coughs. Propolis, made by bees to build their hives, is thought to be antimicrobial and an antioxidant. Many Russians believe that soup has health benefits and eat it at least once a day. In many areas, tap water is not safe to drink. Consequently, many Russians believe that water is generally unhealthy and do not drink much of it; instead, they use bottled water or filtered water for cooking and tea. (Mack & Surina, 2005); however, many poor Russians cannot afford bottled water and instead use tap water even in areas with notoriously bad water, such as St. Petersburg.

Today, Russians are more health savvy. Goldstein points out that "Muscovites today are very sophisticated and tuned into health issues—but now you are also seeing eating disorders, which you never saw before. There are now low-fat products on the market, but I don't think all Russians can afford to buy them" (D. Goldstein, personal communication, March 25, 2008).

 ### GENERAL HEALTH AND NUTRITIONAL INDICATORS SUMMARY

In 2003, adults of both genders, 15 years of age or older, consumed over 10 liters per person of alcohol yearly, and over 48% of adults used tobacco (WHO, 2008). Statistics on the nutritional status of children in the Russian Federation are not well-defined; however, the birth rate in 2007 was 11 per 1000 population and the infant mortality rate was 13 per 1000 live births. The percentage of infants from 2001 to 2007 with low birth weight (less than 2500 grams) was 6%. The maternal mortality rate per 100,000 live births from 2001 through 2007 was 24. The mortality rate of children under 5 years was 15 per 1000 live births; this was an improvement from 1990 when it was 27 and from 1970 when it was 40 (United Nations Children's Fund [UNICEF], 2008).

 ### COMMUNICATION AND COUNSELING TIPS

Recommendations to clients should include gradual reduction of alcohol, sodium, and fat, especially saturated fat. Macro- and micronutrient intake can be estimated from a food diary, a daily recording of intake over a predetermined time frame. An explanation of "The Plate Method" (50% nonstarchy vegetables, 25% grains/starches, 25% lean protein) may help give better visual estimates of portion sizes (Raidl et al., 2007). Lists of acceptable snacks, including yogurt, kefir, or fruit, should be given to clients. It also may be valuable to provide lists of healthy alternatives to common foods and recipes. When expense is an issue, cost comparisons can be made. Suggestions for different types of exercise also can be given, depending on availability. Gradual lifestyle changes and frequent follow-ups should be encouraged to monitor progress.

Nutrition handouts that have been translated into Russian, including "30 'My Pyramid' Steps to a Health-ier You," are available from the University of Florida, IFAS Sarasota County Extension (Henneman, n.d.).

PRIMARY LANGUAGE OF FOOD NAMES WITH ENGLISH TRANSLATION

The primary language of food names with English translation is given in Table 27-1.

TABLE 27-1 Primary Language of Food Names with English Translation

Russian Transliteration	English Translation	Russian Transliteration	English Translation
Blinchiki	Thin pancakes or crepes	*Pirozhki*	Smaller stuffed pie
Bliny	Pancakes with fillings	*Plaveny syr*	"American"-style cheese
Borscht	Russian beet soup	*Prostokvasher*	Thick and sour milk
Brynza	Salted sheep's milk cheese	*Rassolnik*	Kidney and pickle soup
Chai	Tea	*Rossiyskiy*	Semisoft cheese
Golubtsy	Stuffed cabbage	*Ryazhenka*	Sour breakfast drink
Kasha	Buckwheat groats; porridge	*Shashlyk*	Shish kebab
Khleb	Bread	*Shchi*	Cabbage soup
Kholodets	Pig knuckles	*Smetana*	Sour cream
Kisel	Puréed fruit	*Sol*	Salt
Kotlety	Ground-beef patties	*Sushka*	Sweet bread
Krendel	Pretzel-like bread	*Tvorog*	Cheese curds, similar to Farmer's cheese
Kulebiaka	Large filled pie	*Ukha*	Russian fish soup
Kulish	Cylindrical Easter bread	*Vareniki*	Boiled and filled dumplings
Kvas	Fermented beverage	*Zakuski*	Russian appetizers
Kvashenaya kapusta	Sauerkraut	*Zalivnoe*	Meat and vegetables with gel
Paskha	Easter cheese cake	*Zharkoe*	Meat and vegetable stew
Pelmeni	Boiled and filled dumplings		
Pirogi	Stuffed large pie		

FEATURED RECIPE

Moscow-Style Beet Soup (Borscht)

2 lbs. beef shin or beef chuck with bone

9 cups water

3 medium beets, peeled and cut in half

1–1½ tbsp. salt (to taste)

2 medium potatoes, peeled and cubed

1 small carrot, scraped and grated

Half medium head of cabbage (¾ lb.) shredded

1 ripe tomato, coarsely chopped

6 tbsp. tomato paste

4 black peppercorns

Freshly ground black pepper

2 tbsp. wine vinegar

1 tsp. sugar

1 bay leaf

1. Simmer the meat in water for 30 minutes.
2. Add the beets and salt. Boil for 10 minutes more.
3. Remove the beets from the broth and grate coarsely.
4. Return the beets to the pot and add the remaining ingredients, except for the bay leaf and sour cream.
5. Simmer the soup until done (about 1.5 hours).
6. Remove from the heat and add the bay leaf.
7. Let the soup cool to room temperature, then chill overnight.
8. Next day, skim off the fat and reheat. Put a slice of meat and a dollop of sour cream into each bowl.

Yields 3 quarts

From: Goldstein (1999)

More recipes are available at http://nutrition.jbpub.com/foodculture/

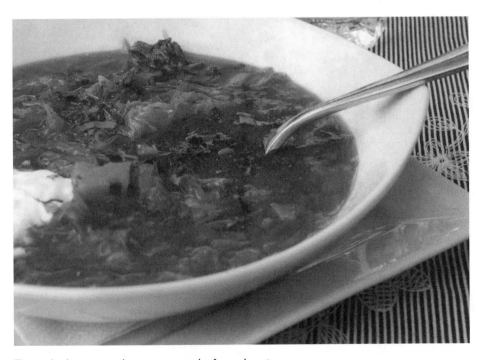

Borscht is a popular soup made from beets.

REFERENCES

Goldstein, D. (1999). *A taste of Russia*. Montpelier, VT: Russian Life Books.

Henneman, A. (n.d.). *30 "my pyramid" steps to a healthier you.* (Translated into Russian by the University of Florida). Retrieved March 31, 2008, from http://sarasota.extension.ufl.edu/fcs/nutrusukrain.shtml/

Mack, G.R., & Surina, A. (2005). *Food culture in Russia and central Asia*. Westport, CT: Greenwood Press.

Raidl, M., Spain, K., Lanting, R., Lockard, M., Johnson, S., Spencer, M., et al. (2007). The healthy diabetes plate. [Electronic version]. *Preventing chronic disease*. Retrieved June 15, 2008, from http://www.cdc.gov/pcd/issues/2007/jan/06_0050.htm/

Schultze, S. (2000). *Culture and customs of Russia*. Westport, CT: Greenwood Press.

Stakhnevich, J. (2007). *The everything learning Russian book*. Avon, MA: Adams Media.

United Nations Children's Fund (UNICEF). (2008). *The state of the world's children* 2009. Retrieved April 19, 2009, from http://www.unicef.org/publications/index_47127.html/

World Health Organization. (2003). *The world health report 2003—Shaping the future*. Retrieved March 28, 2008, from http:/www.who.int/whr/2003/en/

World Health Organization. (2006). *Highlights on health in the Russian Federation 2005*. Retrieved March 28, 2008, from http://www.who.int/countries/rus/en/

World Health Organization. (2008). *World health statistics 2008*. Retrieved April 19, 2009, from http://www.who.int/whosis/whostat/en/

CHAPTER 28

Vietnam

Rachel Fisher, MS, MPH, RD

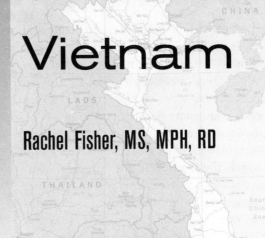

CULTURE AND WORLD REGION

The Vietnamese culture is a mix of native traditions as well as influences from the many nations that have occupied its borders over time. Reflected in the Vietnamese way of life are the religious and philosophical teachings of Animism (belief that spirits inhabit nature), Buddhism, Confucianism, and Taoism, which have coexisted in Vietnam for centuries. From these teachings, the Vietnamese have created a diverse mosaic of adapted and blended philosophies. Despite myriad influences in Vietnam, the culture has retained several core values. These values include harmony, duty, honor, self-control, education, and family allegiance (Hunt, 2002; Nguyen, 1985).

A desire for balance is manifested in many aspects of society and serves as the basic tenet of traditional Vietnamese culture (Jamieson, 1995). Balance, or harmony, is based on the theory of yin and yang, two opposing and, at the same time, complementary aspects

of any one object or process. It is believed that when a proper balance of yin and yang is maintained, positive outcomes are inevitable.

Besides maintaining harmony, Vietnamese culture teaches its members to carry themselves with honor. It is their duty to never bring disgrace upon their family. The Vietnamese are generally modest and reserved in both speech and mannerism. Emotions are kept to oneself, and a hasty word or action is often viewed with disdain. As a result, Vietnamese may be considered reserved or unresponsive by American standards.

Honor and respect also come with education in Vietnamese culture. Individuals who have attained a high degree of intellectuality are well regarded. In the traditional social system, the scholar was at the top of the hierarchy, followed by the farmer, the artisan, and the tradesman (Hunt, 2002). In addition to education, respect is earned by leading a virtuous life.

Family is of paramount importance to the Vietnamese and contributes to a strong sense of collectiveness.

Individuals are taught to put the needs of their family above those of their own. The social identity of an individual is directly tied to his or her membership and position in the family. The traditional Vietnamese family is a hierarchically structured and well-integrated unit that includes not only the extended members but also those who are deceased and those not yet born (Cima, 1989). Historically, the father has been the decision maker and ultimate provider, although elder relatives often share authority. Children also have specific roles and are expected to abide by filial piety, a virtue in Confucian thought whereby utmost love and respect is shown for parents, elders, and ancestors (Jamieson, 1995).

The importance of family is evidenced in celebrations and formal offerings given to honor the dead on the day on which the family member died. In Vietnamese, these days are known as *ngay gio*, and they are considered by many to be more significant than birthdays (Davis, 2000a). Deceased family members are also honored during Tet, a holiday of great importance in Vietnamese culture. In the United States, it would be likened to Christmas, New Year, Easter, and the Fourth of July combined (Crawford, 1969). Tet, which starts on the first day of the first lunar month, marks the beginning of a new year and the coming of spring. It symbolizes rebirth, family, and relaxation. To prepare for this holiday, care is taken to make sure the interior of the home is in impeccable condition, as the house should not be cleaned during Tet (one would not want to sweep out any good luck). Detailed attention is also given to preparing culinary specialties. Both receiving guests and eating are important components of the holiday. Dishes of traditional foods are prepared and placed on the family altar for ancestors (Crawford, 1969). It is common even today for Vietnamese families, even the most Westernized living in Vietnam or abroad, to maintain an ancestral altar in their home to make offerings to the deceased (McLeod & Nguyen, 2001).

Names also have a significant place in Vietnamese culture. In some cases, a person may have a secret name that is known only to that person and his or her parents (Crawford, 1969). It is thought that this name cannot be revealed, lest the person risk being exposed to evil spirits. Most Vietnamese names consist of a family name, a middle name, and a personal given name, although the order of these names is reversed from what is familiar in the American tradition. The American name of Robert John Smith would be Smith John Robert in Vietnamese style. It is most respectful to address a Vietnamese person by Mr., Mrs., or Miss. The family name is not often used, so when addressing

Smith John Robert, it would be most appropriate to say Mr. Robert.

Although the Vietnamese culture is steeped in tradition, many changes have taken place over the past decades. Aspects of family structure, religious practice, medical treatment, social interaction, industry, diet, and even dress have been altered in the wake of war and economic modernization. Vietnamese culture continues to evolve as the country opens to the West and a balance between modernity and tradition is sought.

Vietnam stretches like a big "S" on the eastern coast of the Indochinese Peninsula in Southeast Asia. It is bordered by China to the north, Laos and Cambodia to the west, and over 1800 miles of coastline (Gulf of Tonkin, the South China Sea, and the Gulf of Thailand) to the east and south. The total land area of Vietnam is 128,066 square miles (Embassy of Vietnam, n.d.), which is about the size of New Mexico.

Vietnam is marked by widely diverse terrain with level land covering no more than 20% of the country (Cima, 1989). Thickly forested mountains as well as fertile low-lying plains are found in the north. Low-lying plains are also found to the south in the Mekong Delta region, which leads the country in rice production. Between the larger delta regions of the north and south, mountain regions and high plateaus characterize the long slender part of Vietnam. Major cities include Hanoi (the capital) and Hai Phong in northern Vietnam, Da Nang in the central region, and Ho Chi Minh City (formerly Saigon) in the south.

Vietnam has a tropical monsoon climate with significant rainfall and high humidity; however, due to evident differences in elevation and latitude, the climate can vary considerably across the country. Northern Vietnam has four distinct seasons characterized by large shifts in temperature (averaging 10–15°C [50–59°F] in winter and 30–36°C [86–97°F] in summer). Southern Vietnam is consistently warm year round (averaging 26–29°C [79–84°F]) with only two major seasonal variations: the wet season and the dry season (Embassy of Vietnam, n.d.).

 LANGUAGE

Vietnamese, the country's official language, is spoken by the vast majority of people, although dialects differ in the northern, central, and southern regions. There is debate among scholars as to the origin of the Vietnamese language, but it is most widely thought to be part of the Austro-Asiatic family of languages, which includes various languages spoken in mainland Southeast Asia (e.g., Khmer in Cambodia, and Mon in Myanmar and Thailand). The greatest influence of any single language, however, has been that of traditional Chinese (Cima, 1989).

Throughout history, the Vietnamese have used a variety of writing systems. *Chu nom*, the first script to express Vietnamese, was developed around the 9th century by borrowing and adapting Chinese characters. The written language evolved again during the 17th century when Christian missionaries, wanting to learn Vietnamese but unable to spend the years of study required to master the character-based system, devised a system using Roman letters called *quoc ngu* (Cima, 1989). *Quoc ngu* gradually replaced *chu nom*, and by the end of the 19th century it had become the common method of writing the Vietnamese language.

The Vietnamese language is a tonal language, and each syllable can be pronounced in one of six tones. To indicate different pronunciations, diacritical marks are placed above or below letters. The meaning of a word depends on the pitch in which the word is stated. If the tone is misrepresented or omitted, it may produce a meaningless syllable or even a word that is completely different from the one intended.

CULTURE HISTORY

According to legend, the founder of the Vietnamese nation was the son of Lac Long Quan (Dragon Lord of Lac), also known as the prince of the sea. Lac Long Quan was the descendent of a mythical Chinese ruler considered to be the father of Chinese agriculture. During his reign as king in the land of the Red River Delta, Lac Long Quan married Au Co, a Chinese immortal. She bore him 100 eggs from which came 100 babies, all of whom were male. Because Lac Long Quan was from the Dragon line and liked to dwell on the coast, and Au Co was from the Fairy Line and fond of the highlands, the two separated to their respective lands, each taking with them 50 sons. Lac Long Quan is regarded as a cultural hero and is given credit for bestowing his knowledge of agriculture onto his people and teaching them how to cultivate rice. His eldest son succeeded him as the ruler of Vietnam's first dynasty, the Hung Dynasty, which began in 2879 BC, and is thus considered the founder of the Vietnamese nation (Encyclopedia Britannica Online, n.d.).

The Hung Dynasty was overthrown in around 300 BC by the Chinese, beginning a long history of Chinese domination and cultural influence. After centuries of resistance, a successful revolt enabled Vietnam to reestablish its independence, and by 939 AD, a Vietnamese general had established himself as king of an independent Vietnam. During their independence, the Vietnamese expanded their territory southward into the lands of the Hindu-influenced regions of the Cham and the Khmer. The contact with these civilizations widened the Vietnamese perspective and provided another source of cultural influence.

Another strong set of influences came by way of European missionaries and merchants, who began to arrive in the early 16th century. Early missionaries are credited with perfecting a Romanized system of writing for the Vietnamese language called *quoc ngu*, which because of its simplicity, led to a high literacy rate and a surge of Vietnamese literature. The Vietnamese government looked upon the missionaries and their converts with great disdain, afraid that their communities were breeding grounds for rebellion. In an attempt to rid the country of French missionaries, the government established laws that forbade the practice of Christianity. The missionaries responded to these edicts by pressuring the French government to use military power and establish a protectorate over Vietnam. In 1857, Emperor Napoleon III agreed that an invasion was the best course of action, although missionaries were only the initial justification for the bloody battles that ensued (Cima, 1989). Military and economic interests became the primary reason for French presence in Vietnam. A Treaty of Protectorate, signed in 1883, formally placed Vietnam under French colonial rule.

Under French rule, the Vietnamese were prohibited from traveling outside their own districts unless they carried identity papers. They were also prohibited from publishing, meeting, or organizing into any group. Education declined rapidly. By 1925, it was estimated that not more than 1 in 10 children received a formal education (Cima, 1989). Resistance developed as a result of the social tensions created by colonialism. In 1930, the Indochinese Communist Party was established and became dedicated to overthrowing colonialism and building socialism.

The Vietnamese declared independence at the end of World War II, but French rule continued until 1954, when communist forces took control of the North. By 1956, Vietnam had split into two opposing political units, North and South Vietnam. The communist Democratic Republic of Vietnam (North Vietnam) sought to reunify Vietnam under its authority. A brutal war erupted between North Vietnam and the Republic of Vietnam (South) that lasted until 1975. The United States provided both military and economic support to South Vietnam, but the North Vietnamese forces eventually overran the South. Vietnam was reunified under the Socialist Republic of Vietnam. Even though peace had returned, Vietnam faced dire economic problems inflamed by conservative leadership policies. An exodus of hundreds of thousands of Vietnamese began.

In 1986, a set of economic reforms (*Doi Moi*) were launched in an effort to modernize the economy. In the past 10 years, leadership has shown an enhanced commitment to economic liberalization and structural reform. Increased production and better living standards have followed, although Vietnam still remains one of Asia's poorest countries (McLeod & Nguyen, 2001).

FOOD HISTORY WITHIN THE CULTURE

Both Vietnam's history and geography are reflected in the assortment of flavors and food preparation techniques seen in the Vietnamese kitchen. The various ruling or conquered nations of Vietnam have had significant impact on the cuisine over the centuries. Chinese influence is highly evident, illustrated by the fact that Vietnam is the only Southeast Asian country where people eat primarily with chopsticks, a technique learned from the Chinese. The Hindu-influenced Cham and Khmer territories of Southeast Asia offered the flavors of coconut milk, curry powder, five-spice powder, and oyster sauce. European missionaries and merchants also imparted particular culinary pleasures on the Vietnamese cuisine, such as bread, ice cream, and pastries; however, the expense of some of the non-native ingredients used in French cooking, such as butter, restricted an expansive adoption of the cuisine. Even American influence, by way of restaurants that serve hamburgers and fried chicken, is seen today in urban areas such as Ho Chi Minh City.

The three regions of Vietnam (north, central, and south) share the main characteristics of Vietnamese cuisine, particularly the use of rice as a principal ingredient. Dating back to the birth of the nation and the mythical Lac Long Quan, significance has been placed on rice. According to a 2000 report published by the Food and Agriculture Regional Office for Asia and the Pacific, rice is the staple food of the Vietnamese people, providing 80% of the carbohydrate and 40% of the protein intake in the diet (Bong, 2000). Another

fundamental component of Vietnamese cuisine is fish sauce (*nuoc mam*). It is used both as a condiment and as an ingredient in many dishes. Tropical fruits, fresh vegetables, noodles, stir-fry, soups, and grilled or fried foods wrapped in herb leaves, lettuce, or rice paper are also commonly eaten. Other distinctive characteristics include the use of aromatic herbs and condiments such as bittersweet caramel sauce, which provides a rich color to savory foods (Nguyen, 2006a).

Beyond these similarities, there are noticeable regional differences (Freeman, n.d.; Nguyen, 2006a). Due to physical proximity, northern Vietnam shares the most similarities with Chinese cuisine. In the north, spices are mild; black pepper and ginger are used more commonly than chilies for heat. In addition to fish sauce, which is also used in other regions of Vietnam, soy sauce is consumed in the north. Central Vietnamese dishes are earthy and spicier due to the use of ground chilies. The dishes are known for their beautiful presentation and portions, which may be considered small and dainty to some people. Southern cuisine, on the other hand, tends to be served in larger portions. Foods are often sweeter and more garlicky than foods to the north and may be flavored with coconut milk, turmeric, and curries. A large portion of Vietnamese émigrés have been from the south, so much of the Vietnamese food abroad has had the most influence from this region (Nguyen, 2006a).

The careful search for balance of yin and yang is embodied in Vietnamese cuisine. Foods are meticulously prepared and eaten in relationship to this theory (Thai, 2003). Even how much to consume when invited to a meal requires a search for equilibrium in yin and yang. Emptying one's plate gives the illusion of greed and eating too little implies a lack of manners.

All foods are considered to have yin or yang properties. Yin pertains to whatever is cold, fluid, humid, passive, somber, interior, deficient, and feminine in essence like the sky, moon, night, water, and winter. Yang pertains to whatever is hot, luminous, active, exterior, excessive, and masculine in essence like the earth, sun, fire, and summer (Dang, n.d.; Thai, 2003). The interactions between ingredients are taken into consideration during the preparation of each dish. For example, dishes with yin ingredients such as cabbage (*cai bap*), lettuce (*rau cai*), and fish (*ca*) require the addition of a condiment or spice with yang characteristics, such as ginger (*gung*). The Vietnamese may also turn to food to cure dysfunctions caused by the loss of balance in yin and yang in the human body. If one has an illness of yang nature, such as constipation, foods with yin characteristics (i.e., black-bean compote) would be advised (Dang, n.d.).

Changes in economic reform over the past decade have had a dramatic impact on the food supply and the nutritional status of the Vietnamese. The gross domestic product has increased significantly, and the rapid economic growth has brought about advances in agricultural production and animal husbandry, improving the food supply and contributing to national food security (Hop, 2003; Hop, Mai, & Khan, 2003). A reduction in the malnutrition rate has been observed in Vietnam, although childhood malnutrition still remains relatively high, especially in rural areas.

At the same time that dietary improvements have been made, the country faces another burden. Overweight, obesity, and nutritionally related chronic diseases, such as diabetes, have recently increased (Cuong, Dibley, Bowe, Hanh, & Loan, 2007; Khan & Khoi, 2008; Nguyen, Beresford, & Drewnowski, 2007). Prior to 1995, the prevalence of overweight and obesity was so low that there was little report of this problem; however, according to the results of a 2004 cross-sectional study of adults living in the urban areas of Ho Chi Minh City, the age-standardized prevalence of overweight and obesity was 26.2 and 6.4%, respectively (Cuong et al., 2007). These estimates were based on the Asian-specific body mass index (BMI) cutoff values

(overweight: BMI 23–27.4 kg/m^2; obesity: BMI ≥ 27.5 kg/m^2). Other studies have shown similar results. Changes in diet and lifestyle, especially among urban populations with an increased income, are thought to contribute to these increases in overweight and chronic disease. Chips, soda, ice cream, and fast-food restaurants, once novelties and featured only in Western media, are now found easily in urbanized areas of Vietnam. Dietary patterns have been shifting from a traditional diet rich in cereals, tubers, vegetables, and limited animal-based foods to diets rich in meat, eggs, milk, fat, and sugar. Vietnam now faces a dual challenge of combating undernutrition as well as the rising rates of overweight.

MAJOR FOODS

Protein Sources

Aquatic animals, whether caught from the sea, river, or rice paddy, have consistently been the primary protein source and are eaten fresh, dried, or salted. For most of Vietnam's history, meat has had little role in the cuisine, although it has become much more common in contemporary society. According to results from

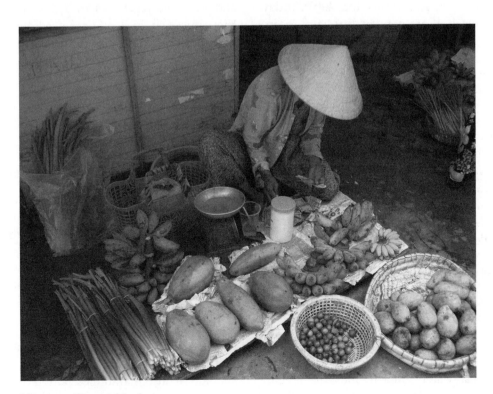

Vietnam Street Market

Observations from the Author (Rachel Fisher)

Fast food in Vietnam is primarily street food. It is often a highly refined system designed to cater exactly to the needs and tastes of an incredibly mobile populace. A friend of mine, who recently spent 6 months traveling through Southeast Asia, had many stories to share regarding her encounters with this "fast" cuisine in Vietnam. One thing that intrigued her was the number of fresh baguette sellers that would set up their baskets along busy intersections. This allowed drivers on motorbikes (10 years ago it would have been bicycles) to pull up and literally reach out to the sidewalk seller, get a bag of fresh bread, and be on his or her way in a matter of seconds. Baguette sellers were often seen jockeying for position, trying to get the most coveted spots where people stuck in traffic were within easy reach.

Another "fast" food that caught the attention of my friend was what she affectionately referred to as the "squid bike." The Vietnamese love dried squid as a snack. Squid sellers attach a large cart to a motorbike or to the back of a bicycle. The cart includes a vertical platform to hang the dried squid, a charcoal brazier on the table-like portion of the cart, and a roller, which is used to flatten the heated squid before serving it. The squid bike would be out all night, driving up and down streets, and people would just wave down the driver, and he would prepare fresh, hot dried squid before their eyes.

Another way to wave down food is from women employed by local markets who sell produce beyond the walls of the market stalls. These women, with shoulder poles and two baskets, walk through their neighborhoods announcing the goods of the day. When stopped, they put their baskets down on the sidewalk and package up fresh produce on the spot. People working in local shops are able to put together whole meals this way, simply by waiting for food to pass by their door!

In areas such as Hanoi and Ho Chi Minh City, fast food is beginning to take on a more Westernized existence. Chains such as Kentucky Fried Chicken can now be found alongside these mobile food carts and snack shops. The "squid bike" my friend found so endearing may soon find competition from a pizza delivery bike or the drive-thru windows now selling hamburgers.

national surveys, meat consumption of the Vietnamese population was 24.4 grams/person per day in 1987 and 51.0 grams/person per day in 2000 (Hop, 2003). Today, chicken, pork, and beef are popular. Specialty meats, such as rabbit, goat, venison, and dog, are also eaten on occasion, generally during celebratory occasions with friends and family (Nguyen, 2006a).

 Starch Sources

Rice is the primary starch in the Vietnamese diet. There are two basic types: glutinous or "sticky" rice, and regular long-grain rice. Rice flour is also used to make noodles, which are commonly eaten. Over the years, Vietnamese have also cultivated a taste for French bread, which they use to make Vietnamese sandwiches called *banh mi.*

 Fat Sources

Vegetable oils, coconut milk, and coconut oil (high in saturated fat) are used.

 Prominent Vegetables

Soy, mung beans, water spinach, mustard greens, Chinese and Japanese eggplants, cucumbers, jicama, Chinese celery, daikon, cabbage, bok choy, potatoes, shallots, and squash are popular vegetables. Pickled and preserved vegetables are also an important part of Vietnamese cooking and are used for giving contrast to texture and flavor.

 Prominent Fruits

Green papayas (unripened), bananas, oranges, grapefruits, lemons, mangoes, jackfruits, durians, and pineapples are the main fruits consumed.

 Spices, Seasonings, and Condiments

Lemongrass, ginger, Chinese five-spice powder, curry powder, dried red chili flakes, ground turmeric, star anise, cilantro, mint, Thai basil, Vietnamese coriander, garlic, fish sauce, shrimp sauce, oyster sauce, tamarind liquid, rice wine, caramel sauce, rice vinegar, and soy sauce are the most common spices/condiments.

 Beverages

Throughout history, green tea has been a favorite among Vietnamese. Alcoholic beverages, such as rice-based liquor, have also maintained popularity. Traditionally, due to the prevalence of soups and broths, beverages were not served with meals, although this has changed with modern trends (McLeod & Nguyen, 2001). There has been a rise in the popularity of soda, beer, and coffee. Coffee is served black or with sweetened, condensed milk and can be hot or iced. Soy milk is also a common beverage.

 ## Desserts

Vietnamese sweets are meant to refresh rather than satiate. Going from north to south, desserts become progressively sweeter, reflecting changes in regional preferences. Popular desserts include fresh fruits, candies made from tropical fruits, puddings, sweet soups, and a variety of cakes (e.g., *banh trung thu*), which have a glutinous rice crust stuffed with sweet sesame paste. More contemporary desserts are Western-style frosted cakes made from wheat flour, eclairs, and ice cream, which is a favorite among the youth.

 ## FOODS WITH CULTURAL SIGNIFICANCE

According to legend, *banh chung*, a traditional dish always served at Tet, can be traced back to the national founder of Vietnam, King Hung. One of his sons made a square cake to symbolize the earth and gave it to him in honor of spring. This square cake, *banh chung*, has been served at Tet ever since. It is made from wrapping green leaves (e.g., banana or lotus) around sticky rice, pork, green pepper, and peas. The harmony of the ingredients is thought to help the blood circulate and prevent disease (Business-Vietnam Open Market, n.d.).

 ## TYPICAL DAY'S MENU

Breakfast is usually eaten in the home with the entire family present before departing for work or school; however, given the faster pace of life as Vietnam industrializes, breakfast may be eaten on the go. Common breakfast foods are rice gruel (*chao*) with meat or fish added to it; *pho bac*, a soup with rice noodles, beef broth, dried shrimp, bits of meat, ginger, fresh bean sprouts, coriander, mint, onions, and lemon (also commonly eaten for lunch or dinner); and *xôi*, steamed glutinous rice, wrapped in a lotus leaf (McLeod & Nguyen, 2001).

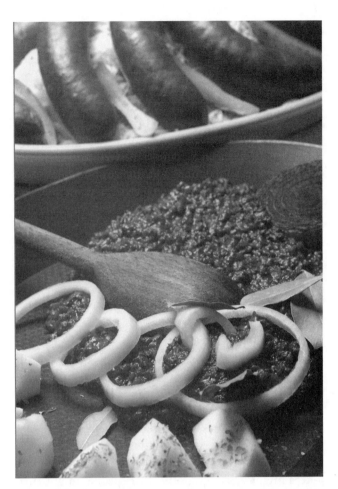

Blood/black pudding is sausage made with animal blood.

Lunch might consist of a Vietnamese sandwich, called *banh mi*, which is served on a baguette with mayonnaise, cold cuts, pickled daikon and carrot, and cucumber slices, and is garnished with coriander and black pepper. *Banh mi* is popular among urbanites who do not go home for lunch and can patronize roadside stalls. In the countryside, lunch tends to resemble breakfast and may consist of rice gruel flavored with shrimp paste or salted eggplant. Dessert, *do trang mieng*, which literally means "something to wash the mouth," is usually a piece of fresh fruit (McLeod & Nguyen, 2001).

Dinner is generally the most elaborate meal of the day and usually consists of *canh*, a meat/seafood dish, a vegetable, and rice. *Canh* refers to an everyday soup that is made with water (not stock) to which meat, vegetables, and herbs are added (Nguyen, 2006a).

All dishes are communal except for rice, which is usually served in individual bowls. Like lunch, if there is dessert, it usually consists of fresh fruit, green tea, and perhaps candy. On special occasions pudding or a Western-style cake might be served.

HOLIDAY MENUS

Holiday menus usually include foods that are only reserved for special occasions, such as *banh chung*, which is served during Tet. Instead of *canh*, *sup* would likely be served. *Sup*, a name derived from the French *soupe*, is often served as a starter course for formal meals. Instead of a water base, it starts with a rich meat broth (Nguyen, 2006a).

HEALTH BELIEFS AND CONCERNS

Within the traditional Vietnamese health-belief system, there are three major causative categories of illness: physical, metaphysical, and supernatural (Davis, 2000b). Health is considered be a balance between physical, moral, as well as internal and external forces. Treatment of an illness or symptom depends on the suspected cause. If the nature of the illness is considered physical or organic in nature, Western healthcare providers might be sought; otherwise, people might turn to shamans (healers), rituals, or herbal medicines.

Metaphysical causes of disease are rooted in the theory of yin and yang. Excessive emotion, an imbalanced diet, a disproportion of hot and cold energy, or the presence of an ill wind (*phong*) all cause disturbances in yin and yang (Davis, 2000b). Bad wind that has entered the body is considered a common cause of illnesses such as headaches, muscle aches, coughs, fevers, upper-respiratory infections, and sore throats. Several methods are used to restore balance and ultimately health in the body. *Cat le* and *cao gio* are two methods to treat wind diseases that involve skin dermabrasion. Rubbing or pinching of the skin is used to bring bad blood to the surface, allowing wind to escape. Other treatments used to reset balance include moxibustion (burning portions of the body), cupping (the application of suction cups to the skin in order to improve the circulation of chi), and coining (the rubbing of metal over the skin). Such treatments may leave visible marks on the skin for several days (Uba, 1992). Misunderstandings of these traditional practices, which can be labeled as physically abusive acts, can have serious repercussions for Vietnamese families living in Western cultures.

GENERAL HEALTH AND NUTRITIONAL INDICATORS SUMMARY

Vietnam's rapid economic growth over the past two decades has brought about many positive changes in health and nutrition. Improvements have included expanded vaccination programs, reductions in poverty and hunger, effective control of malaria, and improvements in maternal and child health. For example, between 1990 and 2007, infant mortality rates (under 1 year) decreased from 40 to 13 per 1000 live births. During the same time period, the under-5-years mortality rate decreased from 56 to 15 per 1000 live births. Also, compared with other countries in the region, Vietnam has achieved a smaller rate (7%) of infants with low birth weight (United Nations Children's Fund [UNICEF], 2008).

Despite economic progress and resulting improvements, however, Vietnam continues to face many health challenges related to disparities across subpopulations. The gap between the richest and poorest quintiles continues to rise. The noticeable disparities seen among rural and ethnic minority populations living in mountainous regions, where adequate access to basic social services is limited, are of particular concern. For example, according to data reported by United Nations Children's Fund (UNICEF, 2008), maternal mortality rates are four times higher in the northern mountainous regions than in the more populated lowlands.

Furthermore, there are striking differences in poverty rates among individuals living in different geographic locations across the country. Although the overall poverty rate in Vietnam fell from 58.1% in 1993 to 24.1% in 2004, poverty rates vary significantly across populations. In 2004, the poverty rate among urban populations was 10.8% compared with a poverty rate of 27.5% among rural populations. Among ethnic minorities, the poverty rate was 69.3% in 2004 (Leipziger, Wodon, Yepes, Categories, & Fay, 2003).

Child undernutrition is another area where Vietnam continues to face challenges. In 2007, stunting[1] affected 36% of children under 5 years, whereas 8% of children the same age suffered from wasting[2] (UNICEF, 2008). The highest rates occur in rural and ethnic minority populations. Deficiencies in key nutrients, such as iron, vitamin A, zinc, and iodine, still persist,

---

[1] Stunting: moderate and severe; below minus two standard deviations from median height for age of reference population.
[2] Wasting: moderate and severe; below minus two standard deviations from median weight for height of reference population.

although efforts to curb these deficiencies have made some progress. In 2007, 95% of children received vitamin A supplementation, and as a result, xerophthalmia is no longer prevalent in Vietnam, although dietary intake of vitamin A is still low, and marginal vitamin A status is common among certain subpopulations, increasing children's vulnerability to deficiency. The addition of iodine to salt has also improved nutritional outcomes by reducing prevalence of cretinism, dwarfism, and goiter. In 2007, 93% of households consumed iodized salt (UNICEF, 2008).

COMMUNICATION AND COUNSELING TIPS

Poor communication and lack of cultural understanding are common barriers to effective counseling between Western health professionals and Vietnamese patients. Some Vietnamese may be reluctant to seek care from those who practice Western medicine, especially if they believe the source of their illness is an imbalance in yin or yang or another cause not recognized by the Western model of health care (Uba, 1992). Depending on previous exposure to Western medicine, when they do seek care, they may be very unfamiliar with medical procedures. For example, some patients may expect the provider to diagnose and treat their illness on the first encounter and may become frustrated if this does not happen. It is also believed by some Southeast Asians that Western drugs and dosages may not be appropriate for them. Consequently, while they may politely accept the physician's prescription, they will either choose not to fill it or they will not take all of the prescribed dosage. In some cases, they will also stop taking the medication if their symptoms subside. Thorough and clear explanation of Western diagnostic techniques and treatments may help Vietnamese patients unfamiliar with these concepts. When a treatment decision has to be made, it may be worthwhile to consider involving other family members due to the high value placed on family in Vietnamese culture.

Vietnamese are taught to remain silent and listen attentively when speaking with an authoritative figure. As a result, patients may not ask questions, even when they do not understand. Counseling sessions should be as thorough as possible to ensure comprehension. It is also important to note that disagreeing with an authority figure is frowned upon, so a patient may respond positively to a question, even when a negative response would more accurately reflect the truth.

To encourage favorable rapport with a patient, it is important to be aware of the nonverbal gestures that may have different meanings in Vietnamese and Western cultures.

In the Vietnamese culture, it is not considered respectful to look directly into the eyes of an authority figure. Patients will often avert their gaze during a discussion. Looking directly into the eyes of the opposite sex is especially discouraged because it may be interpreted as a sign of passion. Health professionals should be mindful not to pat a patient's back, especially one who is senior in age or status, as this will convey disrespect. It is also disrespectful to put one or both hands on the hips or in the pockets while talking, to point to other people, or to beckon with an index finger. This may be especially threatening to children (Hunt, 2002).

COMMON FOOD NAMES WITH ENGLISH AND PHONETIC TRANSLATION

Common food names with English and phonetic translation are given in Table 28-1.

TABLE 28-1   Common Food Names with English and Phonetic Translation

English	Vietnamese	Phonetic Translation
Spices/Herbs/Condiments		
Cilantro	*Ngò*	N-gaw
Thai basil	*Húng quế*	Hoong quay
Curry powder	*bột cà-ri*	Boht kah-ree

(continues)

TABLE 28-1   Common Food Names with English and Phonetic Translation (Continued)

English	Vietnamese	Phonetic Translation
Chinese five-spice powder	bột ngũ vị hương	Boht n–goo vee hoong
Ginger	gừng	Goong
Garlic	Tỏi	Toy
Caramel sauce	nước mầu/nước hàng	Nook moh/nook hahng
Shrimp sauce	mắm ruốc/mắm tôm	Mahm ru-ook/mahm tohm
Fish sauce	nước mắm	Nook mahm
Coconut milk	nước cốt dừa	Nook koht zu-ah
Protein Sources		
Eggs	trứng	Troong
Fish	Cá	Kah
Beef	thị bò	Teet baw
Chicken	Gà	Gah
Pork	thịt heo	Teeth heh-ao
Vegetables		
Onion	hành tây	Haan tay
Mung beans	đậu xanh	Doh saan
Shallot	hành tím	Haan teem
Shiitake (Chinese black mushrooms)	nấm đông cô/nấm hương	Num dong koh/num hoong
Banana leaves	lá chuối	Lah chu-oy
Rice and Noodles		
Chinese egg noodles	Mì	Mee
Flat rice noodles	bánh phở	Baan fuh
Round rice noodles	Bún	Boon
Rice paper	bánh tráng	Baan trahng
Rice, cooked long grain	Cơm	Kuhm
Rice, steamed glutinous/sticky	xôi	Soy

Compiled with permission from A. Nguyen, www.vietworldkitchen.com

FEATURED RECIPE

According to Andrea Nguyen, cookbook author, "Every good Vietnamese cook needs to master this dipping sauce. It's used in many dishes to bring all the elements together." This sauce is likely to be used to add final flavor to foods wrapped in lettuce or herbs, which are not salted and therefore need a little lift to heighten the overall eating experience.

Nuoc Cham (Basic Dipping Sauce)

3 tbsp. lime juice (1 fat, thin-skinned lime)

2 tbsp. sugar

½ cup water

2½ tbsp. fish sauce

1 small garlic clove, finely minced (optional)

1–2 Thai chilies, thinly sliced, or 1 tsp. chili garlic sauce (optional)

1. Make lemonade: combine the lime juice, sugar, and water, stirring to dissolve the sugar. Adjust the flavors to balance out the sweet and sour.
2. Add the fish sauce and any of the optional ingredients. Taste again and adjust the flavors to your liking. When it's a light honey or amber, it may be close to finished.

Yields ¾ cup

Adapted with permission from A. Nguyen, www.vietworldkitchen.com

---

More recipes are available at http://nutrition.jbpub. com/foodculture/

REFERENCES

Bong, B.B. (2000). Bridging the rice yield gap in Vietnam. In M.K. Papademetrio, F.J. Dent, & E.M. Herath (Eds.), *Bridging the rice yield gap in the Asia-Pacific region*. Food and Agriculture Organization (FAO) of the United Nations Regional Office for Asia and the Pacific.

Business-Vietnam Open Market. (n.d.). *All about Vietnam: Traditional festivals*. Retrieved March 5, 2008, from http://www.bvom.com/resource/vn_cultural.asp?pContent=Traditional_Cuisine/

Cima, R.J. (Ed.). (1989). *Vietnam: A country study*. Washington, DC: GPO for the Library of Congress.

Crawford, A.C. (1969). *Customs and culture of Vietnam*. Rutland, VT: Charles E. Tuttle Company.

Cuong, T.Q., Dibley, M.J., Bowe S., Hanh T.T., & Loan T.T. (2007). Obesity in adults: An emerging problem in urban areas of Ho Chi Minh City, Vietnam. *European Journal of Clinical Nutrition, 61*(5), 673–681.

Dang, A.T. (n.d.). *Yin–yang in Vietnamese culinary art*. Retrieved March 8, 2008, from http://www.limsi.fr/Individu/dang/webvn/enourriture.htm/

Davis, R. (2000a). The convergence of health and family in the Vietnamese culture. *Journal of Family Nursing, 6*(2), 136–156.

Davis, R. (2000b). Cultural health care or child abuse? The Southeast Asian practice of cao gio. *Journal of the American Academy of Nurse Practitioners, 12*(3), 89–95.

Embassy of Vietnam. (n.d.). *Learn about Vietnam*. Retrieved March 21, 2008, from http://www.vietnamembassy-usa. org/

Encyclopedia Britannica Online. (n.d.). *Legends and early history of Vietnam*. Retrieved March 10, 2008, from http://www.britannica.com/eb/article-52724/Vietnam#509928. hook/

Freeman, N. (n.d.). *Ethnic cuisine: Vietnam*. Retrieved March 10, 2008, from http://www.sallys-place.com/food/cuisines/vietnam.htm/

Hop, L.T. (2003). Programs to improve production and consumption of animal source foods and malnutrition in Vietnam. *Journal of Nutrition, 133*, 4006S–4009S.

Hop, L.T., Mai, L.B., & Khan, N.C. (2003). Trends in food production and food consumption in Vietnam during the period 1980–2000. *Malaysian Journal of Nutrition, 9*, 1–5.

Hunt, P.C. (2002). An introduction to Vietnamese culture for rehabilitation service providers in the U.S. *The Center for International Rehabilitation Research Information and Exchange (CIRRIE) Monograph Series*. Retrieved March 12, 2008, from http://cirrie.buffalo.edu/monographs/vietnam.pdf/

Jamieson, N.L. (1995). *Understanding Vietnam*. Berkeley: University of California Press.

Khan, N.C., & Khoi, H.H. (2008). Double burden of malnutrition: Vietnam perspectives. *Asia Pacific Journal of Clinical Nutrition, 17*(S1), 116–118.

Leipziger D., Wodon Q., Yepes T., Categories J., & Fay M. (2003). Vietnam, achieving the millennium development goals. In *The Role of the Infrastructure*. Hanoi. Retrieved December 10, 2009, from http://citeseerx.ist.psu.edu/viewdoc/summary?doi=10.1.1.2.8048

McLeod M.W., & Nguyen T.D. (2001). *Culture and customs of Vietnam*. Westport, CT: Greenwood Press.

Nguyen, A.Q. (2006a). *Into the Vietnamese kitchen: Treasured foodways, modern flavors*. Berkeley, CA: Ten Speed Press.

Nguyen, A.Q. (2006b). *Phonetics for common Vietnamese ingredients*. Retrieved March 9, 2008, from http://www.vietworldkitchen.com/features/phonetics-ingredients.pdf/

Nguyen, A.Q. (2007). *Read, learn, cook, and eat! Basic dipping sauce*. Retrieved March 9, 2008, from http://www.vietworldkitchen.com/recipes/basics/nuoccham.htm/

Nguyen, M.D. (1985). Culture shock: A review of Vietnamese culture and its concepts of health and disease [Cross-cultural medicine]. *West Journal of Medicine, 142*, 409–412.

Nguyen, M.D., Beresford S.A., & Drewnowski, A. (2007). Trends in overweight by socio-economic status in Vietnam: 1992 to 2002. *Public Health Nutrition, 10*, 115–121.

Thai, H.C. (2003). Traditional Vietnamese medicine: Historical perspective and current usage. Retrieved March 21, 2008, from http://ethnomed.org/clin_topics/viet/trad_viet_med.html/

Uba, L. (1992). Cultural barriers to health care for Southeast Asian refugees. *Public Health Reports, 107*(5), 544–548.

United Nations Children's Fund (UNICEF). (2008). *The state of the world's children, 2009: Maternal and newborn health*. Retrieved April 21, 2009, from http://www.unicef.org/sowc09/index.php/

Africa

Food, Cuisine, and Cultural Competency for Culinary, Hospitality, and Nutrition Professionals discusses eight prominent regions in Africa:

ALGERIA

Algeria is in northern Africa, bordering the Mediterranean Sea, between Morocco and Tunisia. Algeria has the eighth-largest reserve of natural gas in the world and is the fourth-largest gas exporter; it ranks 15th in oil reserves. Sustained high oil prices in recent years have helped improve Algeria's financial and macroeconomic indicators. The government's continued efforts to diversify the economy by attracting foreign and domestic investment outside the energy sector, however, has had little success in reducing high unemployment and improving living standards.

BOTSWANA

Botswana is located in southern Africa, north of South Africa. It has maintained one of the world's highest economic growth rates since independence in 1966, although growth fell below 5% in 2007–2008. Through fiscal discipline and sound management, Botswana has transformed itself from one of the poorest countries in the world to a middle-income country with a per capita gross domestic product (GDP) of $13,300 in 2008. Two major investment services rank Botswana as the best credit risk in Africa. Diamond mining has fueled much of the expansion and currently accounts for more than one third of GDP and for 70–80% of export earnings. Tourism, financial services, subsistence farming, and cattle raising are other key sectors. On the downside, the government must deal with high rates of unemployment and poverty. Unemployment officially was 23.8% in 2004, but unofficial estimates place it closer to 40%. The HIV/AIDS infection rates are the second highest in the world and threaten Botswana's impressive economic gains.

ETHIOPIA

Ethiopia is in East Africa, west of Somalia. Its poverty-stricken economy is based on agriculture, which accounts for almost half of the GDP, 60% of exports, and 80% of total employment. The agricultural sector suffers from frequent drought and poor cultivation practices. Coffee is critical to the Ethiopian economy, with exports of approximately $350 million in 2006, but historically low prices have seen many farmers switching to chat (a tropical evergreen plant whose leaves are used as a stimulant) to supplement income. Drought struck again late in 2002, leading to a 3.3% decline in GDP in 2003. Normal weather patterns helped agricultural and GDP growth recover during 2004–2008.

KENYA

Kenya is located in East Africa, bordering the Indian Ocean, between Somalia and Tanzania. A severe drought from 1999 to 2000 caused water and energy rationing, which reduced agricultural output. As a result, the GDP decreased by 0.2% in 2000. Despite the return of strong rains in 2001, weak commodity prices limited Kenya's economic growth to 1.2%. Growth lagged at 1.1% in 2002 because of erratic rains. The global financial crisis on remittance and exports reduced GDP growth to 2.2% in 2008, down from 7% the previous year.

NIGERIA

Nigeria is in West Africa, bordering the Gulf of Guinea, between Benin and Cameroon. Oil-rich Nigeria has undertaken several reforms over the past decade. Based largely on increased oil exports and high global crude-oil prices, the GDP rose significantly in 2007 and 2008. Nigeria, like many other African countries, has an extremely high mortality rate due to AIDS.

RWANDA

Rwanda is in Central Africa, east of Democratic Republic of the Congo. Rwanda is a poor country with about 90% of the population engaged in mainly subsistence agriculture. It is the most densely populated country in Africa and is landlocked with few natural resources and minimal industry. The primary exports are coffee and tea. Despite Rwanda's fertile ecosystem, food production often does not keep pace with population growth, which makes food imports necessary.

SUDAN

Sudan is located in northern Africa, bordering the Red Sea, between Egypt and Eritrea. Until the second half of 2008, Sudan's economy boomed on the back of increases in oil production, high oil prices, and large inflows of foreign direct investment. The GDP growth registered more than 10% per year in 2006 and 2007. Agricultural production remains important, because it employs 80% of the workforce and contributes a third of the GDP. The Darfur conflict, the aftermath of two decades of civil war in the south, the lack of basic infrastructure in large areas, and a reliance by much of the population on subsistence agriculture mean that much of the population will remain at or below the poverty line for years, despite rapid increases in average per capita income.

WEST AFRICA (GHANA, SIERRA LEONE, AND LIBERIA)

West Africa includes Ghana, Sierra Leone, and Liberia, among other countries. Ghana borders the Gulf of Guinea, between *Cote d'Ivoire* (Ivory Coast) and Togo. Ghana is well endowed with natural resources and has roughly twice the per capita output of the poorest countries in West Africa. Even so, Ghana remains heavily dependent on international financial and technical assistance. Gold and cocoa exports are major sources of foreign revenue. The domestic economy continues to revolve around agriculture, which accounts for about 35% of the GDP and employs about 55% of the workforce, mainly small landholders. Sound macroeconomic management along with high prices for gold and cocoa helped sustain GDP growth in 2008.

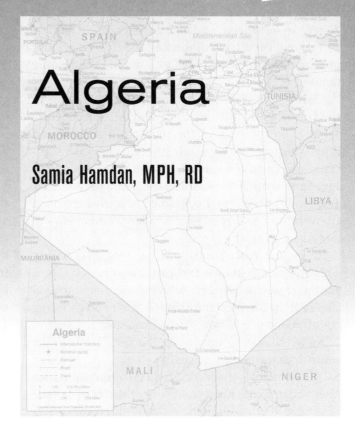

CHAPTER 29

Algeria

Samia Hamdan, MPH, RD

CULTURE AND WORLD REGION

Algeria is a historically fascinating country. Its mosaic culture has evolved from an infusion of native countrymen and some of the world's most powerful civilizations. The culture, customs, and religions of Algeria have incorporated the influences of conquest and trade but amazingly remain rooted in traditions dating back to the nation's earliest existence. Algerian cuisine is no exception. The Algerian diet, like that of most North African countries, is healthy and rich in fresh fruit, vegetables, salads, pulses, bread, olive oil, fish, poultry, broiled meat, spices, and herbs. Its collection of ancient cultural dietary traditions makes Algerian cuisine one of the most unique and intriguing.

Over 33 million people live in Algeria according to the latest population census. Most Algerians live in the northern region surrounding the Mediterranean coastline. Interestingly, over 90% of Algerians live along the Mediterranean on only 12% of the country's land. Al-

most half of the population is composed of urban residents, and this trend continues to grow as many flock to the city to find work. Adequate housing is a major issue in urban areas. In fact, Algeria has one of the world's highest per-housing-unit occupancy rates, according to the United Nations Development Program. Public officials have announced a 1.5-million-unit housing shortage. Moreover, almost 2 million people still live in the Sahara Desert area. They rely heavily on agriculture as a means to survive. These native nomads and *Bedouin* migrate between various pockets of vegetation and water, with the sheep and goats they herd.

The majority of Algerians are Arab in ethnicity, with approximately 20% of Berber descent. Almost all Algerians are Sunni Muslim. Only 1% of the population is of Christian or Jewish faith. Some estimate that the number of non-Muslim residents could be as little as 5000 or fewer. Of those Algerians practicing Christianity, most follow the Roman Catholic, Methodist, and Evangelical faiths.

Arabic culture and customs revolve around the family unit. They are extremely warm, generous, and hospitable people. House guests are treated with high respect, and often served a healthful array of snacks. Visitors are typically served one or more of juices, tea, coffee, desserts, fruit, and nuts during a visit. Comfort and enjoyment during dinners and visitations are important and almost regarded as a duty to the hosting family.

Food is cherished as an important contributor to the family's structure, bonding, and interdependence. Woman do the bulk of the cooking in Algeria and often cook together with their sisters, daughters, mothers, aunts, and other extended female family members. Mealtime is often a casual and gregarious experience, and food is served and consumed at a leisurely pace. Conversation and relaxation are key components to any Algerian meal.

Algeria is located in the northwest region of Africa. This area is also known as the *Maghreb*, which means sunset region in Arabic. Situated on the southern shores of the Mediterranean Sea, Algeria's neighboring countries include Morocco to the west, and Tunisia and Libya to the east. Countries that border Algeria to the south include Mali, Mauritania, Niger, and Western Sahara. Algeria is the second largest country in Africa after Sudan and is nearly four times the size of Texas.

Because of its location on the Mediterranean Sea, Algeria is opportune to trade and tourism; however, the majority of the country's terrain is high plateau and desert. The Sahara Desert covers a vast majority of Algeria and is one of the hottest and driest parts of the world. Temperatures are extreme and can reach over 100°F during the day, and below 32°F at night. Because approximately 80% of Algeria is composed of desert terrain, sparse land is available for vegetation. In fact, only 3% of the land can be cultivated.

Algeria also has a mountainous terrain in the north and is susceptible to severe earthquakes and mudslides, as well as floods during the country's rainy season. The Tellian and Atlas mountain ranges spread across the country from east to west. Fortunately, between the Mediterranean Sea and the mountain ranges, lies a narrow strip of coastal land that is fertile. Due to the area's moderate climate, the land receives adequate rainfall making the area opportune to agricultural production. Wheat and barley are the primary crops that flourish in Algeria's subtropical climate. Rice, however, cannot be grown well in this region and therefore is consumed less than wheat products. The mild climate also allows Algerians to grow dates,

olives, potatoes, and citrus fruits, including lemon and lime. Sheep and cattle are also prominent agricultural products. Algeria's major agricultural trading partners include France, the United States, and Canada. Algeria's chief agricultural imports include wheat, dry cow milk, and corn, and its primary exports include dates, corn oil, and wine. France, Libya, and Spain receive the bulk of Algeria's exports.

LANGUAGE

The official language of Algeria is Arabic. Berber dialects are also spoken throughout the nation. In fact, Berber is known as the national language and Arabic the official language. French is also commonly spoken among Algerians as a second language. Because Algeria was under French rule between 1830 and 1962, the influence of French culture and language is significant. It is not uncommon to hear French words interwoven into Arabic conversation. Bi- and trilingualism are not uncommon in Algeria.

CULTURE HISTORY

Algeria is culturally rich and diverse. Historically, ancient civilizations influenced the country's culture and politics through conquest and trade. Native Algerians were ethnically identified as Berber since the 5th century BC; however, historical shifts impacted the culture and identity of the nation's people indefinitely. Over the next several centuries, Algeria was occupied and invaded by numerous civilizations, including the Phoenicians, Romans, Vandals, Byzantines, Arabs, Turkish, and French. The most significant cultural impact on Algerians took place during the Arab invasion, between the 8th and 11th centuries AD, when the Arabic language and Islamic religion were introduced to Algerians. Arab and Islamic culture, customs, religion, politics, and food were profoundly imprinted on the Algerian people.

The second notable influence occurred during the French occupation. Algeria was occupied under French rule for over 100 years. Algerians were moved off of their own land and forced to give up their farmlands and agricultural livelihoods to the French rulers. In 1954, the National Liberation Front, a major Algerian nationalist party, began revolting against the French to regain rights denied under the occupation. The nation finally achieved its independence on July 5, 1962.

Although the French rulers left Algeria, as did over a million French citizens, the influence of French culture settled, with language, politics, food, and socialist ideals determining the way of life in Algeria.

Algeria is currently governed as a republic. Its laws are based on Islamic and French law, which reflect the nation's influence under various historical invasions. Algeria is a multiparty state with 10 parties representing the nation's parliament. The National Liberation Front continues to dominate politics in Algeria.

 ## FOOD HISTORY WITHIN THE CULTURE

Throughout its history, the Algerian diet has evolved to become one of the world's most diverse and interesting cuisines. The present Algerian diet can trace its roots back to the food patterns of the Berber countrymen. The Berber began producing wheat as early as 30,000 BC. When the Carthaginians occupied the North African region, they introduced the creation of semolina from wheat. This was a landmark moment in Algerian diet history, as it led to the Berber's invention of couscous. Couscous, pronounced *kesksou* in the Algerian-Arabic dialect, is a low-fat complex carbohydrate made from semolina and wheat flour. Due to its versatile uses, its popularity spread all the way from Morocco to Egypt, to sub-Saharan Africa, and to other parts of the Middle East. The word couscous most likely came from the Berber word *seksou*. Other theories speculate that the word comes from *kiskis*, which means steamer pot in Arabic, or that it possibly even derived from the sound that comes from the steam rising during cooking. Couscous is now Algeria's national dish and is served in a variety of ways. A bed of couscous is often served warm as a main entree, with meat, vegetables, and legumes atop. *Smen*, a fermented butter product often used in baking and cooking, was also introduced by the Berber. Dates, a fruit of cultural significance, are also rooted from this era.

The Algerian diet later expanded to include more foreign foods during the French occupation. A variety of Western-inspired foods flourished in the Algerian *souk*, or marketplace. New foods, flavors, and recipes were introduced during French rule, and even after Algeria achieved independence. A major diet change included the addition of more dairy products into cooking. Milk, cheese, fresh butter, whipped cream, and sour cream were not prominent, and some not even native to the traditional cuisine of Algeria, but

are now frequently used. Margarine, a culinary invention of France, is also a popular fat used in Algerian households and restaurants. Margarine is increasingly replacing *smen* in Algerian cooking, as it is inexpensive and relatively shelf-stable.

The preparation of pastries and desserts has also changed through French influence. Fruit and flower waters, such as orange and rose waters, respectively, were traditionally used in recipes. Instead, vanilla is used more often now to flavor desserts. Even the shapes and designs of traditional Algerian desserts have adopted French-style cuisine. *Baklawa*, a dessert made of filo dough, nuts, and honey typically cut into squares or diamonds, can now be found in the Algerian market as a round tart shape with a lattice crust. Packaged pastas have replaced homemade pastas in many recipes. Loaves of French bread have infiltrated the Algerian *souk*. French-style sidewalk cafes are plentiful in the urban areas of Algeria.

Eating is a sensual experience for Arabs. Food is typically eaten with the hands, using two fingers and a thumb. Bread is used to scoop up portions of salads, soups, and stews, and their remaining juices. The hands are freely used in food preparation, although utensils are widely available in the region. Measurements are visual and usually "eyeballed." With the addition of a vast array of spices and fresh foods, meals are often fragrant, colorful, and tender. Mealtime appeals to all the senses. Food is traditionally served on brass, silver, or copper trays set on the floor or a low table, while the family members are seated on cushions that surround the food. Dishes are often served as *mezes* or family style. After the main course, family members leave the dining area to continue socializing in the living room or other common area, but dinner is not yet complete. Hot tea and coffee are often served after the meal, along with a display of fresh fruits, tree nuts, and lavish desserts.

 ## MAJOR FOODS

 ### Protein Sources

Meat is a major contributor to the protein intake among Algerians. Beef, chicken, sheep, and goat meat are all prepared and eaten in various dishes. Pheasant, duck, goose, quail, and pigeon are also popular protein sources. Pork, because of its forbidden consumption under Islamic law, is generally not consumed.

Seafood is fresh and plentiful. The Mediterranean Sea offers a delectable variety of local fish and shellfish. Bass, swordfish, tuna, sea bream, monkfish, sardines, and red and gray mullet are usually eaten. Fish is typically fried, grilled, broiled, or added to stews, couscous dishes, and soups. Scallops, crabs, mussels, shrimp, lobster, squid, and octopus are added to various stews and soups, or prepared by broiling or frying.

Tagine is a popular savory stew that includes any choice of meat, poultry, or fish, and an infused combination of any nuts, spices, and vegetables. The heavy clay pot that *tagine* is cooked in is also called *tagine*. It has a round base and cone- or dome-shaped cover that is removed when the dish is served. A grain dish is usually served with *tagine*.

Other sources of protein are widely available. Dairy products, such as milk and eggs, are also popular protein sources. In fact, milk also provides almost 200 calories to the daily intake of Algerians. Tree nuts are also native to the North African region. They are often added to savory main entrees as well as to desserts and pastries. Walnuts, hazelnuts, almonds, pistachios, and pine nuts are favorites in this region.

 Starch Sources

Wheat, from which couscous is made, is a staple in the Algerian diet. Chicken couscous is a favorite dish in Algeria and often served during times of celebration and festivity. Today, couscous is often packaged and sold in the "instant" variety type, typically prepared by boiling water and adding the couscous to allow the granules to soak up the liquid and soften; however, couscous is traditionally steamed, and the hands are used freely to spread and massage water into the granules. Butter or margarine is generously added. This process is lengthy and requires care, but the finished product is generally thought to be superior in texture and taste than the instant product. Couscous has become popular in Western diets in recent years due to the growth of vegetarianism and low-fat diet recommendations.

Wheat is the nation's primary crop and the highest source of caloric intake for Algerians. It is imported in triple the amount that the nation produces, according to the United Nations Food and Agricultural Organization (2004). Wheat flour is used in versatile ways. Hard durum wheat is native to the Algerian region and is highly suitable for making various breads that are consumed with most Algerian meals. Flour is also used to make filo dough, a flaky, delicate product used to prepare desserts. Potato and corn are also eaten, as is imported rice, but in lower quantity.

Pulses are also popular in Algeria. Their use is versatile and they are often added to variations of soups, purées, dips, salads, and stews. Fava beans, chickpeas, and lentils are most commonly used in recipes.

 Fat Sources

Oils and dairy fats are used in a variety of cooking and food-preparation methods. Like most Mediterranean countries, olive oil is essential to Algerian cuisine. It is a key ingredient in marinades, sauces, and dressings, and is often used in frying. *Smen* is still used for baking and cooking but is more frequently replaced with margarine or butter. Milk and cheese are often consumed at breakfast. A traditional white cheese made with salt preserves is commonly eaten.

 Prominent Vegetables

Vegetables and salads are plentiful in the Algerian diet. A wide variety of vegetables from starchy to colorful to pungent are included and regarded as an essential component to any entree, soup, or salad. In fact, vegetables are often added to main entrees rather than served as a side dish, as is typically done in Western cuisines. Root vegetables, such as potatoes, turnips, parsnips, and carrots, are frequently added to main dishes. Zucchini, eggplant, bell pepper, tomato, cucumber, onion, garlic, lettuce, okra, and spinach grow well in this region and are also included in a variety of dishes. Salads are often prepared as part of an Algerian meal and could include fennel, artichoke, cardoon, leek, and legumes. Olives are a vital component and served as a side garnish with most meals.

 Prominent Fruits

The array of fruits in Algeria is lush and colorful. Bananas, oranges, peaches, lemons, mangoes, melons, figs, watermelons, pomegranates, dates, grapes, and apricots are abundant. Fruits are also versatile in Algerian cuisine and are eaten whole or added to salads, soups, stews, or *tagines*. Juices from fruits are used to enhance the flavor of both sweet and savory main dishes. Orange juice is used in a variety of foods, including soups, sauces, cakes, and pastries, whereas lemon and lime are added to meat and poultry marinades.

Spices, Herbs, and Condiments

Herbs and spices are treated with great respect in Algerian cooking. They are often used to create flavorful and aromatic dishes. Among the popular herbs used in Algerian cuisine are flat-leaf parsley, cilantro, oregano, wild marjoram, thyme, mint, and basil. The wide range of spices commonly used reveal the rich, savory flavors of Algerian cuisine. Fresh mint is used to prepare a traditional favorite, mint tea. Commonly used spices include cumin, cinnamon, ginger, saffron, coriander, paprika, allspice, aniseed, sesame seeds, caraway, cloves, turmeric, cilantro, chili peppers, and garlic. A less familiar spice to Westerners is *sumac*, which is finely ground and added in light quantities to provide a sour flavor to many salad dressings and dishes, and is used to marinate meat, fish, and chicken before cooking. Interestingly, despite the vast array of spices used in Algerian dishes, the food is considerably bland compared with many other tropical African dishes. For those with spicy taste buds, fiery condiments are added at the table to each person's individual taste.

Condiments are also essential to the Algerian diet. *Harissa*, a hot chili paste made of garlic and chili peppers, is often added to stews or stirred into soups. It is also commonly eaten with couscous dishes. *Tahini*, a crushed sesame seed paste, is also a popular condiment added to many dishes and is also used in sauces and dips. (*Tahini* is commonly known as the creamy ingredient used to make hummus.) *Ras el Hanout* is a spice mix created in various ways by individual spice merchants, and can contain up to 20 spices depending on the merchant selling them. *Zahtar* is ground thyme powder, made with *sumac* and sesame seeds. It is often used as a dip with olive oil and eaten with pita bread as an appetizer.

Rosewater and orange water are also favorites in Algerian cuisine. They are often used to add aroma and taste to many desserts. Lemon preserves are also popular in Algeria and are added to a variety of dishes. Pomegranate, a considerably exotic fruit to Westerners, is native to the region and used to add a sweet-and-sour flavor as a garnish to appetizers or fruit salads.

Beverages

Beverages are an essential part of any social gathering in Algeria. Coffee and tea are often served to houseguests and at various social outings. It is very common for people to leisurely congregate at coffee shops and drink strong Arabic coffee flavored with cardamom. Mint tea (*etzai*) is an extremely popular drink made with green tea, water, and fresh mint leaves. Both coffee and tea are served in a brass teapot, known as an *ibrik*. Alcohol is forbidden under Islamic law and is generally not consumed; however, the wine industry flourished under French influence, and wine is now a major export of Algeria. Thibarine and boukha are popular liquors made using figs.

Desserts

In Western cuisine, it is typical to serve dessert at the end of a meal, especially dinner; however, in Algeria desserts are saved for special occasions, holidays, and other celebrations. Pastries, such as *baklawa*, are often served during festivities. Stuffed dates are a popular dessert that is made by opening the date and adding ground nuts and sugar. Fruit, however, is readily available and eaten regularly.

TYPICAL DAY'S MENU

Breakfast (*fatour al-sabah*) often features coffee or tea. Eggs and cheese are often served at breakfast. Bread is served, and it is used to scoop portions of food. Porridge made of millet or chickpea flour is also typically served at breakfast. Fruit is also often served.

Lunch (*al-ghada*) is typically the biggest meal of the day. Salads and soups are often served as appetizers, along with bread. A rich and savory lamb or chicken *tagine* stew with vegetables is commonly served. A warm seasoned helping of couscous is typically served with the *tagine*, providing a major source of grain and carbohydrates to the meal. Dinner (*al-acha*) is usually a smaller meal. It could consist of bread and a few appetizers, such as soup or salad; otherwise a small meal, a poultry or fish dish without accompaniments, is typically eaten.

HOLIDAY MENUS

Food plays a central role in most holiday festivities. Religion is important to Algerians and central to holiday celebrations. Ramadan is the most holy month for Muslims and marks Allah giving the Qur'an (Muslim holy book) to the prophet Mohammed. During the month of Ramadan, Muslims abstain from eating and drinking anything (even water) from dawn until dusk. Many people wake up and eat a light breakfast before dawn. At sunset, the daily fast is broken usually with water and dates. Evening meals are large and families gather together to eat a variety of appetizers, bread, meal or poultry stews, and dessert. Coffee and tea may also be consumed. *Eid ul-Fitr* marks the end of Ramadan. This is a special holiday and people typically dress in their best clothing. In the morning, the community gathers to pray at the mosque. This is followed by various social gatherings. Families visit each other to rejoice, exchange gifts, reward children with money, gifts, and candy, and to feast on a delectable array of desserts.

For many Algerians, meat is an expensive delicacy and not prepared on a daily basis; however, during *Eid ul-Fitr*, typically a whole lamb or sheep is roasted for the entire family to share in a feast. Desserts, such as stuffed dates and *baklawa*, are prepared in mass quantities. *Khtayef* is a popular holiday dessert, made similar to a pancake, stuffed with walnuts, honey, sugar, and cinnamon, and folded. The holiday menu may typically include additional chicken stew dishes, olives, fresh fruits, dates, fresh baked flatbread or French loaf, and a variety of salads.

Another major religious holiday is *Eid ul-Adha*, the Feast of Sacrifice. This holiday marks the pilgrimage of Muslims to the holy city of Mecca, Saudi Arabia. Algerians also celebrate national and regional holidays. Algerians celebrate their independence on July 5. Labor day is celebrated November 1. Regional celebrations also take place in Algeria's fertile coastal lands. The harvest of dates, tomatoes, and cherries are all celebrated.

Observations from the Author (Samia Hamdan)

My experience with Algerian cuisine has given me a deep appreciation for preparing the country's national dish. I once gave couscous the same regard as I did rice. I thought of it as a simple grain that I could cook by just adding boiling water; however, its traditional preparation is actually much more intricate and sensual, and the final product reveals the delicateness and rich flavor for which this dish is known. In writing this chapter, I felt the best way to fully understand and appreciate the food was to take an Algerian cooking class. We were tasked with preparing an "Algerian couscous" dish that included root vegetables, lamb, and spices.

The couscous preparation was the most involved. We first soaked the grains with drops of water and then massaged them until each one soaked up the water. The couscous was then steamed for 20 minutes. This was followed by adding a whole stick of butter. To allow the butter to fully spread to each granule, we massaged the couscous with our hands for at least 5 minutes, allowing the butter to melt and spread. Then we steamed the couscous again, and mixed the grains around with our hands again. The couscous was steamed yet a third time before it was ready to be served. The final product was incredibly fluffy and flavorful. I have never tasted a more delectable couscous dish.

GENERAL HEALTH AND NUTRITIONAL INDICATORS SUMMARY

Although Algeria borders the Mediterranean Sea, there is a general shortage of fresh water supply. In addition, nutritional deficiencies, crowded living conditions, lack of proper sanitation, and little access to modern health care contribute to various infectious and chronic diseases.

Although Algerians generally eat a healthful diet, overnutrition and malnutrition are coexistent public health problems. Algeria is not immune to the obesity epidemic that is growing worldwide. The World Health Organization (2002a) estimates that almost half of Algerian women are overweight (using the body mass index measure of 25 kg/m² or greater). Over one third of men are overweight, and 15% of children under 5

years are overweight. While the protein and fat intake among Algerians has remained steady since 1979, daily caloric intake increased by over 300 calories per day according to the United Nations Food and Agricultural Organization (2004). On the other hand, malnutrition is still afflicting the nation's children. Over 20% of children in Algeria under 5 years are stunted in growth for their age, and 10% are underweight for their age. Because so little of Algeria's land is cultivatable, food must be imported to adequately feed its citizens. As the price of corn and wheat rise, the nation could face increasing challenges in securing food for its people.

COMMUNICATION AND COUNSELING TIPS

Traditional Algerian cooking is healthy and varied. Most of the cooking relies heavily on vegetables, legumes, and grains. Meat is expensive and typically considered a luxury. Olive oil, a beneficial monounsaturated fat, is a primary ingredient used in traditional Algerian cooking; however, as Western cooking influences the Algerian diet, more unhealthy fats, such as margarine and trans fat, find their way into Algerian cooking. In providing nutritional counseling, one may recommend reducing the amount of fat in cooking, opting to use olive oil rather than butter or margarine. Algerians who have migrated to western societies may find meat, such as beef and lamb, more readily available and more affordable. Heart disease is one of the major causes of death in some Western societies, and it is wise to recommend lower consumption of red meat, which tends to be high in saturated fat and cholesterol.

Effective counseling may also include encouraging the continued use of legumes, fruits, and vegetables, because they are rich in fiber, vitamins, minerals, and antioxidants. The 2005 Dietary Guidelines for Americans (United States Department of Health and Human Services, 2005) recommend consuming more variety and quantity of fruit and vegetables for a healthful diet. Pork and alcohol are forbidden by Islamic law, and these should be considered during counseling, because over 99% of Algerians are Muslims.

Physical activity is also important for a healthy lifestyle. In traditional Algerian society, women spend more time in the home cooking and caring for children. Encouraging activity in and outside the home is a great way to add more physical activity. Walking can be recommended as an activity outside the home. Adults should accrue an hour of activity each day.

PRIMARY LANGUAGE OF FOOD NAMES WITH ENGLISH AND PHONETIC TRANSLATION

The primary language of food names with English and phonetic translation is given in Table 29-1.

FEATURED RECIPE

There are many variations and preparation methods for Algerian couscous. Typically, seven vegetables are used in a stew.

TABLE 29-1 Primary Language of Food Names with English and Phonetic Translation

Arabic Transliteration	Phonetic Translation	English Translation	Arabic Transliteration	Phonetic Translation	English Translation
Seksou	Sik-su	Couscous	*Merquez*	Mer-kez	Spicy lamb sausage
Mechoui	Mesh-wee	Charcoal-roasted meat, typically lamb	*Chorba*	Shor-bah	Soup with meat or chicken and vegetables
Tagine	Ta-geen	Stew: clay pot to make stew	*Harrissa*	Har-eesa	Hot chili paste
Souk	Suuk	Marketplace with open stalls	*Khtayef*	Khi-tah-yif	Dessert made of flour, honey, nuts, sugar, and cinnamon
Smen	Smen	Fermented butter			

All food names are Arabic in Algerian dialect, which may be mixed with Berber and French.

Algerian Couscous with Lamb and Vegetables

For couscous:

1 lb. package couscous (non-instant)	1 tsp. rosewater
1 stick of unsalted butter	⅔ cup cold water
Salt to taste	

1. Pour unprepared couscous into large round shallow pan. Slowly stir in ⅔ cup of cold water. Couscous will clump. Rub couscous with clean hands to break up the clumps and drop back into the pan. Continue until all granules are separated and have soaked up all the water. Allow to sit until dry.
2. Place couscous in colander and steam for 20 minutes. Occasionally stir with a fork.
3. Place couscous back into pan and add stick of butter. Allow butter to melt. Rub couscous with hands throughout to allow grains to soak up butter.
4. Add rosewater and rub the grains with hands throughout.
5. Place couscous back in colander and steam for another 30 minutes. Occasionally fluff couscous with a fork.
6. Pour couscous onto a large wooden or earthenware dish.
7. Spoon vegetable and meat stew over the center of the couscous. Serve hot.

For vegetable and meat stew:

2 lbs. lamb shoulder, cut into chunks	1 eggplant, chopped
1 large onion	1 can chickpeas, drained
⅔ tsp. black pepper	2 tomatoes
⅔ tsp. red pepper	2 zucchini, chopped
⅔ tsp. cinnamon	¼ cup raisins
1 tsp. salt	1 tbsp. cilantro, chopped
1 tsp. saffron	
2 carrots, chopped	
2 turnips, chopped	

1. Place lamb chunks into large stockpot. Add the onion, black pepper, red pepper, saffron, cinnamon, and salt.
2. Add water until meat is covered. Heat until boiling. Cover and simmer for 45 minutes or until meat is brown.
3. Add carrots, turnips, zucchini, and eggplant. Simmer for another 20 minutes.
4. Add tomatoes, raisins, chickpeas, and chopped cilantro. Simmer for 15 minutes.
5. Use a slotted spoon to serve lamb and vegetables over a bed of couscous. Serve hot.

Courtesy of Elena Simanovskaya Fields

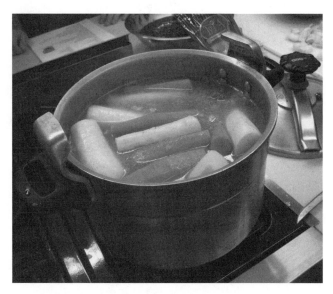

Algerian Couscous with Lamb and Vegetables (in preparation)

Courtesy of Elena Simanovskaya Fields

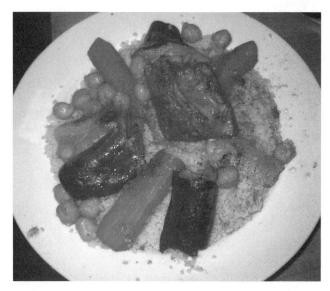

Algerian Couscous with Lamb and Vegetables (the finished dish)

Courtesy of Elena Simanovskaya Fields

Algerian Mint Tea

6 cups water

3 tbsp. loose green tea

Handful of mint sprigs

Sugar or honey to taste

1. Heat water until it boils.
2. Add green tea to a teapot. Add boiling water to teapot. Let tea steep for 3 minutes.
3. Add 2–3 fresh mint sprigs to teapot. Let tea steep for 2–3 minutes.
4. Pour tea into teacups and add mint leaf as a garnish. Add sugar or honey as desired.

More recipes are available at http://nutrition.jbpub.com/foodculture/

REFERENCES

Central Intelligence Agency. (2007). *Algeria.* Retrieved February 1, 2008, from https.cia.gov/library/publications/the-world-factbook/geos/g.html/

Hachten, H. (1970) *Best of regional African cooking.* New York: Hippocrene Books.

Mackley, L. (1998). *The book of North African cooking.* New York: Berkeley Publishing Group.

Magharebia. (2005). *Couscous: Long-term Maghreb staple still going strong.* Retrieved December 10, 2009, from http://www.magharebia.com/cocoon/awi/xhtml1/en_GB/features/awi/features/2005/01/11/feature-01/

Marks, C. (1994). *The great book of couscous.* New York: Donald I. Fine, Inc.

Menzel, P., & D'Aluisio, F. (2005). *Hungry planet: What the world eats.* Napa, CA: Material World Books.

United Nations Food and Agriculture Organization. (2004). *Algeria.* Retrieved March 20, 2008, from http://www.fao.org/countryprofiles/index.asp?lang=en&iso3=DZA&subj=4/

United States Department of Health and Human Services. (2005). *The dietary guidelines for Americans, 2005.* Retrieved February 11, 2008, from http://www.health.gov/DietaryGuidelines/dga2005/document/default.htm/

United States Department of State Bureau of Near Eastern Affairs. (2007). *Background note: Algeria.* Retrieved March 18, 2008, from http://www.state.gov/r/pa/ei/bgn/8005.htm/

United States Library of Congress. (1993). *Algeria.* Retrieved March 10, 2008, from http://lcwe2.loc.gov/cgi-bin/

Winget, M., & Chalbi, H. (2004) *Cooking the North African way.* Minneapolis, MN: Learner Publications Company.

World Health Organization. (2002a). *Algeria & overweight & obesity.* Retrieved March 30, 2008, from http://www.who.int/infobase/report.aspx?rid=114&iso=DZA&ind=BMI/

World Health Organization. (2002b). *Core health indicators: Algeria.* Retrieved March 30, 2008, from http://www.who.int/whosis/database/core/core_select.cfm/

Zadi, F. (2007). *Changes in Algerian and North African recipes over the last 30–40 years.* Retrieved March 1, 2008, from http://www.chefzadi.com/algerian_cookbook/index.html/

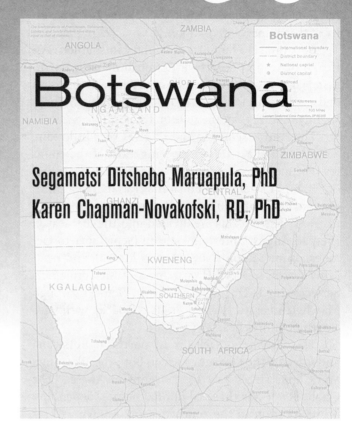

CHAPTER 30

Botswana

Segametsi Ditshebo Maruapula, PhD

Karen Chapman-Novakofski, RD, PhD

 CULTURE AND WORLD REGION

The people of the republic of Botswana are called Batswana, the singular of which is Motswana. Tswana is a tribe or ethnic group, although the word is also used as an adjective for the country (e.g., Tswana culture). Most people in Botswana are Tswana. The Tswana people themselves are comprised of about 8 tribes, although 20 or more tribes reside in Botswana. The four major urban areas are Gaborone, which is the capital, Francistown, Lobatse, and Selebi-Phikwe. With the Kalahari Desert occupying the west and central section of the country, it is easy to understand why most of the population lives in east.

All types of housing are available in Botswana, but the traditional *rondavel* is seen more frequently in rural and urban areas outside the main cities. With walls made of cow dung and mud and a thatched roof, the *rondavel*'s fireplace is the center of the one-room

dwelling. Extended families may spread over several *rondavels*. Within the cities and larger urban towns, many styles of architecture can be found, from colonial to modern and most everything in between.

One consistent aspect of daily life is the area chief, and the *kgotla* or community center. The *kgotla* is an open-air raised porch, often with a thatched roof, that provides a neutral locale for discussions and decisions. Although the political structure has changed, tribal chiefs continue to be consulted on nearly every aspect of life. Disputes are settled by the chief in the *kgotla*.

Health service delivery in Botswana is the primary responsibility of the state, although private health care is emerging. Botswana is divided into 23 health administration districts to serve the health needs of the population. In each health district, there is a district health team headed by a medical officer to provide health and educational services to residents of the district. Each district has either a district hospital or primary healthcare hospital to serve the health needs of the area. There is either a health post or clinic in each village. Patients are referred from health post to clinic to district hospital, and finally to one of the three referral hospitals in the country according to the severity of their illness or condition.

Botswana is a landlocked country in southern Africa. It shares its borders with Zimbabwe in the northeast, Namibia in the west, and South Africa in the south and east. With a total area of 585,000 km², Botswana is slightly smaller than the state of Texas.

The land is semiarid and receives very little rain, with the Kalahari Desert covering most of the country. The mean annual rainfall varies from a maximum of 650 mm in northern Botswana (Kasane) to a minimum of less than 250 mm in the central and southern districts. The seasons are divided into the dry season (May to August), pre-rainy season (September to October), rainy season (November to March), and postrainy season in April (Department of Meteorological Services, 2003). During the summer, October through March, temperatures are near 40°C (104°F), with winter temperatures near 26°C (79°F).

The Okavango Delta is in northern Botswana and is fed by the Okavango River. Both the Okavango and Chobe rivers have their origins in Angola. The Chobe River has three additional names, depending on its location in the country, being known as Linyanti when first entering Botswana from Angola, then Itenge, and finally Chobe/Linyanti Swamp. In the east the Hardveld consists of sandstone and granite and is bordered by the Shashe and Limpopo rivers. In the northwest the Tsodilo Hills form the basis for Drotsky's Caverns.

Botswana was previously known as the Bechuanaland Protectorate prior to being granted independence by Great Britain in 1966. The country is governed through a parliamentary system with the president as the head of state, and three arms of the government (legislature, judiciary, and executive branches). The country is divided into 15 districts with some additional subdivisions for ease of administration. Administration of cities and towns is by clerks, whereas council secretaries head the district councils. Each district has a commissioner who represents the central government (Government of Botswana, 2008).

The primary export is diamonds, which contribute about 80% of the country's revenue. Although the cattle industry has many more people employed, the economic contribution is still a distant second to the diamond industry.

LANGUAGE

The two official languages of Botswana are Setswana and English, but about 20 more languages and even more dialects are spoken by the different tribes. These languages, which include Ikalanga, Sekgalagadi, Seyei, Sembukushu, Sesobea, and Seherero, and many Sesarwa dialects, are spoken in northeastern, northern, and western Botswana.

CULTURE HISTORY

The Khoisan are believed to be the first inhabitants of Botswana. There is evidence of their existence dating from 17,000 BC to 1650 AD. The Khoisan obtained their food from hunting and gathering, and moved from place to place in small groups in search of the food commodities in the northern part of the country, especially around the lakes. By 100 BC, they had begun herding cattle, a practice adopted from East Africa (Parsons, 1999).

During 1200–1400, Tswana dynasties came into being, especially the Tswana dynasty that included several tribes (Hurutshe, Kwena, and Kgatla). These tribes displaced others, such as the Khalahari and the Yeyi, that they found in the area during the 1700s. The Tswana states included the Ngwaketse chiefdom, the Kwena, the Ngwato, and the Tawana. These kingdoms, however, were also attacked by other tribes during the Difaqane wars. After the wars, the Ngwaketse, Kwena, Ngwato, and Ngwato (Tawana) were strengthened again. The country became known as the Bechuanaland Protectorate, under British rule, so that the British could keep a pathway open to northern lands to ensure the expansion of the British Empire. The protectorate was the predecessor to modern Botswana (Parsons, 1999).

FOOD HISTORY WITHIN THE CULTURE

Although the staples in the Setswana diet have remained, their processing and use has changed. Batswana initially processed their grains by hand grinding the cereals on a big stone (*lelwala*) using a small stone, and then moved to hand stamping the cereals in a mortar using a pestle. Currently, grain-milling companies exist in many villages, which enables villagers to take their grain for milling. Some of the milling companies are big commercial ventures that mill the grain and sell it to food chains.

Food-preparation methods have also changed. Many traditional dishes have become extinct; for example, boiled sorghum grain (*lohata*) and sorghum boiled from the husk. A lot of young Batswana are not aware of the many fiber-rich traditional foods, because these have been replaced by processed foods such as rice and pastas. Currently, there is a move to revive the traditional Tswana diet, which was high in fiber, through hosting of events such as *letlhafula*, where traditional foods are showcased, traditional food-recipe competitions, and others. Food-preparation methods have also changed at funerals. Whereas food cooked at funerals used to have no salt added, today's funeral food has salt and other spices.

Another change that has occurred is the preservation of leftovers. Traditionally, leftover foods were mixed with water and fermented to make *motsena*, which could be eaten as a breakfast food or a snack for the children sent outside the home to look after the cows and goats. Leftover bread was dried (*dikwakwala*) and stored for later use.

Botswana used to have a lot of food taboos, but only occasionally are such taboos observed today. Traditionally, children were expected to not eat certain foods; for example, girls were not supposed to eat meat from birds but boys were expected to eat such meat. Pregnancy was also associated with food taboos; for example, a pregnant woman could not drink fresh milk. Other taboos were associated with the types of meat different genders could or could not eat. At wedding celebrations, it is still common for men alone to consume the *mokoto* meat dish (made by cooking different meats including organ meats) to the exclusion of women (Grivetti, 1976).

 MAJOR FOODS

The most widely consumed food items are tea, sorghum, and maize meal (Maruapula & Chapman-Novakofski, 2006); use of millet has greatly diminished. Different sorghum and maize varieties are consumed in a Tswana diet and may vary from region to region. Traditional vegetables and fruits are seasonal and occur in abundance after the rainy season (and are less common during the dry season). Meat and milk, two delicacies, are other food items consumed by Batswana.

 Protein Sources

Batswana consume various protein sources, which include meats, poultry, milk and other dairy products, worms, and legumes. The primary sources of protein are legumes, often mixed together with starches, such as *samp* (cracked maize) and sorghum. Recently, soy has been introduced into the diet as soy milk or cereal mixtures, but it is consumed by primary school students as part of the school feeding program and some religious sects. Common legumes include beans (*dinawa*), bambara nuts (*ditloo*), and lentils (*letlhodi*). Legumes can be boiled and eaten on their own or mixed with sorghum, maize, and groundnuts. Legumes can also be boiled and eaten while still in their pods.

Meat consumption seems to be low, because only 29% of households consumed meat at least once a day according to the National Micronutrient Survey of 1996 (Maruapula & Chapman-Novakofski, 2006). Furthermore, another study by Maruapula and Chapman-Novakofski (2007) revealed, for many ethnic groups in Botswana, meat consumption to be below the two to three servings per day recommended by U.S. Dietary Guidelines (U.S. Department of Health and Human Services, 2005).

Beef, however, is a national favorite, because cattle are the predominant livestock in Botswana. Beef is cooked many ways, including *seswaa* or *chotlho*, a preferred meat dish made of shredded or pounded beef cooked for special occasions such as weddings and funerals. The beef is cut into pieces and cooked until it is very tender. At the tender stage, the bones are removed and the meat is stirred with a large wooden spoon, and the gravy that was removed earlier is put back into the pot to make the meat juicy. Goat meat is second to beef, followed by mutton, and pork is consumed by a small percentage of people. Beef, goat, chicken, and lamb are ingredients in many favorite recipes both at home and in restaurants.

Serobe is yet another meat dish made from the stomach (*mogodu*), intestines (*mala*), and other organs such as kidneys, heart, and liver. These ingredients are cut into pieces and boiled together. After cooking, they are shredded into very small pieces. *Serobe* can be eaten with sorghum or maize stiff porridge, or with bread. Chicken is also eaten and is often cooked boiled, fried, or as a stew. Guinea fowl (*lesogo*) and other wild birds are no longer commonly eaten. Game meat from various types of animals is also not commonly eaten except in parts of the country with game reserves. (Many hotels in areas near game reserves serve game meat.)

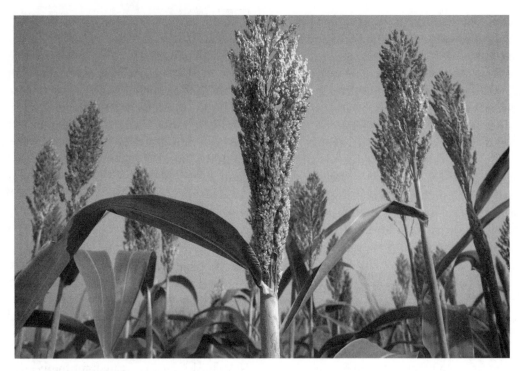

Sorghum is a staple in Botswana.

Biltong (*segwapa*) is dried beef, which is a result of the traditional method of preserving meat. Batswana did not have refrigeration facilities; hence, to preserve large amounts of meat, the meat was cut into strips and sun-dried. The dried meat would then be cut into pieces or pounded and boiled and served with sorghum and maize-meal hard porridge or samp. When cooking the biltong, ingredients such as tomatoes, potatoes, and onions enhance the taste. When pounded groundnuts are added to the biltong, this is referred to as *segwapa dobi*, a dish that is common in northern Botswana. Another method of preserving meat used mainly in the Kgatleng district is to cut it into small pieces, boil it, and then dry it for later use. The meat is called *kuhnwa*.

Phane from mopane worm (caterpillar) is a common protein source especially in northeastern Botswana. It is harvested from the mopane tree by women and children and is eaten fresh or dried. *Phane* can be boiled, fried, or stewed. It is common to see women and children along the highway that links southern and northern Botswana selling this delicious and nutritious caterpillar.

Madila (sour milk) is also a common food item, made from fermenting fresh milk. It can be consumed on its own or served with the different types of porridges, and some melons and squashes.

 Starch Sources

Starch sources in Botswana include sorghum, maize, bread, mealie-rice, and millet. Foods such as rice and different types of pasta have been adopted as part of the diet especially in urban and semi-urban areas. Sorghum meal and maize meal are diet staples that are often made into thin porridges (*motogo*) or stiff porridges (*bogobe*). The boiling water/starch mixture is then cooked slowly over low heat until the desired consistency is reached. Fresh milk, sour milk, or fruit (melon) may be added.

Fermented soft or stiff sorghum meal porridges (*motogo* or *bogobe jwa ting*) are common in southern Botswana. *Ting* is a culture made by mixing a small amount of mealie meal with warm water and allowing it to ferment for a few days. The culture is then used to provide the sour taste when cooking the soft or stiff porridge.

Sorghum mealie meal can be cooked with fruits and, in particular, melon, which gives the dish its characteristic flavor. This dish has become common at wedding celebrations. Sorghum can also be cooked with milk, a dish called *logala*. Some traditional methods of cooking sorghum are no longer common. For example, the nonmilled sorghum grain could be boiled alone (*lohata*) or mixed with beans and oil and salt added to taste, and the dish could be served with milk. Also, the grain could be partially milled and cooked alone or with beans and served with milk. Partially milled sorghum is used in place of rice in stews by some creative people.

Maize can be boiled or roasted and eaten as a snack. Roasted or boiled maize is common and sold when farm products are harvested in spring (*letlhafula*). Sweet reed is another commercialized food item found in markets during spring. It is similar to sugar cane, except that it is much thinner and sweeter.

Bread has become more prominent in the diet in the past decade. Yeast-type breads can be purchased in groceries or bakeries in urban areas. Homemade breads include *matlebekwane* (steamed bread or dumplings), *diphaphatha* (flat cakes) and *magwinya* (fat cakes), and *mapakiwa* (buns).

 ## Fat Sources

Traditional fat sources came from meat and milk. The peritoneum of the slaughtered animal (caul of fat or *lomipi*) has always been a good source of fat for Batswana, who use the fat to fry meat and flavor vegetables, samp, and other items. Some tribes made butter from milk (*room*) and used the butter as a fat source. Melon seeds and peanuts, which were eaten as snacks or used as flavorings in vegetables and meats, were also

good sources of fat; however, the vegetable oil (cooking oil), margarines, and spreads available in grocery stores have replaced the traditional *lomipi* and *room* as the fat sources in Botswana today. Many poor households with malnourished children are provided with cooking oil as part of their food basket by the government in attempts to increase body weight.

 ## Prominent Vegetables

Prominent vegetables in Botswana include the traditional types that are usually gathered from the wild fields or in plowing fields, and those bought from commercial enterprises such as street vendors or grocery stores. Various plant leaves (*morogo*) are eaten, and they include bean leaves (*Vigna unguiculata: morogo wa dinawa*) and pumpkin leaves (*lebobola*), as well as wild vegetables such as *rothwe*, *thepe* (*Amaranthus thunbergii*), and *delele* (similar to okra). Bean and pumpkin leaves can be boiled and spiced with salt and flavored with a little oil to be eaten with the various types of sorghum and maize porridges. Many of the traditional vegetables are available only during the wet seasons and therefore are preserved by sun-drying for later use. The dried vegetables are later reconstituted with water, and oil, spices, and any nondried vegetables are added, and the mixture is boiled to make the vegetable gravy.

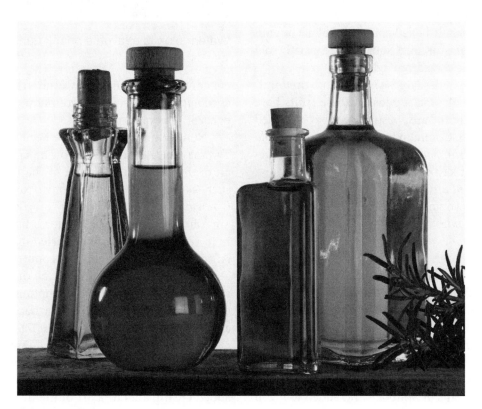

Cooking Oil

In northern Botswana it is common to cook bean or pumpkin leaves with pounded groundnuts or melon seeds (*morogo wa dobi*). Pumpkins are also grown in the country and common during the harvest season. Dried seeds from pumpkins and melons can be roasted and eaten as snacks or pounded and added as a flavoring to vegetables. Spinach, onions, carrots, tomatoes, and cabbage and squash (*makgomane magashu* or *maraka*) are the modern vegetables that are often available, especially in urban areas, and eaten with sorghum or maize-meal porridges. "Gravy" can mean a boiled vegetable mixture rather than the meat-based type of gravy common in the Western world.

 ### Prominent Fruits

Many varieties of melons are available; some are cultivated and others grow wild. Melons that are grown include watermelon and wild melon (*lerotse* or *lekatane*). Watermelon (*legapu*) is a national favorite during spring (*letlhafula*) and is eaten as a snack. The fruit is sold in markets or by street vendors during *letlhafula* and in grocery stores in urban areas. Many people eat watermelon as a dessert. The wild melon can be boiled and eaten with or without milk, cooked with sorghum, or used as a flavoring in vegetables. Batswana make jam from both the watermelon and the ordinary melon. *Makgomane* (squashes) are also another traditional fruit, which are usually boiled and served alone or with either fresh milk or sour milk. Squashes are usually sold in markets and are considered a delicacy.

Wild-fruit varieties are seasonal and predominantly consumed as snacks. Most of these fruits have nuts or shells inside and are not suitable to be consumed by young children. Common fruit varieties are *morula* (*Sclerocarya caffra*), *moretlwa* (*Grewia flava*), *mogorogorwana* (Monkey orange: *Strychnos cocculoides*), *milo* (*Vangueria infausta*), *mokgomphatha* (*Grewia flavescens*), *morojwa* (*Azanza garckeana*), *mogorogorwane* (*Strychnos cocculoides*), *meretologa* (*Zemina spp.*), and *mongongo* (*Ricinodendron rautanenii*). *Mongongo* is a large wild fruit found in the Kalaharai Desert, and like many Botswana fruits, it has an edible part and a kernel that is rich in fat and proteins and is an important component of the !Kung San group in Botswana (Nerd, Aronson & Mizrahi, 1990). Another versatile fruit is the *morula*, which can be used to produce juice, jam, and beer. The *morula* kernel can also be cracked to produce a tasty protein- and oil-rich nut that can be cooked with beans or pounded and added to green vegetables as a flavoring, and to improve their nutri-

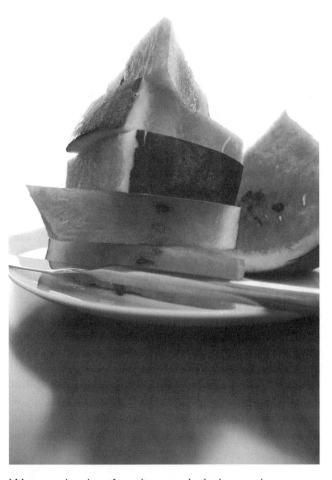

Watermelon is a favorite snack during spring.

ent content. There are many other fruit varieties, such as *mopipi* and *mopenoeng*, commonly eaten in various parts of Botswana.

Nontraditional fruits have been adopted into the Tswana diet. A child will know an apple, a banana, or an orange better than some of the indigenous fruits such as *moretlwa* (*Grewia flava*) or *mokgomphatha* (*Grewia flavescens*). A variety of Western-type fruits are found in many grocery stores but predominantly in towns. Such fruits are imported mainly from South Africa and other neighboring countries, and have become an important feature of the diet. A few limited studies have shown fruit consumption to be low among certain groups of Batswana (Maruapula, 1996; Maruapula & Chapman-Novakoski, 2007).

Another item in the modern Tswana diet is fruit salad, which can include apples, pineapples, raisins, and others. Fruit salads are consumed alone or with added cream, and are part of the menu for many restaurants and for people who can afford it.

Spices and Seasonings

Salt and white pepper are the typical spices. In addition, *morula* nuts, melon, sweet melon, and pumpkin seeds are used to flavor many vegetable, bean, grain, and meat dishes. Recently, however, many spices, such as curries, chili pepper, aroma salt, and others, have been adopted from Indian and other cuisines. Beef and chicken curry stews have become a common dish at many celebrations.

Beverages

Black tea is the most widely consumed beverage after water in Botswana according to some surveys (Maruapula, 1996; Maruapula & Chapman-Novakofski, 2007). Tea has become a social drink that is offered to visitors in most households. Tea is usually consumed by adults and used to be drunk with fresh milk from goats and cows, but ultra-temperature (highly pasteurized) milk or powdered milk has replaced fresh milk. Fresh milk obtained from the family's *kraal* of goats and cows is another beverage that used to be available for children in many households. For many households today, however, the family *kraal* has disappeared and has been replaced by the supermarket, the quick-service shop of a filling station, or the convenience store in the village as the source of milk. Consequently, many children believe that the store is the source of milk, not the goat or cow. Goat's milk was usually boiled before drinking and cow's milk was consumed straight from the cow.

Botswana also has a number of herbal and medicinal teas, including *mosukujane* (mint tea), *kgomodimetsig* (another mint tea), *galalatshwene* (from a plant that smells like lavender), *mokwalane* (from *mokolwane* fruit), and *sengaparile* (*Herpagophytum procumbens* or African penicillin or devil's claws). A newer product in the beverage category is *motlopi* coffee, made from *motlopi* root. This coffee is produced by a group of women in the Kgalagadi district who sell it to improve their livelihoods. All these teas and coffee are believed to have medicinal powers. Another beverage that is no longer common is made from boiling melons and saving the juice part and drinking it either warm or cold (Government of Botswana, 2008).

In addition to tea and milk, Botswana has a wide range of fermented beverages obtained from grown plants and wild plants. Sorghum beer (*bojalwa jwa setswana*) is a popular beverage among adults. The beer that is culturally prepared by women in the Tswana

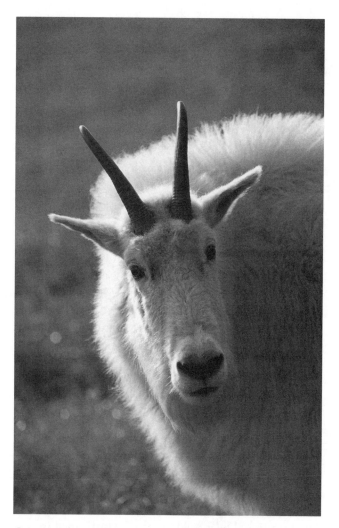

Goat milk is often boiled before drinking.

homestead has also been commercialized as Chibuku and is sold in big trucks all over the country. Some traditional beers mimic the hard liquors that are sold in commercial markets, and a common type is *khadi*, which is prepared from various ingredients depending on the location. One type is made from *greweria* berries (*mogwana*). In addition to being a social drink, the traditional beer has been brewed for sale by many Batswana women. Such beer sales have been used to supplement the family's income and put food on the table, and were used to pay school fees for children prior to the time when schooling was free. Other beers are made from fruit trees such as *moretlwa* and *morula*. *Morula* juice is another beverage that used to be common in spring (*letlhafula*), and this has also been turned into a commercial product.

Ginger beer is a nontraditional beverage that has taken the country by storm and is a favorite at weddings and funerals. It is made from ground ginger

(*Zingiber officinale*) that is mixed with water, brown sugar, malt, and some fruits, such as apples and pineapples, which are all fermented. This product has also been commercialized and even patented, and is sold in stores throughout the country.

There are many commercialized drinks on the market today and they include the "fizzy drinks" such as the many sodas found in supermarkets, yogurt drinks, *mageu* (a fermented maize-meal drink), as well as bottled water.

 ## Desserts

Desserts are not common in a traditional Tswana diet, but are instead a Western influence. A typical Setswana household does not serve dessert but only a meal and a beverage (usually tea or water). Most restaurants and some affluent households do serve dessert as part of the menu. Also, desserts are a common feature at wedding celebrations, and custard, jelly, and trifle are the favorites. Watermelons, which used to be eaten as snacks in a Setswana diet, have now become a part of the dessert menu. In fact, some people seem to equate a good wedding celebration with whether they are served dessert.

 ## FOODS WITH CULTURAL SIGNIFICANCE

The traditional beer holds a lot of significance in Setswana culture. Beer from new sorghum (*molomo*) is taken to the *kgotla* (traditional meeting place) after the harvest (*thobo*). It is also part of the proceedings during *dikgafela*, when grains are taken to the chief to fill his supply. The grains are used to ensure food for the visitors in the community and for members of the community who are unable to fend for themselves. Traditional beer is also important at wedding celebrations and funerals.

Another common food at weddings and funerals is *seswaa* (shredded/pounded beef), which is a cultural icon. *Segwapa* (biltong) is also a national favorite and is in fact served in the national airline as a snack to local and international passengers. *Dikgobe* (samp and beans) is also a common feature at the celebrations of marriage and death. It is one of the two starches, in addition to sorghum, that make up the accepted menu at funerals. Ginger beer is also the flagship beverage of weddings and funerals, because it is an inexpensive beverage to make and is enjoyed by the many guests at such occasions.

 ## TYPICAL DAY'S MENU

A typical day's menu includes three meals: the morning meal (*sefitlholo*), mid-day meal, and the evening meal (*selalelo*). The morning meal usually comprises a sorghum soft porridge, bread, and tea or coffee. The soft porridge may be served with fresh or sour milk, or with sugar. Sometimes this meal may be just tea for poor families. The mid-day meal is usually larger than the morning meal and includes a starch component such as sorghum, millet, or maize stiff porridge, a vegetable (*morogo* relish), and meat. The starch component may also be samp (*dikgobe*) or beans, or one of the newly introduced carbohydrates such as rice, pasta, and others. Salads also may be served. In many towns and villages, it is now common to eat this meal from street vendors and restaurants, and many grocery stores also sell cooked food. The evening meal is also light like the morning meal. It may consist of sorghum soft porridge or leftovers from the mid-day meal. Bread and a beverage may also be consumed as the evening meal.

 ## HOLIDAY MEALS

Batswana used to have important celebrations such as *letsema*, a festival when the chief initiated the plowing season, *letlhafula*, a festival to signify the end of harvest; and *dikgafela*, a festival when community members took a part of their produce to the chief. Due to the interactions with other cultures, however, Batswana have started to celebrate holidays such as Christmas, New Year's Day, and Easter. The typical Christmas menu is rice, served with beef (or sometimes chicken), vegetables, some salads, and dessert.

 ## HEALTH BELIEFS AND CONCERNS

Many Batswana believe in both traditional and modern medicine. In traditional medicine, there are several types of practitioners, such as *dingaka* (traditional doctors) and spiritual healers. *Dingaka* might "throw bones" to determine the problem and give potions to alleviate it, or they might be told of the problem and use herbs for healing it. The doctor who throws bones to determine the problem might also give the client medicine to protect him- or herself from all sorts of ills, including bewitchment. The traditional healer (male or female) learns his or her craft from another healer, especially his or her parent. Spiritual healers use the Christian Bible (and particularly water that has been blessed) to heal people, and also ashes from burnt bones (*sewasho*). Some Batswana believe that they can be bewitched, and that all illness is due to witchcraft; hence, the need to protect themselves using the traditional doctors.

Despite the faith in traditional medicine, most Batswana also use modern doctors and would visit a health facility if they were ill. There are others who use only modern medicine or use only traditional medicine. (Barbee, 1986).

GENERAL HEALTH AND NUTRITIONAL INDICATORS SUMMARY

According to UNICEF (2007), 10% of Batswana infants were in low-birth-weight categories from 1998 to 2005, a rate similar to that of many other poor countries such as Barbados, Bulgaria, Guatemala, Kenya, and Qatar; however, this was still considered near the mean in terms of the world. Thirty-four percent of infants are exclusively breastfed for the first 6 months of life in Botswana, with only 62% receiving vitamin A supplementation. Only 66% of the population consumes iodized salt. Underweight, for children under 5 years, in the moderate to severe category is 23% (UNICEF, 2007). The life expectancy of a Botswana citizen is now 35 years due to the AIDS epidemic. This rate has fallen by 29 years since 1990, when life expectancy was 64 years.

COMMUNICATION AND COUNSELING TIPS

Counseling the Batswana in the area of food and nutrition is still relatively new and in the process of development; thus, many "dos" and "don'ts" have not been developed fully. Traditionally, one of the "don'ts" might be not to look an adult in the eye when talking to him or her, because this is perceived as being disrespectful. Batswana also have totems in the form of animals that signify the tribe to which they belong, and it may not be culturally proper to offer a person a food item that is part of his or her totem. Some Batswana believe in sorcery, and therefore, explaining a diet-related cause of a disease might take longer to assimilate, because the person might believe that he or she is bewitched.

PRIMARY LANGUAGE OF FOOD NAMES WITH ENGLISH TRANSLATION

The primary language of food names with English translation is as follows:

Food Names	English Translation
Bogobe jwa Mabele	Sorghum hard porridge
Motogo wa mabele	Sorghum soft porridge
Dikgobe	Samp and beans
Setampa	Samp from maize
Ting	Fermented sorghum
Legapu	Watermelon
Lerotse/lekatane	Melon
Seswaa	Pounded beef/ shredded beef
Segwapa	Biltong
Mageu	Fermented maize drink
Roi bos	Bush tea/red tea
Longana/galalatshwene	Herbal tea
Madila/maheri	Sour milk
Mandombi/matlebekwane	Dumplings
Raese	Rice

FEATURED RECIPE

Bean Leaves Vegetable

2 cups water
½ cup dried bean leaves
1 tbsp. vegetable oil
1 tbsp. peanut butter or pounded peanuts

1. Mix water and the dried bean leaves, boil together.
2. Add the oil and salt to taste.
3. Add the peanut butter or pounded nuts after the bean leaves are cooked.
4. Serve with sorghum or maize stiff porridge.

More recipes are available at http://nutrition.jbpub.com/foodculture/

REFERENCES

Barbee, E.L. (1986). Biomedical resistance to ethnomedicine in Botswana. *Social Science Medicine, 22*(1), 75–80.

Department of Meteorological Services. (2003). *Botswana's climate.* Retrieved August 31, 2008, from http://www.weather.info.bw/

Government of Botswana. (2008). *Republic of Botswana.* Retrieved August 31, 2008, from http://www.gov.bw/

Grivetti, L.E. (1976). *Dietary resources and social aspects of food use in a tswana tribe.* PhD Dissertation. Department of Geography, University of California at Davis.

Maruapula, S.D. (Ed.). (1996). *Micronutrient malnutrition in Botswana.* Food and Nutrition Unit, Family Health Division, Ministry of Health. Gaborone, Botswana: Government Printers.

Maruapula, S.D., & Chapman-Novakofski, K. (2006). Poor intake of milk, vegetables, and fruit with limited dietary variety by Botswana's elderly. *Journal of Nutrition for the Elderly, 25*(3/4), 61–72.

Maruapula, S.D., & Chapman-Novakofski, K. (2007). Health and dietary patterns of elderly Batswana. *Journal of Nutrition Education and Behavior, 39*(6), 311–319.

Nerd, A., Aronson, J.A., & Mizrahi, Y. (1990). Introduction and domestication of rare and wild fruit and nut trees for desert areas. In J. Janick & J.E. Simon (Eds.), *Advances in new crops* (pp. 355–363). Portland, OR: Timber Press.

Parsons, N. (1999). *Botswana history pages.* Retrieved August 31, 2008, from http://www.thuto.org/ubh/bw/bhpindex.htm/

UNICEF. (2007). *The state of the world's children 2007: Women and children, the double dividend of gender equality.* Retrieved April 14, 2009, from http://www.unicef.org/sowc07/statistics/tables.php

U.S. Department of Health and Human Services. (2005). *Dietary guidelines for Americans, 2005* (6th ed.). Washington, DC: U.S. Government Printing Office.

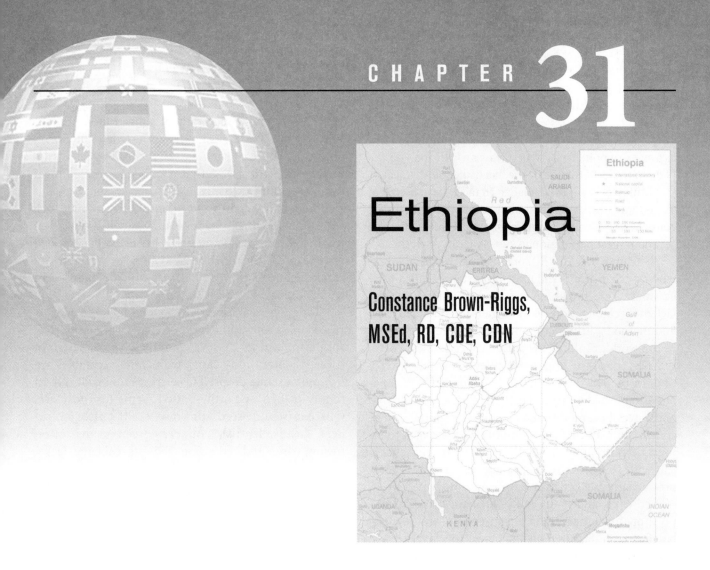

CHAPTER 31

Ethiopia

Constance Brown-Riggs, MSEd, RD, CDE, CDN

 CULTURE AND WORLD REGION

Africa is a land of great contrast and diversity. There are several hundred ethnic groups throughout Africa, each with their own religion, attitudes, beliefs, practices, and way of life. Ethiopia, located on the Horn of Africa, is no exception, with high mountains and great plateaus, 2000–3000 m above sea level, to grasslands, jungles, and deserts. There are seven major ethnic groups in Ethiopia: Oromo, Amara, Tigraway, Somalie, Guragie, Sidama, and Welaita.

Most traditional African religions are based on the belief of a supreme god, and that spirits of dead ancestors can intercede with prayer request. Prayers and sacrifices are offered for good health and fertile land. Religious ceremonies are also conducted to commemorate a person's passage from childhood to adulthood.

Islam is practiced by one third of Ethiopians. Sixty percent of Ethiopians are Christians who belong to Orthodox or Protestant churches. A growing number of Africans are combining the religious practices and beliefs of Islam or Christianity with traditional African practices. Their churches are called syncretic African churches.

Historically, Islamic tradition has permitted the practices of polygyny and arranged marriage. The bride's family was required to give a dowry to the bridegroom. Polygyny continues in Ethiopia today; however, dowries and arranged marriages are less common.

Households in Africa are made up of extended family, which provides security, financial assistance, and social life. Women in rural areas traditionally stay home to care for the family. Forty percent of Ethiopian households are headed by women. The first rains of the growing season, the planting of crops and the harvest, births, marriages, funerals, and curing of the sick are celebrated in community ceremonies. These community gatherings strengthen family ties and religious beliefs.

Hospitality is a hallmark of Africa, with traditional meals served on a communal platter in the center of a large table, and fingers used to scoop up the food. A jug or dish of water is passed around to enable family and guests to wash their hands before eating. Traditionally, as a show of politeness, a guest leaves a little food on the plate to indicate that he or she has had enough to eat.

Ethiopia is slightly smaller than twice the size of Texas, and ranks 34th in size compared with other countries. With over 70 million people, Ethiopia has the second largest population in sub-Saharan Africa.

The majority of Ethiopians live in rural areas where agriculture is the most important sector of the economy. Traditional farming predominates due to the lack of mechanization. Most farmers use outdated tools and methods. Ethiopia is one of the poorest countries in the world, ranking 169 out of 174 countries. Forty-five percent of the population lives below the poverty line. In the late 1400s and early 1500s, after Europeans established trading posts in Africa, gold, ivory, and slaves became the most valuable exports. Today, coffee is most critical to Ethiopia with exports totaling $350 million in 2006. Other exports include chat (a leaf with psychoactive properties), leather and leather products, pulses, gold, livestock and processed meat, oilseed cake, and fruits and vegetables. Principal imports are machinery and transport equipment, miscellaneous manufactured goods, petroleum, natural gas, and durable and nondurable consumer goods, as well as medical and pharmaceutical products.

LANGUAGE

Ethiopia has nearly 80 languages and approximately 200 dialects. Amharic, English, and Tigrigna are the national languages.

CULTURE HISTORY

The ancestors of all humanity are thought to have evolved in the fertile plains of the Nile Valley in Africa. Most scientists believe that the earliest *Homo sapiens* were hunters and gatherers who lived in Africa about 2 million years ago. Many centuries later, agriculture became the primary means of obtaining food. Coffee, *noog* (an oil plant), *ensete* (a banana-like plant), millet, sorghum, and *teff* (a type of grain) were cultivated in Ethiopia.

FOOD HISTORY WITHIN THE CULTURE

The earliest known centrally organized food-production system was established along the Nile 15,000 years ago. Agriculture continues to be the leading economic activity in Africa. The first starches for agricultural purposes came into use in 5000 BC, when sorghum and rice were cultivated in the Sahel region. In 4000 BC, the climate of the Sahara became much drier, causing increased desertification of the area. The climate change forced the inhabitants to move to West Africa's tropical climate. By 3000 BC, yams and oil palms were being cultivated in West Africa.

Today, African crops are divided into two categories: staple crops and export crops. Corn, millet, rice, sorghum, wheat, cassava, potatoes, yams, legumes (peas, peanuts, and beans), fruits, and vegetables are Ethiopia's staple crops. These crops are produced on family-owned or family-rented farms for local use. Oilseeds (sesame seed, sunflower seed), pulses (chickpeas, beans, lentils), potatoes, green beans, okra, melon, white and red onion, shallots, cabbage, leeks, beetroot, carrots, green chili, tomatoes, and lettuce are the main export vegetables. Orange, mandarin grapefruit, mango, guava, lemon, and lime are major export fruits.

Livestock are also part of the agricultural economy in Ethiopia, which has the largest livestock population in Africa. Ethiopia is estimated to have 27 million cattle, 24 million sheep, and 18 million goats.

MAJOR FOODS

Good eating in Africa is based on simple preparation that makes the most of what is available. For that reason many people think of African food as "poor man's food": simple stews, grilled meats, fish, steamed vegetables, side dishes, and an assortment of breads. *Wat*, which means stew, is a traditional Ethiopian dish prepared with chicken (*doro*) or beef (*sik sik*). Ethiopia is the only country in African never to be colonized by a foreign power; therefore, the food in Ethiopia is uniquely Ethiopian, characterized by chilies and spices that are used to flavor dishes. *Injera*, traditional Ethiopian bread, is made from *teff*. It has a spongy texture with a slightly sour taste and is served at every meal.

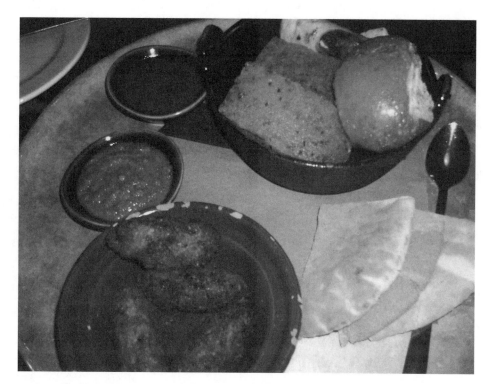

Akara Shrimp Fritters, Mealie, Honey, and Pita Bread
Courtesy of the author

 Protein Sources

Cattle, sheep, chicken, and goat are common sources of protein in Ethiopia, although meals tend to be light on meat, heavy on starch, and laden with fat. Beef is usually reserved for holidays and special occasions. Pork is generally forbidden because most Ethiopians are either Muslim or Orthodox Christian. Eggs are used mainly for sale and chickens are killed for feast. In East Africa beef, goat, chicken, and sheep are available sources of protein, although, as on much of the continent, meat is eaten sparingly. Fish is available in the lakes but is not considered a staple of the Ethiopian diet.

Black-eyed peas or pigeon peas, chickpeas, cowpeas, beans, legumes, lentils, and groundnuts (peanuts) are primary sources of protein. The most common in Ethiopia are chickpeas, field peas, lentils, and broad beans. Legumes are sometimes toasted whole and eaten as a snack with coffee.

Most meats are very tough and therefore require slow-cooking techniques such as stewing or braising.

 Starch Sources

Starch is the foundation of the African diet resulting in a high-fiber, high-carbohydrate intake. Potatoes, sweet potato, maize (corn) meal, and *teff* are staples of East Africa. Maize is the foundation of many dishes throughout Africa. The names may be different, but the basic ingredient, maize, remains the same. Mealie pap is common in southern Africa, *ugali* in East Africa, and *fufu* in West Africa. *Ugali* and *fufu* can also be made from manioc, sorghum, millet, wheat, rice, plantain, green bananas, and yams. *Injera*, bread, is a staple of Ethiopia.

 Fat Sources

Most fat used in African cooking is made from vegetables, seeds, or coconut. Ethiopians use a flavored clarified butter called *niter kebbeh*. Onions, garlic, ginger, and spices give *niter kebbeh* its unique flavor.

 Prominent Vegetables

Green leafy vegetables are plentiful in every country in Africa. Collard greens, mustard greens, bush greens, spinach, cress, pumpkin leaves, and cassava leaves are among the many varieties. Kale is the primary leafy green vegetable in Ethiopia. It is inexpensive and available most of the year. Green vegetables are traditionally steamed or boiled with spices, onions, and tomatoes.

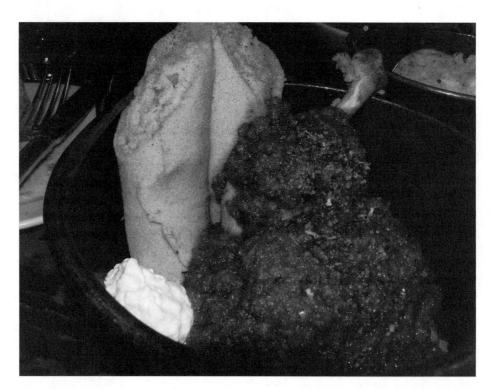

Doro Wat, a spicy chicken stew, served with cottage cheese and *injera* bread.
Courtesy of the author

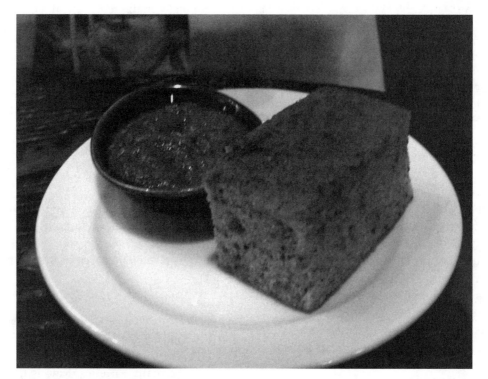

Mealie bread made from dry field corn accompanied with shrimp chili dip.
Courtesy of the author

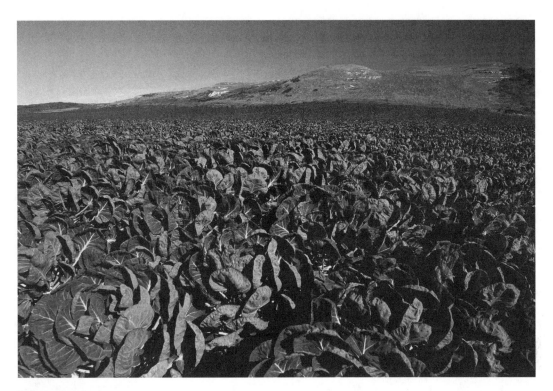

Fresh Spinach
Courtesy of the author

Traditional greens provide a rich source of vitamins and minerals to the African diet.

Other popular vegetables include green beans, okra, melon, white and red onion, shallots, cabbage, leeks, beetroot, carrots, green chili, tomatoes, and lettuce. Vegetables are also served in soups and sauces.

 Prominent Fruits

Fruits are eaten on a seasonal basis throughout Africa. They are also used as sauces or served as *sambals* (spicy chili-based condiments). Typical fruits available in Ethiopia include banana, oranges, pawpaw, mandarin grapefruit, mango, guava, lemon, and lime. The availability of fruit is limited in the central highlands.

 Spices and Seasonings

African food is rich in flavor as a result of a large variety of spices and seasonings. Chilies, ground sesame seeds, melon seeds, and cotton seeds, as well as fresh and dry mushrooms are found in various spice blends. Cumin, caraway, clove, cinnamon, ginger, nutmeg, and saffron are also commonly used. *Berbere* is a common spice blend that is used in many Ethiopian dishes. Each Ethiopian family has its own unique recipe for *berbere*.

Traditional *berbere* can take 3–4 days of preparation. Dried chili forms the base for this spice blend to which garlic, ginger, fresh sacred basil, and roux are added. See a recipe for *berbere* at the end of this chapter.

 Beverages

Highly sweetened hot tea and coffee are popular beverages served throughout Africa. Coffee originated in Ethiopia and is used primarily in the highlands. Sweetened coffee is reserved for those who can afford to buy sugar. The Oromo ethnic group is known to add a small amount of salt. Because tea is imported to Ethiopia and is more expensive than coffee, it is considered a beverage of prestige. As in other areas of Africa, Ethiopians drink highly sweetened tea with added spices, such as roux or mint. For those who cannot afford tea, coffee leaves are used in much the same way as tea leaves. Locally made beer and wine are other common beverages. *Tella* is a local beer served during the week and *tejj*, Ethiopia's national drink, is reserved for feasts such as weddings or the breaking of a fast. *Tejj* is a sweet wine made from honey. It is considered polite to fill a glass of tejj until it overflows, and to serve the second glass as soon as the first is finished.

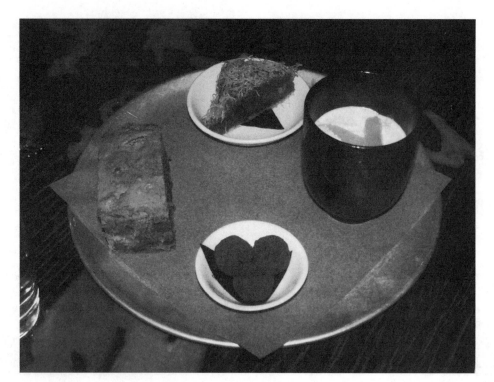

Congo Bar, Baklava, Mango Couscous, and Tamarind Balls
Courtesy of the author

 Desserts

There is no cultural tradition for dessert in Ethiopia; however, there are pastry shops that sell frosted cakes and other desserts. Chocolate cake, the most popular dessert, is usually served at feasts and given as gifts. Meals in Africa typically end with fresh fruit such as pineapple slices, orange wedges, mango chunks, or bananas sprinkled with sugar or honey. Occasionally, fried pancakes or cookies are served. Baked goods seldom grace the table because most Africans do not have ovens.

 FOODS WITH CULTURAL SIGNIFICANCE

Wat is Ethiopia's national dish. It is placed on top of *injera* bread and served in a large basket. Typically, the food is eaten with the fingers by tearing off pieces of *injera* and dipping it into the *wat*. Coffee is sacred in Ethiopia. When Ethiopians drink coffee, it is in a traditional way known as a "coffee ceremony." The coffee is roasted, ground, and placed in a coffee pot with boiling water. When ready, it is served to people in little cups, up to three times per ceremony. The elderly, guest, and husband are served first during a ceremony. Other family members and friends are served last. Ethiopian Orthodox Christians do not eat any food of animal origin during fasting holidays.

 TYPICAL DAY'S MENU

Traditional African cooking methods include steaming food in banana or corn-husk leaves, boiling, frying in oil, or grilling over an open fire. For most Africans lunch serves as the main meal of the day. It usually includes a mixture of vegetables and legumes, and occasionally meat is included.

Injera fit-fit is a typical Ethiopian dish eaten for breakfast. It is a combination of shredded *injera*, *berbere*, onions, and clarified butter. *Dulet* is another popular breakfast food. It is a spicy mixture of tripe, liver, beef, and peppers with *injera*. *Gonfo*, a traditional porridge, may be served for breakfast or on special occasions such as the birth of a child. The mother and guest eat the porridge. On occasion, *injera* is eaten as a snack and the very poor may eat it with *berbere* as a meal. Most meals consist of some type of *wat* and *injera*. The main ingredients in the *wat* are legumes, meat, fish, chicken, vegetables, or tubers. Sometimes, leftover *wat* is served for breakfast.

Qolo, a combination of toasted cereal, legumes, or sunflower seeds is eaten as a snack with coffee. It can also serve as a main meal.

 ## HOLIDAY MENUS

The first rains, crops, births, weddings, puberty, death, and visitors are all occasions for celebration in Africa. Wealth and status determine the foods that will be served. Wealthy individuals may slaughter animals for the celebration and poorer families may simply have larger quantities of everyday foods.

No doubt you're familiar with Kwanzaa, but you may be surprised to know that Kwanzaa is not a holiday celebrated in Africa. Kwanzaa is a Swahili word that means "first fruits of the harvest." Kwanzaa, a seven-day yearly celebration, runs from December 26 to January 1. Each night, in honor of a family's African ancestors, foods and dishes from places where their ancestors lived are prepared and eaten. However, this holiday is not celebrated in Ethiopia.

Ethiopians who practice the Orthodox Christian religion fast during religious celebrations. During the fast, food of animal origin and water are restricted. Meals can be eaten after 3 PM. There are 250 fasting days yearly in Ethiopia.

Steak tartar is an Ethiopian dish served at weddings and other celebrations. Cow's meat is served immediately after slaughter. It is spiced with a mixture called *awaze* or *mitmitta*. These spice mixtures are reserved for raw meat. *Awaze* is a *berbere* mixture with garlic, ginger, salt, and other spices. *Mitmitta* is a mixture of dried bird's-eye chili, Ethiopian cardamom, black cumin, and bishop's weed, mixed with salt.

 ## HEALTH BELIEFS AND CONCERNS

A discussion of the health beliefs of Ethiopia requires a look at the Ethiopian world view. For many Ethiopians disease, including HIV/AIDS, is a result of witchery and evil. Traditional Ethiopians believe that health is a state of equilibrium between the body and the outside world. They do not believe in chance, bad luck, or fate. They believe that every illness has a specific cause, and

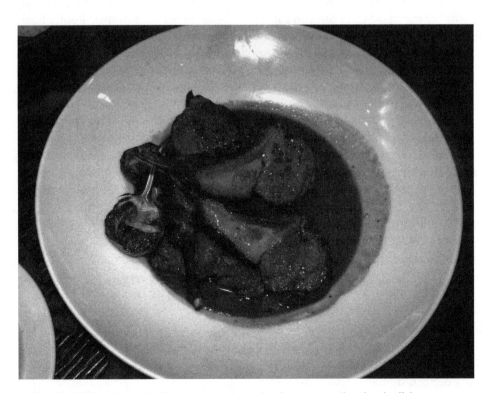

In North Africa, lamb is the centerpiece for important festive holiday celebrations.

Courtesy of the author

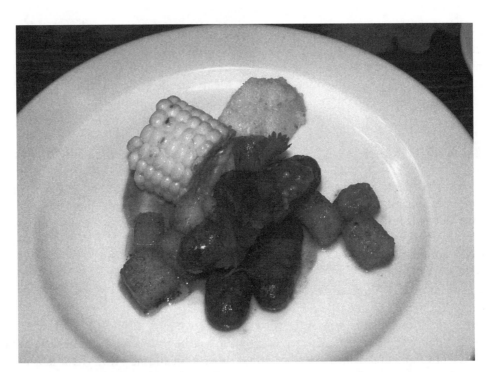

Merquez sausage is used to break the fast after Ramadan. Pictured: merguez sausage, pap, and watermelon.

Courtesy of the author

in order to cure the illness, the cause must first be determined. Ethiopians believe that excess sun can cause headache, eye disease, earache, and other health conditions. Children are given uvulectomies, lower-incisor extractions, and eyelid incisions to prevent disease or in response to disease. Many Ethiopians consult both traditional healers and biomedical professionals for the same condition.

 ## GENERAL HEALTH AND NUTRITIONAL INDICATORS SUMMARY

The economic stability of a nation depends much on the health and overall well-being of its population. In 2005, Ethiopia's infant mortality rate stood at 77 per 1000 live births, and the under-5-years mortality rate was 123 per 1000 live births. The infant mortality rate declined by 20.6% over the 5-year period 2000–2005 from 97 deaths per 1000 live births to 77, and the under-5-years mortality rate decreased by 25.9% from 166 deaths per 1000 live births in 2000 to 123 live births in 2005.

Malnutrition is defined by the World Health Organization as "the cellular imbalance between supply of nutrients and energy and the body's demand for them to ensure growth, maintenance, and specific functions." Protein energy malnutrition affects 11% of the children in Ethiopia. Public health experts assess stunting as the preferred indicator of nutritional status. Stunting is defined as low height for age and is associated with retarded physical growth. The malnutrition rate in Ethiopian children is among the highest in the world; however, data from 2000 to 2005 show that there has been improvement in the nutritional status of Ethiopian children. The percentage of stunted children fell by 10%, and the percentage of children underweight declined by 19%.

Infant mortality and low birth weight can be directly correlated to maternal nutritional status. Low weight gain during pregnancy results in low-birth-weight infants, predisposing them to cognitive impairment, developmental delays, and early mortality. Three in ten Ethiopian women ages 15–49 years are thin or undernourished.

 ## COMMUNICATION AND COUNSELING TIPS

There are several greeting styles in Africa depending upon the ethnic heritage of the person you are meeting. When dealing with foreigners, most Ethiopians

FEATURED RECIPE

Berbere
(Americanized version)

Paprika

Chopped red pepper

Salt

Crushed ginger root

Crushed cloves

Cinnamon

Nutmeg

Crushed cardamom seeds

Allspice

Crushed black peppercorns

Crushed fenugreek

Coriander seeds

Mix together equal amounts of the ingredients listed. Moisten the mixture with a small amount of water until a paste is formed. Use as a flavoring for stews and soups.

More recipes are available at http://nutrition.jbpub.com/foodculture/

shake hands while maintaining eye contact and smiling. The handshake is much lighter than in Western cultures. Some women do not shake hands and merely nod their head, so it is best to wait for a woman to extend her hand. Men kiss a woman they know well on the cheek in place of a handshake. Elders should be greeted first, and greetings are leisurely including time for social discussion and exchanging pleasantries. It is also customary to bow when introduced to an elder or person with a more senior position.

Ethiopians are humble, soft-spoken people, and they respect those qualities in others. They tend to be nonconfrontational, and rather than say something that might embarrass you, they will give what they believe to be the expected response.

Counseling tips are as follows:

- Enquire about lactose intolerance and culturally determined food practices.
- Develop and use culturally relevant educational materials.

- Recommendations for change should be action oriented.
- Avoid making assumptions based on ethnic identification or stereotypes. Determine if the individual is a recent immigrant and ask questions regarding religious beliefs.
- Ask questions about cultural beliefs and practices. It should not be assumed that one's level of education would preclude him or her from adhering to many traditional Ethiopian cultural beliefs.
- It is important to assess all these areas even when the health professional and patient share a cultural or ethnic identity.
- Group discussions and role playing are more effective than lectures.

REFERENCES

Brazzaville. (2004). *Roundtable to discuss Africa's nutrition situation.* Retrieved March 27, 2008, from www.afro.who.int/press/2004/regionalcommittee/pr2004090202.html

Brown-Riggs, C. (2006). *Eating soulfully and healthfully with diabetes.* Bloomington, IN: iUniverse, Inc.

CIA—The World Factbook. (2009). *Ethiopia.* Retrieved August 19, 2009, from https://www.cia.gov/library/publications/the-world-factbook/geos/et.html/

Food in South Africa. (2008). Retrieved March 27, 2008, from http://www.foodbycountry.com/Kazakhstan-to-South-Africa/South-Africa.html/

Gibbon, E. (1999). *Staple dish recipes review.* Retrieved March 27, 2008, from http://www.congocookbook.com/staple_dish_recipes/index.html/

Grolier Incorporated. (2004). *Encyclopedia Americana 2004: International edition* (30 volumes, pp. 256–320). Danbury, CT: Scholastic Library Publishing.

Hodes, R. (1997). *Cross-cultural medicine and diverse health beliefs. Ethiopians abroad.* Retrieved August 23, 2009, from http://www.pubmedcentral.nih.gov/articlerender.fcgi?artid=1303953/

Kepos, P., & Garces, J. (2008). *Nutrition and well-being A to Z: Diets of Africans.* Retrieved March 27, 2008, from http://www.faqs.org/nutrition/A-Ap/Africans-Diets-of.html/

Kwintessential. (2008). *South Africa: Language, culture, customs and etiquette.* Retrieved March 27, 2008, from http://www.kwintessential.co.uk/resources/global-etiquette/south-africa-country-profile.html/

Kwintessential. (2009). *Ethiopia: Language, culture, customs and etiquette.* Retrieved August 23, 2009, from http://www.kwintessential.co.uk/resources/global-etiquette/ethiopia.html/

McHenry, R. (Ed.). (1992). *The New Encyclopedia Britannica* (15th ed., Vol. 15). Macropedia (birds through chemical) (pp. 131–132). Chicago: Encyclopedia Britannica, Inc.

Meredith, M. (2006). *The fate of Africa: A history of fifty years of independence*. New York: Public Affairs.

Reader, J. (1999). *Africa: A biography of the continent*. New York: Vintage.

Samuelsson, M. (2006). *The soul of a new cuisine: A discovery of the foods and flavors of Africa*. New York: Wiley.

Shashshidar, H.R., & Grigsby, D.G. (2009). *Malnutrition*. Retrieved April 23, 2009, from http://emedicine.medscape.com/article/985140-overview/

Teller, C.H., & Alva, S. (2008). *Reducing child malnutrition in sub-Saharan Africa: Surveys find mixed progress*. Retrieved April 25, 2009, from http://www.prb.org/Articles/2008/stuntingssa.aspx/

UNICEF. (2007a). *The state of the world's children 2007: Women and children, the double dividend of gender equality*. Retrieved April 23, 2009, from http://www.unicef.org/sowc07/statistics/tables.php

UNICEF. (2007b). *Ethiopia world fit for children report*. Retrieved August 23, 2009, from http://www.unicef.org/worldfitforchildren/files/Ethiopia_WFFC5_Report.pdf/

U.S. Embassy Ethiopia. (2009). *Guide on how to do business in Ethiopia*. Retrieved August 23, 2009, from http://ethiopia.usembassy.gov/doing_business_in_ethiopia.html/

Williams, J.A. (1962). *Africa: Her history, lands and people, told with pictures*. Lanham, MD: Rowman & Littlefield.

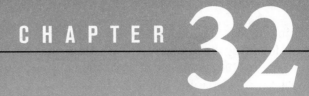

CHAPTER 32

Kenya (Western)

Marilyn Massey-Stokes, EdD, CHES, FASHA

Anna M. Love, PhD, RD, CHES

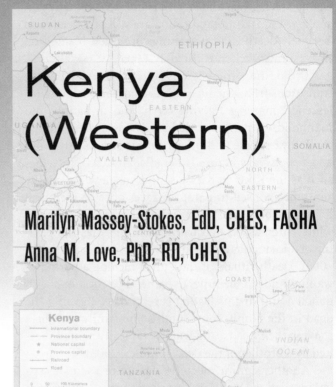

CULTURE AND WORLD REGION

Kenya is a country of grassland prairies, mountain ranges, coastal regions, and desert. It is not only diverse in geography, but also in ethnicity, culture, cuisine, health beliefs, and political climate. This chapter explores these characteristics with respect to the western region of the country and contrasts them with other areas of Kenya. Tribes that comprise the greatest population of the area surrounding Lake Victoria are emphasized.

Kenya is located on the east coast of Africa and borders Somalia, Ethiopia, and Sudan to the north, Uganda to the west, Tanzania to the south, and the Indian Ocean to the east. Kenya covers an area of 225,000 square miles (582,646 km²) and is roughly the size of Texas (Embassy of Kenya, 2006) or approximately twice the size of Nevada (Central Intelligence Agency [CIA], 2008). The estimated total population in 2006 was 35,553,000 (World Health Organization [WHO], 2008b).

Kenya is a land of the *wabenzi* (the upper class) and the *wananchi* (the middle to lower class and those who are unemployed) (Sobania, 2003). Kenya is a multi-ethnic country, partly due to the influx of more than 250,000 refugees from Somalia, Ethiopia, Eritrea, Sudan, Rwanda, Burundi, and the Congo (CIA, 2008; Sobania, 2003). Although the majority of the population belongs to Bantu-speaking tribes, there are also minorities such as Indians, Arabs, and Europeans (Kenyaology, 2008; Sobania, 2003).

In terms of religion, the vast majority of Kenyans are Christian (78%), with estimates for the percentage of Kenyans who are Muslim or adhere to indigenous beliefs varying greatly (CIA, 2008; U.S. Department of State, 2006). In addition, local churches play an important role within communities of western Kenya and are particularly effective channels of communication for health interventions (Muruli et al., 1999). Precolonial religious beliefs among the Luhya tribe were that a High God, *Were*, existed, as did ancestral spirits who had the power in everyday life to cause illness and death. In the 30 years following the first arrival of American Quaker missionaries in 1902, approximately 50,000 Luhya had converted to Christianity, although the belief in ancestral spirits was, and is, still prominent. Witchcraft, sorcery, and traditional healing are still practiced, and untimely deaths and poisonings are often blamed on sorcery and witchcraft (Bradley, 2005).

In addition to religious and traditional beliefs, transitions from one life stage to another, such as adolescence, marriage, giving birth, and initiation into manhood/womanhood, hold great meaning among the Luhya people and others in this region. Attitudes and beliefs vary across tribes. For instance, in tribes such as the Kikuyu, Kipsigis, and Luo, a white chalky substance is used to paint the faces of tribe members for special occasions such as rites of passage. The color white, often associated with death, signifies the passing of one stage as a person moves to another (Sobania, 2003). Death rituals of the Luhya include a period of wailing prior to the funerals, funeral celebrations with dancing and drums lasting several days, burying the dead in the family compound, some family members shaving their heads, and widows typically being inherited by a brother of the dead (Bradley, 2005).

Another significant cultural practice is female genital mutilation (FGM), or female circumcision. FGM is widely practiced by the Gusii and Kipsigis people as well as by some Luhya subtribes (Bradley, 2005; Tannaka, 2000). It is a deleterious traditional practice that results in a wide variety of dire health outcomes, including hemorrhage, infections, and child and maternal morbidity/mortality (Skolnik, 2008; WHO, 2008a). Furthermore, FGM is strongly linked to deeply ingrained cultural beliefs about feminine identity and value (F. Njororai, personal communication, March 10, 2008) as well as the normative culture surrounding marriage (Sobania, 2003).

Farming is the primary occupation in western Kenya. Crops may be food and/or cash crops. Major food crops in this region include maize, sorghum, millet (Ogoye-Ndegwa & Aagaard-Hansen, 2006), sweet potatoes, and bananas, plus tree crops such as avocado, guava, mango, papaya, and local fruit trees. Beans, cowpeas, cassava, English potatoes, kale, okra, pumpkins, soybeans, onions, and tomatoes serve as supplemental crops (Conelly & Chaiken, 2000). Contemporary crops that have fared well in the Western Province include green beans, red beans, bananas, groundnuts (peanuts), *sukuma wiki* (similar to collard greens), cabbages, potatoes, and cassava. Cash crops now include tea, coffee, sugar cane, cotton, sunflower seeds, French beans, and eucalyptus trees (Conelly & Chaiken, 2000).

All the major food crops have a twofold value for farmers because not only do they provide food for consumption, but their stalks, leaves, and vines can also be used to feed livestock such as cattle, goats, sheep, chickens, ducks, and turkeys that are maintained by many farming families (Conelly & Chaiken, 2000). Agro-diversity, which includes multiple cropping and other mindful strategies, such as the use of polyvarietal cultivation and incorporating livestock and cash crops into the agricultural system, has been promoted in western Kenya to "maximize the utility of small parcels of land" (p. 37) and to promote food and economic security for farming families (Conelly & Chaiken, 2000). In addition, fishing, petty trade, shopkeeping, casual trade, and migratory work help supplement household incomes (Lindblade, Odhiambo, Rosen, & DeCock, 2003; Ogoye-Ndegwa & Aagaard-Hansen, 2003, 2006). The trading that historically took place in local markets is now conducted in one of nearly a dozen urban centers in the Western Province (Bradley, 2005).

The Luhya and other ethnic groups of western Kenya are a patrilineal society; men own most of the land and women have usufruct rights (Conelly & Chaiken, 2000; Muruli et al., 1999). Men often migrate to urban areas to find work; therefore, the women are left on their own to manage both farming and caring for the family (Muruli et al., 1999; Whyte & Kariuki, 1997). Given this trend, women are estimated to be responsible for 75% of all food production in Africa (Sobania, 2003).

Traditionally, in groups such as the Luo people, women keep house, do the gardening, gather firewood, prepare meals, and take care of the children (Lindblade et al., 2003). In other words, men are usually considered the main "breadwinners" and women are viewed as the primary caregivers in the home; however, it is important to avoid placing people in stereotypical gender roles. For example, although nutrition is often considered a "women's issue," men's decision-making power affects family nutrition both directly (e.g., their decisions regarding how to allocate resources) and indirectly (e.g., their influence on women's actions and decisions). This is particularly relevant for places such as western Kenya where nutrition interventions aimed at reducing child malnutrition have been proven effective by encompassing both men and women (Johnson-Welch, n.d.).

A related point worth mentioning is that polygamy is often practiced in marital situations within western Kenya, although it varies among ethnic groups. For example, according to Whyte & Kariuki (1997), 37% of women in the Luo-speaking districts are co-wives who share their husbands, in contrast to 16% in the Luhya-speaking Busia district. Polygamy can affect the dynamics of the male and female roles and cultural practices within households and compounds. Among the Luhya, nuclear family units, which consist of a husband, wife, and their children, typically live together in a compound. The addition of other family members to the compound may occur, provided the relationship does not interfere with beliefs. For instance, it is forbidden for mature relatives one generation apart to live in the same house. This results in grandmothers and older children occupying the one house with parents and younger children in another house (Bradley, 2005). This also facilitates the passing down of stories and life lessons from grandmothers to grandchildren. According to Sobania (2003), a typical rural family compound includes a parent's house, perhaps a grandparent's house, places to cook, and structures for sheltering animals.

The World Bank (2008a) classifies Kenya as a low-income country. Low-income countries are those with a gross national income per capita of $935 or less (World Bank, 2008b). According to Sobania (2003), 42% of Kenyans live below the poverty line. As a developing country in sub-Saharan Africa, Kenya faces tremendous challenges in dealing with public health problems such as HIV/AIDS, malaria, diarrheal disease, and tuberculosis (CIA, 2008; WHO, 2008b).

Kenya's political environment has been marked with instability. Recent news headlines from across the world have depicted political chaos, civil wars, rioting, and other forms of violence, along with stories about refugees (e.g., from Somalia and Sudan) and internally displaced persons. The African Development Bank and the World Bank noted in a joint statement that they are deeply concerned that political instability could force 2 million Kenyans into poverty and negatively impact the transit routes/business transactions with other countries in East Africa (World Bank, 2008c). In addition, Kenya has been placed on the Tier 2 Watch List due to lack of efforts to combat severe forms of trafficking in men, women, and children (CIA, 2008). Despite the political turbulence, Kenya remains a top travel destination for tourists from all over the world.

Kenya has seven administrative provinces besides greater Nairobi, its capital. The western region of Kenya,

the most densely populated part of the country (JamboKenya, 2008a), includes the following regions: Nyanza Province surrounding the southeast side of Lake Victoria located on the Ugandan border; the Western Province surrounding the northeast side of Lake Victoria; and the Rift Valley along the rest of the Ugandan border from north of the Western Province (World66, 2008a). Western Kenya is primarily composed of four ethnic groups—the Luhyia (Luhya), Luo, Kisii (Gusii), and Kalenjin (Muruli et al., 1999; Sobania, 2003)—with smaller populations of Maasai and Kikuyu tribes (CIA, 2008; Sobania, 2003). The Luo is the largest ethnic group in the Nyanza Province, with some Kisii, Kuria, and Luhya also residing in this region. The Luo represent the third largest ethnic group in Kenya, estimated to number approximately 3 million people (Encyclopedia Britannica Online, 2008; Ogoye-Ndegwa & Aagaard-Hansen, 2006), or 13% of the total Kenyan population (CIA, 2008). The Western Province is predominantly inhabited by the Luhya, the second largest ethnic group in Kenya (Encyclopedia Britannica Online, 2008), and 14% of the total Kenyan population (CIA, 2008). The Luhya are composed of 18 subtribes in Kenya, 1 subtribe in northern Tanzania, and 4 subtribes in Uganda (Jenkins, 2003). Luhya is an abbreviated form of Abaluhya, loosely translated as "those of the same hearth" (Encyclopedia Britannica Online, 2008). The Kikuyu tribe represents the largest population in Kenya (22% of the total population) and inhabits mostly the Rift Valley (CIA, 2008; Sobania, 2003).

Western Kenya has been described as "a gentle plateau" that is typically hot and humid with abundant year-round rainfall (JamboKenya, 2008b). This part of Kenya is considered the agricultural focal point with productive farmland in the north and tea plantations in the south (JamboKenya, 2008a). Western Kenya has the world's second largest freshwater lake (covering 67,483 square miles), Lake Victoria, which serves as a border between Tanzania, Uganda, and Kenya; however, because international water travel no longer exists between the three countries, Kenya only owns a 3785-km^2 corner of the lake (JamboKenya, 2008c). Another key geographical area in western Kenya is the Mt. Elgon range, the fourth highest in Kenya, known for its daily torrential rains (JamboKenya, 2008d).

Kisumu, the third largest city in Kenya (JamboKenya, 2008c; World66, 2008), once was a major port on Lake Victoria (JamboKenya, 2008c; Microsoft Encarta Online Encyclopedia, 2008) and is approximately a 7-hour drive (1 hour by air, 14 hours by rail) from

Nairobi (iExplore, 2008). Kisumu offers other interesting assets, including Impala Park (game sanctuary, animal orphanage, and home to the rare sitatunga antelope), Hippo Point (excellent viewing of hippo and beautiful Lake Victoria sunsets), Kisumu Musuem (featuring traditional customs and crafts), and Kisumu market (with Kisii soapstone carvings) (JamboKenya, 2008c).

 LANGUAGE

Due to Kenya's diversity, there is more than one language spoken in the country. The Luhya people of western Kenya are culturally and linguistically related to neighboring Bantu-speaking peoples (e.g., in Uganda). Each subtribe has its own traditional language and customs, and the indigenous language is spoken almost exclusively in the home. The most commonly spoken languages among the subtribes are Swahili (or Kiswahili) as the national language and English as the official language (CIA, 2008; Jenkins, 2003).

 CULTURE HISTORY

"Kenya's history dates to the Stone Age, making Kenya one of the countries in the world that possesses the largest and most complete record of man's cultural development" (Embassy of Kenya, 2006, p. 1). There is widespread evidence of tools used during the Iron Age through the precolonial period up to the present; however, the type of inhabitants who lived in Kenya between this early period and the 19th century is unclear (Embassy of Kenya, 2006). Arab colonies exported spices and slaves from Kenya's coast as early as the eighth century (World Almanac & Book of Facts, 2005). According to Sobania (2003), Bantu-speaking agriculturists moved into East Africa from the west before 1000 CE when East Africa's plains became occupied by herding communities (ca. 1000–1300 CE). International exploration and trade by Arab, Chinese, and Portuguese explorers occurred over the next 500 years until the Imperial British East Africa Company was established in 1888. Kenya and Uganda were split into the countries we know them as today in 1898 (Sobania, 2003). Kenya, formerly known as British East Africa (CIA, 2008), won independence on December 12, 1963, four years after the end of the turbulent Mau Mau uprising (World Almanac & Book of Facts, 2005).

 FOOD HISTORY WITHIN THE CULTURE

Historically, crops such as millet, bananas, sugarcane, and yams were most prevalent until the colonial period when tea, coffee, and sisal (a hemp fiber made from an agave-like plant) became key cash crops. Additionally, beans, maize, and potatoes were harvested in the highlands of Africa with pineapple, peanuts, and rice grown as predominant crops in the west. Rice was particularly popular around Lake Victoria (Sobania, 2003).

In many developing countries, such as Kenya, food and nutrition security are often threatened due to climatic conditions (e.g., periods of drought) (Ogoye-Ndegwa & Aagaard-Hansen, 2003), crop diseases (DeVoe, 2008), and high poverty levels (Sobania, 2003); therefore, food-consumption patterns can be influenced by these factors. For example, plants are major food sources for farmers in tropical countries such as Kenya. The Luo people in western Kenya depend on many plant products for subsistence and for cash income (Johns & Kokwaro, 1991). Numerous traditional vegetables contribute to food and nutrition security in western Kenya; however, caution must be exercised because some plants have toxic effects (Ogoye-Ndegwa & Aagaard-Hansen, 2003).

 MAJOR FOODS

Influenced in part by Arabian, Asian, Indian, and British foods, East African cuisine is often vegetarian, with meats consumed on special occasions and by those who can afford them. With the mixture of these influences, even the manner of eating depends on where the dish originates. Traditional foods are eaten with the right hand, whereas European foods are eaten using forks and knives (Microsoft Encarta Online Encyclopedia, 2008).

 Protein Sources

Protein foods include milk, legumes, fish, meat, chicken, and eggs. Other than milk, protein-rich foods are not frequently consumed. Although there can be seasonal variations, meat and fish are generally consumed only once or twice (at most) a week, and beans are usually eaten less than twice a week. Although milk is consumed more frequently, it is often consumed in very small amounts (e.g., in tea or to make a sauce for

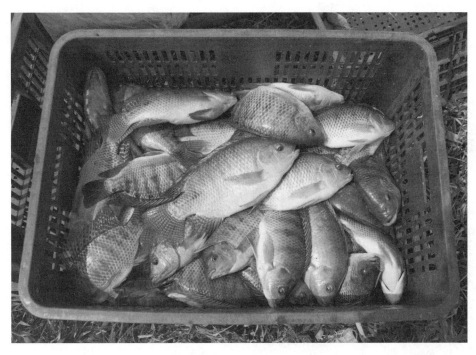

Tilapia is the most common fish garnered from Lake Victoria.

stewed vegetables) as opposed to being drunk in a cup (Conelly & Chaiken, 2000).

Some variation in protein intake is seen depending on the region. For instance, cattle are raised on the northern plateaus of Kenya's Rift Valley. Cattle indicate wealth and are considered a "gift of the gods," particularly by the Maasai tribe. In contrast, fish and seafood are primary sources of protein in the diets among Kenyans living along the coast of Lake Victoria (Kittler & Sucher, 2004). The most common fish from Lake Victoria are tilapia, which are either eaten fresh, or salted and dried to be taken to other regions for trade. The Asian influence in Kenya's cuisine is evident in dishes such as *mchuzi wa samaki* (fish in a curry sauce) and *kuku na nazi* (chicken prepared using coconut milk) (Sobania, 2003).

 Starch Sources

Ugali, a thick maize meal, is the national food of Kenya (Kittler & Sucher, 2004; Whyte, 1997) and a foundational food for most meals. This maize (or sometimes sorghum) meal may have different names depending on its consistency. *Posho* is made by cooking maize with water into porridge; however, if this will be served as the main meal, *posho* is added to boiling water to make the thicker, heavier mixture *ugali* (Sobania, 2003). Fats,

broth, or other condiments are not typically added, so the nutritional content of *ugali* is somewhat low (Conelly & Chaiken, 2000). It can be eaten either with meat, fish, stewed vegetables (e.g., tomatoes and onions sautéed in a little fat), or beans, or with both meat and vegetables; and sometimes it is eaten with milk, either sour or fresh (Conelly & Chaiken, 2000; Oniang'o & Komokoti, 1999).

Additionally, *uji*, a thin breakfast porridge made from maize or sorghum, is a starchy food consumed in western Kenya that is thin enough to be drunk like a liquid or can be eaten from a bowl like soup (Sobania, 2003). Cassava is another very important staple food that is classified as a starch. Its leaves are typically eaten as a vegetable in parts of Asia and Africa, providing vitamins and protein. Nutritionally, cassava roots are comparable to those of potatoes, except that they have twice the fiber content and higher levels of potassium (University of Bath, 2008). High-carbohydrate foods are used as fillers in the diets of most western Kenyans to offset times when vegetables and meats are not bountiful. In addition, *kitumbua* (fried bread), *mandazi* (doughnut-like sweet bread), and *samosas* (or *sambusas;* thin triangular pastries stuffed with either meat or potatoes) are examples of Asian influence, provided by the Indian Ocean trade routes, in the Kenyan diet (Sobania, 2005).

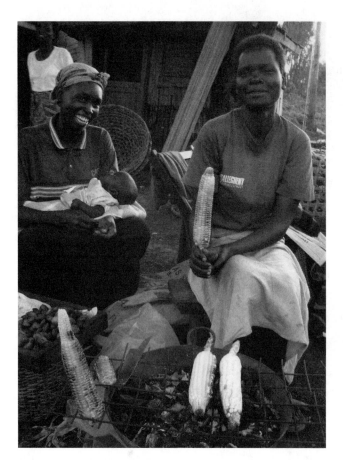

Ugali, a thick maize meal, is the national food of Kenya.

Fat Sources

Milk is being used more often to make butter, but in urban areas Kimbo is the primary commercial cooking fat, with lard used to a lesser degree (Sobania, 2003). Cooking oil also plays a key role in modern, daily meal preparation (Ogoye-Ndegwa & Aagaard-Hansen, 2006).

Prominent Vegetables

Seasonality is a key factor in determining the availability of traditional vegetables because there are almost twice as many vegetables ($n = 72$) available during the wet season as opposed to the dry season ($n = 38$). Dominant traditional vegetables include *apoth* (*Conchorus trilocularis*), *boo* (*Vigna inguiculata*), *atipa* (*Asystasia mysorensis*), *akeyo* (*Gynandropsis gynandra*), and *osuga* (*Solanum nigrum*) (Ogoye-Ndegwa & Aagaard-Hansen, 2003).

There are a wide variety of leafy vegetables in western Kenya; some are locally grown and others come from other parts of Kenya and are found in local mar-

kets. The most important and widespread of these leafy vegetables are *omboga* (*Amaranthus hybridus L.*), *kabich* (*B. oleracea L. var. capitata L.*), *apoth* (*Corchorus olitorius L.*), *mitoo* or *mutoo* (*Crotalaria brevidens Benth. Var. intermedia*), *Akeyo* or *alot dek* (*Gynandropsis gynandra Briq.*), *bo* (*Phaseolus coccineus L.*), and *osuga* (*Solanum nigrum L.*) (Johns & Kokwaro, 1991). These leafy vegetables typically supplement cultivated staples by adding protein, vitamin A, ascorbic acid, folic acid, and minerals to the diet (Fleuret & Fleuret, 1980, as cited in Johns & Kokwaro, 1991). Furthermore, the Luo people believe that the leafy, traditional vegetables protect against gastrointestinal problems (Frison, Cherfas, Eyzaguirre, & Johns, 2004).

According to a study of the Luo people (Ogoye-Ndegwa & Aagaard-Hansen, 2003), "there are two main methods of cooking vegetables: 'aruda' (literally: 'stirred'), and 'aboka' (literally: 'fermented')" (p. 79). Vegetables to be consumed immediately are cooked "aruda" (i.e., seasoned with salt and soda [sodium carbonate] mixture) to "soften and detoxify the vegetables" (p. 79). If soda carbonate is not available, wood ash from the fireplace is mixed with water in very small amounts. Furthermore, milk is often used to initiate fermentation. Vegetables commonly prepared this way include *apoth*, *boo*, and *atipa*.

Cooking vegetables *aboka* requires a longer process, often well over 2 days, to soften the vegetables and reduce bitterness for consumption. No salt is used; instead, milk is added to them and they are cooked several times. Approximately 28 vegetables are typically cooked *aboka*, including *akeyo* (*Gynandropsis gynandra*), *osuga* (*Solanium nigrum*), and *alika* (*Amaranthus spp.*). There are 11 vegetables that may be cooked either *aruda* or *aboka*, or a mixture of the two, including *nyayado* (*Senna occidentalis*), *it rabuon* (potato leaves), and *okuuro*. "A vegetable that is cooked aboka may be mixed with the ones cooked aruda, and if an aruda vegetable is the predominant one, the dish is stirred and becomes aruda and vice versa." (Ogoye-Ndegwa & Aagaard-Hansen, 2003, pp. 79–80).

Another significant vegetable is the sweet potato, which is increasing in importance in Kenya and other areas of sub-Saharan Africa due to its ability to be cultivated for both food security and income production (Hagenimana & Low, 2000). It is important to note that new, high-yielding, orange-flesh varieties of sweet potato should be promoted due to their ability to reduce vitamin A deficiency, which is particularly important to children's health. In addition to cooking orange-flesh sweet potatoes, western Kenyan women have

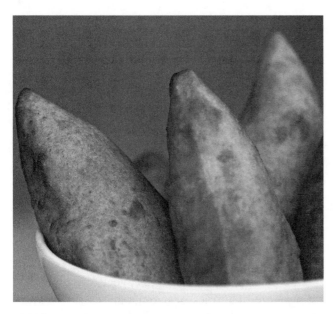

Mandazi, doughnut-like sweet bread, is evidence of the Asian influence in the Kenyan diet.

been taught to substitute orange-flesh sweet potatoes for wheat flour in either boiled, mashed, or flour form to significantly raise the beta-carotene content in other common food products, such as *chapati*, *mandazi*, and small buns. Not only can these enriched food products be eaten at home, they also can be profitable for selling in rural markets (Hagenimana & Low, 2000).

In addition, irio (*kienyeji* in Swahili) is a Highland dish served hot made by mashing potatoes and corn together. In some areas, this same name "applies to a mixture made with a green vegetable such as peas and potatoes or beans" (Sobania, 2003, p. 115). On the streets of urban centers, grilled roasted corn on the cob and deep-fried yams served with a squeeze of lemon juice and a pepper mixture called *pilipile* can be purchased from street vendors (Sobania, 2003).

 ### Prominent Fruits

Papayas, mangoes, pineapples, guavas, *matoke* (plantains), and bananas are common fruits in Kenya, although plantains (the starchy relatives of the banana) must be cooked prior to eating (Sobania, 2003). Plantains are used in stews, fritters, custards, and wine (Kittler & Sucher, 2004). People in western Kenya are knowledgeable about edible wild plants; for example, the Luo primarily eat wild fruits as snacks. Although these plants usually do not make major dietary contributions, they are important as supplementary and emergency foods. Examples of edible wild fruits

include *asaye* (*Aframomum mala K. Schum.*), *ochuoga* (*Carissa edulis [Forsk.] Vahl*), *yago* (*Kigelia Africana [Lam.] Benth.*), and *olemo* (*Xiamenia Americana L.*) (Johns & Kokwaro, 1991).

 ### Spices and Seasonings

Examples of spices used by the Luo include the underground parts of a cultivated edible plant called *tanguas* (*Zingiber officinale Roscoe* or ginger) and the fruit of another cultivated edible plant called *pilipili* (*Capsicum frutescens L.* or chili pepper). They also use a wild root or tuber called *munyu* (*Cissus rotundifolia Vahl*) (Johns & Kokwaro, 1991). Other Kenyan spices include onion, pepper, turmeric, coriander, cinnamon, cloves, and ginger (Gardner, 1993). Additionally, coconut milk, chili peppers, and curry powder (a blend of coriander, cumin, turmeric, and cinnamon) are used to flavor food throughout East Africa (Kittler & Sucher, 2004).

 ### Beverages

Most of the beverages in this region are universal, of which the most popular is tea (Oniang'o & Komokoti, 1999). The tea, consumed as the only breakfast item, is usually sweetened with sugar purchased from local shops (Conelly & Chaiken, 2000). Sugar and milk are often brewed into the tea by adding them to the cold water prior to boiling to make old-fashioned Kenyan tea. This has become popular to bottle and export as *chai* (Swahili for tea), or even *chai masala* (tea is brewed, then steeped with milk and spices such as ginger or cardamom) (Sobania, 2003).

In western Kenya, particularly in the urban areas, bottled colas are available; and *pombe*, the term that refers to any alcoholic beverage, can be brewed commercially or at home. In addition, *maziwa* (milk) is a staple in the western Kenyan diet as in most of Kenya. *Maziwa mala* (sour milk) is sometimes served cold on *ugali* with a side of cooked greens (Sobania, 2003). Other drinks include coffee, cocoa, colas, various fruit juices, and traditional porridge made from maize, millet, and/or sorghum flour (Oniang'o & Komokoti, 1999).

 ### Desserts

Western Kenya is not laden with the elaborate desserts seen in many other regions of the world. Fruits are often eaten instead of desserts (Food in Every Country, 2007), and custard desserts that have a British flare are served in restaurants with local fruits (Sobania, 2003).

FOODS WITH CULTURAL SIGNIFICANCE

It is important to understand the concept of culture in order to better understand foods with cultural significance. In basic terms, culture can be considered "behavior and beliefs that are learned and shared" (Miller, 2004, as cited in Skolnik, 2008, p. 98). Culture encompasses multiple domains, including the family, social groups beyond one's family, communication, religion, art, and music (Miller, 2004, as cited in Skolnik, 2008). With regard to the culture of western Kenya, food represents social status, and generally the type of food consumed or the way it is prepared indicates a particular level of social status. In addition, new foods often have been associated with privileged circumstances (Barthes, 1997, as cited in Ogoye-Ndegwa & Aagaard-Hansen, 2003).

Generally, people who reside in western Kenya use wild plants for both food and medicine (Johns & Kokwaro, 1991; Ogoye-Ndegwa & Aagaard-Hansen, 2003). For instance, most of the traditional vegetables used by the Luo are considered to be medicinal and are used in a variety of ways: treating simple wounds; dealing with *chira* (a curse or an illness caused by breaking social rules and customs related to cultivation, marriage, and sexuality), spirit possession, and the evil eye; and creating love potions and protective charms (Ogoye-Ndegwa & Aagaard-Hansen, 2003).

Food and cultural beliefs are intertwined in all cultures. For example, in a study by Ogoye-Ndegwa & Aagaard-Hansen (2003), the Luo expressed negative attitudes toward vegetables. They considered it "undignified to serve vegetables to a visitor" and referred to vegetables as "the caterpillar's bed" (p. 74). In addition, the Luo considered it culturally unacceptable for a man to pick vegetables and to cook; men who cook were usually referred to as "women" (p. 79). The Luo also held certain beliefs about avoiding kitchen garden vegetables. For example, they believed that a menstruating female (who is considered culturally unclean) should not enter the kitchen garden to pick vegetables; if she did, the vegetables would wither (Ogoye-Ndegwa & Aagaard-Hansen, 2003).

Additionally, according to Ogoye-Ndegwa & Aagaard-Hansen (2003), many Luo traditional foods "are considered to have low status" (p. 84); however, an interesting contradiction is that traditional vegetables, such as *osuga* (*Solanium nigrum*), *akeyo* (*Gynandropsis gynandra*), *mito madongo* (*Crotaliaria brevidens*), and *ododo* (*Amaranthus hybridus*), are often served in large hotels. Furthermore, some of the traditional vegetables are highly nutritious. For example, *ododo*, *akeyo*, and *osuga* reveal higher iron, beta-carotene, and protein content when compared with recently introduced cabbages such as *sukuma wiki* (Ogoye-Ndegwa & Aagaard-Hansen, 2003). In addition, *akeyo* (also referred to as *alot dek*, which means "vegetable food") may have been historically the most important of the leafy vegetables currently eaten by the Luo (Johns & Kokwaro, 1991).

Mixing traditional vegetables during cooking depends on abundance and taste (i.e., some of them are very bitter); however, some vegetables, such as *it kipopyo* (papaya leaves) and *bwombwe matindo* (*Cyphostemma orondo*), are thought to be poisonous and are used minimally in mixtures. As Ogoye-Ndegwa & Aagaard-Hansen (2003) explain, "For example, goats die soon after eating large quantities of it omuogo (cassava leaves), and it is believed that it is equally dangerous for human beings too if not taken minimally. Besides, other species of omuogo are known to be so poisonous that those who have eaten them, usually during famine, have been reported to die from poisoning" (pp. 80–81).

Another noteworthy food-culture phenomenon found across the world is earth-eating (geophagy), the purposeful and regular ingestion of earth (e.g., soil and clay). Geophagy is common in Africa, where it appears to be culturally accepted among women, particularly during pregnancy, and among children (Geissler, 2000). Earth-eating is particularly common among school-age children in western Kenya (Geissler, Mwaniki, Thiong'o, & Friis, 1997). Although nutrition professionals tend to view geophagy as maladaptive or as a symptom of metabolic dysfunction (Johns & Duquette, 1991), earth-eating is an ordinary social and cultural practice among many traditional cultural groups, such as those who reside in western Kenya (Geissler, 2000).

TYPICAL DAY'S MENU

Mashed beans, lentils, corn, plantains, and potatoes are foods frequently seen in East Africa (Kittler & Sucher, 2004). Another popular food is *sukuma wiki*, which "is Swahili for 'stretch of the week' and is a stew of leftover meats and vegetables" (Kittler & Sucher, 2004, p. 191). A literal translation for this dish is "push the week" (Sobania, 2003). The vegetables in this stew are usually kale or collard greens made with onions and tomatoes (Sobania, 2003). In addition, starch sources, such as cooking bananas, roasted or boiled maize cobs, and sweet potatoes, are often consumed as side items to *ugali* (Conelly & Chaiken, 2000).

Plantains can be steamed and served with tea for breakfast, or boiled and then fried for lunch or dinner (Sobania, 2003). While taro greens and other leafy vegetables (such as kale) are often served with local grains, papaya and eggplant are side dishes (Kittler & Sucher, 2004; Sobania, 2003). Prepared foods are often served in hollowed-out gourds called *calabash* (African Studies Center, n.d.). Dining out is most often done at food kiosks in urban areas. Common fare at these kiosks generally includes a traditional Highland dish made with maize and beans that is served with a variety of beef, chicken, goat, or mutton. Additionally, *nyama choma* (roasted meat) may be available for those who can afford it. The indoor alternative to these street kiosks is a *hoteli* (restaurant), typically serving a reasonably priced lunch, which often is the main meal of the day (Sobania, 2003).

 ## HOLIDAY MENUS

Holidays celebrated in Kenya include New Year's Day (January 1), Easter weekend in April (Good Friday through Easter Monday), Labor Day (May 1), *Eid ul-fitr* (festival celebrated by Muslims marking the end of Ramadan, typically in the tenth month of the Islamic calendar), Christmas (December 25), and the traditionally British holiday, Boxing Day (December 26). Other holidays specific to Kenya are Moi Day, Kenyatta Day, Madaraka Day, and Jamhuri. Moi Day (October 10) signifies when Daniel arap Moi became president. Kenyatta Day (October 20) signifies when Mzee Jomo Kenyatta was arrested for opposing British rule in 1952. Madaraka Day (June 1) commemorates when Kenya attained internal self-rule in 1963 prior to its Independence Day (December 12, 1963). Independence Day, also called *Jamhuri*, is a national holiday and considered the most important day of the year.

These holidays are most commonly celebrated with feasts. For example, a lunch feast is the meal of celebration for Christmas in Kenya. *Nyama choma* (roasted meat) is the dish most commonly used for celebrations and feasts (Sobania, 2003). Meat feasts are also held when elders or warriors decide it is time to do so, but typically they correspond to celebrating a rite of passage; and, as in many cultures, the cut of meat and who is allowed to eat the choice cuts is "strictly regulated by custom" (Sobania, 2003, p. 122). According to Sobania, no ceremony or social gathering is complete without

beer. In fact, the Kipsigis drink from a communal beer pot as part of their ceremonies. Beer is also considered repayment to those who provide neighborly assistance with crops or other projects on the compound in times of need (Sobania, 2003).

 ## HEALTH BELIEFS AND CONCERNS

According to Tanaka (2000), the Gusii people of western Kenya do not perceive distinct differences between illness, disease, or misfortune. Although they believe that diseases can be caused by a variety of factors, when a person becomes sick or dies, they often point to a supernatural cause. Supernatural causes of disease can include *chisokoro* (ancestral spirits), *ebirecha* (evil spirits), and witchcraft. For example, mental health problems, infertility, chronic wounds, and epilepsy are linked to witchcraft and the evil eye. The Gusii also believe that illness and disease can be caused by breaking cultural taboos, lying, sexual offenses (particularly adultery), and naturalistic causes (e.g., bad air). The Gusii's preferred method of treatment for illnesses and diseases depends on the disease types and their causes. They either use traditional healing methods, modern Western medicine, or a combination of the two. Hospitals and clinics are primary sources for medical attention, but community health workers and traditional healers are also used by the Luhya and other tribes (Bradley, 2005).

The Kipsigis, a clan among the larger Kalenjin ethnic group, also possess traditional health beliefs. For example, a common belief is that drinking boiled water too frequently causes stomach illness. In addition, pregnant women should not eat eggs, sweet potatoes, chicken, sugarcane, or honey, because eating these foods will make the baby too big and therefore cause birth complications (Tanaka, 2000).

Another belief among western Kenyans that is related to health and nutrition is the notion of *ledho* or *heru*, which is used to explain thinness and failure to thrive in very young children. As Whyte and Kariuki (1997) explain, "If a breastfeeding mother becomes pregnant, it is thought that the nursing child is in a dangerous relationship to the child in its mother's womb. It is weaned immediately 'for its own good'... [and] some mothers even avoid holding the 'displaced' child, in order to protect it from ledho caused by contact with its unborn sibling" (p. 137).

Furthermore, many peoples (including the Luo) associate fatness (e.g., "big bellies") with "wealth and good health" (p. 244) and leadership positions, whereas

TABLE 32-1 Communication "Do's and Don'ts"

Verbal Communication Do's	Verbal Communication Don'ts
Address the eldest member of the family first.[a]	Tell clients what to do; instead, respect their independence and discuss what works well for others who are in similar situations (more indirect).[b]
Tailor information to the client by first asking more open-ended questions, then reinforcing client response and elaboration. This demonstrates a caring attitude and creates trust.[c]	Ask direct questions about sensitive topics (e.g., sex, child birth, or child care) among the Luo; instead, use metaphors and stories to convey health message, or keep discussion general.[b]

Nonverbal Communication Do's	Nonverbal Communication Don'ts
When eating *ugali*, use the right hand to break off the dough and form it into a scoop, which can then be used to eat other foods.[d]	Point finger at someone from the Kipsigis tribe.[e]
Wear clothes that cover legs and shoulders in Muslim regions (mainly coastal Kenya).[a]	Eat with the left hand (considered improper).[d]
Recognize the high status of elders in the community,[b] and establish strong rapport with communities before attempting major behavior changes.[f]	Photograph without permission.[a]
Arrange for male field workers to talk to men and female field workers to talk to women among the Luo (fits most tribes in this region).[b]	Approach Luo women before establishing rapport with Luo men and elders in the community.[f]
Smile and shake hands, but act in less formal manner to establish trust.[c]	

Sources are as follows:
[a]Best of Kenya (2005) [c]Kim, Odallo, Thuo, & Kols (1999) [e]Tanaka (2000)
[b]Blount (1972) [d]Food in Every Country (2007) [f]Southall (1972)

thinness is linked with sickness and a lack of resources to eat well (Ogoye-Ndegwa & Aagaard-Hansen, 2006); however, it is noteworthy that this standard does not apply to women, partly because women traditionally have not been considered for leadership positions. Also, extreme thinness is associated with *chira* (a type of curse) (Whyte & Kariuki, 1997) and HIV/AIDS (Ogoye-Ndegwa, 2005, as cited in Ogoye-Ndegwa & Aagaard-Hansen, 2006).

Another common belief among Kenyans is that there are various types of *chira* (curse) that affect both children and adults. Almost all cases of *chira* are linked to some violation of cultural principles governing sexuality and/or seniority. *Chira* (*ishira* in the Luyha languages) also can occur due to carelessness in adhering to the proper separation of sexuality between generations. For example, one common belief is that it is un-acceptable for a grandmother who is still sleeping with her husband to hold her grandchild (Whyte & Kariuki, 1997). There are also a variety of possible causes of *chira* in children, including these two examples from a study of Luo people: (1) when a midwife (*jacholo*) who has assisted in delivery has intercourse with her husband within the required 3-day abstinence period; and (2) if two women who are still breastfeeding engage in a fight (Olenja, 1991).

Among the Luo, hunger is symbolically associated with internal parasitic worms in the human body destroying external predators (ogres); therefore, the "sound" of intestinal muscular contractions is interpreted as a sign of hunger because "the worms are hungry and crying for food" (Ogoye-Ndegwa & Aagaard-Hansen, 2006, p. 241). In addition, the Luo view naming as a culturally significant activity. According to Ogoye-Ndegwa and Aagaard-Hansen (2006, p. 234), "Naming practices show that famine, food, and food-related activities and observances are an important lens in understanding and constructing local history and defining cosmic relationship among the Luo."

 ## GENERAL HEALTH AND NUTRITIONAL INDICATORS SUMMARY

Nutritional deficiencies negatively impact both child and adult health by contributing to increased rates of disability, illness, and death, as well as adversely affecting long-term growth and development (Skolnik, 2008). Furthermore, high rates of malnutrition adversely affect Kenya's economic growth by reducing human capital and potential. In Kenya as a whole, child mortality rates and malnutrition remain high, and efforts to reduce the two have been complicated by the HIV/AIDS epidemic that has left numerous children orphaned and at increased risk for malnutrition (Kabubo-Mariara, Ndenge, & Mwabu, 2008).

Improving the nutrition of children is of utmost importance in attaining Millennium Development Goals (MDGs), particularly those related to child health (United Nations, 2008). Kabubo-Mariara et al. (2008) asserted that helping women attain at least a secondary education would make a tremendous difference regarding child nutrition and help achieve MDGs related to child health and nutrition. Because women are the primary caregivers, their level of education markedly impacts the health and well-being of their children, including their nutritional status. For example, the more educated Kenyan women are, the more likely they are to breastfeed their babies at least up to 6 months. In addition, they are more likely to take proactive steps toward providing better nutrition to their families, such as preparing orange-flesh varieties of sweet potato that are rich in vitamin A (Hagenimana & Low, 2000).

It is important to note that UNICEF (2007) has identified nutritional indicators for the world's children. For 1996–2005, these indicators for Kenya were as follows: 13% of children were exclusively breastfed for at least 6 months, 84% were breastfed with complementary foods at 6–9 months, and 57% were still breastfeeding at 20–23 months. In addition, for 1998–2005, 10% of Kenya's infants were born with low birth weight. For 1996–2005,

20% of children under 5 years suffered from moderate and severe underweight, 4% suffered from severe underweight, 6% suffered from moderate and severe wasting, and 30% suffered from moderate and severe stunting. In addition, in 2004, the vitamin A supplementation coverage rate for young Kenyan children between 6 and 59 months was 63%, and 91% of households consumed iodized salt between 1998 and 2005.

 ## COMMUNICATION AND COUNSELING TIPS

There are many considerations in communicating with people from western Kenya that vary by tribe. For instance, in the Kipsigis people, it is considered taboo to point directly at somebody because it might cause disease (Tanaka, 2000). It is also considered impolite to ask a guest to leave. When guests leave, the host may walk with the departing guests well past the front door, escorting them for part of their trip home (Sobania, 2003). In addition, tales using animals as metaphors are popular in western Kenya. These tales are used to pass along moral stories and other wisdom to younger generations, often by a Senior Mother or *Ma Mkubwa* (Sobania, 2003).

One guiding principle in working with people from western Kenya is to establish a rapport with elders and clergy or "diviners" first and gain their approval before communicating with the target or priority population. Another guiding principle is that cultural competence must be carefully practiced when working with health beliefs different from one's own to prevent loss of trust in members of that community. The ancient Greek physician Hippocrates' well-known rule, "First, do no harm" (Greek Texts, 2005), should be considered by those working with tribes that hold traditions sacred, particularly when their beliefs and/or practices conflict with those of the health professionals. Airhihenbuwa (1995), creator of the PEN-3 model for culturally appropriate health education, details identifying health behaviors as positive, negative, or existential, meaning that they may be indigenous to the culture but do not actually harm the person; therefore, cultural competence is a prerequisite for understanding health beliefs and health behaviors in order to work more effectively with a particular person.

TABLE 32-2   Primary Language of Food Names with English and Phonetic Translation

Swahili	English Translation	Phonetic Translation
Sukuma wiki	Push the week	Soo-KOO-muh wee-kee
Nyama choma	Roasted meat	NYAH-mah CHO-mah
Mchuzi wa samaki	Fish and curry	SHOO-zee wah Suh-MAH-kee
Kuku na nazi	Chicken with coconut	Koo-koo na NAH-zee
Kienyeji	Native way or indigenous to the country	Kyen-YEH-jee

Matoke (Plantains)

12 plantains (ripe or unripe as desired)

Salt to taste

Curry powder

Spring onions (chopped)

3 tbsp. butter (optional)

Seasonings (optional):

Royko® Mchuzi

Knorr® cubes

Pepper

1. Peel the plantains and cut into pieces.
2. Put in a deep saucepan and add 3 cups of water, adding more if necessary until cooked.
3. Add salt and curry powder to taste, then spread the onions over the plantains with the desired seasonings.
4. Bring to a boil and then cook on medium-low heat until the pieces are soft and fully cooked.
5. Remove from the heat. If there is more liquid than desired, drain it off. Serve hot or cold mashed or unmashed.

Variations:

Plantains can be cut into smaller pieces and deep-fried (especially if they are almost ripe).

Plantains can be roasted over the heat, wrapped in aluminum foil, or baked in the oven.

Yields 6 servings

Recipe courtesy of Fletcher Njororai

More recipes are available at http://nutrition.jbpub.com/foodculture/

FEATURED RECIPE

Matoke bananas are cooked and eaten as a main meal with vegetables and soup, meats, chicken, or fish. They can be mashed on their own or with sweet potatoes.

REFERENCES

African Studies Center. University of Pennsylvania. (n.d.). Accessed July 22, 2008, from http://www.sas.upenn.edu/African_Studies/Cookbook/Kenya.html/

Airhihenbuwa, C. (1995). *Health and culture: Beyond the western paradigm*. Thousand Oaks, CA: Sage Publications.

Best of Kenya (2005). *Frequently asked questions*. Accessed July 23, 2008, from http://www.bestofkenya.com/faq.htm/

Blount, B.G. (1972). The Luo of South Nyanza, western Kenya. In A. Molnos (Ed.), *Innovations and communication* (pp. 275–280). Nairobi, Kenya: East African Publishing House.

Bradley, C. (2005). Luyia. In *Encyclopedia of world cultures* (Vol. 9): *Africa and the Middle East* (pp. 202–206). Retrieved March 22, 2008, from http://www.gale.cengage.com/servlet/ItemDetailServlet?region=9&imprint=000&titleCode=M40E&cf=e&type=4&id=226742

Central Intelligence Agency (CIA). (2008). *The world factbook: Kenya*. Retrieved April 18, 2008, from http://www.cia.gov/library/publications/the-world-factbook/geos/ke.html/

Conelly, W.T., & Chaiken, M.S. (2000). Intensive farming, agrodiversity, and food security under conditions of extreme population pressure in western Kenya. *Human Ecology, 28,* 19–51.

DeVoe, D. (2008). *Preventing a Great Lakes food crisis*. Retrieved April 18, 2008, from http://crs.org/kenya/crop-control/

Embassy of Kenya. (2006). *Kenya*. Retrieved May 20, 2008, from http://kenyaembassy.com/geninfo.html/

Encyclopedia Britannica Online. (2008). *Luo*. Retrieved April 18, 2008, from http://www.britannica.com/EBchecked/topic/351643/Luo/

Food in Every Country (2007). *Kenya*. Retrieved July 22, 2008, from http://www.foodbycountry.com/Kazakhstan-to-South-Africa/Kenya.html/

Frison, E.A., Cherfas, J., Eyzaguirre, P.B., & Johns, T. (2004). *Biodiversity, nutrition, and health: Making a difference to hunger and conservation in the developing world*. Keynote address to the Seventh Meeting of the Conference of the Parties to the Convention on Biological Diversity (COP 7). Retrieved April 18, 2008, from http://www.cbd.int/doc/speech/2004/sp-2004-02-09-cop-02-en.pdf/

Gardner, A. (1993). *Karibu: Welcome to the cooking of Kenya*. Nairobi, Kenya: Kenway.

Geissler, P.W. (2000). The significance of earth-eating: Social and cultural aspects of geophagy among Luo children. *Africa: Journal of the International African Institute, 70,* 653–682.

Geissler, P.W., Mwaniki, D.L., Thiong'o, F., & Friis, H. (1997). Geophagy among school children in western Kenya. *Tropical Medicine and International Health, 2,* 624–630.

Greek Texts. (2005). *Hippocrates*. Retrieved August 14, 2008, from http://greek-texts.com/library/Hippocrates/index.html/

Hagenimana, V., & Low, J. (2000). Potential of orange-fleshed sweet potatoes for raising vitamin A intake in Africa. *Food and Nutrition Bulletin, 21,* 414–418.

iExplore. (2008). *Kenya travel tips: Do's and don'ts*. Retrieved May 14, 2008, from http://www.iexplore.com/res/d.jhtml?destination=Kenya&type=Do's-and+Don'ts/

JamboKenya. (2008a). *Locations: western Kenya*. Retrieved March 27, 2008, from http://www.jambokenya.com/jambo/location/wkenya.htm/

JamboKenya. (2008b). *Geography: Western Kenya*. Retrieved March 27, 2008, from http://www.jambokenya.com/jambo/kenya/geogrph4.htm/

JamboKenya. (2008c). *Locations: Lake Victoria and Kisumu*. Retrieved March 27, 2008, from http://www.jambokenya.com/jambo/location/victoria.htm/

JamboKenya. (2008d). *Locations: Mt. Elgon region*. Retrieved March 27, 2008, from http://www.jambokenya.com/jambo/location/mtelgon.htm/

Jenkins, O.B. (2003). *People profile: The Luhya of Kenya*. Retrieved April 18, 2008, from http://strategyleader.org/profiles/luhya.html/

Johns, T., & Duquette, M. (1991). Detoxification and mineral supplementation as functions of geophagy. *American Journal of Clinical Nutrition, 53,* 448–456.

Johns, T., & Kokwaro, J.O. (1991). Food plants of the Luo of Siaya district, Kenya. *Economic Botany, 45,* 103–113.

Johnson-Welch, C. (n.d.). *Linking agriculture and nutrition: The human dimension*. Retrieved April 28, 2008, from http://www.cipotato.org/vitaa/Proceedings/VITAA-paper-ICRW-jsedit-back%20to%20Carmen-20Mar2002.pdf/

Kabubo-Mariara, J., Ndenge, G.K., & Mwabu, D.K. (2008). Determinants of children's nutritional status in Kenya: Evidence from demographic and health surveys. *Journal of African Economies,* 1–25. doi:10.1093/jae/ejn024/.

Kenyalogy. (2008). *Population and culture*. Retrieved May 21, 2008, from http://www.kenyalogy.com/eng/info/pobla.html/

Kim, Y.M., Odallo, D., Thuo, M., & Kols, A. (1999). Client participation and provider communication in family planning counseling: Transcript analysis in Kenya. *Health Communication, 11*(1), 1–19.

Kittler, P.G., & Sucher, K. (2004). *Food and culture*. Belmont, CA: Thomson/Wadsworth.

Lindblade, K.A., Odhiambo, F., Rosen, D.H., & DeCock, K.M. (2003). Health and nutritional status of orphans <6 years old cared for by relatives in western Kenya. *Tropical Medicine and International Health, 8,* 67–72.

Microsoft Encarta Online Encyclopedia. (2008). *Kenya*. Retrieved May 20, 2008, from http://encarta.msn.com/encyclopedia_761564507/Kenya.html/

Muruli, L.A., London, D.M., Misiko, M., Okusi, K., Sikana, P.M., & Palm, C.A. (1999). *Strengthening research and development linkages for soil fertility: Pathways of agricultural information dissemination* (Project report to IDRC). Kenya: Institute of African Studies, University of Nairobi.

National Standard Research Collaboration. (2008). *Vitamin A (retinol)*. Retrieved August 30, 2008, from http://www.nlm.nih.gov/medlineplus/druginfo/natural/patient-vitamina.html/

Ogoye-Ndegwa, C., & Aagaard-Hansen, J. (2003). Traditional gathering of wild vegetables among the Luo of Western Kenya: A nutritional anthropology project. *Ecology of Food and Nutrition, 42,* 69–89.

Ogoye-Ndegwa, C., & Aagaard-Hansen, J. (2006). Famines and famished bodies in a food deficit locality among the Luo of Kenya. *Food & Foodways, 14,* 231–247.

Olenja, J. (1991). Factors which influence child health with specific reference to nutrition in Siaya district western Kenya. *Journal of Tropical Pediatrics, 37*, 136–139.

Oniang'o, R.K., & Komokoti, A. (1999). Food habits in Kenya: The effect of change and attendant methodological problems. *Appetite, 32*, 93–96.

Skolnik, R. (2008). *Essentials of global health.* Sudbury, MA: Jones and Bartlett.

Sobania, N. (2003). *Culture and customs of Kenya.* Westport, CT: Greenwood Press.

Southall, A.W. (1972). The Luo of South Nyanza, western Kenya. In A. Molnos (Ed.), *Innovations and communication.* Nairobi, Kenya: East African Publishing House.

Tanaka, K. (2000). *Medical anthropological study in western Kenya and its implications for community health development* (IDCJ Working Paper Series No. 55). Tokyo: International Development Center of Japan.

UNICEF. (2007). *The state of the world's children 2007: Women and children, the double dividend of gender equality.* Retrieved April 14, 2009, from http://www.unicef.org/sowc07/statistics/tables.php

United Nations. (2008). *Millenium development goals 2015: Make it happen.* Retrieved April 19, 2009, from http://www.un.org/millenniumgoals/

University of Bath. (2008). *What is cassava?* Retrieved May 21, 2008, from http://www.bath.ac.uk/bio-sci/cassava-project/about.html/

U.S. Department of State. (2006). *Kenya: International religious freedom report 2006.* Retrieved April 18, 2008, from http://www.state.gov/g/drl/rls/irf/2006/71307.htm/

Whyte, M.A. (1997). The social and cultural contexts of food production in Uganda and Kenya. In T.S. Weisner, C. Bradley, & P.L. Kilbride (Eds.), *African families and the crisis of social change* (pp. 125–134). Westport, CT: Bergin & Garvey.

Whyte, S.R., & Kariuki, P.W. (1997). Malnutrition and gender relations in western Kenya. In T.S. Weisner, C. Bradley, & P.L. Kilbride (Eds.), *African families and the crisis of social change* (pp. 135–153). Westport, CT: Bergin & Garvey.

World Almanac & Book of Facts. (2005). *Kenya.* Retrieved February 8, 2008, from http://www.worldalmanac.com/

World Bank. (2008a). *Data and statistics: Country classification.* Retrieved July 17, 2008, from http://web.worldbank.org/WBSITE/EXTERNAL/DATASTATISTICS/0,,contentMDK:20420458~menuPK:64133156~pagePK:64133150~piPK:64133175~theSitePK:239419,00.html/

World Bank. (2008b). *Data and statistics: Country groups.* Retrieved July 17, 2008, from http://web.worldbank.org/WBSITE/EXTERNAL/DATASTATISTICS/0,,contentMDK:20421402~pagePK:64133150~piPK:64133175~theSitePK:239419,00.html/

World Bank. (2008c). *Joint statement by the African Development Bank and the World Bank on the situation in Kenya.* Retrieved July 17, 2008, from http://web.worldbank.org/WBSITE/EXTERNAL/NEWS/0,,contentMDK:21618245~pagePK:34370~piPK:34424~theSitePK:4607,00.html/

World Health Organization (WHO). (2008a). *Health risks and consequences of female genital mutilation.* Retrieved May 21, 2008, from http://www.who.int/reproductive-health/fgm/impact.htm/

World Health Organization (WHO). (2008b). *Kenya.* Retrieved May 21, 2008, from http://www.who.int/countries/ken/en/

World66. (2008). *Western Kenya travel guide.* Retrieved March 27, 2008, from http://www.world66.com/africa/kenya/westernkenya/

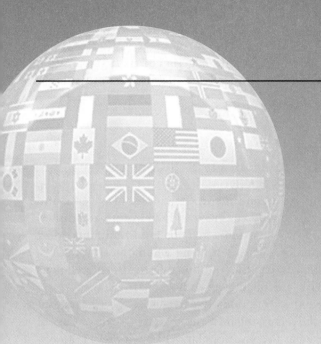

CHAPTER 33

Nigeria

Titilayo O. Ologhobo, BS, MPH Candidate
Jeffrey I. Harris, DrPH, MPH, RD, LDN

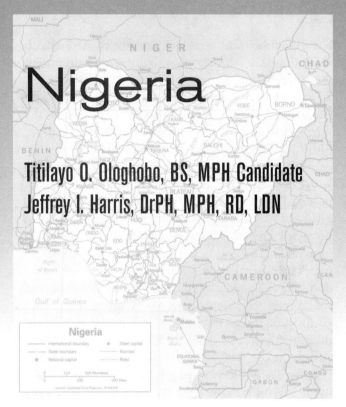

 ## CULTURE AND WORLD REGION

Nigeria, with an estimated area of 923,768 km² and a population of about 130 million people, is situated in the western part of sub-Saharan Africa. It is a culturally diverse nation as evidenced by the various languages spoken, the various dialects that exist within the same local language, the lifestyles that highlight various tribal classifications, and a variety of local cuisines. Food in Nigeria plays an important role in distinguishing one tribe from another as well as serving as a source of pride to Nigeria's many ethnic groups. Each ethnic group has its distinct taste and flavor. Nigerians, although diverse in their cuisine based on geographic region and local culture, generally possess a strong affinity for locally made foods, which tend to be rich in spices, palm oil, and boiled vegetables/leaves, and high in carbohydrates, fat, and fiber.

Nigeria is located in the western part of the African continent along the Gulf of Guinea, and shares its borders with the Republic of Benin in the west, Cameroon in the east, and Niger and Chad in the north. Nigeria is a federal republic that consists of 36 states with Abuja as the nation's capital.

 ## LANGUAGE

English, which was selected to aid the cultural and linguistic unity of the country, is the official language of Nigeria (Refugee Health: Immigrant Health, 2004). Three major indigenous languages, Hausa, Yoruba, and Ibo, are spoken by three major tribes, and about 500 dialects are spoken by different ethnic groups (Refugee Health: Immigrant Health, 2004). Pidgin, a blend of indigenous and English languages, is common in the southern and eastern parts of Nigeria. Pidgin English was created when the British sailors needed to communicate with local merchants (Countries and Their Cultures, 2007). Presently, pidgin is commonly spoken by people who have little or no formal education in English (Countries and Their Cultures, 2007).

CULTURE HISTORY

Nigeria is the most populous country in Africa with more than 250 ethnic groups, but the most dominant are Hausa (29%), Yoruba (21%), Ibo (18%), Ijaw (10%), Kanuri (4%), Ibibio (3.5%), and Tiv (2.5%) (World Factbook, 2007). The Hausa people are located in the northern part of the country, and 90% of them are Muslims. The Yoruba people are located in the western part of the country, and are predominantly Christians with a small percentage of Muslims and traditional believers. Traditional believers are people who believe in a variety of local deities and herbal doctors who are popularly known as Babalawo. The Babalawos prepare local and herbal concoctions that are locally known as juju. Their practices are similar to witchcraft and voodoo. The Ibo people are located in the eastern part of the country, and are predominantly Christians. Other ethnic groups, such as Delta, Edo, Tiv, Ibibio, Kanuri, Jukun, Nupes, and Ijaw, are located in the southern part of the country.

The Neolithic Nok people were the first inhabitants in Nigeria from 800 BC to 200 AD, and they flourished in Jos where they made terra-cotta sculptures (Infoplease, 2007). Jos, one of the most important tourist destinations in Nigeria, is the capital of Plateau State, which is located in the central part of Nigeria. In the 8th century, the Kanem Bornu Dynasty was founded and reigned in the north, and was a major influence on the development of the nation of Nigeria. By the 11th century, Islam was introduced, and the Kanuri, Fulani, and Hausa people migrated to northern Nigeria. Due to the trans-Sahara trade with the North Africans and Arabs, the Kanem Borno Empire began to convert to Islam (Infoplease, 2007). The northern people founded the Sokoto Caliphate, which ruled the region until it was taken over by the British. In the 19th century, Britain influenced and controlled Nigeria until it gained independence on October 1, 1960. The civilian government was, however, short-lived because the country came under military rule in 1966. Later, a democratic government emerged ending 16 years of military rule. On May 20, 1999, the new civilian president was inaugurated, but 8 years into civilian rule, there were religious conflicts that threatened the stability of the country (Infoplease, 2007). These clashes were between Muslims and Christians in northern

Nigeria. In April, 2007, Nigeria had its first transition from one democratically elected president to another (Infoplease, 2007).

FOOD HISTORY WITHIN THE CULTURE

Food plays a vital role in the culture of Nigeria, and each ethnic group has its own food history and dishes, depending on customs, religion, and traditions. Most ceremonies, such as naming ceremonies, weddings, engagement parties, traditional festivals, and religious holidays, are incomplete without sharing a meal.

Food is traditionally eaten with the fingers, but with the increasing influence of foreign cultures use of cutlery has become popular. Although there is an obvious effect of western influence on Nigerian culture, some traditional values have endured (Countries and Their Cultures, 2007). For instance, using the left hand to eat, smelling food that has already been prepared, declining to offer foods to guests when they visit, and talking when eating, are considered impolite.

A TYPICAL NIGERIAN'S EATING HABITS

Most families in the rural areas stick to traditional foods and preparation techniques, whereas families in the urban areas consume more canned, frozen, and packaged foods (Countries and Their Cultures, 2007). Staple crops, such as rice, yam, and cassava, are the base of the Nigerian diet and are often eaten with tomato stews and vegetable soups. In all ethnic regions, white rice, boiled yam, bread, and boiled beans are often eaten with tomato stew as a main meal, served with beef, chicken, turkey, or fresh fish. A typical Nigerian family eats three square meals per day. Table 33-1 shows a typical day's menu for an average Nigerian in all geographic regions.

REGIONAL VARIATIONS OF NIGERIAN CUISINES

Most eating habits and Nigerian cuisines are similar among ethnic groups, but there are slight variations among urban/rural areas and geographic regions. In most urban areas, a typical Nigerian meal at any time of the day consists of a one-course meal and fruits,

TABLE 33-1   A Typical Day's Menu for an Average Nigerian in All Regions

Breakfast	Lunch	Dinner
White bread/boiled yam, fried eggs/tomato stew, tea/coffee or cereal, *ogi/pap* (cereal made from maize)	Rice, beef/chicken/fish stew or pounded yam, *egusi* (melon soup), *efo* (vegetable soup, juice)	Dodo (fried plantain), fish/egg stew or boiled beans, *moin-moin* (steamed bean cake)

such as oranges, grapes, bananas, pineapples, and watermelon, are served as appetizers, whereas most meals in the rural areas consist of one-course meals with no appetizers. Pounded yam served with melon-seed soup (*egusi*) or spinach soup (*efo*), and *amala* served with okra soup, melon-seed soup, or spinach soup, are mostly consumed by the Yoruba people in western Nigeria. *Eba* (soft dough made with processed cassava called *gari*) served with pumpkin-leaves soup, palm-kernel soup, or okra soup is consumed by the Ibo, Ijaw, Delta, and Edo tribes located in eastern and southern Nigeria. All of the aforementioned dishes are also served with either beef, *pomo* (made from cow skin), or dried fish. *Moin-moin* (steamed bean cake) is common among the Hausa and Yoruba tribes in the northern and western parts of the country, and it is eaten as a main course served with either *ogi* or *pap* (a cereal made from soaked maize) or *gari*. In the north, especially among the Muslims, pork is forbidden. Beef in a roasted form, called *suya*, and *balangu* (roasted meat made from sheep and goat), both of which are common in the northern part of the country, have become delicacies. In all ethnic regions, pepper soup made from ox tail, or the offal of sheep or goat, may serve as the appetizer to a main meal. In eastern Nigeria, where the Ibo people predominantly reside, *Isi-ewu* (goat-head pepper soup) is served with vegetables and is usually eaten as a main meal.

MAJOR FOODS

Protein Sources

Legumes and peas, particularly black-eyed peas, are important sources of protein for Nigerians of low socioeconomic status, providing from 20 to 30% of protein in the diet. Other plant sources of protein include groundnuts and legumes such as cowpeas, soybeans, benne seed, coconut, African locust bean, and palm nut (Muhammad & Amusa, 2005). Sources of animal protein include meat, poultry, fish, pork, bush meat, snails, shrimps, termites, eggs, cheese, and milk.

Starch Sources

Starch sources include grains, such as maize, rice, guinea corn, sorghum, and millet; fruits, such as plantain and banana; and root tubers, such as yam, cocoyam, sweet potato, Irish potato, and cassava.

Fat Sources

Fats as sources of fatty acids include oils such as groundnut, soybean, sesame, and palm, all of which are usually used in cooking. Most Nigerian soups are prepared with a lot of fats and oils (Alade, 1985), but due to growing health concerns, sesame oil, sunflower oil, and olive oil are now more commonly used.

Prominent Vegetables

Most fruits and vegetables are rich in water-soluble vitamins, including the B vitamins and vitamin C, photochemicals, and substantial amounts of fiber (Alade, 1985). The common vegetables consumed are tomatoes, spicy red peppers (commonly called *rodo*), bell peppers, carrots, coconuts, pumpkin leaves, green leaves, okra, spinach, bitter leaves, ginger, garlic, onions, and cabbage.

Prominent Fruits

Common fruits are mango, orange, sugarcane, grape fruit, tangerines, banana, pineapple, African pear, cashew fruit, avocado pear, almond fruit, watermelon, African apple, pawpaw, pitanga, cherry, and African apricot.

Spices, Seasonings, and Condiments

Ndukwu and Ben-Nwadibia (n.d.) described spices and condiments as products of plants that are mostly used for seasoning and enhancing the taste of food, but it is sometimes believed that they have medicinal properties

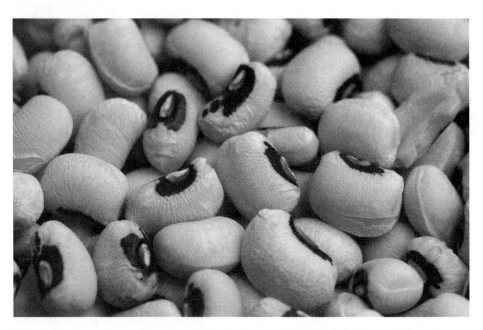

Black-eyed peas provide 20 to 30% of protein in the Nigerian diet.

and are therefore used in the treatment and management of diseases. In Nigeria, the commonly used spices and condiments include pepper, salt, curry, thyme, bouillon cubes, ginger, nutmeg, clove, basil leaves, red pepper, and chili pepper.

 ## Beverages

Palm wine, a natural juice from palm trees, is a favorite drink throughout Nigeria, especially in the south where the trees grow wild. Burukutu (BKT) is a local beer brewed from *dawa* (millet) and is very popular in the north. Another local drink, *zobo*, is also common in northern Nigeria. It is made from a flower called *Hibiscus sabdariff* (Kolawole & Maduenyi, 2004), which is boiled to remove the reddish color before sugar and other flavorings are added.

 ## Desserts

Dessert is not common in Nigerian culture, but appetizers, such as soups, pastry snacks, and finger foods, are common accompaniments to a Nigerian meal.

 ## FOODS WITH CULTURAL SIGNIFICANCE

The Ibo people in eastern Nigeria celebrate the New Yam festival, which is locally called the *Iri-ji*. Yams are one of the highly regarded root tubers, and a symbol that is integrated into social, cultural, economic, and religious aspects of life (Ukachukwu, 2007). This festival symbolizes the abundance of yam produce, and it is believed that the New Year must start with fresh or new yams. During the festival, only dishes of yam are served, and the leftover yam, which is known as the "old yam," must be thrown away.

The Yoruba people in western Nigeria place great importance on naming ceremonies, and honey and salt play significant roles in the naming of a child. Honey symbolizes that the child will be as mighty as the ocean, and salt is used as a reminder that life has adversity.

In many other tribes, the breaking and eating of kola nut plays a significant social role during festivals, engagement parties, traditional marriages, reconciliation, and burial ceremonies (Afrimedia Project, 2004). On these occasions, kola nut offered or shared signifies friendship, respect, hospitality, and mutual understanding (Afrimedia Project, 2004). Palm wine is a symbolic drink that also signifies hospitality, respect, and mutual understanding, and plays a social role during traditional wedding ceremonies, festivals, heralding events, and libation (Falconer, 1990).

 ## TYPICAL DAY'S MENU

Nigerians have a wide choice of where and what to eat, ranging from local and international cuisine, which

Observations from the Author (T.O. Ologhobo)

Upon my arrival in the United States in 2005, I had a few acculturation issues in terms of adjusting to American cuisines. I hardly went to restaurants because the meals were completely different from the traditional dishes that I grew up eating in Nigeria. I was not impressed by the few meals I had tasted, so I made an assumption at that time that most of the meals in the United States were bland and not well seasoned. I also noticed the differences between main-course meals and side dishes in the United States and Nigeria. A meal from a Nigerian's perspective consists of carbohydrates as the main dish, and meat (beef, chicken, or fish) as the side dish, whereas in the United States, the main meal consists of mostly meat, with carbohydrates as the side dish. Living in the United States for 3 years, and my perspective on American cuisines has changed. I have adjusted to these differences, but I still prefer spicy foods and only prepare Nigerian meals, or go to restaurants that serve spicy dishes.

Another difficulty I had with regard to American cuisines is the concept of well done vs medium rare. Nigerians eat everything well done. We believe that if the food is not cooked completely, the chances of becoming ill increase. My first experience with this was when I ordered eggs sunny side up and the waitress returned with runny eggs. I was highly upset and asked for the eggs to be scrambled instead. My experience in that restaurant made me realize that the Nigerian notion of well-done fried eggs is completely different from the American perspective. I am still trying to get used to the concept of rare and medium-rare food.

hotels and restaurants especially in the major cities offer, to the quick-service chains that are now becoming a common feature in the cities. The favorite roadside restaurants called *bukateria* serve locally prepared dishes. These restaurants are often patronized by people of modest income, but occasionally by wealthier people also, because such restaurants offer the best local cuisine.

 HOLIDAY MENUS

There are two major religions in Nigeria: Christianity and Islam; 40% of the people are Christians, 50% are Muslims, and the remaining 10% are traditional believers or have other beliefs (World Factbook, 2007). The Christian holidays include Christmas and Easter, and the foods consumed during these occasions are

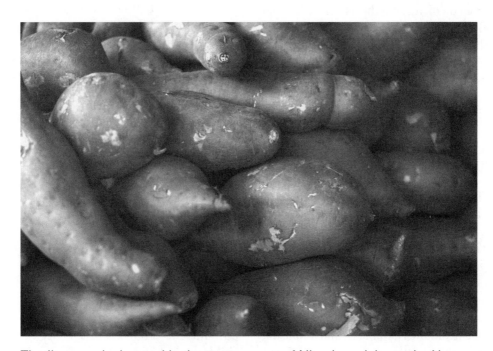

The Ibo people, located in the eastern part of Nigeria, celebrate the New Yam festival that is locally called the *Iri-ji*.

chicken, turkey, *moin-moin*, fried plantain, fried rice, and jollof rice. On Good Friday, most Christians avoid any kind of meat and eat fish instead, because they believe that meat is unwholesome for this day. The Muslim holidays include *Eid ul-Fitr*, which marks the end of the Ramadan; *Eid el-Kabir*, which marks the end of the hajj season; and *Eid el-Maulud*, which marks the birthday of Mohammed. Most foods consumed on Muslim holidays are similar to those eaten on Christmas and Easter except on *Eid el-Kabir*, when rams are killed and cooked to mark the day.

There are four major secular holidays in Nigeria: New Year's Day (January 1), Workers' Day (May 1), Children's Day (May 27), and National Day (October 1), but New Year's Day is the major feasting day (Countries and Their Cultures, 2007). The dishes prepared on New Year's Day include jollof rice, fried rice, *moin-moin*, fried plantain, and pounded yam with melon-seed soup.

 ## HEALTH BELIEFS AND CONCERNS

Modern and herbal forms of medicine are common in Nigeria, but herbal medicine is sometimes preferred to modern health practices because often it is effective and has little or no side effects (Countries and Their Cultures, 2007). Traditional believers and rural dwellers engage in herbal medicine, but the use of traditional healing methods and herbs have become widespread even among urban dwellers. Based on the health and cultural beliefs, vegetables, fruits, and spices are used to treat illnesses (Refugee Health–Immigrant Health, 2004), and most families have their personal remedies for minor health problems (Countries and Their Cultures, 2007). Ndukwu and Ben-Nwadibia (n.d) describe the medicinal uses of some commonly used spices and vegetables as follows:

1. Scent leaf. This is locally known as *efinrin* and is used as an anticonvulsant. It is also used to cure colds, fever, chest pain, and diarrhea.
2. Basil leaf. This is locally known as *esewon, efinrin po*, and *efinrin ajija*, and its juice is used as an anthelmintic.
3. Thyme. Generally known by the same name, thyme is used as a sedative, antiseptic, and anthelmintic.
4. Onion. It is locally known as *alubosa* and *alubarha*, and it is used to treat asthma, convulsion, ulcers, skin infections, and eye infections.

5. Garlic. It is locally known as *ayun* and is used to cure fevers, constipation, asthma, nervous disorders, and skin infections.
6. Nutmeg. Generally known by the same name, nutmeg is used to treat diarrhea and rheumatic pains.
7. Curry. It is used to cure diarrhea, dysentery, vomiting, herpes, and fever.
8. Chili pepper and red pepper. They are locally called *ata-jije, bini-isie*, and *ose-oyinbo*, and they are used to cure cold, fever, dysentery, malaria, and gonorrhea.
9. Ginger. It is locally known as *jinja, aje, orin*, and *atale*, and it is used to treat toothache, influenza, asthma, liver infections, cold, and cough.

A study by Obute (n.d.) described the ethnomedicinal use of some fruits and plants commonly consumed in southeastern Nigeria, which include:

1. Neem plant. It is locally known as *dogoyaro* and is used to treat chicken pox, malaria, ulcer, and eye infections.
2. Pawpaw. The unripe fruit is used as a diuretic agent and also for eczema and razor bumps. Johns, Booth, and Kuhlein (1992) state: "Barren women should be restricted from papaya because it is a delicacy for worms, and sterility is thought to be caused by worms."
3. Lime. It is used to cure colds, stomach cramps, and fever.
4. Lemon. It is used for weight loss, diarrhea, ulcer, and insect bites.
5. Palm oil. It is locally known as *epo* and is used as an antidote for poison and to treat skin infections.
6. Bitter kola. It is used as a stimulant and also to treat throat infections.
7. Cassava. The roots are used to treat eye infections.
8. Pumpkin leaf. It is locally known as *ugu* and is used to treat anemia.
9. Bitter leaf. It is used to treat hemorrhoids and diarrhea.

FORBIDDEN FOODS IN NIGERIA

Apart from the use of foods and plants for medicinal purposes, some foods that are rich in nutrients are considered as forbidden foods, and are generally avoided by immune-compromised people (e.g., pregnant women, children, and the elderly) (Onuorah & Ajayi, 1985). There are no scientific or nutritional facts that support these prohibitions, but they are based on cultural beliefs, many of which still persist in rural areas, and have a great impact on health status. Onuorah and Ajayi (1985) explain why some foods are avoided.

1. Eggs. Children should not be given eggs because they will become thieves.
2. Snails. Pregnant women should avoid snails because their babies will salivate and have slow speech.
3. Gizzard of chicken. It is believed to make men impotent and women infertile.
4. New yam. It must be eaten only after the New Yam festival.
5. Dogs. Pregnant women must not eat dogs because their babies will behave like dogs. Even though eating dogs is considered a taboo, some tribes, such as the Akwa Ibom and Ibibio, eat dog meat because it is believed to enhance their sex lives.
6. Pork. Muslims stay away from pork because it is considered an unclean animal.
7. Castor oil. It is believed to cause waist pain.
8. Sugar. It is generally believed that high intake of sugar could cause hemorrhoids and diabetes as well as reduce sperm count.

 GENERAL HEALTH AND NUTRITIONAL INDICATORS SUMMARY

The nutritional status of Nigerians was unfavorable before 1999 and the establishment of a democratic government, which led to significant remediation work to help Nigerians improve their nutritional profile. Recently, the Nigerian government has enacted initiatives to improve the nutrition of their people.

Nigerian children have suffered the most due to poor prevalence of breastfeeding, inadequate calories per person, crop failure, and lack of iron, vitamin A, and iodine-containing foods. Compared with the rest of the world, Nigeria ranks high in infant mortality, iron-deficiency anemia, stunting, and wasting. With lack of safe water in some areas and poor immunity due to nutritional inadequacy, children are at high risk of infectious disease. With more women entering the workforce, both parents and children are getting a high proportion of calories from convenience foods high in fat, sodium, and sugar, and low in fiber. These developments increase the probability that many Nigerian children will not reach their productive potential.

As previously mentioned, vitamin A, iron, and iodine deficiency are very common in Nigeria. Recent efforts, such as public health efforts to promote iodized salt and fortifying sugar, flour, and oil with vitamin A and iron, are sure to improve the nutritional status of the population. For example, most recent data show that 97% of Nigerian households use iodized salt.

In Nigeria there are significant disparities in nutritional status between urban and rural as well as north and south. People living in the north and rural areas have a greater prevalence of nutritional problems.

Nigerians are optimistic that recent public health efforts and governmental policies will improve things over time. For instance, in 1995 the National Policy on Food and Nutrition was drafted, and it was launched in 2002. Measures to improve national data collection have been implemented. Also, the National Committee on Food and Nutrition was established to oversee national efforts to improve food security and nutrition in Nigeria.

Even though much improvement is needed, Nigerians have much to be encouraged about in terms of nutrition. With increased globalization and relaxation of trade restrictions, Nigerians will have greater access to nutritive foods and, as a result, have greater earning capacity.

 COMMUNICATION AND COUNSELING TIPS

In a country with more than 200 languages, English is the most common language and the best mode of communication. For uneducated people, other languages, such as Yoruba, Ibo, Hausa, and pidgin, are used to communicate. Methods of communicating with the public include radio messages, television advertisements, posters, newspapers, billboards, and magazines. Some communication tips for foreigners and indigenes of Nigeria are as follows:

1. Be respectful of other religious views and cultures.
2. Be attentive and avoid interruption.
3. Use nonverbal communication methods such as nodding.
4. Use simple sentences and native languages, if necessary.
5. The one-on-one counseling visit is an effective approach.

The primary language of common foods with English translation is given in Table 33-2.

TABLE 33-2 Primary Language of Food Names with English Translation

Nigerian Names	English
Iresi	White rice
Obe Ata	Pepper soup
Efo	Vegetable soup
Egusi	Melon
Ila	Okra soup
Ewa	Beans
Moin-moin	Steamed bean cake
Isu	Yam
Dodo	Fried plantain
Gari	Dried processed cassava
Iyan	Pounded yam
Jollof	Jollof rice
Amala	Soft dough made from yam flour
Banga	Palm kernel soup
Edikikong	Water leaves and pumpkin leaves soup
Eba	Soft dough made from gari
Fufu	Soft dough made from cassava flour
Gbegiri	Bean soup
Ikpekere	Fried unripe plantain
Isi-ewu	Goat-head soup
Akara	Fried bean cake

Moin-Moin

2 cups black-eyed peas
2 tomatoes
½ onion
2 red peppers
1 cup water
1 tbsp. vegetable oil
2 boiled eggs (optional)
4 oz. corned beef (optional)
4 oz. diced meat (optional)
salt, bouillon cubes, spices (to taste)
banana leaves (optional)

1. Rinse black-eyed peas and soak in water over night.
2. After soaking, rub the peas together between hands to remove the skin, and rinse to wash off skin. Do this and sieve repeatedly until all the skin is removed.
3. Add red peppers and onion to the skinless black-eyed peas, and blend/grind together to form a thick paste.
4. Add water and vegetable oil to form a smooth watery paste.
5. Add corned beef, diced meat, fish, or eggs to the mixture, based on preference.
6. Add salt, bouillon cubes, and other spices to taste.
7. Scoop mixture into muffin/tin pans and place in a pot partially filled with water. (The mixture can also be wrapped in banana leaves and stacked in the pot. Racks are used to keep the pans out of water.)
8. Allow to steam for 45–60 minutes.

More recipes are available at http://nutrition.jbpub.com/foodculture/

REFERENCES

Afrimedia Project. (2004). *The cola nut and HIV/AIDS*. Retrieved December 30, 2007, from www.sti.ch/fileadmin/user_upload/Pdfs/Report__E_Colanut.doc/

Alade, I. (1985). The classification of Nigerian foods: A review. *Food and Nutrition Bulletin, 7*, 2.

Boomie, O. (1998). *Motherland Nigeria*. Retrieved December 19, 2007, from http://www.motherlandnigeria.com/

Countries and Their Cultures. (2007). Retrieved January 2, 2008, from http://www.everyculture.com/Ma-Ni/Nigeria.html/

Countries of the World. (2007). Retrieved April 4, 2008, from http://www.theodora.com/wfb/

Falconer, J. (1990). *The major significance of "minor" forest products: The local use and value of forests in the West African Humid Forest Zone*. Rome: Dickerson Studio.

Infoplease. (2007). *The Columbia electronic encyclopedia* (6th ed.). New York: Columbia University Press. Retrieved January 5, 2008, from http://www.infoplease.com/search?fr=ipce6&query=Nigeria+and+History&in=encyclopedia&x=10&y=9/

Johns, T., Booth, S.L., & Kuhnlein, H.V. (1992). Factors influencing vitamin A intake and programs to improve vitamin A status. *Food and Nutrition Bulletin, 14*, 2.

Kolawole, J.A., & Maduenyi, A. (2004). Effects of Zobo drink (Hibiscus sabdariffa water extract) on the pharmacokinetics of acetaminophen in human volunteers. *European Journal of Drug Metabolism and Pharmacokinetics, 29*(1), 25–29.

Muhammad, S., & Amusa, N.A. (2005). The important food crops and medicinal plants of northwestern Nigeria. *Research Journal Agriculture and Biological Sciences, 1*(3), 254–260.

Ndukwu, B.C., & Ben-Nwadibia, N.B. (n.d.). *Ethnomedicinal aspects of plants used as spices and condiments in Niger Delta area of Nigeria*. Retrieved January 10, 2007, from http://www.siu.edu/~ebl/leaflets/niger.htm/

Obute, G.C. (n.d.). *Ethnomedicinal plant resources of southeastern Nigeria*. Retrieved January 4, 2007, from www.siu.edu/~ebl/leaflets/obute.htm/

Okediran, A., Daney, A.H., & Olujide, M.G. (2007). Counseling and innovative literacy approaches as strategies for preventing STDs and HIV/AIDS incidence among person with disabilities. *Journal of Human Ecology, 222*, 115–121.

Onuorah, J. U., & Ajayi, O. A. (1985). Riboflavin content of breast milk in lactating Nigerian women: Its implications for child welfare in developing countries. *Nutrition Reports International*, 31, 1211–1217.

Refugee Health–Immigrant Health. (2004). Retrieved January 12, 2008, from http://www.baylormag.com/story.php?story=005610

Travel Notes. (2008). Retrieved April 4, 2008, from http://www.travelnotes.org/Africa/index.htm/

Ukachukwu, C.M. (2007). The sacred festival of Iri-ji Ohuru in Igboland, Nigeria. *Noradic Journal of African Studies, 16*(2), 244–260.

UNICEF. (2007). *The state of the world's children 2007: Women and children, the double dividend of gender equality*. Retrieved April 14, 2009, from http://www.unicef.org/sowc07/statistics/tables.php

World Factbook. (2007). *Nigeria*. Retrieved February 11, 2010, from http://www.cia.gov/library/publications/the-world-factbook/geos/ni.html

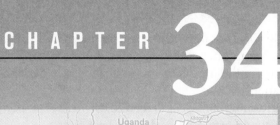

CHAPTER 34

Rwanda

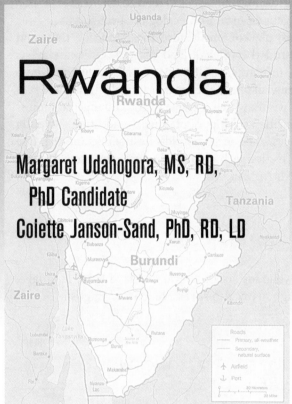

Margaret Udahogora, MS, RD,
  PhD Candidate
Colette Janson-Sand, PhD, RD, LD

 CULTURE AND WORLD REGION

Rwanda is a landlocked country in sub-Saharan Africa bordered in the north by Uganda, in the east by Tanzania, in the south by Burundi, and in the west by Democratic Republic of Congo. The earliest inhabitants of the region, approximately 2000 years ago, were the Twa, or pygmies, who were hunters and gatherers. Immigration of an agricultural group, known today as the Hutus, began to clear forests in order to grow their crops. Another major migration brought in a predominantly cattle-farming people known as Tutsi. The Hutus and Tutsis organized themselves into small camps or states with the Tutsi taking on a nobility role due to their cattle-raising wealth and the Hutus, being farmers who tilled the soil, taking on a subservient role. The Hutu and Tutsi were able to remain free of European colonization until the 1885 Berlin Conference, when the land became a German colony. During

World War I, it was occupied by Belgium. After the war, it became a Belgian League of Nations mandate, along with Burundi, under the name of Ruanda–Urundi. The mandate was made a United Nations Trust Territory in 1946. The Tutsi had long held a dominant role, and there had always been tension between the Tutsi and the Hutu. Belgium initially supported Tutsi dominance but eventually encouraged power sharing between Hutu and Tutsi. Ethnic tensions led to civil war, forcing many Tutsi to leave the country. Rwanda became an independent nation on July 1, 1962, under Hutu rule.

In October 1990, Tutsi rebels who had fled the country invaded in an attempt to overthrow the Hutu-led Rwandan government. A peace treaty was signed in August 1993, calling for a coalition government, but after the downing of a plane, which killed the presidents of both Rwanda and Burundi, ethnic violence erupted. The genocide of 1994, which resulted in the killing of

800,000 Tutsi along with some Hutu sympathizers, left the country in political, social, and economic ruin. Roughly 1 million people were killed (about 10% of the population).

As Rwanda continues to rebuild itself, it has turned to its geographical and ecological beauty as a means to boost its economy. Called the "land of a thousand hills" and the "Switzerland of Africa," Rwanda has begun to market itself as a tourist destination where one can visit one of the most beautiful wildlife reserves in the world, which is home to the endangered mountain gorilla and hippopotamus. In addition, Rwanda produces some of the world's best coffee and tea, due to cultivation at high altitude, in a consistent climate and rich African soil.

 ## LANGUAGE

All Rwandans speak Kinyarwanda, a tonal language, although many also speak French and English.

 ## FOOD HISTORY WITHIN THE CULTURE

Historically, the Hutus were among the earliest inhabitants of what is now Rwanda. They came mostly from central and western Africa and made up the majority of the population and were farmers. Tutsis who most likely migrated slowly from Ethiopia and Egypt raised cattle but were vegetarian because they believed that eating meat was taboo and caused one to be cursed by God who would then cause their cattle to disappear, leaving them destitute. The Hutus grew grain and legumes and traded them for meat from the Tutsis. The third cultural group, the Twas (pygmies), made up only a small percentage of the population and were the original inhabitants of the area. The Twas were hunter-gatherers and meat eaters, primarily of game and sheep. Both the Hutus and Tutsis looked down on the Twas because consuming sheep was considered taboo by both cultures. The Tutsis remained vegetarian until the late 1800s when the Germans colonized the area and the Tutsis slowly adopted the German meat-eating culture. In the 1940s the Belgians took over the country and also introduced some European foods, which have been adopted into the diets of both the Tutsis and Hutus.

 ## MAJOR FOODS

 ## Protein Sources

Meat, poultry, fish, and eggs are served at most meals, along with legumes. Meats include goat (a favorite), beef, lamb, pork, and rabbit. Meat tends to be consumed in small amounts, primarily in soups and stews. Milk is consumed in tea and used in cooking certain dishes, but buttermilk is consumed as a beverage. There are several varieties of beans available, either fresh or dried. Soybeans are popular and versatile. Peanuts as well as peanut powder and peanut butter are ingredients in many dishes.

 ## Starch Sources

Sorghum, maize, and wheat are the primary grains, which are made into flour and used to make breads such as corn cakes and donuts, and porridge. Other popular starches include rice, taro, cassava, and finger millet. Starchy vegetables include plantains, referred to as cooking bananas, yams, sweet potatoes, and white potatoes.

 ## Fat Sources

All types of oils are used in cooking. Among the most common oils are soybean, corn, sunflower, palm, coconut, and olive oil. Both butter and margarine are used as spreads and in cooking.

 ## Prominent Vegetables

Typical vegetables include carrots, spinach, celery, tomatoes, eggplant, green beans, squash, onions, green peppers, leeks, kale, and cabbage. Squash leaves, amaranthus, and cassava leaves are also popular.

 ## Prominent Fruits

A variety of tropical fruits are popular, especially mango, guava, passion fruit, papaya, banana, and pineapple. Citrus fruits include oranges, lemons, and tangerines. Strawberries and avocado are also popular. Many fruits, including bananas, are made into juices.

 ## Spices and Seasonings

Rwandan food is fairly plain; however, salt, black pepper, cayenne pepper, and chilis are commonly used, as are herbs such as chives.

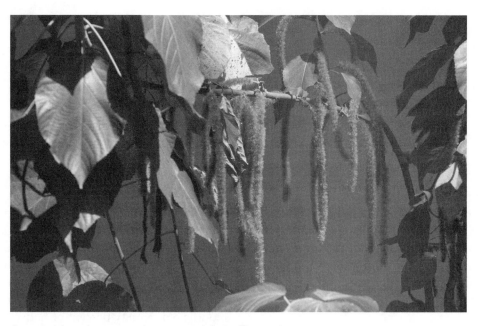

Amaranthus is a popular vegetable in Rwanda.

 Beverages

Tea, coffee, and fruit juices are commonly consumed, as are sorghum and banana beer. Soft drinks are also popular.

 Desserts

Rwandans eat a variety of fruits for dessert, either singly or as part of a fruit salad.

 TYPICAL DAY'S MENU

Breakfast

Breakfast may be simple, such as bread with butter or margarine and some jelly, porridge, and tea with milk; or a more substantial meal consisting of the latter along with a boiled egg or omelet. Sometimes donuts are served instead of bread. Fruit almost always completes the meal.

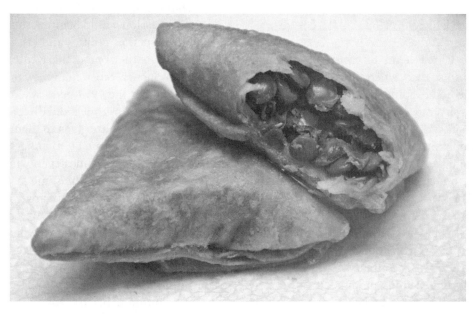

Sambusa with Lentils.

Lunch

Several small dishes of the following make up a typical lunch: baked fish or a stew composed of red meat, along with either plain rice or a rice pilaf. Vegetable accompaniments are usually baked, boiled, or fried sweet potato, plain or sautéed amaranthus with or without beans, and often a peas-and-carrots medley.

Dinner

Typically called supper, dinner tends to be a lighter meal and may consist of a number of small dishes such as meat stew, a thick cassava porridge, and sautéed cassava leaves. Also typical is *igisafuriya,* fried, baked, or boiled plantains, eggplant sautéed with beans, fish stew, and peanut butter sauce.

 ## HOLIDAY MENUS

Rwandans celebrate both secular and religious holidays with song and dance, and the fare for celebrations is generally similar. One popular food that is sure to be served is a goat brochette cooked over a fire or coals. Goat stew and roast chicken are also popular offerings, as are *sambusas.* A variety of vegetable dishes, such as sautéed green beans, white potatoes, plantains, or sweet potatoes, are served along with a fruit salad. Beverages include various local beers, especially sorghum and banana beer, but imported beers are also served, as are juices and soft drinks.

 ## HEALTH BELIEFS AND CONCERNS

People from rural areas tend to consult traditional healers and may do so even when they seek treatment from Western medicine. Some commonly held beliefs include eating raw liver to treat anemia and consuming squash and papaya seeds to treat intestinal parasites.

Fish heads and animal brains are fed to children to increase their intelligence and boys are often fed the testicles of animals to increase their virility. Goat milk is essential in treating kwashiorkor and only children with this form of malnutrition are allowed to consume it. Milk from a cow that has just calved is thought to cause diarrhea by some and constipation by others. Women who breastfeed are often encouraged to consume the local beer to help stimulate milk production; however, a breastfeeding woman is told to avoid cold drinks, which are considered to hinder milk production.

 ## GENERAL HEALTH AND NUTRITIONAL INDICATORS SUMMARY

Low birth weight, defined as weighing less than 2500 g at birth, affects 9% of newborns in Rwanda (UNICEF, 2007). Ninety percent of the nation's children are exclusively breastfed during the first 6 months of life. Sixty-nine percent of infants 6–9 months old are breastfed with complementary food, and 77% remain breastfed at 20–23 months of age.

Twenty-three percent of the nation's children below 5 years suffer from being moderately to severely underweight (UNICEF, 2007). Being severely underweight affects 4% of Rwanda's children. Moderate to severe wasting was found in 4% and stunting in 45% of this particular population. The nation has a 95% vitamin A supplementation coverage rate for children 6–59 months old. Ninety percent of households in Rwanda consume adequately iodized salt.

Seventy-four percent of Rwanda's total population uses improved drinking-water sources (UNICEF, 2007). Specifically, 92% of the population in the nation's urban areas and 69% of the rural population has access to improved drinking-water sources.

 ## COMMUNICATION AND COUNSELING TIPS

The traditional greeting is a firm handshake usually done by grasping the right forearm with the left hand while shaking hands with the right hand. A typical counseling session would begin with small talk, avoiding subjects such as politics and ethnicity. Discussing family and whether one is married or has children is a common opener. Since many Rwandans lost family members during the 1994 genocide, one should show empathy for their loss but avoid discussing particulars. Rwandan last names are given to them and are not typically family names. In fact, members of a family may all have different last names even when they have the same father, and having the same last name does not indicate that they are related in any way.

Most Rwandans find direct eye contact to be rude or impolite and will look away when speaking with someone of authority. Emotions are kept under control, especially anger, and avoiding conflict is very important.

As is common in conventional counseling, it is important to develop a trusting relationship at the beginning of any encounter. The authority figure of the household should be acknowledged and informed of the purpose of the counseling session and then he or she can allow or decline the intervention. Typically, healthcare workers are perceived as knowledgeable and nutrition and health messages are generally well received; however, Rwandans are very wary of giving too much personal information, such as socioeconomic barriers, which might reveal too much about their private life. Identifying barriers to change may be difficult, but sensitivity to cultural norms, beliefs, and values can go a long way in developing a trusting relationship in which an individual may be more willing to share information.

PRIMARY LANGUAGE OF FOOD NAMES WITH ENGLISH AND PHONETIC TRANSLATION

The primary language of food names with English and phonetic translation is as follows:

Rwandan Names	English
Amagi (Ahmahgee)	eggs
Amakaroti (AhMahKahRowTee)	carrots
Amandazi (AHmahndAHzi)	donut
Amashaza (AhMahShahZah)	peas
Amavuta (AhMahVooTah)	butter, margarine, oil
Amazi (AhMahZee)	water
Avoca (AhVohKah)	avocado
DoDo (DohDoh) or Isogi (EeSohGee)	amaranthus
Ibeyeri (EeBeeYehRee)	beer
Ibihaza (EeBeeHahzah)	squash
Ibijumba (EeBeeJoomBah)	sweet potato
Ibikoro (EeBeeKohRoh)	yam
Ibirayi (EeBeeRAIYee)	white potato
Ibishyimbo (EeBeeHeemBoh)	beans
Ibisusa (EeBeeSooSah)	squash leaves
Icunga (EeCoonGah)	orange
Icyayi (EeKEYyahYee)	tea
Ifi (EeFee)	fish
Igitoke (IGeeToeGee)	plantains
Ihene (EeHenAy)	goat
Ikawa (EeKAHwah)	coffee

Rwandan Names	English
Ikigori (EeKeyGorEe)	corn
Ikinyamunyu (EeKinYahMuhnYoo)	cooking bananas
Ikinyobwa (EeKinYohBwah)	peanut
Imineke (EeMeeNAYkay)	bananas
Imyembe (EemYehmBee)	mangoes
Inanasi (EeNahNahSee)	pineapple
Indimu (In DeeMoo)	lemon
Inkoko (EenKohKoh)	chicken
Inshyushyu (Een ChiuChiu)	milk
Intama (EenTahMah)	sheep
Intore (EenTohRee)	eggplant
Inyama (EenYahMah)	meat
Inyanya (EenYAHNyah)	tomatoes
Inyumbati (EemYoomBahTee)	cassava
Ipapayi (EepahPahYee)	papaya
Ishu (EeShoo)	cabbage
Isombi (EeSohmBee)	cassava leaves
Isukari (EeSooKAHree)	sugar
Kayk (Keke)	corn cake
Marakuca (MahRahKooKah)	passion fruit
PiliPili (PeeLeePeeLee) or *urusenda* (OoRooSenDah)	hot chilis
Pinari (PeeNahRee)	spinach

(continues)

Rwandan Names	English
Puwaro (PewWahRoh)	leek
Ubuntunguru (OoBooToonGooRoo)	onions
Uburo (OoboorOh)	finger millet
Ugali (OoGahLee)	cassava porridge
Umubimba (OomooBimBah)	green beans

Rwandan Names	English
Umucelli (OomooCHELLee)	rice
Umukati (OoMooKAHtee)	bread
Umunyu (OoMoonYoo)	salt
Umutobe w'imbuto (OomooToeBay WeemBooToe)	fruit juice

FEATURED RECIPE

Igisafuriva (Ee-GEE-Sah-Foo-REE-Vah)

1 chicken, cut into pieces

1 lb. plantains

4 tbsp. vegetable oil

1 large onion, thinly sliced

4 large tomatoes, diced and mashed

3 tbsp. tomato paste

4 stalks of celery, cut into thin rounds

1½ tsp. salt

1 hot pepper

1. Fry chicken in oil until browned and cooked through.
2. Remove and add sliced plantains.
3. Cook until slightly golden.
4. Remove and add onion.
5. When golden brown, add remaining ingredients.
6. Return chicken and plantains to the pot. Simmer for 15–20 minutes to blend flavors.

More recipes are available at http://nutrition.jbpub.com/foodculture

REFERENCES

Adekunle, J.O. (2007). *Culture and customs of Rwanda.* Westport, CT: Greenwood Press.

Anonymous. (2007). *Culture of Rwanda.* Retrieved December 10, 2007, from http://www.everyculture.com/No-Sa/Rwanda.html/

Bisangua, A. (1997). *Sins of the flesh.* Retrieved April 10, 2008, from http://wwwsatyamag.com/dec97/sins.html/

Food and Nutrition Technical Assistance II Project. (2008). *National guidelines and protocol for food and nutritional support and care for people living with HIV/AIDS in Rwanda, 2006.* Retrieved March 21, 2008, from http://www.fantaproject.org/publications/rwandan_guidelines2006.shtml/

UNICEF. (2007). *The state of the world's children 2007: Women and children, the double dividend of gender equality.* Retrieved April 14, 2009, from http://www.unicef.org/sowc07/statistics/tables.php

Vansina, J. (2004). Antecedents to modern Rwanda: The Nyiginya Kingdom. In T. Spear, D. Henige, & M. Schatzberg (Eds.), *Africa and the diaspora: History, politics, culture.* Madison: University of Wisconsin Press.

CHAPTER 35

Sudan

Ahlam Badreldin Ibrahim Al Shikieri, PhD

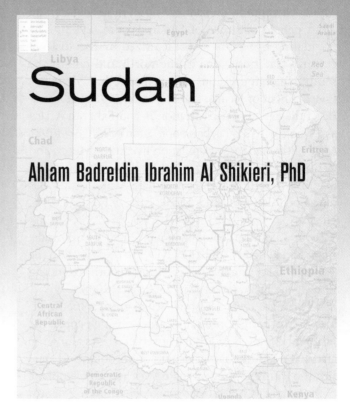

 CULTURE AND WORLD REGION

Sudan is the largest country in Africa and covers an area of about 2.5 million km², or nearly 10% of the total area of Africa (Department of Statistics, 1991). This includes an estimated 12% area devoted to agriculture and 18% to forestry (Biegler, 1998). Sudan is located in the northeastern part of the continent and extends from about latitude 3–23° north and from longitude 22–39° east. It is 2100 km from north to south and about 1800 km from east to west. Moreover, Sudan shares borders with eight countries: Egypt and Libya to the north; the Central African Republic, Chad, and Zaire to the west; Kenya and Uganda to the south; and Ethiopia to the east; the Red Sea forms part of the eastern borders (Department of Statistics, 1991).

Northern Sudan consists of six regions: Khartoum, which is the capital, the northern region (northern and Nile provinces), eastern region (Kassala and Red Sea provinces), central region (Blue Nile, White Nile, and

Gezeira provinces), Kordofan (North Kordofan and South Kordofan provinces), and Darfur (North Darfur and South Darfur provinces) (Department of Health and Statistics, 1993). Southern Sudan consists of three regions: Equatoria (eastern Equatoria and western Equatoria provinces), Upper Nile (Upper Nile and Jonglei provinces), and Bahar El Ghazal (Bahar El Ghazal and El Buheyrat provinces) (Department of Statistics, 1991).

Sudan gained its independence from Britain and Egypt in 1956. The legal system in Sudan is based on a mix of English common law and Islamic law; however, the constitution and legal systems have been thrown out and changed with each coup of the government.

Currently, *Shar'ia* (Islamic law) is implemented in the northern areas (Sudan, 2008). The climate in northern Sudan is dry (with minor variations) and characterized by high temperatures and little rainfall. In contrast, southern Sudan is humid with milder temperatures and heavy rains. Sudan therefore has rain forest vegetation in the south and savannah woodland, semidesert, and desert vegetation in the north.

Sudan has a population of 33.5 million people, 84% of whom live in urban areas (Awad, Eltayeb, & Capps, 2006). The population is made up of mostly black and Arab people (Culture of Sudan Forum, 2008). The population of Sudan is characterized by two distinct cultural traditions, one in the north and one in the south; regional divisions reflect these ethnic divisions (Department of Health and Statistics, 1991). Sudan reflects the extent of urbanization in sub-Saharan Africa as a whole with 32% urban population (UNICEF, 1998). Most of the Sudanese population live in Khartoum and Central Sudan (Department of Statistics, 1991). There are different ethnic groups in Sudan: Arabs form 49.1% of the population, Dinka 11.5%, Nuba 8.1%, Beja 6.4%. Nuer 4.9%, Azande 2.7%, Bari 2.5%, Fur 2.1%, Shilluk 1.7%, and Lotuhu 1.5% (Sudan Net, 2008). The Azande, Bor, and Jo Luo are "Sudanic" tribes in the west, and the Acholi and Lotuhu live in the extreme south, extending into Uganda (Bureau of African Affairs, 2008).

There are several distinct tribal groups: the Kababish of northern Kordofan, a camel-raising people; the Ja'alin and Shaigiyya groups of settled tribes along the rivers; the seminomadic Baggara of Kordofan and Darfur; the Hamitic Beja in the Red Sea area; the Nubians of the northern Nile area, some of whom have been resettled on the Atbara River; the Nuba of southern Kordofan; and Fur in the western reaches of the country (Bureau of African Affairs, 2008).

LANGUAGE

The official language of Sudan is Arabic, although many native languages, such as Nubian, Ta Bedawie, Beja, Fur, Nuban, Ingessana, and other local Sudanic languages, and diverse dialects of Nilotic and Nilo-Hamitic, are spoken. In all, there are more than 100 different indigenous languages spoken in Sudan (Culture of Sudan Forum, 2008). The populations in the south of the country, along with government officials throughout the country, speak English (Sudan, 2008). In general, they are more closely linked to population groups farther south than to those in northern Sudan (Department of Statistics, 1991). Furthermore, the religious affiliation in Sudan is mainly Sunni Muslim (73%), with animist/traditional beliefs forming 16.7%, Christian 9.1%, and other religions (1.2%) (Sudan Net, 2008). The majority of people in southern Sudan practice traditional religions.

FOOD HISTORY WITHIN THE CULTURE

Between 1990 and 1992, Sudan had a modest shortage of food supply; total dietary energy of 10.9%, which was similar to the average for Africa as a whole (10.2%) (Food and Agriculture Organization, [FAO], 1996). This indicates a need for an increase in total food supply to attain dietary-energy sufficiency (FAO, 1996). In 1990–1992, the main sources of dietary energy were sorghum and millet (38.4%) followed by wheat (18.4%). Millet, along with sorghum, is especially important in western Sudan, whereas wheat, consumed mainly as bread, is of increasing importance to the diet in urban areas and in the north. Cassava, yams, and sweet potatoes are the main staples in the southern region. In many areas of the south, maize and milk contribute substantially to the diet, and in some tribal areas, as much as 40% of all food consumed are milk and dairy products.

In terms of total protein availability, at 63 g per person/day, Sudan compared favorably with the average for Africa as a whole (57 g per person/day), but not with developed countries such as the United Kingdom (UK) (92 g per person/day) (FAO, 1996). The percentage of energy from dietary protein in Sudan was 11.7% per person/day, which was similar to both Africa (10%) and the UK (11.2%) from 1990 to 1992 (FAO, 1996). The percentage of energy from protein in Sudan was below the recommended level of 15–17% (World Health Organization, [WHO], 1990).

In 1990–1992, the total fat supply was 62 g per person/day, which was higher than the rest of Africa (47 g per person/day) and 2.3-fold lower than the UK (144 g per person/day) (FAO, 1996). In terms of percentage of energy from fat, Sudan had on average 26.4%, Africa as a whole had only 18.5%, and the UK had 39.5% (FAO, 1996). This could indicate that Sudan's fat supply was within the recommended 30% energy from fat (WHO, 1990). The animal fat supply fell from 30 g (37%) in 1979–1981 to 26 g (42%) per person per day in 1990–1992, but it was threefold higher than the averages for Africa in general in the same period (FAO, 1996).

Figure 35-1 shows the changes in the per capita energy, protein, and fat supply between 1969 and 1994. This was despite the supply of milk, which doubled while there was only a small increase in the supply of cereals, pulses, and eggs (FAO/AGROSTAT, 1996). Over the same period, there was a substantial decline in the per capita supply of vegetables and fruits. The supply of meat, fish, sweets (sugar and honey), and fats and oils decreased. Figure 35-2 shows the per capita supply of food groups (kilograms per year) between 1969 and 1994.

In Sudan, large households are common, with a national average of 6.6 members in the household. Urban households are larger than rural households, with 7.5 and 6.2 members, respectively, and a range of between one and more than nine people (Department of Statistics, 1991). One third of urban households are composed of nine or more members compared with one fifth in rural areas. Urban men tend to be more educated than their rural counterparts (Department of Statistics, 1991). Women who reside in urban areas have considerably more education than those in rural areas. In general, however, Sudanese women are less educated than men (Department of Statistics, 1991). Men's literacy rate was 58% and women's rate was 35%

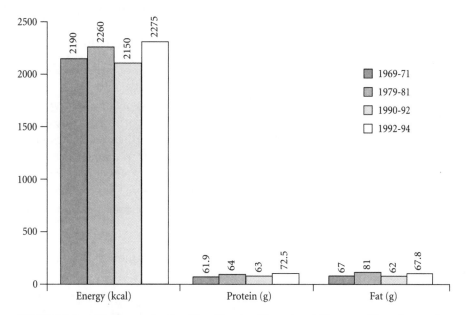

FIGURE 35-1   Changes in the Per Capita Supply of Energy, Protein, and Fat in Sudan

Source: FAO (1996); FAO/AGROSTAT (1996).

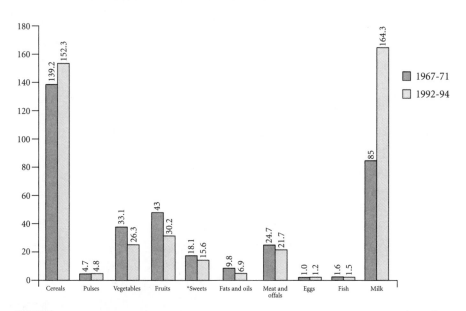

FIGURE 35-2   Changes in the Per Capita Supply of Food Groups (kg/y) in Sudan

Source: FAO/AGROSTAT (1996).

(UNICEF, 1998). In comparison with the whole of sub-Saharan Africa, Sudanese men and women had lower literacy rates than other areas (66 and 47%, respectively) (UNICEF, 1998).

 MAJOR FOODS

 Protein Sources

Nomads in the north rely on dairy products (from cows, sheep, goats, and camels), and meat from camels (FAO, 2005; Culture of Sudan Forum, 2008) is sometimes the main source of energy, protein, and other nutrients. The main protein sources in the country are cereals, milk, eggs, lamb, beef, fish, and poultry (FAO, 1996, 2005). In addition, Sudan has many livestock, producing large amounts of beef and veal (227,000 metric tons), mutton, and goat meat (141,000 metric tons). Mutton and beef are favored over other types of meat (FAO, 2005). Beef is the commonly consumed meat (85% of meat consumption), and lamb is also consumed. Poultry is the least produced meat (66,000 metric tons) (FAO, 2009), and there is a small catch of freshwater fish (32,000 metric tons); thus, the consumption of fish is low. Most of the fish eaten is inland freshwater fish, whereas sea fish is consumed only along the Red Sea coast (FAO, 2005).

 Starch Sources

Sudan produces large amounts of sorghum (2,828,000 metric tons), significant amounts of wheat (378,000 metric tons) and millet (349,000 metric tons), and small amounts of maize (36,000 metric tons) and rice (1000 metric tons) (FAO, 2009). Wheat and rice are not exported, but small amounts of the others are (sorghum 184,000, millet 27,000, and maize 5000 metric tons). Wheat has recently displaced sorghum as the staple food (Musaiger, 2000) because increased prices put sorghum beyond the reach of many poor people. In addition, the country grows sugarcane (4,394,000 metric tons) and beans (5000 metric tons). Cassava, yams, and sweet potatoes are the main starch sources consumed in the south (FAO, 2005).

 Fat Sources

Among a variety of oilseed crops grown, groundnut, cottonseed, and sesame seed are produced in large amounts (305,000, 239,000, and 197,000 metric tons,

respectively) with relatively small amounts of sunflower seed (26,000 metric tons) (FAO, 2009). Groundnuts and sesame are the main sources of local vegetable oils (FAO, 2005). The other types of oils used are peanut, sesame, corn, and sunflower. Sesame oil is used mainly as a garnish for the broad-beans dishes (Shikieri, Landman, Armstrong, & Sutherland, 2002). The Sudanese use ghee moderately and mainly for cooking certain sweet dishes such as sheiria and suksukania, and sometimes for preparing egg omelets.

 Prominent Vegetables

Large amounts of vegetables and fruits are produced (953,000 and 820,000 metric tons, respectively). The prominent vegetables are shown in Table 35-1. Okra is eaten in dried form. Tomatoes and onions are eaten in urban areas. Other vegetables not listed in Table 35-1 include carrots, potato lettuce, spinach, cabbage, sugar beet, parsley, green chilies, cauliflower, and broccoli. Legumes, grown and consumed mainly in northern Sudan, include beans, peas, and cowpeas. The consump-

TABLE 35-1 Names of Prominent Vegetables in Sudan

English Name	Arabic Transliteration
Okra	Bamia
Onion	Basal
Pigeon pea	Adasi
Hot pepper	Shatta
Jews' mallow	Molkhia
Cantaloupe, snake cucumber, etc.	Shamam, tibish, agour
Pumpkin	Gara
Tomato	Tamatin
Haricot beans	Fasulia
Pea	Pisilla
Purslane	Rigla
Radish	Figil
Eggplant	Bazingan
Cowpea	Lubia hilo

Compiled from Ahmed & Mohammed (2008).

tion of fresh vegetables, especially green leafy varieties, is limited.

Prominent Fruits

The prominent fruits in the country include pineapple, grapefruit, orange, banana, grapes, watermelon, mango, strawberry, mandarin, dates, guava, pomegranate, and sugar melon (New Partnership for Africa's Development [NEPAD] & FAO, 2005). Most of these fruits are seasonal (FAO, 2005). The consumption of fruit, with the exception of dates, is limited.

Spices and Seasonings

The commonly used spices in Sudan are given in Table 35-2.

Foods with Cultural Significance

As in some Arab countries, such as neighboring Egypt (Jerome, 1997), people in Sudan eat from communal dishes. In one meal there could be up to five people eating together from more than three foods and/or dishes (Shikieri et al., 2002). People do not use forks and knives and only use spoons for eating certain foods, such as rice and porridge. Also, in some families, men eat separately from women and children.

In addition, women generally eat meals at home, because most of them are not employed and therefore not obliged to eat outside the house, as are men. Most Sudanese men (75%) have breakfast, but not the other meals, away from home. Men are always served first and given the best of everything (Shikieri et al., 2002).

In studies conducted by Shikieri and coauthors (2002) and Shikieri and Osman (2004), for the commonly consumed foods in Sudan (n = 124 and 100, respectively), bread accounted for 52–55% by weight of total cereals consumed daily, equivalent to a medium-size portion of a Sudanese French breadstick (see Table 35-3 for a list of portion sizes). Also, few amounts of fresh fruit, equivalent in edible portion to ~1.5–2 medium bananas, were consumed daily (Shikieri et al., 2002). No one reported consuming whole-grain cereals or fatty fish; only lean local fish, such as Nile perch or Tilapia *nilotica*, were consumed.

Different regions in the country have various methods of cooking foods and/or dishes. For instance, in southern Sudan, the traditional Nuer foods *kop* (a grain-based, steamed dough ball later cooked with greens and meat) and *wal wal* (a similar grain-based dough rolled into balls and steamed, and served with milk or yogurt-milk) are consumed regularly and prepared with sorghum or corn flour (Willis & Buck, 2007). Moreover, they have a dish known as *kajaik*, which is made with dried fish. The fish is ground, and water, onion, and spices are added to the powdered fish and put on a fire. Dried okra powder is added to thicken the mixture. This dish is usually eaten with the *kop*. Table 35-4 gives the sources of cereals, legumes, fruits, and vegetables classified by the different regions of Sudan.

In western Sudan, a porridge made of millet, *damerga*, is usually consumed with locally cooked dishes. Millet flour is ground using the hand, and water is added. The dough is left for fermentation after which it is shaped into small balls and left to dry. Once needed, a ball is taken, mixed with water, and put on a fire to make porridge. This porridge is usually eaten with meat stew, *mulah kaldee* or *mullah akdar*. The latter stew consists of minced meat, spices, water, and oil thickened with dried okra powder. A plant known as *kawal* is then dried, ground, and added to the meat stew.

TYPICAL DAY'S MENU

In a typical day, black tea with milk (mostly whole milk) and sugar is consumed between 5:30 AM and 11:00 AM, followed by breakfast between 9:00 AM and 12:30 PM. Breakfast is served with an average of three foods and/or dishes (range of one to seven foods/dishes).

TABLE 35-2 Commonly Used Spices in Sudan

English Name	Arabic Transliteration
Black cumin	*Kamoun aswad (habat elbaraka)*
Galangal	*Quronjal*
Cumin	*Shamar (kamoun akdar)*
Black pepper	*Filfil aswad*
Red pepper	*Filfil ahmar (shata)*
Cinnamon	*Girfa*
Clove	*Grounful*
Coriander	*Kozbara*
Cardamom	*Houbahan*
Ginger	*Zanjabeel*

TABLE 35-3 Portion Size of Commonly Consumed Foods and/or Dishes in Sudan (Average of Eight Measurements with a Calibrated Scale)

Food/Dish	Small Portion (g)	Medium Portion (g)	Large Portion (g)	Food/Dish	Small Portion (g)	Medium Portion (g)	Large Portion (g)
Baked beans dish	80[c]	171	262[d]	Egg (raw)	50	62	74
Baklava, sweet, filled with nuts		26		Eggplant salad with peanut butter	12[a]	19	26[b]
Banana (peeled)	60	72	84	Eggplant stew	95[c]	150	204[d]
Beef soup with dried okra powder	58[c]	149	240[d]	Falafel	8	12	15
Beef stew	58[c]	134	210[d]	Fish (tilapia nilotica, fried)	75	98	120
Biscuit for tea (homemade)		16		Flour (any type, powder)	87[e]		124[f]
Biscuit, plain (locally made)		9		Fried meat cubes	3	17	30
Bread				Fruit salad	26[b]		95[c]
Toasted		43		Ghee	12[a]	19	25[b]
French stick	63	72	81	Gorasa bread	107	253	399
Turkish toast		91		Green chilies (piece)		2	
Round	75	89	103	Guava (whole, raw)		66	
Bread crumbs (powdered)	5[a]	8	10[b]	Honey	7[a]	12	17[b]
Broad beans, cooked	125[c]	240	355[d]	Jam	13[a]	21	29[b]
Cake (homemade)		78		Jews' mallow stew	88[c]	187	286[d]
Carrot				Kisra bread (piece, cooked)		76	
Raw, whole	23	41	58	Lamb intestine (marara)	99[c]	209	318[d]
Raw, sliced		2		Lentil soup	58[c]	134	210[d]
Cheese (Sudanese, white, shredded)	10[a]	17	24[b]	Lettuce			
Chicken				Chopped		6[b]	
Breast, boiled	28	54	80	Whole leaf		14	
Leg, boiled		42		Macaroni			
Cucumber				Boiled	56[c]	104	152[d]
Raw, chopped		15[b]		Sheiria	15[a]	23	30[b]
Slices	2 thin	4	5 thick	Mango	80	215	350
Raw, whole		109		Mashed okra stew	99[c]	196	292[d]
Custard (dessert)	99[c]		160[e]	Mashed spinach stew	62[c]	129	196[d]
Dates (dry, raw)	5	8	11	Meat powder (Sharmout)		35[c]	

TABLE 35-3   Portion Size of Commonly Consumed Foods and/or Dishes in Sudan (Average of Eight Measurements with a Calibrated Scale) (Continued)

Food/Dish	Small Portion (g)	Medium Portion (g)	Large Portion (g)	Food/Dish	Small Portion (g)	Medium Portion (g)	Large Portion (g)
Milk				Sausage (Loli company, one cooked piece)	15	20	25
Fresh (from cow)	139[e]	205	270[f]				
Powdered	4[a]	6	8[b]	Soup, beef or mutton	55[c]/ 133[e]	131/ 197	207[c]/ 260[f]
Minced beef stew with dried okra powder	85[c]	194	303[d]	Squash stew	109[c]	191	273[d]
Minced meat	12[a]	18	2[b]	Sugar (white granulated)	116[e]	174	232[f]
Okra powder		43[c]		Sugar melon			
Olive (black)		6		Cubes		14	
Onion powder		41[c]		Slices		37	
Onion (raw, whole)	27	79	131	Whole		309	
Onion ring (fine slice)		1		Sweet		5	
Peanut butter	11[a]	23	34[b]	Tahania sweet	7[a]	11	15[b]
Pepper				Tea (powder)	2[a]	4	5[b]
Green or red (fine slices)		2		Tomato (raw)			
Whole	13	24	34	Chopped		17[b]	
				Sliced	5	7	9
Pepsi cola	250 ml	350 ml	1 L	Whole	50	68	87
Porridge	80[c]	105	130[d]	Tuna fish		25[b]	
Potato chips (thinly sliced)		2		Vegetable oil	3[a]	7	11[b]
Potato dish with minced meat	108[c]	202	295[d]	Vegetables, stuffed			
				Aubergine		146	
Potato stew	128[c]	195	261[d]	Courgette		112	
Purslane stew	67[c]	139	211[d]	Green pepper		55	
Rice (boiled)	102[c]	175	247[d]	Tomato		83	
Rice pudding		30[b]		Watermelon (square piece)		64	
Rocket leaf		1		Whole okra stew	99[c]	174	257[d]
Samosa		24		Yoghurt	144[e]	210	275[f]
				Zucchini dish	95[c]	150	204[d]

From Shikieri et al. (2002).

[a]Teaspoon

[b]Tablespoon

[c]Small cooking spoon

[d]Large cooking spoon

[e]Small cup

[f]Large cup

TABLE 35-4   Sources of Cereals, Legumes, Fruits, and Vegetables Classified by Region

Region	Cereals	Legumes	Fruits	Vegetables
Nile, north, Khartoum	Wheat, sorghum, maize	Chickpea, broadwing, and haricot beans	Dates, citrus, mango, banana	Potatoes, onions, garlic, spices, leafy vegetables
Tokar and Gash deltas	Sorghum			Watermelon, tomatoes, leafy vegetables
Other riverine areas and water sources	Sorghum	Chickpea	Banana, guava, citrus, mango	Onions, tomatoes, okra, eggplant, leafy vegetables
Gezira, Managil, White Nile projects	Sorghum, wheat	Pigeon pea, wing bean, groundnut	Citrus, guava	Onions, tomatoes, okra, eggplant, leafy vegetables
Kassala, New Halfa, areas south of Red Sea	Sorghum, wheat	Pigeon pea, wing bean, groundnut	Citrus, banana, guava	Onions, tomatoes, okra, eggplant, sweet potatoes, pepper, leafy vegetables
Darfur, Kordofan (rain fed)	Millet, sorghum	Pigeon pea, cowpea, groundnut		Okra
Darfur, Kordofan (valleys)		Broad beans, chickpea, pigeon pea	Mango, citrus, guava, dates	Tomatoes, okra, onions, pepper
Gebel Mara area	Millet, sorghum, wheat	Broad beans, chickpea, pigeon pea, cowpea	Mango, citrus, guava	Potatoes, sweet potatoes, onions, garlic, okra, pepper, leafy vegetables
Central Sudan (e.g., Gedarif, South Blue Nile areas)	Sorghum, maize	Pigeon pea, cowpea		Okra
Khartoum State		Snap bean, green peas, pigeon peas, broad beans	Mango, citrus, guava, banana	All vegetables

Compiled from Magboul & Mohamed (2002).

These dishes include cooked broad beans, bread, jam, meat stews, egg, or yogurt.

Lunch, the main meal of the day for which all the family gathers, is served between 2:00 and 5:00 PM and consists on average of three foods and/or dishes (range of one to six foods/dishes). Traditional dishes (including vegetable stews with meat), vegetable salads, and fruits are consumed. The last meal of the day is supper (dinner), which is served between 5:30 and midnight and served with two foods and/or dishes (range of one to five foods/dishes). The foods served for supper are similar to those given for breakfast (Shikieri et al., 2002; Culture of Sudan Forum, 2008). Table 35-5 shows the nutritive values (selected nutrients) of selected dishes.

 HOLIDAY MENUS

There are four main religious occasions in Sudan for which special foods and drinks are served. For instance, at the Eid ul-Adha, the Feast of the Great Sacrifice that comes during hajj, it is customary to slaughter a sheep and give some of the meat to people who cannot afford it themselves (Culture of Sudan Forum, 2008). Certain beverages are consumed during this Eid, namely *sharbout*, which is made of fermented dates, and *abyad damirak* from fermented rice. During Ramadan, a special fermented drink called *holo mour* is consumed. It is prepared locally in most households. Other drinks consumed during the holy month and also on normal days include hibiscus (*karkadi*), tamarind (*aradeb*),

TABLE 35-5   Nutritive Values of Traditional Sudanese Foods and Dishes (per 100 g)

Foods and Dishes	Energy (kcal)	Protein (g)	CHO (g)	Fat (g)	SFA (g)	MUFA (g)	PUFA (g)	Cholesterol (mg)	Weight Loss (%)
Whole okra stew with beef	129	5.6	3.9	10.6	3.0	4.4	2.5	17.9	2.4
Mashed okra stew with beef	112	5.8	3.3	8.6	2.7	3.5	1.5	20.3	28
Potato stew with beef	155	5.0	10.1	10.9	2.9	4.6	2.7	17.1	38.5
Purslane stew with beef	129	6.7	11.4	6.6	2.0	2.9	1.6	11.2	11
Aubergine salad with peanut butter	189	2.6	3.1	19.1	3.7	7.3	8	0	35
Rice	250	2.3	27.6	15.7	3.2	5.9	4.9	0	9
Beef soup	228	11.9	3.5	18.5	6.1	7.9	3.1	53.8	52.6
Lamb soup	201	13.4	2.3	15.2	7.7	6.6	1.1	58.6	53
Lamb stew	175	8.3	34.9	15.1	6.5	6.3	2.2	35.6	60
Beef stew	195	8.4	4.4	16.4	4.8	7.1	3.0	32.6	60
Falafel	472	12.3	35.7	32.7	5.8	13.0	11.6	0	36
Mashed Jews' mallow stew with beef	136	8.6	6.3	9.5	2.8	3.9	1.4	21.7	28
Jews' mallow stew with beef	139	7.4	7.2	9.5	2.6	4.4	2.0	15.8	34
Lentil soup	307	15.8	41.4	10.0	1.9	3.6	3.4	0	23.6
Minced beef stew with dried okra powder	228	7.1	9.8	19.0	4.4	8.3	4.2	17.7	40
Beef soup with dried okra powder	195	9.3	10.8	13.5	3.7	5.5	2.3	34.6	52.6
Stuffed vegetable dish	223	2.4	18.0	17.3	4.1	2.8	6.6	21.0	15.7
Fermented fish stew	214	16.7	4.1	14.5	2.9	5.7	4.6	30.6	37
Fried lamb	279	15.1	0.1	24.5	11.3	11.0	2.9	73.2	76
Chicken stew	133	13.1	2.0	8.3	1.9	3.8	2.1	35.2	49
Courgette stew with beef	128	3.8	3.0	11.2	2.9	5.4	2.5	17.8	36
Fried Nile perch	151	11.5	4.3	9.6	1.8	4.5	2.8	66.4	42

(continues)

TABLE 35-5 Nutritive Values of Traditional Sudanese Foods and Dishes (per 100 g) (Continued)

Foods and Dishes	Energy (kcal)	Protein (g)	CHO (g)	Fat (g)	SFA (g)	MUFA (g)	PUFA (g)	Cholesterol (mg)	Weight Loss (%)
Homemade cake	346	7.6	42.2	17.3	4.1	5.9	4.3	91.5	5
Kidney bean stew with beef	253	12.7	27.5	10.7	3.0	4.6	2.8	16.5	42
Gorasa bread	371	11.5	78.8	2.0	0	0	0	0	15
Zalabia	534	8	52.9	33.5	6.0	15.4	9.2	0	39
Fried beef	261	16.3	0.3	21.3	7.4	10.2	2.6	76.7	76

CHO: carbohydrates; *SFA:* saturated fatty acids; *MUFA:* monounsaturated fatty acids; *PUFA:* polyunsaturated fatty acids
From Shikieri et al. (2002).

Grewia tenax (*godaim*), and *Adansonia digitata* (*gongolaiz*) juices. All these drinks are prepared by soaking the leaves or seeds in water. After 2–3 hours, a sieve is used to obtain the clear liquid after which sugar is added and the juice is drunk cold.

The Eid al-Fitr, or Breaking of the Ramadan Fasting, is another joyous occasion and involves a large family meal. Fish is usually consumed on day one. The birthday of the Prophet Muhammad is primarily a children's holiday, celebrated with special desserts: pink sugar dolls and sticky sweets made from nuts and sesame seeds (Culture of Sudan Forum, 2008). Sheep are usually killed for feasts or to honor a special guest. The intestines, lungs, and liver of the animal are prepared with chili pepper in a special dish called *marara*. The ritual of hospitality is as important in Sudan as it is in other Arab countries (Zaroug, 2008). In many places around the country, cooking is done in the courtyards outside the house on a tin grill called a *kanoon*, which uses charcoal as fuel.

 HEALTH BELIEFS AND CONCERNS

Some traditions affect children's health negatively, including the way food is served. As noted previously, the best food is given to the men, who are served first, and then women and children share what remains. In addition, some Sudanese women believe that breastfeeding has to be stopped promptly once they know that they are pregnant with another baby. When a child is ill with diarrhea or vomiting, traditional drinks, such as rice water, tea with lemon, and custard drink, will be the first choice of treatment. If no improvements are noticed after several days of suffering, the child will

be taken to a nearby hospital or clinic, which might be thousands of miles away, and it may be too late to help the child. This situation is caused primarily by the low education levels of women, who are responsible for the preparation of food.

Women do not know what constitutes healthy foods and what to feed their family. In a poor country with increased inflation rates, such as Sudan, it is always difficult and not usually possible for one member of the house (the man) to provide food for a family of more than six members. There is also a low level of employment especially among women. This situation is worsened by the fact that there are no current health and/or nutrition education programs in the country, aimed at, for example, increasing the supply of fruits and vegetables, or proper ways of weaning, or even ways to help women improve the family situation (income-generating programs).

 GENERAL HEALTH AND NUTRITIONAL INDICATORS SUMMARY

Low birth weight, defined as weighing less than 2500 g at birth, affects 31% of newborns in Sudan (UNICEF, 2007). Sixteen percent of the nation's children are exclusively breastfed during the first 6 months of life. Forty-seven percent of infants 6–9 months are breastfed with complementary food, and 40% remain breastfed at 20–23 months.

Forty-one percent of Sudanese children below 5 years suffer from being moderately to severely underweight (UNICEF, 2007). Being severely underweight affects 15% of children. Moderate to severe wasting was found in 16% and stunting in 43% of this particular population. Sudan has a 70% vitamin A supplementation coverage rate for children ages 6–59 months. Only 1% of households in Sudan consume adequately iodized salt.

Seventy percent of Sudan's total population uses improved drinking-water sources (UNICEF, 2007). Specifically, 78% of the population in the nation's urban areas and 64% of the rural population has access to improved drinking-water sources.

COMMUNICATION AND COUNSELING TIPS

In northern Sudan, men work outside the home, whereas in western and southern Sudan, women leave the house looking for work, while men are either employed or stay at home. Women's work can sometimes be very hard, such as building, farming, or carrying goods.

Married women usually wear the Sudanese dress called *toub*, which can also be worn by unmarried women; the latter also wear the Islamic dress (*hijab*), which covers their legs, arms, and head. The face is only covered by certain Islamic groups called *Akwan Muslemeen*.

Sudanese men wear the *jalabya*, which is a white or other-colored long, one-piece dress. A special hat (*tageya*) is worn and another piece of cloth (*emaa*) is put on the shoulder or sometimes around the head. Men also wear trousers and shirts.

FEATURED RECIPE

Beef Stew (Damaat Ajalee)

2 cups beef (meat from rib or leg)

1¾ cups red onion, chopped

4¼ tbsp. tomato paste

½ cup oil (peanut or cottonseed)

Spices, garlic, salt

1. Add oil to an empty saucepan and put on fire.
2. Add chopped onion and stir until golden yellow in color.
3. Add meat and water.
4. When meat is cooked (tender), add tomato paste and the remaining ingredients.

More recipes are available at http://nutrition.jbpub.com/foodculture

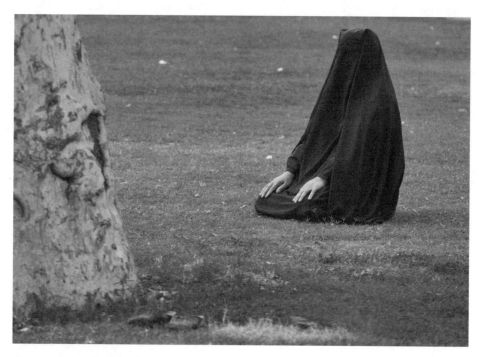

Unmarried women often wear the Islamic dress (hijab) that covers their legs, arms, and head.

REFERENCES

Ahmed, M.K., & Mohammed, E.T.I. (2008). *Indigenous vegetables of Sudan: production, utilization and conservation.* Retrieved March 13, 2008, from www.bioversityinternational.org/publications/web_version/500/begin.htm/

Awad, A.S., Eltayeb, I.B., & Capps, P.A. (2006). Self-medication practices in Khartoum State, Sudan [Electronic version]. *European Journal of Clinical Pharmacology, 62*, 317–324.

Biegler, A. (1998). Country profile. *The Economist Intelligence Unit*, 1997–1998.

Bureau of African Affairs. (2008). *Background note: Sudan.* Retrieved March 11, 2008, from http://www.state.gov/

Culture of Sudan Forum. (2008). *Culture of Sudan.* Retrieved March 11, 2008, from www.everyculture.com/forum/

Daly, M.W., & Forbes, L.E.S. (1994). *The Sudan: Photographs from the Sudan archive.* Reading, UK: Garnet Publication Limited.

Department of Health and Statistics. (1993). Fourth population census of Sudan: Final tabulation. Sudan: Northern states. *Demographic characteristics Khartoum* (Vol. 1). Khartoum: Department of Health and Statistics.

Department of Statistics. (1991). *Sudan demographic and health survey.* Khartoum: Sudan Institute for Resources Development/Macro.

Eltohami, M.S. (2008). *Medicinal and aromatic plants in Sudan.* Retrieved March 8, 2008, from www.fao.org/docrep/x5402e/5402e00.htm/

Food and Agriculture Organization (FAO). (1996). *The sixth world food survey.* Rome: FAO.

Food and Agriculture Organization. (2005). *Sudan nutrition profile. Food and nutrition division.* Retrieved March 13, 2008, from http://www.fao.org/

Food and Agriculture Organization. (2009) *Food balance sheet 1984–1996.* Retrieved April 24, 2001, from http://apps.fao.org/csv_down/

Food and Agriculture Organization/AGROSTAT. (1996). *Food balance sheets 1992–1994.* Rome: FAO.

Jerome, N.W. (1997). Culture-specific strategies for capturing local dietary intake patterns. *American Journal of Clinical Nutrition, 65*, S1166–S1167.

Magboul, B.I., & Mohamed, K.A. (2002). Nutrition activities during the 20th century in Sudan. *Sudan Notes and Records*, Special Issues IN Print.

Musaiger, A.O. (2000). Nutrition situation in the Near East Region. *Nutrition Health*, 143–146.

New Partnership for Africa's Development (NEPAD), and Food and Agriculture Organization (FAO). (2005). *Bankable investment project profile: Smallholder Water Harvesting and Productivity Enhancement Government of the Republic of Sudan.* (Vol 2 TCP/SUD/2909 (I): (NEPAD Ref. 05/12 E).

Sasaki, S., & Kesteloot, H. (1992). Value of Food and Agriculture Organisation data on food-balance sheets as a data source for dietary fat intake in epidemiologic studies. *American Journal of Clinical Nutrition, 56*, 716–723.

Shikieri, A., Landman, J., Armstrong, R., & Sutherland, D. (2002). *The use of 24-hr recall records for the assessment of daily dietary intake in Khartoum, Sudan.* Unpublished paper from A. Shikieri's PhD thesis.

Shikieri, A., & Osman, N. (2004). Dietary fibre intake amongst healthy Sudanese population. Unpublished paper from N. Osman's Master Thesis.

Sudan. (2008). *Menus & recipes from Africa.* Retrieved March 11, 2008, from www.africa.upenn.edu/Cookbook/AS.html/

Sudan Net. (2008). *Sudan: general data of the country.* Retrieved March 9, 2008, from www.sudan.net/

UNICEF. (1998). *The state of the world's children 1997.* London: Oxford University Press.

UNICEF. (2007). *The state of the world's children 2007: Women and children, the double dividend of gender equality.* Retrieved April 14, 2009, from http://www.unicef.org/sowc07/statistics/tables.php

Willis, M.S., & Buck, J.S. (2007). From Sudan to Nebraska: Dinka and Nuer refugee diet dilemmas [Electronic version]. *Journal of Nutrition Education and Behavior, 39*(5), 273–280.

World Health Organization. (1990). *Diet, nutrition and the prevention of chronic diseases.* Geneva, Switzerland: World Health Organization.

Zaroug, M.G. (2008). *Country pasture/forage resource profiles: Sudan.* Retrieved March 13, 2008, from http://www.fao.org/ag/AGP/AGPC/doc/pasture/forage.htm/

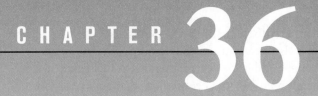

CHAPTER 36

West Africa
(Ghana, Sierra Leone, and Liberia)

Chandra Carty, MMSc, RD

 ## CULTURE AND WORLD REGION

Food is synonymous with culture. Daily rituals and seasonal traditions involve the preparation of culturally specific foods. This chapter discusses the foods and cultures of three West African countries: Ghana, Sierra Leone, and Liberia.

History suggests that some of the native people of Ghana are immigrants from the ancient Ghana (Wagadou) Empire. The foods and cultures of this region are similar in many ways to the indigenous African traditions that were impacted by both colonialism and the presence of missionaries. Sierra Leone and Liberia were both formed during the postcolonial and post-slavery period. The people who lived in these countries introduced new traditions, which included strong influences from the West.

Obtaining historical documentation of the cultural evolution of these countries has been difficult. Information about Africa has been extracted from archeologi-

cal digs, folklore, poetry, and diaries from missionaries and explorers. Written information regarding the food and cultural habits of the peoples is scarce. Archeological digs suggest that hunters and gatherers collected and prepared the indigenous crops, thus giving rise to man's first dietary habits. These indigenous crops were often seeds, berries, and fruits. During the precolonial period, most Africans communicated orally, information that was passed from generation to generation in the forms of storytelling, folklore, and song. Historical accounts of West Africa have been described through the eyes of Christian and Muslim missionaries, various explorers, and political leaders. The missionaries describe the culture as it relates to the indigenous peoples' ability to adapt to foreign religious traditions. The explorers describe West Africa from the perspective of its ability to adapt to specific social, economic, and/or political rules.

Culture is forever evolving as new traditions replace some old ones. The diversity is vast; however, there are distinct similarities, and also West Africans have also been influenced by new cultural norms. Although food is the central theme, the influence on it by social, political, and economical changes are obvious.

Some anthropologists define culture as learned and shared attitudes, values, and ways of behaving (Grunlan, 1988). British anthropologist Sir Edward Tylor defines culture as "that complex whole which includes knowledge, belief, art, morals, law, custom, and any other capabilities and habits acquired by man as a member of society" (Tylor, 1871, p.1). The formation of cultural complexes occur when cultural traits are mixed and combined. The complexity of the cultural evolution that occurred in Ghana, Sierra Leone, and Liberia is beyond the scope of this chapter; however, a brief summary will help the reader understand how the culture and foods have evolved over the centuries. Using Grunlan's (1988) definition of culture as the point of departure, let us explore further the West African culture.

The traditional social and political structure was centered on "Divine Kingship." The kingship represents a religious symbol as well as a sacred institution, which is surrounded by taboos and restrictions. The king was symbolic of the kingdom, and its religious center. The king delegated authority to the chief who in turn was the representative to the people. This form of political or social government was foreign to the explorers and missionaries from the West. In this form of leadership, old or ill kings, or those who were no longer suitable symbols for the nation, were killed. Modern-day Africa may still harbor some of the old traditions. Although the colonists forced a new form of leadership onto Sierra Leone and Liberia, the old traditional rule fought to dominate the social structure. There continues to be ethnic violence; however, the introduction of democratic rule is bringing about another cultural shift.

In African society, the family dominates cultural norms. Children grow up to understand the significance of kinship and family. In this kinship-dominated society, relationships are formed within kinship groups. Compared with the American family, there is less emphasis on individualism and more emphasis on the group. Individuals are taught their roles in the family. An elder teaches the husband and wife what they are expected to do in their family. Respect for an older person is seen in the way persons greet or speak to one another. For example, a younger person would bow the head before speaking to an older person.

There are some similarities as well as vast differences within West African families. For example, some families are monogamous and others are polygamous.

The context of these relationships is difficult for Westerners to understand. The kinship group shares the responsibility of taking care of the widows and divorcees. The women have specific roles; they are usually responsible for food production, food preparation, and trading in the market place. The mother teaches the young girl how to prepare food at a young age. Recipes are not written but are oral. These roles are changing as women assume various roles in the workplace and learn more industrialized ways of food production and preparation. The art of cooking does not have the same emphasis with the younger generation; thus, family leaders may fear that the change in roles will weaken the kinship system.

The African market is an institution that has existed for a long time. Archeological evidence reveals that around the first century AD nomadic Berbers traveled on camels toward the Bilad al-Sudan—the Land of the Black Peoples (Catchpole & Akinjogbin, 1984). Records indicate that pastoralists (herders) traded horses and cattle for rock salt and luxury manufactured goods. These pastoralists bartered the salt and luxury goods for millet and cotton grown by the West African savannah farmers. The savannah farmers were already exchanging their products for gold and kola nuts from the people of the south. A complex trading system thus began along the northern border of the Sahel. These trading centers led to the development of the first West African states along the trans-Sahara. These three centers became the nucleus of the West African Empire: Tekrur, Ghana, and Kanem-Bornu. The modern-day markets are both colorful and lively. They are the central points in some communities and major centers of entertainment. Women are often market salespeople.

The African religions are monotheistic. The indigenous West Africans believed in a single God, the creator of the world. However, belief in that God allowed for subgods; thus, the belief is also polytheistic in nature. Subgods exist alongside the spirits of the people's ancestors. The West Africans worship the gods and spirits. Elaborate rituals and sacrifices are performed, and diviners help people cope with everyday problems. The introduction of Islam, gradually introduced by the Berbers of the Maghrib, changed the religious beliefs of many West Africans. According to Catchpole and Akinjogbin (1984), the first West African royal family to accept the teachings of Islam was the Gao Dynasty. Tekrur, a town on the Senegal River in the West African Empire, was the first Sudanic kingdom to totally convert from a pagan religion to the Muslim religion. The spread of Islam linked West Africa with North Africa and the eastern Sudan. The migration continued, and in 1725 and 1775 the first and second jihads, respectively, spread the teachings of the Prophet Mohammad.

European missionaries introduced Christianity to the coastal areas of the south and gradually spread inland. Muslim missionaries were restricted to the north, although they were penetrating southward into Yorubaland (Nigeria). The Middle Belt remained an area in which Islam and Christianity competed for converts. Missionaries helped to spread Western education and technology.

The African continent is a large plateau. Pre-Cambrian rock, 600–1600 ft. (200–500 m), outlines most of West Africa from the northeast to the southwest. Records suggest that it has been a land area for millions of years. Sand is widespread throughout the interior and lateritic material in the south. The composition of the coast depends on the types of rocks, earth movements, relief, drainage, and climate. There are swells and basins. The winds, long-shore drift, waves, and tides affect the shoreline. The West African coasts are low, sandy, and without natural harbors; however, there are exceptions where a river or a tidal range has allowed an opening. Ports along the coast were very expensive to construct.

The total area of West Africa is about 2.5 million square miles (about two thirds the size of the United States). There are 15 countries that share the land.

Ghana is about 92,100 square miles and has a population of 9.1 million people. Liberia has an area of 43,000 square miles and 1.5 million people. Sierra Leone is 27,900 square miles and has 2.9 million people.

The northern boundary follows the southern limits of the Sahara Desert. The Atlantic Ocean provides the southwest boundary and the Gulf of Guinea the southern boundary. West Africa is composed of three vegetation zones: the sahel, the savannah, and the tropical rain forest. Historians have identified three major time divisions: Early Stone Age (2,500,000–50,000 BC), Middle Stone Age (50000–1500 BC), and Late Stone Age (1500–500 BC).

Two air masses, the Tropical Continental (cT) Air, warm and dusty from the sahara, and the Tropical Maritime (mT) Air, warm and humid from the southwest, are major forces in the climate. The climates affect the food crop. Some of the major climate classifications are:

- Monsoonal, a dry season followed by a long and very wet season. Liberia and interior Sierra Leone fall into the monsoonal category. During the dry season vegetation growth stops for several months. There is less variety of food crops and rice is the main crop.
- Equatorial, rain in every month, with two longer months. South-Central Ghana is included in this zone. Plant growth continues throughout the year. There is high humidity, which is ideal for the lowland rainforest.
- Tropical, one rainfall maximum, becoming shorter inland. Liberia has many tropical areas.
- Mauritanian Coastal, minute winter rainfall.
- Saharan, no regular rain.

West African temperatures vary from the world averages for similar latitudes during the northern hemisphere winter in the north, during the rains in the south, and almost all year in the highlands. Temperatures are higher than the world averages for similar latitudes in April, July, and October in the central and northern areas. High temperatures are common in the south at the end of the dry season. Climatic changes greatly affect the food crops produced in West Africa.

LANGUAGE

There may be over 800 languages in Africa. The Niger-Congo family is the major language group spoken by the three countries in this chapter. This family group is further divided into seven subfamilies. In Ghana, 75% of the population speaks Kwa. The Kwa group consists of subfamilies: Akan, Ga-Adangbe, and Ewe. The Akan is further divided into Asante, Fante, Akwapim, Akyem, Akwamu, Ahanta, Bono, Nzema, Kwahu, and Safwi. The Asante are members of the Twi-speaking branch. Each family group follows these subfamily group divisions. Historically, each category has a traditional group identity. The recipes and other information in this chapter were primarily from the Asante group. In Liberia and Sierra Leone, English is the primary language. Liberia has 16 different indigenous languages. In Sierra Leone there are two major ethnic groups: the Mende, who speak Mande; and the Temne, who speak a West Atlantic language. They also speak Krio, a dialect of several African languages, and English.

CULTURE HISTORY

Information regarding the various indigenous tribes is scarce. Most of the information available is from the colonial period. In 1462, Pedro da Cintra, a Portuguese seaman, recorded his voyage to the West African coast. He named the coast "Sierra Leone" (Lion Mountain). His main interest was gold but later included the search for slaves. European companies, such as the British Royal African Company (1672–1750), traded goods in exchange for West African people (Catchpole & Akinjogbin, 1984).

In his book, Ijagbemi (1976) describes the Koya Temne Kingdom. This large kingdom included all of Sierra Leone during 1787. The Koya people lived peacefully with their neighbors for many years. The fertile soil allowed the people to produce rice, cassava, palm trees, kola nuts, and ginger, as well as other food crops. The women engaged in fishing and the men hunted, reared cattle, and carried out other activities included weaving. The Watering Place was a popular trading port. The district chief protected the Africans as well as Europeans who came to this area to trade. They bartered their slaves, gold, ivory, camwood, and other commodities for European goods such as knives, mirrors, trinkets, rum, and tobacco. The slave trade provided the rulers the wealth needed to live in luxury. According to Koya customs, when a man is elected king he assumes a new name, and it is taboo to refer to him by his old name. According to European historians, the sons of rich Koya men became well-educated traders who competed on an equal basis with European traders. Chief Naimbana became opposed to the slave trade and was instrumental in the formation of Freetown Colony in 1787. Chief Naimbana died in 1793, thus ending the peace between the Koya people and the Freetown Colony.

At the end of the 18th century, Sierra Leone became the location for Britain's partial reparation for the slave trade. Many ex-slaves and discharged African soldiers settled in Freetown, founded in 1792, the main navel base in Sierra Leone. Americans concerned about the growth of freed ex-slaves formed The American Colonization Society in 1816 to reintroduce black Americans to their African roots. The ex-slaves, or Creoles, were shipped to Freetown, Sierra Leone. Mixed blood, higher education, and the combination of African and non-African culture separated the Creoles from their former African brothers. The hostility from the local interior Africans limited their advancement beyond the coast. Constant rivalry between the ethnic groups prevented unity. Colony-protectorate division stifled economic growth until 1961, when the country gained its independence.

In 1822, The American Colonization Society, with the help of King Peter, acquired a strip of land they

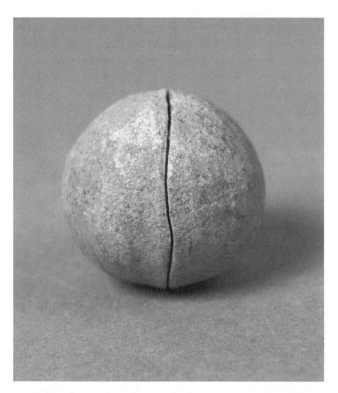

In West Africa, the kola nut is eaten as a stimulant like tobacco or coffee.

called Liberia. The colonists landed at Cape Mesurado and built a capital at Monrovia. This group of unskilled ex-slaves encountered hostility from the Africans and lack of support from the Europeans. Native Africans were excluded from citizenship in the new republic until 1904.

Present-day Ghana derived its name from the ancient Ghana Empire. Information recorded in the Library of Congress suggests that the migration into modern Ghana may have occurred as early as the 10th century AD. Arab writer Al Yaqubi described the Ghana Empire as one of the three most organized states in the region. The kings organized complex trading systems, which attracted North Africans into this region. With the advancement of Islam into the region, Ghana came under attack from its neighbors and was defeated.

Portuguese explorers named the area "Gold Coast," because of the abundance of gold found along the coastline. Vast resources brought other European nations and traders to the Gold Coast (English, Dutch, Swedes, Danes, and Brandenburgers). English companies traded from 1618 to 1820. After this period, trading was controlled by the governor of Sierra Leone until the Gold Coast became a separate colony in 1874. In 1957, this former British colony gained its independence. The new country adapted the ancient name, Ghana.

FOOD HISTORY WITHIN THE CULTURE

The indigenous tribes from the forest regions had a diet that consisted of fruits, insects, rodents, lizards, and fish. Foods introduced during colonization included cassava, sweet potato, groundnut, maize, lima beans, chilies, tomatoes, pawpaw, avocado pear, guava, and pineapple. Early migrants brought varieties of yams, cocoyams, aubergines, citrus fruits, mangoes, and bananas, and varieties of peas, beans, and sugarcane from Asia. Other foods include swamp rice from Asia as well as sisal and cocoa from America.

Most West Africans are farmers. Food shortages occur because the land that could be used to produce food is used to produce cash crops. Although cocoa is the main crop, plantain, maize, cocoyam, and cassava are grown for sale in the neighboring district of Accra-Tema. Cassava is grown in the dry-climatic and poor-soil area. Maize is grown where conditions are wetter, and coconut trees are planted along the coastal sands.

Fishing is the main occupation of the region. In northern Ghana and the Accra plain farmers have herds of cattle; however, poor grazing and water shortage during the dry season limit cattle production. Livestock include, in increasing order of abundance, goats, sheep, cattle, and pigs, with poultry being the most prevalent meat. Farming in the northern savanna region consists of yams, poultry, and livestock. Kola is the oldest cash crop of the forest zone. The kola nut is consumed as a stimulant like tobacco or coffee.

Men and women have distinct roles in farming. The area of land farmed may be limited by the area the men can clear and the women can cultivate. The women process the palm nut and the cassava. With the introduction of machines, the division of labor changes because men usually operate the machines. Women may earn less when machines are introduced.

The market square is the most effective agency for the distribution of manufactured goods and foodstuffs. Yams and cattle come from the north to the south, which in turn supplies fish to the north and central areas. In the towns, food cost is higher. As more people move to the cities searching for work and a better education, the old ways of growing and preparing food are being abandoned. More markets have convenient

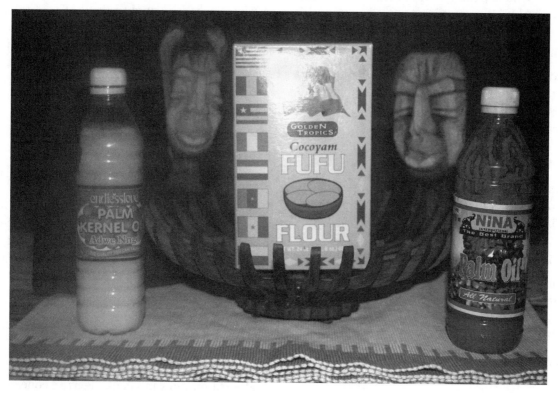

Fufu in a Box
Courtesy of the author

foods such as *fufu* in a box, dried or dehydrated meats, and vegetables. Dried fish is popular and often used in soups and stews.

MAJOR FOODS

Protein Sources

Protein sources include goat, beef, fish, pig (for the non-Muslim people), chicken, guinea fowl, turkey, and snails. Additional sources include among legumes: groundnut (peanut), pigeon pea (Congo pea), cow pea, lima bean (butter bean), and locust bean.

Starch Sources

Starch sources include among cereals: rice, maize, guinea corn, and millet. Additional sources include among roots: cassava and manioc; among yams: white or yellow, water yam, and Chinese yam; and among lesser roots: cocoyam (sweet potato), ginger, and tiger "nuts."

Fat Sources

Fat sources include palm oil (*ngo*), benniseed oil, and angwa (vegetable oil).

Prominent Vegetables

Prominent vegetables include onion, shallot, okra (gumbo), sorrel, African spinach, pepper, chili, tomato, cucumber, gourd, pumpkin, melon, Asiatic aubergine, garden egg, and sugarcane.

Prominent Fruits

Prominent fruits are coconut, mango, papaw, orange, lime, grapefruit, banana, plantain, and pineapple (grown in Ghana).

Spices and Seasonings

Common spices are soya seasoning, hot pepper, and alligator pepper seed.

Beverages

Common beverages are dairy milk and sorrel tea.

Dessert

The common dessert is fresh fruit.

FOODS WITH CULTURAL SIGNIFICANCE

Fufu, which is made from yam or plantain, is a common dish throughout West Africa. It is prepared in a variety of ways depending on the country. In Liberia, *fufu* is eaten with most meals. *Fufu* can be heated slowly to produce *gari* meal. In Ghana, *gari* is eaten as an alternative to *fufu*. Starch is made from the flour and, if it is dropped on heated plates, tapioca is made. It is believed by some people that *fufu* and soup are especially good for a sore throat or if a person is too ill to eat. *Fufu* is also included in most celebrations and holiday meals.

TYPICAL DAY'S MENU

Breakfast consists of corn porridge, lunch consists of yam and cocoyam leaf stew with meat and vegetables, and dinner consists of *fufu* and vegetable soup. Fruits and seeds are consumed as snacks. (Courtesy of Mavis Kwarteg from Ghana.)

HOLIDAY MENUS

A Christmas menu might consist of any of the following: collard greens, jollof rice, fried okra (in Ghana), banku and okra, kanke and fish with ground pepper, beans with red oil and fried plantain, *fufu* and palm nut, peanut butter vegetable soup, jollof rice with meat and vegetables, yam or plantain and cocoyam leaf stew, and rice and vegetable stew.

HEALTH BELIEFS AND CONCERNS

People generally live a long time. Many West Africans believe that if someone is disobedient, or if a witch has put a spell on someone, then that person will die early. They believe that sickness is a curse, and they use leaves and seeds as medicine.

GENERAL HEALTH AND NUTRITIONAL INDICATORS SUMMARY

Malnutrition rates in Ghana, Sierra Leone, and Liberia are among the highest in the world. Sierra Leone has the highest mortality rates worldwide for children

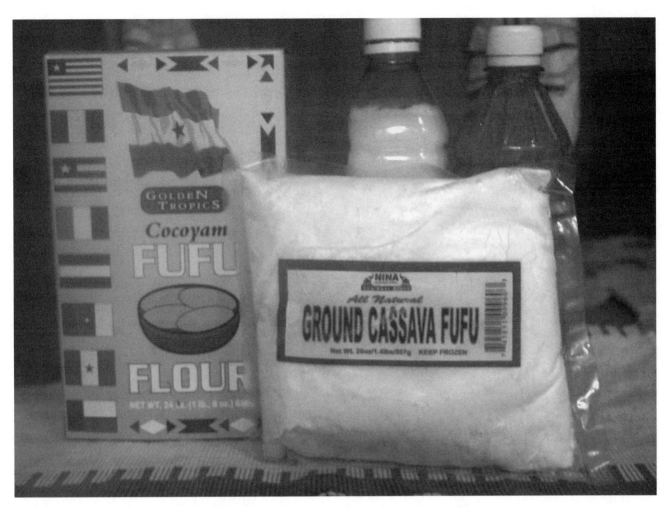

Ground Fufu
Courtesy of the author

under 5 years. Epidemiological studies link malnutrition to child mortality rates. Scientists measure the child's malnutrition by the degree of underweight. The range of underweight varies from mild to severe. The severely underweight child has an increased mortality risk. Sierra Leone and Liberia have the highest infant and child mortality rates (first and fifth, respectively). In Sierra Leone, one child in four dies before the age of 5 years. A survey of recent data sources suggests that 27% of Sierra Leoneans are moderate or severely underweight. Poor feeding practices during infancy and early childhood explain the progression of malnutrition. The malnourished child experiences declining health as well as slow growth and development during the first 2 years.

Vitamin A deficiency is prevalent. The mortality risk increases 1.75 times in a vitamin A-deficient child. An estimated 40% of Sierra Leoneans under 5 years suffer from vitamin A deficiency. In utero, the growing fetus needs iodine for brain development. Research suggests that 3% of babies born to iodine-deficient women suffer from cretinism and 10% suffer from severe mental retardation. A subclinical iodine deficiency has been identified in approximately 25% of the population. If suboptimal feeding practices continue, the risk of stunting growth increases with age. In Sierra Leone, 31.5% of the children demonstrate stunting by the age of 35 months. Anemia has been identified in 68% of women of reproductive age.

Other nutrient deficiencies have been suggested; however, more scientific studies are needed. Animal studies on zinc supplementation during pregnancy shows improvement in infant mortality rates after supplementation. Supplementation with calcium and folate suggest improvement in hypertension in adults and also in infant mortality rates.

See Table 36-1 for a summary of the health indicators.

TABLE 36-1   Summary of Health Indicators

Country	Mortality Rank[a]	Severe Underweight (%)[a]	Moderate/ Severe Underweight (%)[a]	Stunted Growth (%)[a]	Vitamin A (%)[a]	Iodine (%)[a]	Anemia (%)[b]
Sierra Leone	1	9	27	34	40	25	68
Liberia	5	8	26	39	–	–	–
Ghana	42	5	22	30	–	–	–

[a]Data are for children under 5 years.
[b]Data are for women of reproductive age.
Source: UNICEF, 2009.

FEATURED RECIPE

Ghanaian Recipe

Fufu and Vegetable Soup

⅓ cassava, peeled and boiled

2 large tomatoes

2 red bell peppers

1 large white onion

1 (8 oz.) can tomato sauce

1 bouillon cube

Salt to taste

10 oz. diced chicken

1. Combine ingredients and cook until chicken is brown and cassava is tender.
2. To make *fufu*, peel the cassava, soak or boil, and then pound and make into a dumpling. It can be boiled or fried, or dried and ground into flour after peeling or soaking. It can be warmed slowly to produce *gari* meal. If it is dropped on heated plates, tapioca is made.

(Courtesy of Mavis Kwarteg)

More recipes are available at http://nutrition.jbpub.com/foodculture/

REFERENCES

Catchpole, B., & Akinjogbin, I. (1984). *A history of West Africa*. London: Collins Educational.

Grunlan, S.A. (1988). *Cultural anthropology* (2nd ed.). Grand Rapids, MI: Zondervan.

Harrison Church, R.J. (1968). *West Africa: A study of man's environment and man's use of it* (6th ed.). London: Longmans.

Ijagbemi, A. (1976). *Naimbana of Sierra Leone*. London: Heinemann Educational Books.

McCulloch, M. (1964). *Peoples of Sierra Leone*. London: International African Institute.

Reuben K.U. (1978). *A comprehensive geography of West Africa*. New York: Africana.

Salm, S.J. (2002). *Culture and customs of Ghana*. Westport, CT: Greenwood Press.

Smith, I. (1995). The case for indigenous West African food culture. BREDA Series No. 9, Dakar. Retrieved December 23, 2009, from http://unesdoc.unesco.org/images/0010/001055/105546E.pdf

Swartz, B.K. (1980). *West African culture dynamics: Archaeological and historical perspectives*. New York: Mounton.

Tylor, E. (1871). *Primitive culture*. New York: J.P. Putnam's Sons.

UNICEF. (2009). United Nations Population Division and United Nations Statistics. Retrieved December 23, 2009, from http://www.un.org/popin/index.html

Central America and the Caribbean

Food, Cuisine, and Cultural Competency for Culinary, Hospitality, and Nutrition Professionals discusses four prominent countries in Central America and the Caribbean:

COSTA RICA

Costa Rica is in Central America, bordering both the Caribbean Sea and the North Pacific Ocean, between Nicaragua and Panama. Costa Rica's stable economy depends on tourism, agriculture, and electronics exports. Exports have become more diversified in the past 10 years due to the growth of the high-tech manufacturing sector, which is dominated by the microprocessor industry and the production of medical devices. Tourism continues to bring in foreign exchange, as Costa Rica's impressive biodiversity makes it a key destination for ecotourism. Poverty has remained around 20% for nearly 20 years.

HAITI

Haiti is in the Caribbean and is the western third of the island of Hispaniola, between the Caribbean Sea and the North Atlantic Ocean, west of the Dominican Republic. Haiti is the poorest country in the Western Hemisphere with 80% of the population living under the poverty line and 54% in abject poverty. Two thirds of all Haitians depend on the agricultural sector, mainly small-scale subsistence farming, and remain vulnerable to damage from frequent natural disasters, which are exacerbated by the country's widespread deforestation.

GUATEMALA

Guatemala is in Central America, bordering the North Pacific Ocean, between El Salvador and Mexico, and bordering the Gulf of Honduras (Caribbean Sea) between Honduras and Belize. Guatemala is the most populous of the Central American countries, with a gross domestic product (GDP) per capita of approximately 50% that of Argentina, Brazil, and Chile. Coffee, sugar, and bananas are the main products, with sugar exports benefiting from increased global demand for ethanol.

JAMAICA

Jamaica is an island in the Caribbean Sea, south of Cuba. The Jamaican economy is heavily dependent on services, which now account for more than 60% of the GDP. The country continues to derive most of its foreign exchange from tourism. Jamaica's economy, already saddled with the lowest economic growth in Latin America, will face increasing difficulties with the ongoing global recession. The economy faces serious long-term problems: a sizable merchandise trade deficit, large-scale unemployment, and underemployment.

CHAPTER 37

Costa Rica

Katherine L. Cason, PhD, RD

Marta Eugenia Gamboa-Acuna, BS

Yenory Hernandez Garbanzo, BS

 CULTURE AND WORLD REGION

Costa Rica is known as the "Switzerland of the Americas" and is characterized by cultural diversity, with 4,016,000 inhabitants, of whom 94% are European and some Mestizo, 3% are of African origin, 1% Chinese, 1% Amerindian, and 1% from other ethnic groups. Costa Rica's citizens have free access to education, health, and social security. Their life expectancy is between 72 and 75 years, and the literacy rate is approximately 96%. It is estimated that 76.3% or more of Costa Ricans are Roman Catholics; therefore, most of the national and family events are related to Catholic traditions; for example, Christmas, Easter, Saint's Day celebrations, and "Virgin of the Angels" Day (celebrated August 2). In addition, 13.7% of the population is Evangelist, 1.3% Jehovah's Witness, 0.7% other Protestant, 4.8% other religion, and 3.2% practice no religion.

Currently, the cultural life of Costa Ricans, who are also called *Ticos* and *Ticas* (from a diminutive suffix added by Costa Ricans; e.g., *chiquitico* instead of *chiquitito*), is modern and includes going to the cinema, dancing, theater, dominical mass, restaurants, soccer stadiums, libraries, and museums. Nevertheless, Costa Rica still preserves some of the folkloric traditions from its Hispanic roots, such as the national dance called *El Punto Guanacasteco Mascaradas* danced to the rhythm of a *Cimarrona* played during the celebration of the *Fiestas Patronales* (local fairs). In general, the Ticos and Ticas are people of *pura vida* (pure life): friendly, helpful, and educated with some important values that protect their democracy, peace, natural environment, and family units. The father, in most cases, is the provider for the family; however, the role of the woman as mother and wife is very important for maintaining and supporting the stability of the family members.

Costa Rica is located in the isthmus of Central America and extends from the Pacific Ocean to the Caribbean Sea. Along the country's borders are Nicaragua to the north and Panama to the southeast. Its land portion occupies only 0.1% of the world's land mass; however, despite being such a small country, its different microclimates and exceptional tropical weather lead to its having 6% of the world's biodiversity, including more than 800 species of ferns, 1000 species of orchids, 2000 kinds of trees, and 200 species of mammals. Costa Rica is divided into seven provinces: San José, Heredia, Alajuela, Cartago, Guanacaste, Limón, and Puntarenas. In the center of the country, within a valley, is located the capital, San José.

Costa Rica has been officially independent from Spain since September 15, 1821; it is strongly democratic and established its first constitution in 1823. It is the only country in Latin America without an army, which was abolished in 1948. Today, Costa Rica is an open economy that is growing in the telecommunications and technological multinational industries. Most of Costa Rica's direct exports are from tropical flowers and fruits (particularly bananas and pineapples), gourmet coffee, and textiles. Costa Rica is also known worldwide for its tourism, and its 2008 Travel and Tourism Competitive Ranking results (made by the Worldwide Economical Forum) positioned Costa Rica in first place in Latin American tourism.

 LANGUAGE

Spanish is the official language of Costa Rica, although a lot of people speak some English. Also, in Limón, its Caribbean province, people have their own language, which is referred to as Limón Creole English. Moreover, the languages Bribi and Cabecar are understood by an estimated 18,000 people, most of whom are indigenous and live on both sides of the *Cordillera de Talamanca* (the Talamanca Mountain Range).

 CULTURE HISTORY

The first habitants of Costa Rica were probably nomadic hunters, and a variety of indigenous groups include Chorotegas and Talamancas. On September 25, 1502, Cristóbal Colón (Christopher Columbus) arrived in the territory, the first Spaniard to set foot on Costa Rica. After his arrival, other conquerors explored the territory, including Fernández de Córdoba, who named the territory Costa Rica ("Rich Coast") because he believed that it had more gold than all of Spain. In

the 19th century, the Caribbean region received immigrants, especially Africans who went to work during the construction of the railroads and later established homes. Africans also went to the country as slaves of the conquerors. Chinese immigrants also came to the port towns of Limón and Puntarenas and later extended in small numbers to other cities in the country. This mix of populations gives the region a cultural and ethnic uniqueness, the influences of which are evident throughout the country.

 FOOD HISTORY WITHIN THE CULTURE

Costa Rica's cuisine is the result of a combination of indigenous and Spanish cuisines with an African influence. Before the Spanish arrived, the indigenous people hunted local animals and fished. They also took advantage of the different microclimates of the area by growing a variety of plants, the most important of which were beans and corn because of their use as sources of protein and energy, respectively. The foods made from corn included tortillas, corn bread, and tamales. The indigenous people drank a beverage called *chicha*, which was made with corn and fruit juices. Chocolate was also an important beverage, consumed for special occasions such as funerals.

It was only after the first Spanish conquest, between 1502 and 1560, that cattle were settled in Costa Rica's territory. The Spanish also brought a variety of fruits, vegetables, and grains, such as oranges, strawberries, lettuce, sugarcane, rice, wheat, and bread. African slaves also cooked in the houses of the wealthy, bringing Africa's influences into cooking techniques and the use of different ingredients and recipes. One of the dishes often consumed then in Costa Rica, and which exemplifies the influence of Africans, is the *gallo pinto*, which means "speckled rooster." The principal ingredients of *gallo pinto* were white rice and black or red beans. Africans also brought plantain to Costa Rica. Plantain was fried and served as a dessert after lunch. Today, the tradition of eating plantain after lunch continues in most Costa Rican houses.

According to Sedó (2008), some preparations that are considered to be traditionally from Costa Rica are present in other countries as well; however, there are some important differences, mainly in ingredients, preparation techniques, and the inclusion of *culin* marinade. For instance, from the Spanish influence, "the typical Costa Rican *picadillos*" are characterized as less moist and as having finely chopped ingredients (vegetables, onion, sweet pepper, cilantro, garlic, annatto, and some meat). They are served with tortillas, which reflect the aboriginal influence.

Costa Rica's gastronomic traditions also vary depending on the region, and the cuisines from the Central Valley, Guanacaste, Limón, and Puntarenas stand out. Today, changes in the production systems, industry, globalization, and the increase in Central American and South American immigration have impacted the dietary habits of Costa Ricans; therefore, it is more common to find food from Nicaragua, such as *nacatamales pupusas* from El Salvador, *arepas colombianas* from Colombia, and fast-food restaurants from the United States.

 ## MAJOR FOODS

 ### Protein Sources

Costa Ricans eat beef more frequently than others meats (around 1 oz./person per day), followed by chicken and processed pork meat. Other sources of protein are eggs, beans, milk, and cheeses. Most Costa Ricans prefer white cheese known as *queso turrialba*, a fresh cheese, to milk.

 ### Starch Sources

Rice and beans are the basis of Costa Rican meals and are consumed by 97% of the population at least twice per day. Sometimes they are also consumed during breakfast as *gallo pinto*. Bread and pastas are also highly consumed.

 ### Fat Sources

The consumption of fat is related to preparation as well as food sources. Costa Ricans have substituted shortening for vegetable oils, although this change does not imply a reduction in the amount of fat consumed because of the usual consumption of at least one fried preparation per day. The main animal fat sources are eggs and processed meats, particularly bologna and spiced sausage.

 ### Prominent Vegetables

The consumption of vegetables is low in Costa Rica. Usually, less than a cup of shredded cabbage is served during lunch, topped with one or two slices of tomato. Other important vegetables that are consumed are *palmito* (hearts of palm), carrots, cilantro, and some starchy vegetables such as potato, yucca, sweet potato, corncob, *tiquisque*, and plantain. Fried ripened plantains are one of the favorite dishes.

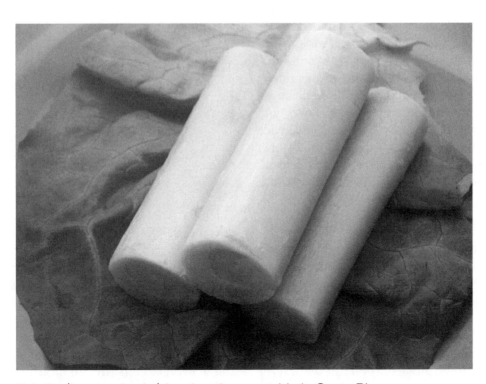

Palmito (hearts of palm) is a favorite vegetable in Costa Rica.

Prominent Fruits

Costa Rica grows a wide variety of exotic and tropical fruit. The most common fruits are banana, watermelon, pineapple, mango, cantaloupe, papaya, and blackberry (most commonly used for beverages). Other important fruits are *pejibaye* (miniature orange coconut, also known as "palm fruit" or "peach palm"), *mammon chino* (small green spheres containing grape-like pulp), *granadilla* (egg-sized fruit), and *guayaba* (guava).

Spices and Seasonings

Costa Ricans use oregano, thyme, *achiote* (a red paste used in a lot of Costa Rican dishes to provide color), cilantro, garlic, onion, black pepper, and sauces such as Tabasco and *Salsa Lizano*. *Salsa Lizano* is a deep-brown condiment that is slightly sweet and has a hint of spiciness (similar to Worcestershire sauce) and is used in the same way that North Americans use ketchup. Its popularity and frequent use in Costa Rican cuisine made the following phrase apt: "*Esté donde esté un tico, siempre habrá Salsa Lizano*" ("Wherever a Costa Rican is, there will be *Salsa Lizano*").

Beverages

Coffee is "Costa Rica's grain of gold" and is traditionally served very strong, with sugar and hot milk. Another warm drink is *agua dulce*, which is made from melted sugarcane. The refreshers in Costa Rica are the natural fruit drinks known as *frescos* or *refrescos*, which are usually made with fresh fruits such as tamarind, blackberries (*moras*), mangoes, Costa Rican guavas (*cas*), star fruit (*carambola*), passion fruit (*maracuya*), and pineapple, and mixed with milk or water and sugar. Other kinds of beverages are the *horchata*, made from rice, peanuts, cinnamon, milk, and cocoa powder; *chan*, made with a seed of a plant; *pinolillo*, a corn–cocoa drink, and *resbaladera*, a rice-and-barley drink.

Desserts

Most of the sweets, marmalades, or conserves in Costa Rica are made from the fruits of the season, which are chopped and mixed with, for example, sugar or brown cane sugar syrup, vanilla essence, cinnamon, nutmeg, and cloves. Carrot candies or *chiverre* (similar to spaghetti squash) are common, as are *cajetas*, handmade candies made from sugar, and different mixes of evaporated, condensed, and powdered milk; *queque seco*, or "dry cake," an orange pound cake; rice pudding; cara-mel or coconut *flan*; corn sweet breads; *mazamorra*, a cornstarch pudding; *milanes*; and *tapitas*, which are chocolate candies.

FOODS WITH CULTURAL SIGNIFICANCE

Regional Variations

The Central Valley is composed of the provinces of Alajuela, Cartago, Heredia, and San José. Most of the inhabitants of Costa Rica live in this valley, which is why the cuisine of the region is often believed to be the only one in Costa Rica. When discussing the typical dishes of the Central Valley, it is important to mention the soups. *Sopa de albóndigas* (meatball soup) and *olla de carne* (beef pot), the soups most often consumed, are a combination of meat and vegetables typical of the region, such as *chayote*, potato, *yucca*, and carrots. This kind of dish represents the junction of the Spanish cuisine (meat) with the vegetables aboriginals once ate. Like soups, *picadillos* are characteristic of the Central Valley. *Casado* ("married"), which is also popular for lunch, includes white rice, beans, *picadillo*, meat, poultry, or fish, and fried plantain. Another important dish is *gallos* (literally translated as "rooster"). *Gallo* is a corn tortilla filled with almost anything, including beef, cheese, or refried beans, so they are similar to what Mexicans call "tacos."

Besides these dishes, dairy products have been an important part of the culinary history of Costa Rica. The country produces two particular types of cheeses: *turrialba* and *palmito*, which are like mozzarella cheese but drier and saltier. Milk has been used to make foods such as eggnog, breads, ice creams, cakes, and *cajetas*. *Natilla*, or sour cream, is a very common product that Costa Ricans eat with *gallo pinto* at breakfast.

Guanacaste

Guanacaste, one of the provinces located in the Pacific north of the country, preserves the dishes of Costa Ricans' pre-Hispanic ancestors. Today *Guanacastecos* (inhabitants of Guanacaste) eat tortillas, *atol* (corn pudding), *mazamorra* (corn pudding served as dessert), *chorreadas* (fried ground tender corn), and *dumb tamal* (corn dough without stuffing). Popular beverages are *chicha*, a fermented drink made from corn, water, ginger, and sugarcane syrup, and *horchata*. Because of its African influence, it is important to mention a frequently prepared dish known as *bajo*,

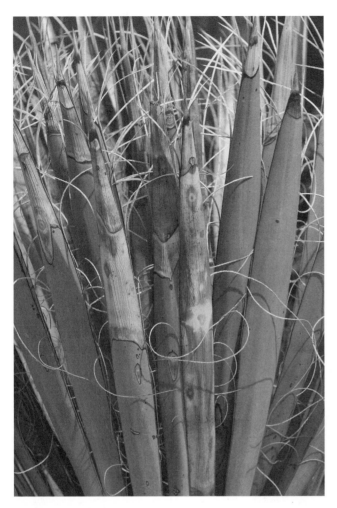

The Yucca Plant

in which meat and plantains are covered with plantain leaves and cooked in water. For sweets, *jocotada* is a typical preserve made from milk and *jocote* (*Spondias purpurea*, a red fruit with a single large seed).

Puntarenas

Puntarenas is a port city located on the Pacific Coast, well-known for its *chuchecas* (seafood). The fried *palometa* fish stands out above the other delights, although the *Chuchequeros*, as the residents of Puntarenas are known, prefer the corvine and pargo fish, clams, squid, crabs, and cambute. Most of these fish are fried with butter, sautéed with oil and garlic, or are included in meals that contain rice, milk soups, cocktails, and ceviche. The *ceviche puntarenense*, one of the most famous dishes, is raw fish or shellfish marinated in citric juices such as lime, lemon, or orange juice, and mixed with chopped onions, cilantro, parsley, celery, red peppers, and other popular condiments such as Tabasco, *Salsa Lizano*, tomato ketchup, and sometimes mayonnaise.

Finally, it is served at cold-room temperature with soda crackers or with fried green plantain made in the form of *patacones*.

Limón

Limón has been a port of entry for different cultures that came mostly from Jamaica, but also from China, India, and Africa. This migration has distinguished the Limonese cuisine from that of the rest of the country. It is characterized by certain condiments: coconut oil and coconut milk (which bring a particular Caribbean flavor and aroma to the food), *Panama* pepper, sweet pepper, onion, tomato, thyme, black pepper, cinnamon, vanilla, nutmeg, curry powder, garlic, and cilantro. The coconut milk is involved in the preparation of the rice-and-beans dish (Limonense's *gallo pinto*), the most representative dish of Limón, which is accompanied by chicken, beef, pork, or fish. Other highly popular foods and drinks of Limón are *paty* (meat pastries scented with hot Panama pepper), *bacalao* with *aki* (*bacalao* prepared with the edible part of the *aki*, coconut oil, onion, tomato sauce, and hot pepper), *rondon* (a mix of palm heart, plantain, green onion, and peppers with fish and other types of meats), turtle meat (with rum, in soups or in *rondon* with coconut milk), *Bon* bread (a round, dark bread made with eggs, spices, and sugarcane molasses), *johnny cake* (round coconut bread), *agua de sapo* or *hiel* (a spicy drink made of ginger, lime, and brown cane sugar), and fruit juices made primarily with papaya, watermelon, banana, guava, and star fruit.

 TYPICAL DAY'S MENU

According to the nutritionist Marcela Dumani, the typical day's menu for Costa Ricans varies depending on the province. Table 37-1 gives some examples of typical day's menus in the Central Valley, the Pacific Coast, and Limón.

 HOLIDAY MENUS

Many Costa Rican holidays are religious. For example, during *Semana Santa* (Holy Week), it is common to cook especial dishes, such as *chiverre empanadas* (turnovers), bean tamales, mustard tamales, and cheese, sugar, and cinnamon empanadas (turnovers). During the Christmas season, Costa Ricans enjoy *fiestas cívicas*, which are similar to the state fairs in the United States. At these fairs, dishes such as *gallos*, tamales (usu-

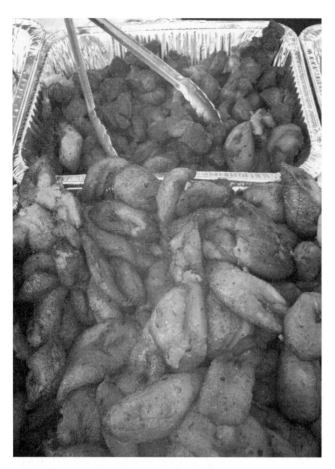

Fried ripened plantains are one of the Costa Ricans' favorite dishes.

ally prepared with flavored cornmeal and mashed potatoes stuffed with chicken, pork, rice, olives, carrots, green peas, and pimentos formed into a rectangle shape and wrapped in banana leaves), *chicharrones*, and *chorreadas* are easy to find. For Christmas dinner, tamales, roasted pork leg, and Christmas cake (a cake made with dried fruits, nuts, and rum) are the most typical dishes prepared. In Costa Rican cities named for a saint, inhabitants of the city celebrate the saint with a kind of fair called *turnos*. The common dishes available at the *turnos* include meat tamales, rice with chicken (rice mixed with pieces of chicken, and vegetables), rice pudding, and *churros* (a cruller). For social activities, such as birthday parties, *quinceaños* (celebration of one's 15th birthday), weddings, and rosaries, *arroz con siempre* ("always rice") is always present. *Arroz con siempre* can include other ingredients, but rice is always present, as in *arroz con pollo* and *arroz con leche*.

 HEALTH BELIEFS AND CONCERNS

Health care in Costa Rica is family based. Either grandmothers or mothers can recommend home remedies made primarily with natural herbs, fruits, and vegetables. For instance, carrot juice mixed with orange juice is thought to be good for vision, chamomile tea is prepared to fight against inflammation (especially during

TABLE 37-1   Daily Menu by Region

Typical Day's Menu	Central Valley[a]	Pacific Coast[b]	Limón
Breakfast	Sweetened coffee, bread, *gallo pinto*, egg, and sour cream	Sweetened coffee, tortilla, *gallo pinto*, egg, meat, or chicken in tomato sauce	Rice and beans, fried cake, sweetened coffee, fried plantains, some meat with coconut sauce
Mid-morning	Some fruit, sweetened coffee, and bread		
Lunch and dinner	Rice, red or black beans, meat (beef or chicken), processed meat, fried plantains, cabbage salad with tomato, and natural fruit drink with sugar	Rice, beans, meat (mostly fried), tortillas, fried plantains, and natural fruit drink	Rice or rice and beans, meat or chicken prepared with Caribbean sauce or fried fish, yucca, green banana, green plantain, *patacones* cabbage salad with tomato, natural fruit drink or *hiel*
Afternoon coffee	Sweetened coffee and bread		*Hiel* and *paty*

[a]San José, Alajuela, and Heredia
[b]Puntarenas and Guanacaste

menstrual periods), and ginseng is thought to be good for the brain. Nutritionist Marcela Dumani has found through her experience working with the Costa Rican community that they generally believe, among other misconceptions, the following:

1. The *guineo* (unripe banana) contains iron.
2. Honey and brown sugar are substitutes for normal sugar and have fewer calories.
3. Regular margarine and oil have fewer calories than butter and shortening.
4. Beans are very fattening.
5. Adults do not need to consume milk.
6. Fruit beverages have enough fruit content.
7. Dietary fiber can come from meats.

 ## GENERAL HEALTH AND NUTRITIONAL INDICATORS SUMMARY

Costa Rica's territory comprises 51,000 km² with an estimated population of 4,509,290 and an annual growth rate of 1.2% (National Institute of Statistics and Census of Costa Rica [INEC], 2009). Among Latin American countries, Costa Rica has one of the highest indices of social development (46.9%), due to improvements in basic health indicators. In a period of 10 years (1987–2007), Costa Rica reduced the country's birth rate to 16.3/1000 population, which is below the average birth rate of Latin America in general (21.0/1000 population). In addition, Costa Rica has managed to increase the life expectancy to 75 years for men and 80 years for women, and to reduce the infant mortality rate and crude death rate, respectively, to 10.1/1000 lives births and 12/1000 population (World Health Organization, 2009). According to the INEC (2009), the primary cause of death among adults is heart attack followed by heart disease.

Costa Rica has worked hard to improve its social conditions. Overall, in Latin America, Costa Rica has one of the highest rankings of human development index (0.834). The adult literacy rate is 95.2%, and the percentage of people who live in extreme poverty has decreased to 3.3% (Costa Rican Ministry of Health, 2008).

With regard to nutritional indicators, the last data available are from the National Nutrition Survey conducted in 1996. Results for the prevalence of anemia shows that 82 preschool-age children, 22 pregnant women, and 211 nonpregnant women were classified with anemia according to criteria recommended by the World Health Organization; thus, anemia was classi-fied as a moderate public health problem caused primarily by iron deficiency followed by folate deficiency. Moreover, anthropometric data were collected among preschool children, school children, and women from 15 to 59 years old. Overall, the results showed a reduced presence of undernutrition and, importantly, increased overweight and obesity. The percentage of preschool children with some degree of undernutrition was 5.1%, and 9.1% were overweight. Among school children the prevalence of undernutrition was 16.5% and overweight 14%. Among adolescent women (15–19 years) the prevalence of undernutrition was 1.4% and overweight 23.2%. Among 20- to 44-year-old women the prevalence of undernutrition was 9% and overweight 45.9%. Among 45- to 59-year-old women the prevalence of undernutrition was 2.5% and overweight 75.9%.

 ## COMMUNICATION AND COUNSELING TIPS

In order to provide the best and most effective service, health providers should have a better understanding of the culture, health beliefs, family roles, and preferred communication styles. In general, Costa Ricans are friendly people to whom family is very important. Gestures such as shaking hands, smiling, and asking about the family are tips that can help health providers to create an environment in which the patient can communicate easily. According to Sedó (2008), some of the information that a healthcare provider should determine includes the province of Costa Rica from which the patient comes, the foods typically consumed, how foods are prepared, and whether the person eats between meals (known in Costa Rica as *pellizcar*). In addition, to know whether it is necessary to work with interpreters or to speak slowly, the healthcare provider must also determine the English level of the patient. The use of pictures, food models, shopping tips, portion sizes, examples of menus, and gestures can facilitate the communication between patient and counselor. It is also important to give the patient recommendations regarding healthier cooking techniques (e.g., baking instead of frying) for the foods they customarily consume.

FEATURED RECIPE

Gallo Pinto is garnished with sour cream, either on top or on the side. You can also eat it with scrambled or over-easy eggs.

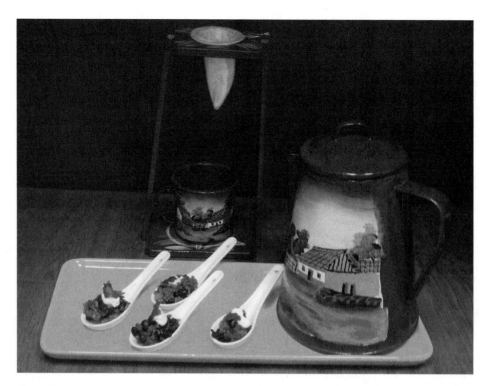

Gallo Pinto
Courtesy of the author

Gallo Pinto (Speckled Rooster)

1 can (approximately 2 cups) black or pinto beans

2 cups cooked white rice

1 small onion, chopped

¼ cup red bell pepper, chopped

¼ cup cilantro, chopped

1 tsp. minced garlic

2 tbsp. *Salsa Lizano* (or Worcestershire sauce)

½ tbsp. canola oil (or olive oil)

Salt to taste

1. Sauté the onion and bell pepper in the oil.
2. Once the onions and peppers are cooked, add the garlic.
3. Let the mixture cook until almost soft and then add the beans, and cook for another 2 minutes.
4. Add the rice, cilantro, and sauce, and cook for about 2 minutes more.

Yields 2–3 servings

More recipes are available at http://nutrition.jbpub.com/foodculture/

ACKNOWLEDGMENTS

The authors thank the following people: Patricia Sedó, Nutritionist, Director of the Human Nutrition Department of the University of Costa Rica; Marcela Dumani, Nutritionist, Human Nutrition Department of the University of Costa Rica; María Isabel Campadabal, Costa Rican chef; and Miguel Barboza, Editorial Director of *Sabores* magazine and Grupo Nación/Producciones Talamanca Verde. We also thank Jeremy Thompson for the recipe and Davis Jaeger for the photo.

REFERENCES

Abarca L., Dumani M., & Elizondo F. (1997). *Alimentación Usual en Seis Grupos de Mujeres de la Gran Área Metropolitana de Costa Rica. Seminario de Graduación.* San José, Costa Rica: Escuela de Nutrición de la Universidad de Costa Rica.

Adams, E., & Sockalingam, S. (1999). *Communication patterns and assumptions of differing cultural groups in the United States.* Retrieved March 4, 2008, from http://www.awesomelibrary.org/multiculturaltoolkit-patterns.html/

Anonymous. (2003). *Why language and culture are important.* Retrieved February 5, 2008, from http://www.diversityrx.org/HTML/ESLANG.htm/

Anonymous. (2007). *Costa Rica.* Retrieved February 12, 2008, from http://www.infoplease.com/ipa/A0107430.html/

Anonymous. (2008). *Costa Rica: General information.* Retrieved January 23, 2008, from http://www.tourism.co.cr/

Boyle, M., & Holben, D. (2006). *Community nutrition in action: An entrepreneurial approach.* Belmont, CA: Thomson Wadsworth.

Costa Rican Ministry of Health. (2008). *Situación de salud en Costa Rica: Indicadores basicos de Costa Rica 2008.* Retrieved on December 23, 2009, from http://www.ministeriodesalud.go.cr/estaindibas.htm/

Coto, A. (2006). *Cocina tradicional de Costa Rica.* San José, Costa Rica: Ediciones Jadine.

Coto, T. (2005). *Las mejores recetas de Costa Rica.* San José, Costa Rica: Ediciones Jadine.

Food and Agriculture Organization (FAO). (2008). *Perfiles de Nutrición por País: Costa Rica.* Retrieved February 9, 2008, from http://www.fao.org/ag/agn/nutrition/cos-s.stm/

Goyan, P., & Sucher, K.P. (2004). *Food and culture.* Stamford, CT: Thomson Learning.

Greenspan, E. (2008). *Frommer's Costa Rica.* Retrieved February 9, 2008, from http://www.frommers.com/destinations/costarica/0219020880.html/

Grupo Nacion/Producciones Talamanca Verde. (2007, September–October). Texts and pictures of Costa Rican recipes. *Revista Sabores* (18th ed.). San José, Costa Rica.

Helmuth, C. (2000). *Culture and customs of Costa Rica.* Westport, CT: Greenwood Press.

Infocostarica Staff. (2007a). *Costa Rica today.* Retrieved January 15, 2008, from http://www.infocostarica.com/history/present.html/

Infocostarica Staff. (2007b). Costa Rica: *Our language.* Retrieved January 15, 2008, from http://www.infocostarica.com/culture/language.html/

Infocostarica Staff. (2007c). *Overview: History of Costa Rica.* Retrieved January 15, 2008, from http://www.infocostarica.com/history/history.html/

Instituto Costarricense de Turismo (ICT). (2008). *Costa Rica: Official promo.* Retrieved January 24, 2008, from http://www.youtube.com/watch?v=V5hA-i-1Ssg/

Meza, N. (2002). *Seminario "Indice glicérico en salud y alimentación humana: Hábitos alimentarios de la población Costarricense."* Retrieved January 30, 2008, from http://www.inciensa.sa.cr/contenido/publicaciones/memorias_pdf/CONTENIDO/7%20Habitos%20aliment%20CR%20.PDF/

Ministerio de Salud. (1996). *Encuesta nacional de nutrición 1996.* San José, Costa Rica: Ministerio de Salud.

Ministerio de Salud. (2006). *Política nacional de alimentación y nutrición 2006–2010.* San José, Costa Rica: Ministerio de Salud.

Museo de Costa Rica. (2008). *Promoviendo la cultura: Costa Rica, información general.* Retrieved January 23, 2008, from http://www.museosdecostarica.com/infocostarica.htm/

National Institute of Statistics and Census of Costa Rica (INEC). (2009). Boletin 03.1 Panorama Demográfico 1987–2007. Retrieved January 7, 2010, from http://www.inec.go.cr/

Palmer, S., & Molina I. (2004). *Costa Rica reader: History, culture, politics.* Duram, NC: Duke University Press.

Ross, M. (2001). *Entre el comal y la olla. Fundamentos de gastronomía costarricense.* San José, Costa Rica: EUNED.

Sedó, P. (2008). *Trabajo comunal universitario: TCU-486 rescate de la cocina criolla Costarricense con la participación de las personas adultas mayores.* San José, Costa Rica: Universidad de Costa Rica.

UNICEF. (2007). *The state of the world's children 2007: Women and children, the double dividend of gender equality.* Retrieved April 14, 2009, from http://www.unicef.org/sowc07/statistics/tables.php

World Health Organization. (2009). *Statistics. Countries: Costa Rica.* Retrieved December 23, 2009, from http://www.who.int/countries/cri/en/

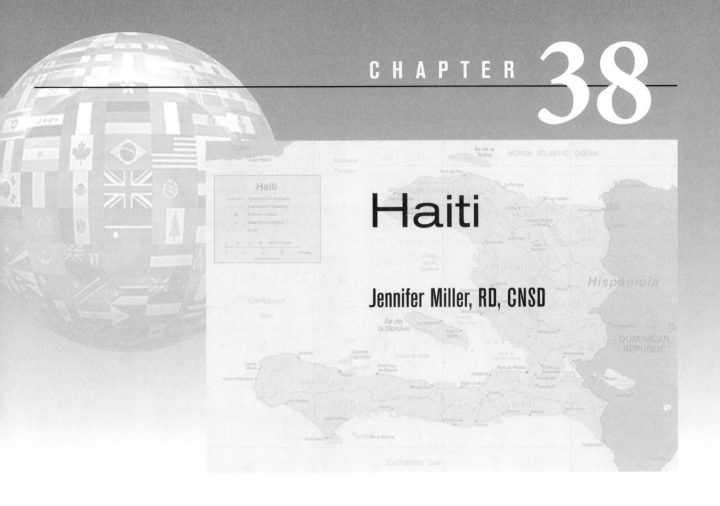

CHAPTER 38

Haiti

Jennifer Miller, RD, CNSD

 ## CULTURE AND WORLD REGION

Haiti is located on the western third of the island of Hispaniola, bordered on the north by the Atlantic Ocean and on the south by the Caribbean Sea. Most of Haiti's population is descended from African slaves who were imported onto the island by Spanish and French colonists. Hispaniola, which is now home to the Dominican Republic and Haiti, was at one time populated by natives called Taino Arawak. In 1492 Christopher Columbus discovered the island and claimed it for Spain. The Spanish set about cultivating the land on a large scale, and eventually forced the natives into servitude on the new sugar plantations. When the population of Taino Arawak declined to the point that there was a labor shortage, the Spanish began to import slaves onto the island from Africa. Several years later, French buccaneers landed on Hispaniola and established a settlement in the northwestern part of the island. They prospered there by a combination of farm-ing and piracy. At the end of the 17th century, Spain ceded the western third of Hispaniola to France. This is now Haiti. The French built up sugarcane and coffee plantations, and continued to import great numbers of slaves from Africa to work on them. These slaves are the ancestors of modern Haitians.

France enjoyed enormous prosperity from the export industry it created, which was dependent on free slave labor. Over the next approximately 100 years, the population in Haiti was divided mainly between slave owners and slaves; however, a class of mulatto *affranchis*, free men who were of mixed African and European descent, developed. The *affranchis* tried to gain equality with the white Europeans, but the Europeans did not regard them as equals. Hostility began to develop among the *affranchis* toward the Europeans, which united them to some degree with the African slaves. During the 1790s the *affranchis* demonstrated against the French, which ultimately encouraged slave rebellions that were led by a self-educated slave,

François Dominique Toussaint. Toussaint was later captured by the army of Napoleon, but his successor as leader of Haitian nationalist forces, Jean-Jaques Dessalines, along with other army generals, continued to fight against the French, and in 1803 France surrendered. On January 1, 1804, Haiti became the first black republic in the world.

Toussaint and Dessalines are considered heroes by Haitians, who are proud of their heritage. As an independent republic, however, Haiti has suffered political unrest and many changes in government. At times the government has been extremely oppressive. The majority of the population of Haiti has remained poor and uneducated.

Haitian culture is stratified along class lines. There is a small wealthy class who live and work in the cities, a small middle class who work in professional jobs, such as teaching and civil service, and a large lower class. The wealthy class, which is about 5% of the population, live in relative luxury and have adopted a Westernized lifestyle. They speak Creole, the dominant but unwritten language of the country, but also read and write in French, and are well educated. This small wealthy class has a disproportionately large influence in government compared with the other classes. The vast majority of the population is lower class, living in slums called shantytowns outside the cities, or in the rural countryside.

Outside of the wealthy class, the population of Haiti has the lowest per capita income in the Western Hemisphere. Poverty in Haiti is related to a number of factors, including overpopulation, unemployment, little industry, high inflation, and a high illiteracy rate. Their spoken language is Creole, an unwritten pidgin version of French. Poor Haitians have limited access to clean water, food, and health care. Many of them are able to get only enough food for one meal per day, which may consist of porridge made from corn, rice, or sorghum. Most preschool-age children suffer from malnutrition. The infant and child mortality rate is extraordinarily high, and the average lifespan for both men and women is approximately 50–55 years.

Religion plays an important role in Haitian life. Roman Catholicism is considered the major religion in Haiti, with up to 80% of the population identifying themselves as Catholic. Many Catholics in Haiti also practice Voodoo religion, however, and Voodoo is probably practiced more than any other religion among rural Haitians. Men and women both play strong roles in Voodoo and are considered equals at the level of Voodoo priesthood. This may contribute to a general

sense of equality between men and women in the lower social strata.

Music, dance, and art are important parts of Haitian culture and life, and are a big part of the many festivals celebrated by people of all classes. Major celebration days include, among others, Christmas, New Year's Day, Haitian Independence Day, Mardi Gras, and the anniversaries of the deaths of Toussaint and Dessalines. Haitians of all backgrounds and ages celebrate with great abandon during their many festivals.

LANGUAGE

French and Creole are the official languages of Haiti. Virtually everyone in Haiti can speak and understand Creole, a spoken but unwritten language. French is spoken only by educated people.

FOOD HISTORY WITHIN THE CULTURE

Haitian cuisine is interesting in its diversity of influences, and in the way that Haiti's history is reflected in them. French, African, and Caribbean flavors and styles of preparation blend together to make Haitian food unique. Heavy use of starches, such as plantain and cassava, comes from African influence, whereas delicate sauces highlight the French contribution to Haitian cooking. The geography of Haiti is reflected in many commonly consumed foods. Fish is eaten most frequently in the coastal areas. Beans and legumes are native protein sources consumed throughout the country. Native foods, such as okra, mangoes, limes, and coconuts, are typical of Caribbean geography. Haiti's history of poverty can be recognized in the use of dried fish, which is necessitated by lack of refrigeration, and in meals that may consist only of manioc flour bread or starchy porridge.

Getting enough food to survive is a challenge for a large percentage of people. In contrast to the culturally rich and well-developed Creole cooking tradition is the scarcity of the most basic food staples for poor rural and urban Haitians, who live on approximately two dollars per day. The average daily calorie intake for an adult is only about 1650 calories. During the past year, riots have broken out in the cities over the rising cost of food. Many people live on a single starchy meal per day, which could fuel civil unrest and political instability.

MAJOR FOODS

 Protein Sources

Protein sources are fish, shellfish, pork, goat, chicken, and beans.

 Starch Sources

Starch sources are rice, corn, millet, yam, and sorghum.

 Fat Sources

Fat sources are pig fat and imported cheese.

 Prominent Vegetables

Prominent vegetables are wild greens, black mushrooms, okra, and lima beans.

 Prominent Fruits

Prominent fruits are citrus fruits, mango, breadfruit, avocado, coconut, and plantain.

 Spices and Seasonings

Common spices are anise, cinnamon, clove, chive, garlic, ginger, leek, lemongrass, mint, onion, parsley, chili pepper, red and green peppers, scallion, and thyme.

 Beverages

Common beverages are clairin (a rum-like drink made from sugarcane), coffee, and soft drinks.

 Desserts

The popular dessert is shaved ice with sweet flavored syrups.

 FOODS WITH CULTURAL SIGNIFICANCE

Conch is a culturally significant food, because the conch shell was used for communication between slaves during their revolts against the French.

 TYPICAL DAY'S MENU

For the average Haitian farmer, breakfast is eaten early in the morning and consists of locally grown coffee and plain bread made from manioc flour. A light snack is eaten around midday, which is usually porridge of corn or sorghum. The main meal of the day is eaten in the late afternoon and is often the same thing eaten at midday, possibly with the addition of a piece of fresh fruit such as pineapple or mango. For people who can afford it, the main meal may consist of rice and beans,

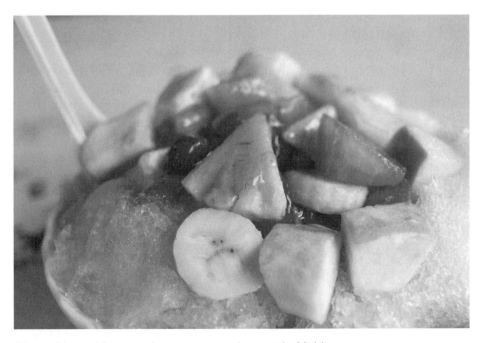

Shaved ice with syrup is a common dessert in Haiti.

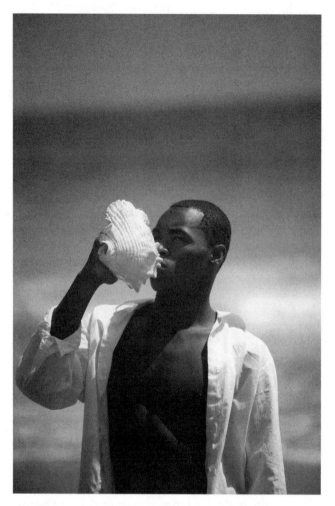

The conch shell was used for communication between slaves during the slave revolts against the French.

and, on Sundays, pumpkin soup. Money permitting, some people will add a small amount of meat to the main dish.

HOLIDAY MENUS

A holiday menu might consist of fried goat or pork, *pikliz* (spicy pickled carrots and cabbage), fried plantains, *pain patate* (sweet potato, fig, and banana pudding), Haitian bread, and pineapple nog.

HEALTH BELIEFS AND CONCERNS

Access to health care in Haiti is limited, and most clinics are located in the cities. The majority of rural Haitians do not see doctors for health conditions. It is common for most Haitians to seek medical care from folk-medicine practitioners or Voodoo priests. As religion plays an important role in daily life, it is common for illness to be seen as related to one's spiritual condition rather than to a cause with a scientific basis. Poor health may also be attributed to causes outside the body, such as cold, wind, and so on. Most Haitians go to a healer seeking treatment for a specific problem and may not understand the concept of disease being chronic.

There are some commonly held health beliefs, such as the concepts of "pedisyon" and "seziman." Pedisyon is the concept that a woman is pregnant but the flow of blood to the baby is redistributed by the body to become menstrual blood, thus ending the pregnancy. It is considered a chronic condition that is demonstrated to have been cured when a pregnancy "resumes" and results in the birth of a baby. Seziman is a condition believed to result from fright and stress in which there is movement of blood to the head resulting in blindness and the possibility of stroke.

Educated Haitians may be more amenable to the use of modern health care and may have a better understanding of the scientific basis of illness and medical treatment. Education and socioeconomic status play important roles in health beliefs and practices, as in most other cultures. It is noteworthy, however, that even among educated Haitians use of alternative or folk medicine is often sought in addition to westernized health care.

GENERAL HEALTH AND NUTRITIONAL INDICATORS SUMMARY

Low birth weight, defined as weighing less than 2500 g at birth, affects 21% of newborns in Haiti (UNICEF, 2007). Twenty-four percent of the nation's children are exclusively breastfed during the first 6 months. Seventy-three percent of infants 6–9 months old are breastfed with complementary food and 30% remain breastfed at 20–23 months of age.

Seventeen percent of Haitian children below 5 years suffer from being moderately to severely underweight (UNICEF, 2007). Being severely underweight affects 4% of children. Moderate to severe wasting was found in 5% and stunting in 23% of this particular population. Only 11% of households in Haiti consume adequately iodized salt.

Fifty-four percent of Haiti's total population uses improved drinking-water sources (UNICEF, 2007). Specifically, 52% of the population in urban areas, and

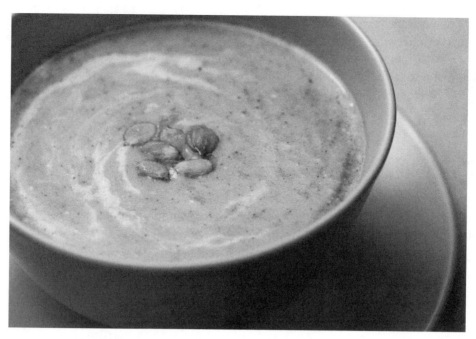

Pumpkin soup is often served on Sundays in Haiti.

56% of the rural population, has access to improved drinking-water sources.

Establishing rapport with Haitians is not particularly different from doing so with other North Americans. Friendliness is appreciated. Personal space needs are similar to what is comfortable for other North Americans. Communication style is generally direct, although modesty is important to Haitians, and they may be less forthright in talking about matters seen as personal. In some cases, an effort may be made to avoid conflict, and some Haitians will appear to agree with a person of higher socioeconomic status even if they are not truly in agreement.

The family dynamic may be relevant in a counseling situation. The ideal social unit for Haitians is the extended family. The man generally holds ultimate authority in decision making, although the woman, especially if she is a mother, is basically responsible for running the home and caring for children. Parents tend to be authoritarian in their discipline and may be forceful with children. Respect for adults is expected of children.

Common health problems among Haitians include diabetes and hypertension. In children, malnu-trition and anemia are frequently seen. HIV is also a big problem in Haiti. When seeking medical attention, Haitians are focused on relief from specific symptoms, and unless well educated, the person may not have a good understanding of the concept of a disease being chronic. For this reason, noncompliance may be an issue with patients.

It is common for Haitians to try home or "folk" remedies before turning to modern health care, and to continue them in addition to it. Black-market or borrowed antibiotics may be used for self-medication. Also, magic or religious treatments may seem preferable to Western medicine. Some traditional methods of health maintenance are beneficial and include maintaining a balance between "heavy" and "light" foods, keeping clean, practicing massage, and breastfeeding infants. Other methods may be less beneficial or even harmful. Purgatives are regularly given to pregnant women and infants. Babies frequently are given baby formula with starchy additives mixed into it.

An interpreter will frequently be needed by English-speaking practitioners. Although patients or parents may feel comfortable having a family member or friend translate (if there is an English-speaking one available), this is a potential cause for conflict within the family; thus, there is a risk that the message may not be translated accurately. For this reason, it is probably best to use an interpreter who is unknown to the family.

It is important to remember that many immigrants and refugees from Haiti are poorly educated and illiterate. For these people, their native language (Creole) is mostly unwritten; therefore, printed instructional materials will be of little use. When working with middle- or upper-class Haitians, printed materials in French may be helpful.

FEATURED RECIPE

Rice with Black Mushrooms

Creole Name: Diri ak Djon-Djon
French Name: Riz aux Djon-Djon

2 cups djon-djon mushrooms or European dried mushrooms

2 tbsp. vegetable or olive oil

3 garlic cloves, crushed and minced

1 small onion, chopped

1 shallot, sliced

2 cups long-grain rice, rinsed with cold water

2 tsp. salt

4 cloves

1 (12 oz.) can cooked lima beans

1 tbsp. tritri (a type of dried fish)

1 or 2 sprigs thyme

1 green Scotch bonnet pepper

1. In a small saucepan, soak mushrooms in 4 cups of water for 10 minutes.
2. Boil mushrooms on low heat for 10 minutes. Strain the mushrooms, reserving the liquid.
3. Add oil to cast iron pot on medium heat. Stir in garlic, onion, and shallot for 2 minutes.
4. Add rice and stir for 3 minutes.
5. Add mushroom water, salt, cloves, cooked lima beans, and tritri. Bring to a boil until water evaporates.
6. Lower heat, stir rice, and place the whole Scotch bonnet pepper and thyme on top of the rice.
7. Cover and cook for 20 minutes.
8. Remove hot pepper and thyme. Stir before serving.

More recipes are available at http://nutrition.jbpub.com/foodculture/

REFERENCES

Kemp, C. (2008). *Haitians*. Retrieved August 24, 2008, from http://bearspace.baylor.edu/Charles_Kemp/www/haitian_refugees.htm

Klarreich, K. (2008). *Food crisis renews Haiti's agony*. Retrieved August 29, 2008, from http://www.time.com/time/world/article.html/

Ng Cheong-Lum, R. (2005). *Haiti. Cultures of the world*. New York: Marshall Cavendish Benchmark.

Pan American Health Organization. (2001). *Haiti*. Retrieved August 24, 2008, from http://www.paho.orgEnglish//sha/prflHAI.htm/

UNICEF. (2007). *The state of the world's children 2007: Women and children, the double dividend of gender equality*. Retrieved April 14, 2009, from http://www.unicef.org/sowc07/statistics/tables.php

Yurnet-Thomas, M. (2002). *A taste of Haiti*. New York: Hippocrene Books.

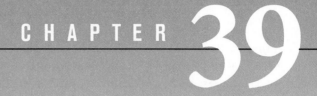

CHAPTER 39

Guatemala

Hugo Melgar-Quinonez, MD, PhD

CULTURE AND WORLD REGION

Guatemala is a multilingual and multicultural country populated mainly by descendents of the Mayan indigenous people (almost 40%), and by *Ladinos* (mixed Mayan and European ancestry) (Instituto Nacional de Estadística, 2006). This broad spectrum of cultures is highly enriched by the diversity within the indigenous population, which comprises people of 21 different Mayan linguistic groups. Guatemala is also the homeland of the *Xinca* people, who are non-Mayan indigenous people living mainly in the southeast. Mayan and non-Mayan indigenous people represent a significant share of the total population, the larger groups being represented by the K'iche' (11.3% of the total population), Q'eqchi' (7.6%), Kaqchikel (7.4%), Mam (5.5%), Q'anjob'al (1.4%), Poqomchí (1%), Achí (0.9%), and Ixil (0.8%) (Instituto Nacional de Estadística, 2002). Along the Caribbean coast live the Garifuna people (around 6000), who are descendents of Caribbean natives and

whose culture also includes African elements. Besides the vast majority of people who identify themselves as natives from Guatemala, the country is home to thousands of European and Asian immigrants, which adds to the multiculturalism of the Guatemalan's eating habits and culinary traditions.

Guatemala is located in the northern part of Central America, bordering Mexico (NW), Belize (NE), Honduras (E), and El Salvador (E). In addition, Guatemala has borders with both the Caribbean Sea (NE) and the Pacific Ocean (S). Despite its size (42,042 square miles), Guatemala is recognized for its great climatic diversity. Its topography consists mainly of mountainous regions and the cool highlands, where the majority of Guatemalans live. The highest mountain peaks reach over 13,000 ft., and some of the main cities, such as Huehuetenango and Quetzaltenango, are located at altitudes between 6000 and 8000 ft. The capital, Guatemala City (almost 3 million inhabitants) (Instituto Nacional de Estadística, 2006), is also located in the mountainous region, at an altitude of approximately 5000 ft. Along the Pacific and the Caribbean coasts the climate is tropical and the terrain is flat. Some of Guatemala's biggest cities, such as Escuintla and Puerto Barrios, are also located near or at the coast. Among the 23 departments that constitute Guatemala, Petén, characterized by its tropical jungle and lowlands, is the largest (13,843 square miles). Petén also contains some of the most impressive Mayan ancient cities. Finally, Guatemala's topography includes a region known as La Fragua Plains in the east that, despite being a semidesert environment, includes major rivers and has been identified as arable for certain fruits.

LANGUAGE

Including Spanish as the official language, which is also the mother tongue of the Ladinos (almost 60% of the population), Guatemalans overall speak 24 different languages.

CULTURE HISTORY

With regard to religious practices and beliefs, Roman Catholicism still represents the predominant religion in Guatemala, but given the strong presence of the Mayan culture, Catholic rituals and ceremonies include elements of traditional indigenous forms of worship. Protestantism and other Christian churches also have an increasing presence in Guatemalan religiosity. Religious festivities are characterized by gastronomic traditions and/or dietary restrictions practiced and observed only or mainly on such occasions. The consumption of certain foods increases during those festivities while the consumption of others decreases. Within the Mayan religious traditions, corn occupies an outstanding position. Besides representing the basic staple food, corn is sacred to the Mayan culture since it is believed that the gods used it as the main substance to create the first human beings. As described in the ancient book *Popol Vuh* (in K'iche language: "Book of the Community"), in the Mayan cosmology the creation of humanity is the result of several trials where different materials were used to form the first human beings, which all failed until maize was utilized. The Maize God also plays a very important role in the world's creation and in sustaining life; thus, maize production has played a central role in the development of the Mayan civilization in different ways. Maize constituted not only the principal sources of nutrients, but also the keystone supporting their vision of the physical and spiritual world.

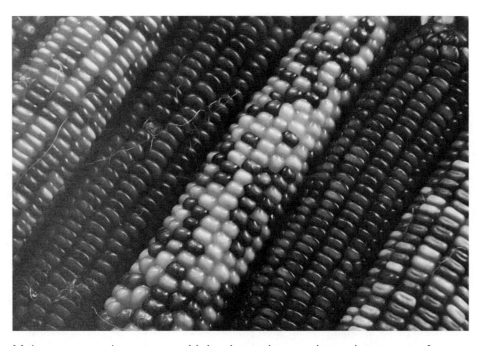

Maize consumption rates are higher in rural areas than urban areas of Guatemala.

Diversity and multiculturalism comprise a very complex framework within which Guatemala developed as a state. Nevertheless, this nation's history has been characterized by confrontation and by very violent and tragic episodes. The encounter between the European *conquistadores* and the indigenous nations populating Guatemala's territory in the early 16th century was far from being sociable and constructive. Like the rest of the continent, Guatemala was conquered due to more-advanced war technologies, accompanied by infectious diseases never experienced by the native people. Additionally, the new arrivals brought with them different religious views that condemned the Mayan spirituality as unsacred and sinful. The survivors of years of war then became the main labor force, working mostly under slavery conditions, used to construct a new nation. After its independence from Spain in 1821, Guatemala became a state where the descendents of the Mayas, although still the majority of the population, represented the most impoverished and disadvantaged group. In 1960, the country engaged in a devastating civil war that lasted almost 36 years. In 1996, peace agreements were finally signed between the Guatemalan government and the rebel groups. Guatemala still struggles with the legacy of the war, and its people are among the poorest in the Western Hemisphere.

Despite an increasing diversification of the economy, Guatemala's domestic production and exports are still dominated by the agriculture, which is a sector that employs almost half of the labor force. Coffee and sugar are two of the main export products along with other agricultural products as well as petroleum and some minerals. A little over 50% of Guatemalans live in rural areas (Instituto Nacional de Estadística, 2006), although urban immigration is a continuous and rapidly growing phenomenon; thus, the diet of the Guatemalans is determined, on one side, by ancestral rural traditions, and on the other side, by the forces of globalization and urban lifestyles. In addition, migration to other countries, especially the United States, has exposed hundreds of thousands of Guatemalans to other socioeconomic environments as well as new cultures. For 2005, the United States Census Bureau (2006) estimated as almost 600,000 the number of Guatemalans living in the United States, which represents almost 5% of the total population of Guatemala. A report released by the International Organization for Migration (IOM, 2007) agencies estimates that by 2007 the number of Guatemalans residing in the United States surpassed 1.5 million. Thousands of Guatemalans reside in Mex-

ico and in Canada as well. It is also reported by the IOM that about 55% of Guatemalan immigrants in the United States are originally from the rural areas, but former residents of Guatemala City represent a large proportion of those sending remittances from the United States. The same document reports that in 2007 Guatemalans in the United States sent to Guatemala over $3.8 billion in remittances, which obviously has a direct impact in the household economics of their families, and therefore in the access to food items. About 40% of these remittances are designated as being for the purchase of food items. In addition, people who invest the money in productive areas do that mainly in trading, restaurants, and in the agricultural sector.

 ## FOOD HISTORY WITHIN THE CULTURE

Guatemala's socioeconomic background represents a determining factor of its population's nutritional status. Based on data by the United Nation's Food and Agriculture Organization (FAO, 2006), undernourishment affects at least 25% of the total population, and Guatemala is among the countries that have recently experienced an increase in the prevalence of this phenomenon. Guatemala's population is very young (41% of Guatemalans are 14 years old or younger) (Instituto Nacional de Estadística, 2006), with a very large proportion of the children suffering from undernourishment. The United Nation's Children's Fund (2007a) reported that about half of the children were suffering from chronic malnutrition; the prevalence among indigenous children reaches almost 70%. Despite the efforts of international and national institutions promoting various strategies against hunger, undernourishment still represents the main public health problem. On the other hand, the rates of exclusive breastfeeding are among the highest in the Americas, especially in the rural areas and among indigenous people: The rate of exclusive breastfeeding among indigenous infants under 5 months is 65% (United Nations Children's Fund, 2007b).

Besides high rates of undernourishment, Guatemalans also suffer the effects of drastic lifestyle changes associated with increasing urban migration and greater access to energy-dense foods higher in refined sugars and fat. A recent report by the FAO office in Guatemala showed that the diet of 75% of Guatemalan families is composed of only five foods: maize tortillas, sweet bread, beans, eggs, and tomato (de Clementi, Villeda, Morrás, & Vivero, 2005). In addition, the same report expresses a concern about the increasing consumption of processed foods. Changing dietary habits, in addition to lower levels of physical activity, are resulting in an increase in the prevalence of diabetes and other chronic diseases such as cardiovascular disease and cancer.

MAJOR FOODS

Protein Sources

Based on FAO data, by 2003 the main sources of protein in the diet of Guatemalans were cereals and beans (FAO, 2008a). Almost 50% of the protein consumed in the country comes from maize and beans (41 and 7%, respectively) (FAO, 2008b). In addition, wheat contributes about 12.5% of the protein consumed in the country. The relative contribution of these foods to the total protein intake among Guatemalans is even higher in the rural areas, where over two thirds of the proteins come from maize and beans (57 and 12%, respectively) (Alarcón & Andrino, 1991, as cited in Serrano & Goñi, 2004).

Black beans (*Phaseolus vulgaris*) are the most commonly consumed legume in Guatemala, with a mean intake among adults of 70 g/day (in urban and rural areas: 81 and 60 g/day, respectively) (Alarcón & Andrino, 1991, as cited in Serrano & Goñi, 2004). Although some statistics show a decrease in the consumption of beans during the past decades, some authors state that at least 77% of Guatemalan families consume beans for breakfast, lunch, and dinner (Bressani, Navarreto, Garcia-Soto, & Elias, 1988). Black beans are prepared in many different ways, including (1) *frijoles parados* (whole cooked beans), (2) *frijoles colados* (puréed- or blended-beans paste, initially very liquid), and (3) *frijoles volteados* (refried-beans paste). These three dishes are prepared at different times of the week, starting with the boiling of the whole black beans and ending with the refried-beans paste as the last stage of the black-beans cooking cycle. In addition to black beans, occasionally Guatemalans consume red and white beans, to which beef or pork are commonly added.

The importance of maize as a protein source has already been mentioned, but it is necessary to add that maize also constitutes a very large proportion of the amount of food consumed by Guatemalans, especially in the rural areas where the daily mean adult intake of maize and its derivates reaches more than 650 g

(Alarcón & Andrino, 1991, as cited in Serrano & Goñi, 2004). In urban areas maize consumption is by far not as high. Given that the protein quality of maize and beans is limited by its low content in some amino acids, their combination on a daily basis provides Guatemalans with a more complete protein intake. Maize is deficient in lysine and tryptophan, and beans are a relatively rich source of these two amino acids. In addition, maize proteins contain good amounts of sulfur-containing amino acids, which are deficient in the legumes (Bressani, Murillo, & Elias, 1974). Traditionally, black beans are consumed with maize tortillas, but the combination of these two staples is expressed in a wide variety of ways. For instance, maize *tostadas* prepared with a black-bean spread are commonly served at parties and celebrations. A maize-based drink known as *atol* (in Mexico this drink is called *atole*), is called *atol shuco* ("dirty *atol*") when prepared with black beans. In some areas of Guatemala thick tortillas are prepared by mixing maize *masa* with cooked black beans. This preparation is known as *tayuyo*. The word *tayuyo* is also used in Guatemala to name bricks that have an especially robust composition called *ladrillos tayuyos* (*tayuyo* bricks), which are known to be stronger than the more commonly produced *adobe* (mud) bricks.

With regard to animal products (meat, eggs, and dairy), it has been reported that eggs have the highest prevalence of consumption (69 and 37% of urban and rural families, respectively, consume eggs on a daily basis) (Alarcón & Andrino, 1991, as cited in Serrano & Goñi, 2004). In addition, the same authors report that the percentage of urban families that consume meats and dairy products on a daily basis is over 60%, whereas less than 20% of rural families consume dairy products, and only about one third of them consume meat on a daily basis. In terms of meat consumption, there are variations determined by the geographical area of residence, besides the obvious limitations given by the economic status of Guatemalans. In the coastal areas the consumption of fish tends to be higher than in the mountainous regions. Some meats are also traditionally consumed in higher or lower amounts during certain times of the year or even during some days of the week. For example, the consumption of red meat decreases during *Semana Santa* (Holy Week, the week before Easter) and during the previous 40 days, a period known as *Cuaresma* (Lent). During this time of the year Guatemalans tend to consume more fish, especially during Fridays. Another example is the consumption of pork, which occurs traditionally on Saturdays. One of the most traditional Guatemalan sayings goes "*A cada coche le llega su sábado*," which literally translates as "To each pig arrives their Saturday." Although it actually means "everybody gets what he or she deserves," it clearly illustrates the tradition of eating pork on that day.

Based on FAO statistics, the consumption of both chicken and beef increased in Guatemala from 1994 to 2003 (24 and 40%, respectively) (FAO, 2008b). In 2003, the average daily beef and chicken consumption per capita was estimated to be 13.7 and 38.4 g, respectively. The increase in chicken consumption goes hand in hand with the development and expansion of one of the most successful Guatemalan restaurant chains. *Pollo Campero* (country-style chicken) is a very popular restaurant company that serves fried chicken all over Guatemala. Founded in 1971, this company currently has over 100 restaurants throughout the country in addition to the restaurants it manages in 10 more countries, including the United States and China. In the United States, this company franchises almost 40 restaurants, which are located in California, Texas, and seven other states, plus Washington, DC. (Pollo Campero, n.d.).

 Starch Sources

Having briefly described its historical development, its complex topography, and its syncretic religiosity, it is not difficult to visualize the food culture of Guatemala as a fusion of eating practices by people from very diverse backgrounds. Despite that, the colorful culinary traditions of this country have their main foundation in the Mayan maize-based culture. Maize tortillas constitute what bread represents in other cultures, and are consumed by almost all Guatemalans' at every meal. Maize represents the keystone of the Guatemalan food culture, providing 40% of the energy intake (FAO, 2008b). Nixtamalization, which is the procedure still used to prepare tortilla dough, was used by the ancient Mayans as well as by other pre-Columbian cultures. It consists of soaking and cooking the corn kernels in an alkaline water solution, which allows easy removal of the hull. The resulting *nixtamal* is then ground into *masa* (maize dough), which can subsequently be used to prepare different foods.

The maize dough is the main component of the steam-cooked tamales, which, among other food items, include olives and raisins, and are wrapped in plantain leaves; these three ingredients are all native to other latitudes. Tamales are considered a special meal in Guatemala, and some variations are consumed on specific days of the week. Despite the strong influence from other cultures, in many Guatemalan households, poor and rich, tamales constitute the central dinner dish for Christmas Eve. Furthermore, tamales, in their many different preparations, reflect the diversity of the Guatemalan culture. In that regard, Guatemalans are used to consuming red tamales (*tamales colorados*) prepared with a tomato-based sauce, black tamales (*tamales negros*), which include chocolate and raisins, *chuchitos* ("little dogs") wrapped in corn husk (*tuza*), and *paches*, which are made from potatoes. Other tamales are made using plants and herbs native to Central America, such as *chipilín* (*Crotalaria longirostrata*) and *loroco* (*Fernaldia pandurata*), which are called *tamales de chipilín* or *tamales de loroco*, respectively. Last but not least, Guatemalans enjoy sweet tamales, such as *tamales de elote* made with sweet corn, and *tamales dulces*, which include fruits and nuts.

Besides its consumption in the form of tortillas and tamales, maize is used to prepare different beverages, the most commonly consumed being the *atol blanco* (maize gruel prepared with water and sugar, with some cooked maize kernels added). Other maize-based drinks are mixed with cacao and/or spices such as *pozol* and *pinol*, and *chilate*, which can be prepared in different ways and is considered a ceremonial drink. In this case, the maize kernels are boiled in water with ashes added. Occasionally, cacao is also added to this drink.

Wheat is another important starch source in Guatemala, especially in the urban areas, where bread is consumed by almost 95% of the families on a daily basis, providing about 17% of the energy consumed (Alarcón & Andrino, 1991, as cited in Serrano & Goñi, 2004). Although recognized worldwide for their "maize culture," Guatemalans are also very proud of their bread, consumption of which is expanding with urban migration. Besides the broadly consumed *pan francés* (French bread), Guatemalan bakers prepare daily a wide variety of *pan dulce* (sweet bread), some of which is named by its shape: *molletes, aviones, hojaldras, champurradas, cubiletes, royales, palitos, semitas, cortadas,* and *rayadas.* In addition, the *shecas* are an important part of the religious traditions in places such as San Pedro Sacatepequez, in the department of San Marcos. As a symbol of solidarity and religiosity, families exchange *shecas* during Holy Week. *Shecas* are prepared in different ways, and some are even filled with marmalade. Perhaps because of its recognition as a nutritious food, the word *sheca* is also used to identify those who are intelligent and clever. It is also used as the nickname for the students and alumni from the Instituto Central para Varones (public high school for male children) located in Guatemala City.

With regard to other energy-dense foods, potatoes have also an important place in Guatemalan food culture. The FAO reports an average annual per capita consumption of potatoes of about 9 kg, which is very low compared with other countries (e.g., Bolivia, 55 kg/per capita per year; Germany, 75 kg/per capita per year) (FAO, 2008a). Nevertheless, potatoes are tightly linked to the food traditions of Guatemala. Potato-based tamales, known as *paches* (flat or short), which are usually prepared on Thursdays only, hold a special place. Although consumed in several regions of the country, *paches* originate from Quetzaltenango. Even though its main component is potato, these tamales are sometimes prepared by mixing wheat or maize flour into the potato dough. *Paches* include some meat as well and are known to be spicy due to the addition of hot peppers.

Rice also has an important presence in the culinary culture of Guatemala, but it is eaten mainly in urban areas, where about 40% of families consume it (Alarcón & Andrino, 1991, as cited in Serrano & Goñi, 2004). When compared with the intake of other cereals, rice has marginal levels of consumption. Despite that, rice is also a common component of tamales, which, as previously mentioned, represent one of the most traditional dishes of Guatemalan food culture. Additionally, rice is sometimes used as a substitute of maize to prepare *atol*. Mixed with chocolate, *atol de arroz* (rice *atol*) is commonly sold during the colder months of the year, especially in cities such as Antigua Guatemala located in the mountainous region of the country. Traditionally, Guatemalans rinse the rice before cooking, which results in nutrient losses in case the rice is enriched with a micronutrient-dense powder. Rice is usually consumed for lunch, and although it is prepared in different ways, Guatemalans like to cook it mixed with finely minced carrots, green beans, and other vegetables.

 Fat Sources

Based on FAO data, about 1% of the energy intake by Guatemalans is provided by animal fat, whereas vegetable oils provide almost 8% (FAO, 2008b). Studies conducted in eastern Guatemala show that, as a percentage of energy consumption, fat among Guatemalan adults comprises 18%, from which less than one third is saturated fat (Stein et al., 2005). Some of the

most traditional foods in Guatemala are fried (*frijoles volteados*) or include fair amounts of fat (tamales). Despite having a fat consumption within the recommendations of international and national agencies, overweight and obesity are on the rise in Guatemala (Gregory, Dai, Ramirez-Zea, & Stein, 2007).

 Prominent Vegetables

Guatemalans consume a wide range of vegetables, many of which are best known in Guatemala by their local names, such as *güisquil* (*Sechium edule*; Mexican *chayote* or chayote squash), and the squash/pumpkin varieties *güicoy* (*Cucurbita Pepo*; squash), *ayote* (*Cucurbita argyrosperma*; pumpkin variety), and *chilacayote* (*Cucurbita ficifolia*; winter squash). The latter three vegetables are prepared in different ways, but mainly in soups or as desserts. *Güisquil* is usually added to certain soups, such as *cocido*, which includes some meat and several vegetables. In addition, *güisquil* is also sliced, dipped in egg batter, and fried. *Güisquil* is one of the foods "offered" to the deceased each year on November 1, All Saints Day. The *güisquil* root, known as *ichintal*, is also served fried in egg batter.

With regard to other vegetables, carrots, peas, red beets, cabbage, and green beans are also widely consumed and usually combined with potatoes as part of some salads. A typical example of these salads is represented by the popular *curtido*, which mixes some or all of these vegetables with oil, vinegar, and some herbs and spices (garlic, onion, oregano, bay leaves, and thyme). *Curtido* is usually prepared at least 1 day before consumption and acquires during the time in-between its characteristic bright purple color. This salad represents the core component of some traditional dishes, such as the Guatemalan *enchilada*, which, regardless of its name, is not spicy and resembles a Mexican *tostada* (crispy corn tortilla) topped with a lettuce leaf, sautéed minced pork, beef or chicken, a generous *curtido* serving, and tomato sauce, grated cheese, and finely minced parsley, as well as a slice of hard-boiled egg.

 Prominent Fruits

Big differences between urban and rural families have been reported with regard to fruit consumption. Despite the great variety of fruits produced in Guatemala, less than 20% of rural adults meet the fruit intake recommendations. In comparison, the proportion of urban adults meeting the recommendations for fruit intake is almost 70% (Alarcón & Andrino, 1991, as cited in Serrano & Goñi, 2004). Banana is probably the most abundant fruit in Guatemala. In addition to the extended consumption of nonnative fruits, such as apples, oranges, mangoes, and pineapples, Guatemala has a wide variety of tropical fruits, some of them consumed in the areas of production. Among those fruits native to Guatemala and the Central American region are some that are little known in the United States, such as the very colorful *pitahaya* (*Hylocereus undatus*). *Pitahaya* is not consumed throughout the whole country, but it is easily found at local markets in the coastal regions and in Guatemala City. This cactus fruit, which is also cultivated in Southeast Asia, is also known as "dragon fruit." The small but sweet fruit of the *nance* tree (*Byrsonima crassifolia*) is widely consumed raw, but also as a dessert. Some places in Guatemala bear this fruit's name, such as the towns Nance Dulce and El Nance in the province of Baja Verapaz. The *jocote* (*Spondias purpurea*: hog plum; known in Mexico as *ciruela*) is another highly valued fruit for Guatemalans. The name of this fruit originates from the Nahuatl word for fruit, *xocotl*. The fruit known in Mexico as *tejocote* (*Crataegus pubescens*: Mexican Hawthorn) is called *manzanilla* in Guatemala (not to be confused with the chamomile flower, also called *manzanilla* in Guatemala) because it resembles a small apple (*manzana* in Spanish). Besides being cooked with sugar as a dessert, this fruit is used to decorate the Christmas tree and the *nacimiento* (crib) with long strings of yellow/orange *manzanillas*. The *jocote marañon* (*Anacardium occidentale*: cashew fruit), which is native to Brazil and known there as *caju*, represents a fruit that is a favorite to many Guatemalans, especially when prepared in beverages. Its seed, the cashew nut, is also widely consumed by Guatemalans and can be bought in small amounts from street vendors who also offer *nances*, *jocotes*, and other fruits and nuts in the streets of cities and towns.

Another native fruit consumed in Guatemala and widely cultivated in tropical countries is the papaya (*Carica papaya*). At the gates of schools and other public places, it is common to see street vendors offering plastic bags filled with slices of papaya, mango, pineapple, watermelon, and mango marinated in lemon juice, and a mix of spices with salt, ground squash seeds, and chili pepper.

 ## Spices and Seasonings

Guatemalan cuisine includes several spices and herbs. Among the most popular ones is the cinnamon used to prepare several desserts. Among a wide variety of hot peppers, the favorite is the small *chiltepe*, which is a round 4- to 5-mm pepper consumed raw, or marinated in vinegar and spices. *Chiltepe* is added in the preparation of some foods, especially seafood dishes such as *ceviche* (raw seafood marinated in lemon juice). Similarly to other foods, some places bear the name of this hot pepper, like the town El Chiltepe in the southeastern province of Jutiapa.

Similarly to other countries in Latin America, Guatemalan culinary culture uses *achiote* (*Bixa orellana*: annatto) as one of its main ingredients, adding a bright red color to several dishes, such as *tamales colorados* (red tamales), *kak'ik* (turkey soup–stew), or *carne adobada* (marinated pork).

Different sauces, including ground-roasted nuts or seeds, chocolate, hot peppers, cilantro, onion, and garlic, are used to prepare meat dishes such as *jocón* (cilantro-based stew), or *pepián* and *pulique* (guaque-pepper-based stews).

 ## Beverages

Lemonade is probably the most popular fresh beverage consumed by Guatemalans, although other fruit beverages made with orange juice, pineapple, watermelon, and so on, are also widely consumed. Soda consumption is on the rise just like in any other developing country with a large urban migration and an improving communication infrastructure (i.e., such improvement facilitates product advertising).

Worldwide, Guatemala is one of the most important producers of coffee, which is consumed by people all over the country. By 2007, Guatemala was exporting over 220,000 metric tons of coffee, representing almost $560 million for the Guatemalan economy, which makes coffee one of the three main export products of the country (Asociación Nacional del Café, 2007). The use of instant coffee is widespread in Guatemala, but some traditional ways of preparation are still in use, such as *café apagado* ("turned-off coffee"). In this preparation ground coffee is added to boiling water, which decreases the water temperature for about 1 minute before boiling again. Exactly at this second boiling point cold water is added to "turn off" the boiling process. Most Guatemalans drink their coffee black with two or more teaspoons of sugar.

The consumption of alcoholic beverages is also widespread, with beer (locally brewed mainly), *aguardiente* (strong sugarcane-based distilled), rum, and other traditional drinks such as *chicha* (fermented sugarcane beverage; also called *boj*) in the province of Alta

Verapaz. The term used in Guatemala to name alcoholic beverages of all kinds is *guaro*, which actually is a distilled drink made from sugarcane. In several regions of Guatemala, people used to produce alcoholic beverages personally, which, because of being illegal, are called *guaro de contrabando* (smuggled *guaro*) or *guaro clandestino* (underground *guaro*). Besides *chicha* and *boj*, *caldo de frutas* (fruit broth), a liquor made of different fermented fruits (e.g., apples and peaches) grown in the Guatemalan highlands, is especially traditional to the town of Salcajá in the province of Quetzaltenango. *Cuxa*, which is consumed in the northwestern mountainous regions, is another traditional alcoholic beverage. Alcoholic beverages are widely consumed during ceremonies and events, and also have religious uses (as part of offerings to divinities and saints). In 2003, the FAO reported a per-capita annual consumption of alcoholic beverages by Guatemalans that was equivalent to 7 kg (FAO, 2008b).

 Desserts

The most traditional desserts in Guatemala, such as the traditional *buñuelos* (deep-fried wheat-flour dough mixed with eggs and sugar, and seasoned with anise), seem to be those of Spanish origin given that the main component is wheat flour. Other desserts, such as *torrejas*, are prepared with fried-batter sweet bread immersed in sugar-based syrup. This dessert is typically consumed during Holy Week. Syrup-based desserts are traditionally prepared using raw brown sugar, cinnamon, and other spices such as pepper and ginger. This syrup (*miel*) is the basis for desserts such as *ayote en miel* (squash), *jocotes en miel* (hog plum), and *nances en miel*. In addition, Guatemalans are proud of their great variety of traditional sweets, which include *canillitas de leche* (milk sticks), tamarind rolls, and coconut balls, among others. Refined sugar provides 17% of the caloric intake through an average daily per capita consumption of almost 100 g (FAO, 2008b).

 TYPICAL DAY'S MENU

It is important to keep in mind that a "typical" menu is not easy to define, because Guatemala has one of the highest rates of undernourishment and food insecurity. Nevertheless, based on the previous description of Guatemala's food culture, and for those who can afford a relatively balanced diet, a typical day's menu is given below.

Tortillas, or sometimes white bread, are served at every meal. For breakfast, beans accompany one or two eggs, coffee is the usual beverage, and a sweet-bread roll is not uncommon. For lunch, rice with minced vegetables accompanies a stew with beef or chicken. Beans are also typical, especially prepared as *frijoles volteados* (refried beans), and lemonade is the most common beverage. A mid-afternoon snack of coffee and sweet bread is not uncommon, especially in urban areas. For dinner, Guatemalan's might again have some bread or tortillas with beans, or leftover food from lunch is served. Because some kinds of tamales are prepared only once a week, dinner will include one tamale (*chipilin tamales* on Wednesday, *paches* on Thursday, and *tamales colorados* on Saturday).

 HOLIDAY MENUS

Besides tamales as a holiday meal for Christmas, *fiambre* is a dish that is prepared only once a year. It is prepared to celebrate the "Day of the Dead," or All Saints Day, and is eaten on November 1 and 2. Although in other Spanish-speaking countries the word *fiambre* is used to name hams and other cold cuts, in Guatemala it is basically a salad that may include up to 50 ingredients. The basis of this salad is the *curtido*. The *fiambre* can be *fiambre colorado* (red) or *fiambre blanco* (white), which does not include red beets. Perhaps its name stems from the variety of cold cuts and sausages that are added to the *curtido*, but it also includes chicken, fish, or even shrimp. Eggs (usually hard-boiled) are also added to the salad and meats, in part to decorate the dish, which can also include different kinds of cheeses and spices. It is no wonder that the word *fiambre* in Guatemala is also used to denominate mixed-up things or complex issues. Given the wide diversity of ingredients that compose this dish, the ways of preparation vary greatly, and many families have their own recipes, which they use year after year for generations. Families meet for lunch on November 1 after having visited the cemeteries where their beloved ones rest. Flowers, and on occasion food and alcohol, are part of the offerings to the deceased.

 HEALTH BELIEFS AND CONCERNS

Beliefs with regard to the health properties of foods in Guatemala are dominated by the cold/hot theory. Fish and avocado are considered cold foods, whereas coffee or hot peppers are considered hot foods. Depending on the weather, one's health status, or one's pregnancy status in the case of women, one should consume or avoid certain types of foods in order to heal or stay healthy. During pregnancy, for example, women should not eat cold foods such as beans, eggs, and milk, even if consumed cooked and warm. The consequences to the nutritional status of women and their infants are obvious, given that such foods are often the only sources of protein available to them. Nevertheless, the list of forbidden foods varies from region to region. The basic idea is to maintain harmony balancing cold with hot foods; consumption of foods that create imbalance can lead to illness.

 ## GENERAL HEALTH AND NUTRITIONAL INDICATORS SUMMARY

In 2008, Guatemala's human development index was 0.696, occupying position 121 of 179 nations listed in the Human Development Report by the United Nations Development Program (2008). With a crude death rate of 6 per 1000 live births, in 2007 the life expectancy at birth for Guatemalans was 70 years. That same year, however, the infant mortality rate and the under-5-years mortality rate were 29 and 39 per 1000 live births, respectively. The mortality rate reached 130 per 100,000 live births and the adult literacy rate was 73%. Data by the United Nations Children's Fund (2007a) indicate that many Guatemalan children still suffer the effects of undernourishment: 49% are stunted and

23% underweight. Furthermore, in 2004 only 18% of children 6–59 months of age were covered with vitamin A supplementation (United Nations Development Program, 2008). The most recent data on anemia by the World Health Organization (2009) indicate that iron deficiency affected over one third of Guatemalan women (Hb < 12 g/dl) and over one fourth of all children 1–5 years of age (Hb < 11 g/dl). In terms of food insecurity, the FAO (2008a) reported that Guatemala continues to have problems in reducing the prevalence of hunger, experiencing an increase in the number of undernourished people from 1.3 to 2 million between 1990 and 1992 and 2003 and 2005.

 ## COMMUNICATION AND COUNSELING TIPS

As previously discussed, Guatemalans constitute a very diverse community, and that presents a challenge to people who think that Latinos, and therefore Guatemalans, are culturally the same group. In fact, people who counsel Guatemalans in the United States might find that some Guatemalans do not speak Spanish as their mother tongue or as their language of preference. The strong roots and identity as Mayan descendents is something that many Guatemalan immigrants bring with them to the United States; thus, it is becoming more common for nutrition educators who teach in Spanish to need an interpreter of one of the

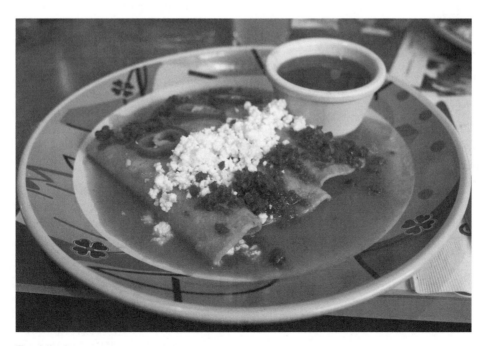

Enchiladas

main Mayan languages. In addition, nutrition counselors should recognize the importance of self-identity among Latinos. Even though the terms "Latino(a)" and "Hispanic" are widely accepted by this community, as well as by other Latin American immigrants, people from Guatemala identify themselves first and foremost as Guatemalans. In either case, the main suggestion for people who work with Latinos in the United States is to exhaustively learn about the specific characteristics of the groups with which they are working. That will allow counselors a better chance to establish trustful and productive relationships with their clientele.

FEATURED RECIPE

Jocón

3 lbs. chicken, pork,
or beef, cut into pieces

2 onions, 1 finely chopped

4 garlic cloves, 2 finely chopped

2 corn tortillas, soaked in water

10 tomatillos

½ cup cilantro, finely chopped

½ cup scallions, finely chopped

1 green bell pepper, finely chopped

2 Serrano peppers, finely chopped

2 bay leaves

½ tsp. salt

½ tsp. pepper

1. Cook the meat in water with 1 onion and 2 garlic cloves; then add salt. Once cooked, remove the meat and set aside.
2. Using the broth, cook the remaining onion and garlic gloves, cilantro, scallions, and bell and Serrano peppers. Once cooked, add the soaked tortillas and blend into a smooth sauce.
3. Add the cooked meat to the sauce. Add pepper and bay leaves, and simmer for about 20 minutes on a medium-low flame. Season with salt, if desired.

Yields 6–8 servings

More recipes are available at http://nutrition.jbpub.com/foodculture/

REFERENCES

Asociación Nacional del Café. (2007). *Cuadro cifras de exportación cinco años 02/07.* Retrieved August 28, 2008, from http://portal.anacafe.org/portal/Home.aspx?tabid=10/

Bressani, R., Murillo, B., & Elias, L. (1974). Whole soybeans as a means of increasing protein and calories in maize-based diets. *Journal of Food Science, 39*(3), 577–580.

Bressani, R., Navarreto, D., Garcia-Soto, A., & Elias, L. (1988). Culinary practices and consumption characteristics of common beans at the rural home level. *Archives of Latin American Nutrition, 18*(4), 925–934.

de Clementi, L., Villeda, B., Morrás, E., & Vivero, J.L. (2005). *Avances en la implementación del derecho a la alimentación en Guatemala.* Work document No. 2. Guatemala: Food and Agricultural Organization.

Gregory, C.O., Dai, J., Ramirez-Zea, M., & Stein, A.D. (2007). Occupation is more important than rural or urban residence in explaining the prevalence of metabolic and cardiovascular disease risk in Guatemalan adults. *Journal of Nutrition, 137*(5), 1314–1319.

Instituto Nacional de Estadística. (2002). *Ethnic group: Censos nacionales XI de población y VI de habitación.* Retrieved August 28, 2008, from http://www.ine.gob.gt/Nesstar/Censo2002/survey0/index.html/

Instituto Nacional de Estadística. (2006). *National results: Encuesta nacional de condiciones de vida 2006.* Retrieved August 28, 2008, from http://www.ine.gob.gt/descargas/ENCOVI2006/Resultados_Nacionales.pdf/

International Organization for Migration & United Nations International Research and Training Institute for the Advancement of Women. (2007). *Remittances survey 2007: Gender perspective* [Encuesta sobre Remesas 2007: Perspectiva de género]. Cuadernos de Trabajo Sobre Migración #24. Retrieved August 28, 2008, from http://www.un-instraw.org/es/docs/remesas/Cuaderno_de_Trabajo_No_24.pdf/

Pollo Campero. (n.d.). *Guatemala.* Retrieved August 28, 2008, from http://www.pollocampero.com/

Serrano, J., & Goñi, I. (2004). Role of black bean *Phaseolus vulgaris* on the nutritional status of Guatemalan population. *Archives of Latin American Nutrition, 54*(1), 36–44.

Stein, A.D., Gregory, C.O., Hoddinott, J., Martorell, R., Ramakrishnan, U., & Ramírez-Zea, M. (2005). Physical activity level, dietary habits, and alcohol and tobacco use among young Guatemalan adults. *Food Nutrition Bulletin, 26*(2 Suppl 1), S78–S87.

United Nations Children's Fund (UNICEF). (2007a). *The Guatemalan children in figures: Statistical summary on the Guatemalan children and adolescents* [La niñez guatemalteca en cifras: Compendio estadístico sobre las niñas, niños y adolescentes guatemaltecos]. Guatemala: UNICEF.

United Nations Children's Fund (UNICEF). (2007b). *The state of the world's children 2007: Women and children, the double dividend of gender equality.* Retrieved April 27, 2009, from http://www.unicef.org/sowc07/statistics/tables.php

United Nations Development Program. (2008). *Statistical update, Guatemala.* Retrieved April 27, 2009, from http://

hdrstats.undp.org/en/2008/countries/country_fact_sheets/cty_fs_GTM.html/

United Nations Food and Agriculture Organization (FAO). (2006). *The state of food insecurity in the world 2006: Eradicating world hunger—taking stock ten years after the World Food Summit*. Rome: Author.

United Nations Food and Agriculture Organization (FAO). (2008a). *The state of food insecurity in the world 2008*. Retrieved April 27, 2009, from http://www.fao.org/docrep/011/i0291e/i0291e00.htm/

United Nations Food and Agriculture Organization (FAO). (2008b). *Consumption data: FAOSTAT*. Retrieved August 28, 2008, from http://faostat.fao.org/

United States Census Bureau. (2006). *Facts for features. Hispanic heritage month: September 15 to October 15, 2006*. Retrieved August 28, 2008, from http://www.census.gov/Press-Release/www/releases/archives/facts_for_features_special_editions/index.html/

World Health Organization. (2009). *Country brief: Guatemala*. Retrieved April 27, 2009, from http://www.paho.org/English/DD/AIS/cp_320.htm/

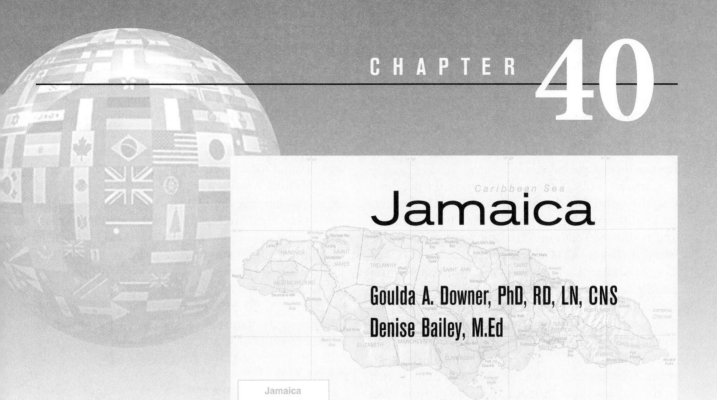

CHAPTER 40

Jamaica

Goulda A. Downer, PhD, RD, LN, CNS
Denise Bailey, M.Ed

 CULTURE AND WORLD REGION

Utter the word "Jamaica" and images of reggae music, white sandy beaches, azure waters, exotic fruity drinks, rum punch, and jerk food comes to mind; however, this Caribbean Island is a lot more than that. Jamaica is a country built on tradition and culture. It is a culture rooted in multiethnic and multiracial traditions. Its unique national motto, "Out of Many, One People," best describes the melting pot that is the Jamaican people. The majority of the population is of African heritage; however, Jamaicans can lay claim to roots from Europeans, East Indians, Chinese, and Middle Easterners. These ethnic groups and their cultures are interwoven into the Jamaican cultural tapestry and have each made significant contributions to Jamaica's unique cultural diversity. It is this amalgam of cultures that has given Jamaica its rich sense of national pride and a distinct heritage that is prominently showcased in its religion, music, dance, family, and food.

Religion is the cornerstone on which Jamaican society is built. It is fundamental to Jamaican culture and thus plays a vital role in the lives of the Jamaican people. It is probably no coincidence that there are more than 100 traditional and nontraditional denominations in Jamaica (Davidson, 2003). The country also lays claim to having more churches per square mile than any other country in the world (Getjamaica.com, n.d.). Music and dance are symbolic expressions of Jamaica's ancestral heritage. They are also fundamental components of everyday life—birth, death, marriage, and social gatherings. In fact, many of the popular artists began their careers singing in the church. Where there is music there is dance. Jamaican dances integrate elements of both their European and African ancestry into a style all their own. Like its music, Jamaican dances tell stories of the history of Jamaica. Historic dances, such as the Kumina, Myal, Dinki-Mini, and Pocomania, are ritualistic and integral parts of worship ceremonies such as all-night vigils and burial services. Other dances include the Quadille, Maypole, and Jonkonuu (John Canoe), and are performed on special occasions. The family is another important component of Jamaican culture. If religion is the foundation of society, then the family is the whole structure. Families are usually very close knit and may include several generations living together in one household.

Jamaica is one of the three islands in the northern Caribbean forming the Greater Antilles. It is the largest English-speaking country in the Caribbean region and is situated south of Cuba and west of Haiti. The island is roughly 4244 square miles (about the size of Connecticut) with a population of 2.7 million (Central Intelligence Agency, 2008). The population is 91.2% black (of West African descent), 6.2% mixed, and 2.6% other or unknown groups (Central Intelligence Agency, 2008). The country's name is derived from an Arawak word "Xaymaca," meaning "land of wood and water" (History of Jamaica, 2008). The country is rich in natural resources including bauxite, gypsum, and limestone. The capital, Kingston, is the largest city and a major commercial and cultural center. The head of state is the governor general, who is appointed by the monarch of England (presently Queen Elizabeth II). The head of government is the prime minister, who is elected by the people (Government of Jamaica, 2007).

 ## LANGUAGE

Language in Jamaica reflects the diversity of the people. English, the official language, is defined as standard British English and is used in the education system, media, and most formal interactions. Most Jamaicans, however, have a language of their own, called Patois (pat-wha). It is a mixture of English, French, Spanish, and African dialects (Creole), and is spoken by many Jamaicans in informal settings. Although most Jamaicans can speak or understand Patois, and it is increasingly being spoken, it is still considered by many to be "bad or broken English" and therefore socially unacceptable in some circles.

 ## CULTURE HISTORY

The Tainos are considered to be the first inhabitants of Jamaica. Originally from South America, they settled in Jamaica around 600–1494 AD. These gentle people lived in simple communities where the men were skillful at hunting and fishing. The women were involved in small-scale farming and grew cassava, yam, corn, and sweet potatoes (Jamaican Gleaner Newspaper Online, n.d.). On May 4, 1494, on his second voyage to the New World, Christopher Columbus arrived on the island of Jamaica. Columbus claimed the island in the name of the King and Queen of Spain. At war with Spain, England seized Jamaica in 1655. The British controlled Jamaica from 1655 to 1962. By the 1700s sugarcane became the main crop for the island and was a very lucrative business for plantation owners. As the plantation economy grew, enslaved individuals were brought from West Africa to harvest sugarcane. The slave trade also became a profitable investment for the colonists. The slave trade was, however, abolished in 1808. After years of rebellion, resistance, and internal strife, Jamaica gained independence from Britain in 1962.

 ## MAJOR FOODS

 ### Protein Sources

Fish and seafood are great sources of protein for Jamaicans. Seafood is abundant and includes favorites such as lobster and shrimp, and fish such as red snapper, blue marlin, king fish, mackerel, and sprat. Chicken, goat, beef, and pork are also good sources of protein. Poultry, meats, and fish are usually prepared curried, jerked, baked, fried, roasted, or stewed, and are plentiful year round.

Red kidney beans, black beans, broad beans, black-eyed peas, gungo peas (pigeon peas), and yellow and green lentils are primary sources of protein for many Jamaican families. Most Jamaicans eat the traditional rice and peas, especially on Sundays and special occasions. Peas, beans, and lentils are also used in stews, side dishes, and soups. During the past two decades, soy and soy-based products have become familiar as a "new" food in the Jamaican diet. This protein-rich food is a staple in many households.

 ### Starch Sources

The base of the Jamaican diet is carbohydrates. Foods high in carbohydrates, such as rice, breadfruit, bananas, plantains, bread and other flour, or baked products and ground provisions (yams, sweet potatoes, dasheen, cocoa, cassava, etc.), are an important component to a healthy, balanced diet, and a great source of fuel for the body; however, adding fats, such as heavy

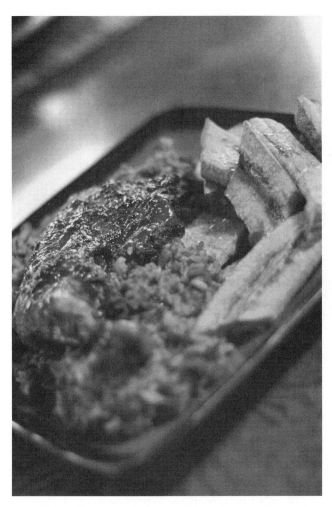

Poultry is served curried (pictured), jerked, baked, fried, roasted, or stewed.

sauces, gravies, butter and margarine, oils, and large portions of meat fats, increases the calorie content and may increase the risk for chronic illnesses, including cardiovascular diseases.

Breadfruit, a round fruit that grows on trees, is an important staple. It can be used as a replacement for rice, bread, potato, and other starches. Breadfruit is boiled, roasted, steamed, fried, baked, or a combination of these cooking methods (e.g., baked and then lightly salted and fried). It is eaten at breakfast, lunch, dinner, or as a snack. Breadfruit chips are a favorite delicacy. Breadfruit is also a good source of vitamin C.

Cassava, a root vegetable, is also known as manioc and yucca. This vegetable is usually boiled. When grated, cassava is used to prepare an island favorite, "bammy," and is enjoyed with fried fish as a favorite breakfast meal. It is also used in puddings and dumplings.

Dasheen is a starchy tuber usually served boiled or as a thickener for soups and sauces. Yams, a tuber of which there are several varieties, are usually prepared boiled, mashed, baked, fried, or roasted. Sweet potatoes can be fried, baked, boiled, mashed, or roasted. They can be used in soufflés, puddings, or even pancakes.

 Fat Sources

Fat is a necessary nutrient and an essential part of the diet for body functioning. Too much fat, however, can cause a myriad of chronic illnesses. In cooking, people enjoy using fat since it gives food its flavor and texture; however, it is also high in calories. Saturated and trans fats are the less healthy fats and should be eaten only occasionally and in moderation. Cheese, whole milk, ice cream, cream, and fatty meats are all high in saturated fats. They are also found in some vegetable oils such as coconut, palm, and other tropical oils. Trans-fatty acids are found in fried foods, commercial baked goods (donuts, cookies, crackers, pastries, etc.), processed foods, and margarines. The typical Jamaican diet is high in fat. Coconut milk and coconut cream is liberally used in many dishes; both are high in saturated fats. Desserts, such as pies, cookies, cakes, pastries—made with lots of butter—and lard are also common. While fruits and vegetables may be the fillings used in pastries, the crusts are usually laden with butter or lard, thus rendering them less healthy, especially when eaten regularly or in large quantities. Furthermore, although cooking methods include grilling and baking, frying, barbecuing, and serving foods with gravy and sauces are also quite common.

 Prominent Vegetables

Jamaicans have access to many vegetables including carrots, tomato, cabbage, cucumber, lettuce, sweet pepper, bok choi, and calaloo (a type of spinach). Steamed vegetables and/or a raw garden salad is a common accompaniment to dinner. The following are some of the vegetables found on a Jamaican table:

1. Calaloo. This is a type of spinach and is similar in texture and flavor. It is typically served as a breakfast dish but is also enjoyed as a side dish. It is a great accompaniment with cod fish or pickled mackerel, and is usually served with boiled green bananas, fried dumplings, breadfruit, rice, bread, or other starchy foods. It is used in the famous Jamaican pepper pot soup, a peppery vegetarian soup made with the leaves of the calaloo and other Jamaican vegetables. It is a good source of folic acid, vitamin C, vitamin A, fiber, and iron.

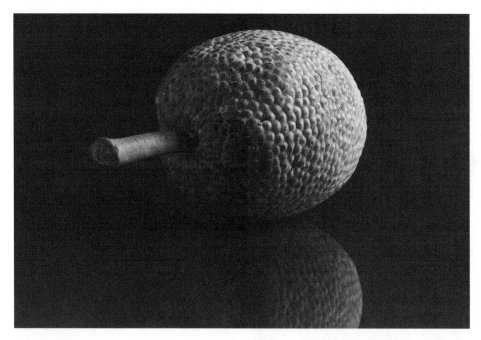

Breadfruit, a round fruit that grows on trees, is an important staple of the Jamaican diet.

2. Okra. This is a finger-shaped vegetable that is served fried as a side dish or used in stews and soups. It is a good source of calcium and vitamin A.

3. Cho-cho. This is light green and pear shaped with small prickles. It is versatile and can be boiled, used in stews and soups, or even used as a substitute for apples in apple pie.

4. West Indian pumpkin or calabaza. These vegetables are members of the squash family. High in vitamin C, with a mild nutty flavor, they are delicious in soups, stews, breads, puddings, and pies. Pumpkin is often added to a mixture of rice, cod, diced carrots, and Jamaican spices, and then cooked down to make a one-pot meal called seasoned rice. Pumpkin can also be boiled, roasted, or eaten with gravy or sauce.

 Prominent Fruits

In Jamaica, fruits are generally inexpensive, abundant, and available year round. These staples are enjoyed fresh or as salads, juices, snacks between meals, and as desserts including pies, tarts, candies, pastries, and a variety of ice creams. Tamarind, papaya, passion fruit, star apple, sweet sop, jackfruit, pineapple, and a wide variety of mangoes, to name a few, are delicacies that are easily available. The following fruits are Jamaican favorites:

1. Guava is a small pear-shaped fruit with lots of seeds. Guava is used in syrups, jams, jellies, candies, ice creams, and as toppings. Guavas can also be used in stews and pies. They are a good source of vitamin C and iron.

2. Naseberry is roughly the size of a peach but looks like a kiwi. The skin is edible and the pulp has a mild, sweet taste. It is used in salads or eaten raw.

3. Mammy apple is a large fruit with an edible tangerine-colored flesh that has a flavor similar to that of the peach or mango.

4. Soursop is a green-skinned spike-covered fruit with a white-pulp interior. The flavor is a combination of sweet and tart, and it makes a nonalcoholic drink or ice cream.

5. Otaheite apple is a pear-shaped fruit with a dark skin and white interior. It is usually eaten raw but can be poached in red wine or made into a drink.

 Spices and Seasonings

Spices and seasonings are the foundation on which cooking is based in Jamaica. Few cuisines mix such a wide range of spices and flavors, which can be interchanged between sweet and savory dishes. Escallion and thyme are popular seasonings in Jamaican cooking and are used in savory dishes. They are essential for the Jamaican cook; they add a mild flavor to dishes. Nutmeg grows naturally throughout Jamaica. The seed is the nutmeg and the outer covering is called mace; both are used in custards, buns (sweet breads), porridge, and many other dishes. Ginger, fresh or powdered, is another favorite of Jamaican cooks. It is used to flavor dishes, is made into ginger beer, candy, and even into wine. Scotch bonnet peppers are to Jamaicans as hot sauce is to Louisiana. This colorful pepper, which comes in a variety of colors (yellow, red, orange, green) is an essential ingredient in Jamaican cooking. These are one of the hottest peppers and are used to give flavor to many dishes. Pimento is another essential ingredient. It is versatile and used in savory as well as sweet dishes. It is used in salads, soups, rice and peas, and desserts such as carrot, spice, and pumpkin cakes. Jamaica is the world's largest producer of pimento. Many of the aforementioned spices are used in the preparation of jerk. The "jerking" of meats has gained worldwide popularity. This spicy seasoning is a special blend of spices used to season meat, fish, poultry, and vegetables.

 ## Beverages

Jamaican cuisine is renowned not only because of its exotic blends of foods, but also because of its memorable beverages. Many of the exotic fruits and vegetables on the island are utilized to create delicious tropical drinks. The juice of carrot, beet, guava, mango, cherry, soursop, lime, seaweed, and passion fruit are popular and refreshing beverages. Sorrel, a traditional Christmas drink, is made from the sorrel flower. The flowers can be dried or used fresh to make this exotic-flavored beverage. Irish or sea moss makes a delectable gelatinous beverage. The dried seaweed is boiled and then blended with condensed milk, nutmeg, and vanilla. Ginger is another all-time favorite used to make ginger beer, which is a nonalcoholic beverage made from grating fresh ginger root and mixing it with sugar and lemon, and then serving it over ice. Variations of ginger beer are also customary. Colas, such as Pepsi and Coca-Cola, along with local Champagne Cola, are also available. Red Stripe, Dragon, and Guinness are national alcoholic beverages. Coffee and tea are also popular nonalcoholic beverages. Jamaica's Blue Mountain Coffee is world renowned.

 ## Desserts

Desserts are an important part of the Jamaican meal. Coconuts, mangoes, guavas, plantains, bananas, and otaheite apples are frequently used in tarts and pies. Dessert could be a simple fare such as fruit with a sim-

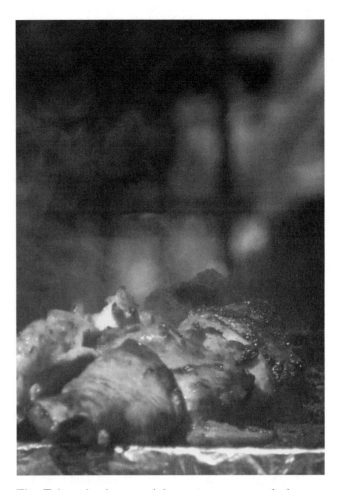

The Tainos had a special way to preserve their meats and fish by adding peppers, spices, and salt, and placing them over a pit—the precursor to the grill. The Maroons later perfected this seasoning and cooking method, which today is referred to as *jerk*.

ple sauce, or a scoop of ice cream; or it could be the dessert of all desserts, "matrimony," which is a mixture of orange sections, star apples, guavas, and sweetened condensed milk. Other popular desserts include sweet potato pudding, gizzards, bread pudding, toto (small coconut cake), plantain tarts, cakes, and a wide array of fruit-inspired ice creams including an island favorite, grapenut ice cream.

 ## FOODS WITH CULTURAL SIGNIFICANCE

Jamaican food is truly a celebration of its diverse culture and eclectic history. Food is the centerpiece of all celebrations—holidays, festivals, births, deaths, marriages, and any other occasion in between. For example, the wedding cake has always been the main attraction of the wedding ceremony. Traditionally, country weddings had "cake parades." On the day of the wedding, married women dressed in white carried the wedding cakes to the wedding location (Tortello, 2004). While this tradition is not practiced today, the traditional cake, made with a mixture of dried fruits soaked in rum, is still served at weddings. The traditional wedding menu may include curry goat, rice and peas, stewed chicken, manish water, and ice cream. Food also plays an integral role in ritualistic ceremonies such as funerals and wakes. The traditional fare at a Jamaican wake or funeral may include curry goat, fried fish, fritters, fried dumplings, hard-dough bread (an unsliced loaf of bread), and beverages including cocoa, coffee, and rum. Little changes in the traditional use of foods have been evidenced over the years.

In Jamaica many foods are considered to have aphrodisiac properties. While some traditional dishes may be served at restaurants, many others are primarily home-cooked dishes or can be purchased at roadside vendors. Manish water and cowcod soup are popular roadside favorites. Manish water is a thick spicy soup made with goat's head, goat tripe, green bananas, and other vegetables. It is a traditional dish at country weddings and other festive occasions. It is said that this soup can cure infertility, impotence, and even the common cold. Cowcod soup, made with bananas, peppers, yams, and penis ("cow's cod"), is another infamous Jamaican specialty. This is said to be the "soup of champions." This soup is purported to not only cure impotency and infertility, but to give added stamina to lovers. Traditional meals continue to grace the tables of many homes, roadside vendors, and restaurants.

The Tainos had a special way of preserving their meats and fish: by adding peppers, spices and salt, and placing them over a pit (the precursor to the grill). The Maroons later perfected this seasoning and cooking method, which today is referred to as "jerk." Cassava was processed into flour and used to make bammy, a pancake-shaped deep-fried cassava bread. Today, bammy is still a staple on the Jamaican table. Pepper pot and its main ingredient, callaloo, were as popular then as it is today. The Spanish brought with them Escoveitch fish, a dish for which fried fish is marinated overnight in a vinegar sauce with onions, carrots, and peppers. They also introduced bean and pea dishes, along with citrus fruits such as oranges, lemons, tamarind, ginger, plantain, coconut, and bananas. The English contributed the patty, a pastry filled with spicy meat. They also introduced sweets and desserts such

as puddings, tarts, pies, jams, marmalade, and pastries. Many other English favorites that are still enjoyed by Jamaicans today include roast beef and corned or salt beef. The Maroons perfected the art of "jerking." Jerk is the process of spicing and grilling meats, poultry, and fish over a low flame. Today, jerk is synonymous with Jamaican cooking. It is usually served with rice and peas and festival bread (made from cornmeal and similar to a "hush puppy"). The African contribution included duckunoo, a pudding made with cornmeal or green bananas, coconut, spices, and sugar. The mixture is tied up in a banana leaf and steamed. Ackee, breadfruit, yams, and other root vegetables were also brought from Africa. These "ground provisions" are the mainstay of the Jamaican diet. East Indians and Chinese introduced exotic curries and spices. Although curry goat is extremely popular, seafood and chicken are just as popular. Curry dishes are essential at parties and functions. The Chinese brought with them sweet-and-sour dishes and hard-dough breads, which have become Jamaican staples.

 ## TYPICAL DAY'S MENU

There are many variations to the Jamaican meal. Generally, Jamaicans eat three meals a day; however, breakfast and dinner are considered the main meals.

Breakfast can be eggs, bacon, and toast, or ackee and salt fish (national dish), fried dumplings, and hot tea. It can also be a larger meal that might include boiled bananas, boiled yams, bread, fried plantains, roasted and fried breadfruit, fried bammy, liver with onions, and herring or mackerel.

Lunch is usually a light snack such as meat patty, bun, fruit, and juice, or a vegetable soup, although for some people lunch may be a main meal as dinner would be for others.

Dinner is usually the largest meal, and the menu typically includes rice and peas, and curry goat or curry chicken; or jerk pork, fish, or chicken, fried plantains or boiled bananas, and a steamed vegetable or raw vegetable salad. Fruit and fruit juice are usually consumed.

 ## HOLIDAY MENUS

Christmas

The Christmas season is one of the most festive times of year. This is the one time of the year when all family members are expected to get together. Family and friends come from abroad to celebrate the season. The Christmas Day breakfast typically includes ham, ackee and saltfish, breadfruit, fried plantains, fried dumplings, boiled bananas, and Jamaican chocolate tea or regular tea/coffee. Christmas dinner is the culinary event of the day. The menu varies depending on each home, but families, rich and poor alike, make this a special meal. Several types of meats are usually served, including baked chicken, roast beef and/or pork, curry goat, or oxtail. Rice and peas, and potato or macaroni salad, are usual accompaniments. Throughout the year, red peas are used with the rice; however, at Christmas red peas are replaced by gungo peas. Christmas cake is another holiday specialty. This cake is made from dried fruits soaked in rum months before the holiday. Sorrel and ginger beer are favorite drinks for Jamaicans at Christmas.

Easter

Easter in Jamaica is synonymous with the bun and cheese. During the Lenten season bun, cheese, avocado, and fried fish (particularly snapper, king fish, and sprat), along with hardo bread, have become quintessential foods for many households. The Easter bun is believed to be relative to the hot cross bun, which is a traditional Good Friday fare for the English. Over the years Jamaicans have adapted the bun into their own cuisine. The bun is a sweet bread baked with lots of spices such as nutmeg, cinnamon, allspice, and mixed fruit. To make the experience uniquely Jamaican, a slice or two of cheddar cheese is placed between two slices of the bun.

HEALTH IMPLICATIONS

Many Jamaican cuisines are rich in fruits and vegetables, beans, peas, and fish (e.g., mackerel, herring, and sardines), all of which are recommended as part of a healthy diet and the prevention of diseases such as cancer and coronary heart disease; however, the ways in which many of these foods are prepared increase the fat content and render them less nutritious.

The proliferation of fast-food restaurants, which are ubiquitous to North America, now exist in the landscape of Jamaica, bringing with them the plethora of breaded, deep-fried, salty, and sugary foods and beverages. With this unhealthful fare, the health implications, including the burgeoning onset of nutrition-related lifestyle diseases such as obesity, hypertension, diabetes, stroke, heart disease, and certain types of cancer, are rapidly becoming a public health crisis in Jamaica. Added to this imported fast food are perennial local favorites such as beef patties, curry goat, oxtail, jerk pork, and stewed tripe. As a result, Jamaica will soon face the health challenges of the Western world. Another less healthful aspect of the Jamaican diet is the fact that it is high in simple carbohydrates, which often includes many refined foods made from flour and white rice. Consumption of more complex carbohydrates, such as whole grains, would be more healthful, and in fact, during the past two decades, these carbohydrates have been gaining in popularity. The key to reducing the amount of fat in the daily diet, whether preparing meals at home or when eating out, is education. It is important to know what low-fat alternatives are available and to make the right choices, such as selecting foods made with unsaturated fats and reducing those high in saturated fats, trans fats, and cholesterol.

HEALTH BELIEFS AND CONCERNS

Roots, tonics, and teas have long been staples in the Jamaican grassroots culture. They are said to be able to cure anything from the common cold to infertility, infidelity, and cancer; therefore, it is no wonder that practitioners of bush medicine purport to treat a wide range of ailments. Many Jamaicans swear by their roots and tonic and would try home remedies before seeking medical assistance. Cerassee tea, for example, is said to be a cure-all for many ailments. Cerassee is a climbing plant native to Africa, the Middle East, and the Mediterranean area. It is used for diabetes, fever, indigestion, cancer, hypertension, worms, dysentery, and malaria. Although Jamaican cerassee is used as an antidiabetic agent, studies have not confirmed this. Rheumatism can be treated with poultices of leaves. Many Jamaicans also believe in the use of fruits and vegetables for their healing properties. For example, the otaheite apple plant can be used as a remedy for diabetes and constipation, papaya helps relieve indigestion, guava leaves treat diarrhea, and tamarind soothes itchy skin and chicken pox. Marijuana can be boiled into a tea for asthma and eye conditions. Research has begun to further investigate and formally document these decades-old claims.

GENERAL HEALTH AND NUTRITIONAL INDICATORS SUMMARY

Estimates in 2008 place Jamaica's population at 2.8 million people. Life expectancy at birth according to United Nations International Children's Fund (UNICEF, 2008) is 72 years. In 2005, there were 313,656 children ages 0–5 years in Jamaica (UNICEF, 2008). The infant mortality rate (ages 0–1 year) continues to be high, at 26 per 1000 live births, while the under-5-years mortality rate stands at 31 per 1000 live births, and the maternal mortality ratio is 110 per 100,000 live births. These numbers are comparable to those of the rest of the Caribbean region. A 2006 survey indicated that infants and under-5-years mortality rates were lowest in the rural areas (UNICEF, 2006).

The nutritional status of children under 5 years for 2000–2007 indicated that 3% of them were suffering from moderate or severe stunting, 4% from moderate or severe wasting, 3% were underweight, and approximately 12% of births were of low birth weight. Approximately 7% of children under 5 years were considered malnourished; however, there was a high prevalence of overweight children in this age group as well (UNICEF, 2008).

A 2005 multiple-indicator cluster survey done by UNICEF (2006) found that approximately 62% of all mothers reported that breastfeeding had been initiated within the first hour of their baby's life, and 84% within the first day. The 2000–2007 figures show that 15% of children less than 6 months were exclusively breastfed, and 36% of infants 6–9 months were being breastfed and receiving complementary food (solids and semisolids). Approximately 15% of children less than 6 months were exclusively breastfed. Twenty-four percent of children 20–23 months were still being breastfed. In general, there is need for improvement both in terms of breastfeeding rates and infant feeding, because both are below global targets.

COMMUNICATION AND COUNSELING TIPS

To understanding how far Jamaica and its people have come since independence is to understand the confident and self-assured attitude of many Jamaicans. In general, Jamaicans are fun-loving, easygoing people. They are hard workers and believe that success can be achieved only through hard work and persistence. From an early age they are instilled with a "can-do" spirit. First impressions are important and set the tone for communication. A greeting using Ms., Mrs., or Mr. is a sign of respect and will yield a favorable response. Maintaining eye contact, yet not staring, is also important because it conveys candor and a sense of trustworthiness. Jamaicans place high value on intellect. They also have a strong sense of culture and national pride. Avoid showing aversion when discussing foods or situations that are unfamiliar to you. If you are unsure, simply inquire, because most Jamaicans are delighted to share information about their culture.

FOOD NAMES WITH PHONETIC TRANSLATION

Food names with phonetic translation are given in Table 40-1. Food names reflect the history of Jamaica's interaction with a variety of cultures and languages. After years of colonialism, the adaptation of many traditional dishes into a cuisine that is "truly Jamaican" has placed Jamaica on the global culinary map.

TABLE 40-1 Food Names with Phonetic Translation

English	Phonetic Translation
Ackee	A–ki, a–kee
Annatto	An–nat–to
Callaloo	Ca–la–lu
Cassava	Cass–ava
Cerassee	Sir–ru–si
Chocho	Cho–cho
Duckunoo	Du–ku–un
Escoveitched	Es–ko–veech
Guinep	Gee–nep
Naseberry	Nees–berry
Ortanique	Or–ta–neek
Otaheite apple	O–ta–he–ti
Pawpaw (papaya)	Paw–paw
Tamarind	Tam–rine

FEATURED RECIPE

Jerk Chicken

8 pieces chicken,
skinless (breast, drumstick)

½ tsp. cinnamon, ground

2 tsp. allspice, ground

2 tsp. black pepper, ground

1 tbsp. hot pepper, chopped

1 tsp. dried hot pepper, crushed

2 tsp. oregano, crushed

1 tbsp. dried basil

2 tsp. thyme, crushed

2 tsp. salt

6 cloves garlic, finely chopped

¼ cup vinegar

1 cup onion, pureed or finely chopped

3 tbsp. brown sugar

3 tbsp. soy sauce (low sodium)

1. Wash chicken with vinegar and pat dry.
2. Preheat oven to 350°F and add all ingredients.
3. Rub seasoning over chicken. Marinate in the refrigerator for 4 hours or more.
4. Evenly space chicken on nonstick or lightly greased baking pan.
5. Cover with aluminum foil and bake 30 minutes.
6. Remove foil, turn chicken, and continue baking for an additional 30–40 minutes or until the meat can be easily pulled away from the bone with a fork. (Breasts may require more cooking time than drumsticks.)

More recipes are available at http://nutrition.jbpub.com/foodculture/

REFERENCES

Central Intelligence Agency (CIA). (2008). *The world factbook: Jamaica.* Retrieved February 15, 2008, from https://www.cia.gov/library/publications/the-world-factbook/geos/jm.html/

Davidson, M. (2003). *Jamaica and religion.* Retrieved February 2, 2008, from http://www.jamaicans.com/culture/articles/

Getjamaica.com. (n.d.). *Jamaica and Jamaican religion: Jamaican religion examined from 1834 to present.* Retrieved January 12, 2008, from: http://www.getjamaica.com

Government of Jamaica. (2007). *Jamaica information service: Bulletin board.* Retrieved January 7, 2010, from http://www.jis.gov.jm/

History of Jamaica. (2008). *Jamaica information service: Bulletin board.* Retrieved January 7, 2010, from http://www.jis.gov.jm/

Jamaican Gleaner Newspaper Online. (n.d.). *Jamaican history I (1494–1692): Columbus to the destruction of Port Royal.* Retrieved February 12, 2008, from http://www.discoverjamaica.com/gleaner/discover/geography/history1.htm/

Statistical Institute of Jamaica (STATIN) with technical support from UNICEF and in collaboration with UNAIDS, UNESCO, and UNDP. (2005). *Jamaica: Monitoring the situation of children and women. Multiple indicator cluster survey, 2005 final report.* Retrieved December 23, 2009, from http://www.unicef.org/jamaica/resources/

Tortello, R. (2004). *Pieces of the past old-time Jamaican wedding.* Retrieved January 12, 2008, from http://jamaica-gleaner.com/

UNICEF. (2006). *The state of the world's children.* Retrieved December 23, 2009, from http://www.unicef.org/sowc06/

UNICEF. (2008). *Country statistics: Jamaica.* Retrieved April 13, 2009, from http://www.unicef.org/infobycountry/jamaica_statistics/

South America

Food, Cuisine, and Cultural Competency for Culinary, Hospitality, and Nutrition Professionals introduces the reader to three prominent countries in South America:

BRAZIL

Brazil is located in eastern South America, bordering the Atlantic Ocean. Brazil is characterized by large and well-developed agricultural, mining, manufacturing, and service sectors. Brazil's economy outweighs that of all other South American countries and is expanding its presence in world markets.

ARGENTINA

Argentina is located in southern South America, bordering the South Atlantic Ocean, between Chile and Uruguay. Argentina benefits from rich natural resources, a highly literate population, an export-oriented agricultural sector, and a diversified industrial base. Although one of the world's wealthiest countries 100 years ago, Argentina suffered during most of the 20th century from recurring economic crises.

PERU

Peru is in western South America, bordering the South Pacific Ocean, between Chile and Ecuador. Peru's economy reflects its varied geography, an arid coastal region, the Andes farther inland, and tropical lands bordering Colombia and Brazil. Abundant mineral resources are found in the mountainous areas, and Peru's coastal waters provide excellent fishing. The Peruvian economy grew by more than 4% per year during 2002–2006, with a stable exchange rate and low inflation. Growth jumped to 9% per year in 2007 and 2008, driven by higher world prices for minerals and metals. Peru's rapid expansion has helped to reduce the national poverty rate by about 15% since 2002, although underemployment and inflation remain high.

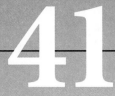
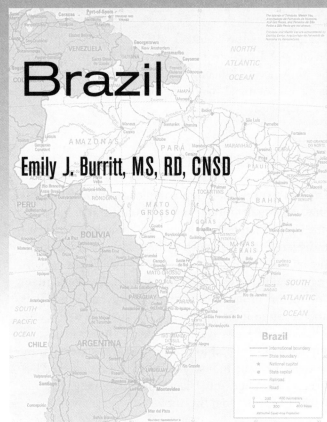

Brazil

Emily J. Burritt, MS, RD, CNSD

 CULTURE AND WORLD REGION

South America is considered part of the New World as discovered in 1498 by Christopher Columbus, when he landed on what is now known as Venezuela. Two years later, Pedro Alvarez Cabral landed on the coast of Brazil. Brazil has since been a melting pot of indigenous people, Portuguese settlers, African slaves, and immigrants. Seventy-five percent of the people in Brazil are Roman Catholic, a religion imported by the Iberian colonists.

Approximately 20% of the population lives below the poverty line, with a higher incidence seen in the indigenous groups. This directly affects food security and the nutrition status of the poor population. Indigenous tribes attempt to maintain a traditional lifestyle, but their existence is endangered by rapid urbanization, industry, and assimilation. Currently, rural populations are relocating to cities looking for better economic opportunities. Eighty-five percent of Brazil-

ians live in urban cities such as Rio de Janeiro and São Paolo. As Brazil continues toward full modernization, shifts in health status as well as food culture are evident. This is illustrated by an increased prevalence of obesity in urban areas, as people adopt a diet higher in processed high-fat and low-fiber foods.

South America is the fourth largest continent and comprises 12 countries: Argentina, Bolivia, Brazil, Chile, Colombia, Ecuador, Guyana, Paraguay, Peru, Suriname, Uruguay, and Venezuela. Three South American territories also exist: the Falkland Islands, French Guiana, and the Galapagos Islands. Brazil, the largest country on the continent, is slightly smaller than the United States, occupying approximately half of South America. It is located in the Western Hemisphere at the equator, with the Atlantic Ocean as its eastern border. The country has a vast landscape and a diverse climate varying from semiarid in the northeast, to wet and hot in the Amazon basin, with the largest portion of the country being tropical. Brazil contains

60% of the Amazon rain forest, which is the largest tropical rain forest in the world.

LANGUAGE

Portuguese is the country's official language and differentiates Brazil from the rest of Spanish-speaking South America. Nheengatu, an Amerindian language, is also recognized in the municipality of São Gabriel da Cachoeira.

CULTURE HISTORY

In order to understand the complexity of Brazilian cuisine, it is important to consider its cultural heritage. In pre-Colombian times, Brazil was home to a variety of indigenous tribes. Following the discovery of the country by Pedro Alvarez Cabral, Portugal began exploring the land and establishing colonies. The Portuguese conquerors brought to Brazil their own cultural beliefs and began to force this way of life onto the natives. In addition, Africans were brought to the continent to supplement the labor force by working as slaves mainly in the sugarcane industry. Acculturation occurred between the indigenous tribes, the Portuguese, and the Africans throughout this time.

In the early 19th century, Brazil gained independence from Portugal. An influx of immigration from European and Asian countries occurred beginning in the 1830s, continuing intermittently until the 1960s. Brazil received immigrants from an array of locales including Japan, Italy, and Germany. Immigrants further shaped the country's cultural habits with an ongoing layering of customs. (Brazil has the largest Japanese population outside of Japan, the largest Italian population outside of Italy, and the largest African population outside of Africa.)

FOOD HISTORY WITHIN THE CULTURE

The traditional diet of the indigenous people was based on maize (corn) and manioc (cassava). Manioc required careful processing to remove toxic hydrocyanic acid. Tribal women masticated and spit the juice of cassava into a jug to make *chicha*, an alcoholic beverage made from fermented cassava, which was widely consumed. Guinea pig and muscovy duck were domesticated by

the Indians and served as a protein source. The majority of natives ate an almost vegetarian diet, as meat was reserved for the elite. Beans also originated in South America, provided protein to the diet, and were found throughout the area. Indigenous people flavored their foods with differing quantities of the native spice capsicum, as well as salt.

The Amerindians ate moderately sized meals two or three times per day depending on geographical location. Women did most of the cooking and ate separately from the men. Natives typically did not talk or socialize during meals and ate sitting on the ground. Most tribes believed in animism and frequently gave offerings or ceremonial tributes to the gods or spirits of hunted animals and food-bearing plants. These traditions began to change and were discouraged with the introduction of European cultural practices.

The Portuguese colonists initially depended on the Indians' food staples but soon began to import plants and animals used in their traditional fare. Moreover, they viewed the native cuisine as inferior to their own. In contrast to the Indians' culture, the colonists favored mealtimes for social interaction and ate large portions of food. The Europeans also introduced frying, a cooking technique not previously used due to lack of cooking oil. Wheat, wine, and olives were mainstays of the Europeans' diet; however, these foods were very difficult to cultivate in tropical regions and were grown successfully only in limited regions of South America. Rice was another grain introduced by colonists that, unlike wheat, flourished in its new environment. Rice remains a significant part of Brazilian cuisine today.

Cows, pigs, sheep, goats, and chickens were transported to the continent via expedition ships. These animals readily reproduced and thrived in their new environment, and therefore were in such abundance that meat was easily available to everyone regardless of economic standing. Meat remains the most important part of a Brazilian meal.

Sugar manufacturing was established in Brazil by the Portuguese early in the 16th century, and sugar became a major export to European countries. During this period, the use of honey faded and sugar took its place as the primary sweetener.

Africans were transplanted from their homeland to South America to work as slaves. They were a large part of the workforce, utilized on sugarcane plantations largely in Brazil; thus, the cuisine of Brazil reflects the influence of the Africans more than any other cuisine in the region. This is evidenced by the use of African ingredients, such as dende oil (palm tree oil), okra, and collard greens, in Brazilian dishes. A combination of the food traditions of the indigenous people, the Portuguese, and the Africans provides the base of Brazilian cuisine today.

MAJOR FOODS

Protein Sources

Meat is the primary source of protein. Recipes for meat and poultry demonstrate the union of the Amerindian and European culinary traditions. Furthermore, the most important contribution to the cuisine, by the Portuguese, was beef, pork, and poultry. Many of the dishes, especially pork, are of Iberian origin. (*Churrascarias* are popular barbeque restaurants that serve unlimited amounts of beef, pork, and chicken to customers, usually for a set price.)

Beef

Beef is the favored source of protein for many Brazilians. Typically, beef is prepared roasted or barbecued, preferably well done. Unlike in the United States, Brazilians consume a broader array of animal parts such as tripe, kidney, and heart.

Pork

Brazilians love pork and it is incorporated into the diet in a variety of cuts and preparations. Pork is used in *feijoada*, a traditional stew with black beans, but it is also used to make *chorizo* and numerous other sausages. Pork legs are roasted or boiled and combined with seasonings such as hot pepper, garlic, or cumin. Pork loin is usually roasted with a sauce.

Poultry

Chicken, being a more affordable protein as compared with beef and pork, is becoming more popular for people with financial limitations. It is usually prepared poached and simmered with various herbs and spices. As with all meats, chicken is used in stews mixed with starchy vegetables and spices.

Fish

Both freshwater fish from the Amazon River, and the saltwater variety from the Atlantic Ocean, are used in Brazilian cuisine. *Surubim* is a preferred type of fish found in the Amazon River. Fish is served fried, grilled, or stewed. *Moqueca*, which originated in the state of Bahia, is a popular fish stew made with coconut milk and dende oil.

Starch Sources

Starches are typically viewed as a side dish but do comprise a large portion of breakfast calories.

Manioc

Manioc (cassava) is a major staple food of Brazil. Manioc is a tuber that comes in two varieties: sweet and bitter. The bitter cassava contains hydrocyanic acid, which is poisonous to humans and requires careful processing to extract the toxins. It has a brown, rough skin and is the source of tapioca. Manioc meal is

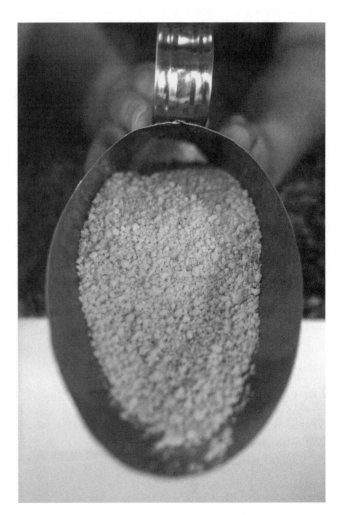
Farofa, lightly roasted flour with a nutty flavor, is served mostly as a flavoring sprinkled over foods.

used to make *farofa* (lightly roasted flour with a nutty flavor), which is consumed mostly as a flavoring sprinkled over foods. In addition, manioc is peeled and then boiled or fried to be served as a side dish.

Corn

Deeply rooted in history, corn is a pervasive ingredient in numerous dishes. *Pamonhas* are traditional tamales made with corn and either milk or coconut milk.

Wheat

Wheat was introduced as a superior grain by the Portuguese and still carries that reputation. Wheat flour is used to make breads, pasta, and desserts.

Rice

Rice grows easily in tropical climates and therefore is readily included in multiple dishes. White rice is cooked to achieve a texture comparable to *al dente* pasta. It is usually served as a side dish accompanying meat and/or vegetables. Assortments of flavors are added depending on the region.

 FAT SOURCES

Lard

Lard was widely used in Brazilian cooking, because historically cooking oils were not easily available. Lard is usually obtained from pork or beef. Only recently has cooking oil become more common, replacing the use of lard, except in the more rural areas.

Dende Oil

The use of dende oil (palm tree oil) was established by the African slaves and is common in the cuisine of Bahia. It provides dishes with a mildly nutty flavor and a golden color.

 Prominent Vegetables

Vegetables are usually boiled. Many of the vegetables could be classified as starches, because Brazilian cuisine includes numerous tubers and root vegetables.

Beans

Beans are used in both savory and sweet preparations. Black (turtle) beans and kidney beans are most com-

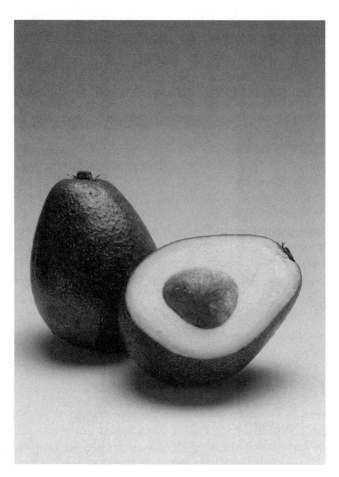

Avocado is enjoyed raw, as a sauce, or even as a flavor of ice cream.

monly consumed. Beans are used in soups, stews, and as a side dish.

Okra

Originally introduced by African slaves, okra is now a commonly enjoyed vegetable. Okra is especially seen in the Afro-Brazilian cuisine of Bahia.

 Prominent Fruits

Fruit is one of the only foods eaten raw. It is consumed fresh, as juice, in salads, and also in stews. The fruits consumed are a combination of native and introduced fruits.

Guava is native to South America and was well accepted by the Portuguese. It is typically eaten raw, dried, or drunk as juice. The fruit has a pink flesh, small seeds, and emits a strong perfume-like aroma.

Papaya is another native fruit that is also eaten raw or drunk as juice. Its silky flesh is orange in color with a delicate, sweet taste. Sometimes meat is wrapped in papaya leaves because the enzymes in papaya act as a tenderizer.

Avocado is enjoyed raw, as a sauce, or even as a flavor of ice cream. Avocado has the largest fat and fiber content of any other fruit, thus giving it high nutritional value.

Bananas, introduced to South America in the early 16th century, quickly became a valuable food resource. Bananas, which are indigenous to Asia, are eaten raw, boiled, or fried. Banana leaves are also used to wrap maize dough for steaming.

Coconut is used in a great variety of ways and is found in both sweet and savory dishes.

 ## Spices and Seasonings

Annatto seed was first used in food as a replacement for saffron by the Iberian colonists. It dyes dishes a golden yellow and lends a light flowery flavor.

Ajicero refers to hot sauce or capsicum sauce. Peppers are well-known to the entire world but are indigenous to South America. The degree of spice use is broad, from bland to spicy, depending on the region. Hot sauce can be found on most tables.

 ## Beverages

Mate, which is commonly consumed in southern Brazil, is a tea made with dried leaves of the Ilex tree and hot water. *Mate* is available in tea-bag form and yields an earthy, grassy flavor. It is traditionally served in a hollowed out gourd and sipped through a straw made of metal.

Coffee was unknown in South America until its introduction in the late 18th century. Most of the coffee plantations on the continent export the majority of their crops; however, coffee (*cafezinho*, the common way to refer to it in Brazil) has gained popularity and is now widely consumed.

The national cocktail specific to Brazil, *caipirinha*, is a sweet-and-sour drink with *cachaça* (an alcoholic beverage made from fermented sugarcane), sugar, and lime.

 ## Desserts

Many Brazilian desserts are, not surprisingly, fruit based and commonly involve fruits prepared in sweet syrup. Additional ingredients of such desserts are milk and sugar, or condensed milk. Egg-based desserts, such as *flan*, are also consumed.

 ## FOODS WITH CULTURAL SIGNIFICANCE

Feijoada, Brazil's national dish, is the foremost culturally significant food. It consists of various meat ingredients, including the ears, tail, and feet of the pig, and

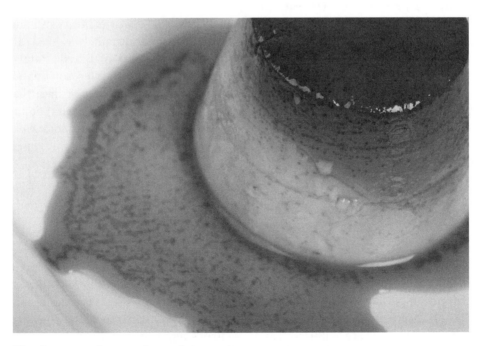

Flan is a popular egg-based dessert.

black turtle beans. Traditionally, the Portuguese colonists discarded such parts of the animal, which were then salvaged by the African slaves and cooked into a stew.

Another culturally significant food in the Brazilian diet is manioc, which represents the history as well as the cultural influences of all peoples, indigenous, colonists, and slaves alike.

 TYPICAL DAY'S MENU

Breakfast is typically a light meal. Foods commonly eaten for breakfast include bread, fruit, and coffee (with or without milk) or *mate*.

Lunch is usually the heaviest meal of the day. This meal almost always includes soup and sometimes this is the only course; however, soup can be followed by meat or fish with rice and beans.

Dinner is typically a lighter meal than lunch and usually includes meat and side dishes of cassava or rice and beans. Leftovers from the main course at lunch are often served at dinner. Dessert is sometimes served after dinner.

 HOLIDAY MENUS

Beginning on the Friday prior to Ash Wednesday is *Carnaval*, a festive annual celebration enjoyed by most Brazilians. *Carnaval* is a time to socialize, eat, and party before the beginning of Lent. Many traditional foods are eaten during this time, especially meat dishes such as *feijoada* and *churrasco*, because customarily meat is not consumed on certain days during Lent. Street foods are popular and many cakes and pies are sold, both savory and sweet, such as *pão de queijo* (Brazilian cheese bread) and pastels (deep-fried pastries). The party would not be complete, of course, without the national drink of Brazil, *caipirinha*, which contains lime, sugar, and *cachaça*.

 HEALTH BELIEFS AND CONCERNS

Limited access to modern Western medicine has perpetuated the ancient ideas on food classifications (humoral theory of Hippocratic–Galenic origin), and the use of medicinal plants. Native Indians, in particular, used medicinal plants to treat a variety of illnesses, and this knowledge is passed verbally through the genera-

tions. Using the humoral theory, foods are separated into two opposing categories, "hot" and "cold." Hot and cold does not refer to temperature, but rather to specific food traits. Moreover, this theory is used primarily during vulnerable times of illness, pregnancy, the postpartum period, and menstruation. Brazilians easily accept alternative medicine as a viable treatment for disease and illness, because this is inexpensive and viewed as effective.

 GENERAL HEALTH AND NUTRITIONAL INDICATORS SUMMARY

Overweight is a sign of well-being for some Brazilians, especially in children. This is a reflection of an elevated mortality rate in children under 5 years. Malnutrition, lack of safe water supply, and low rate of immunization are all factors that affect primarily the poorest populations. Overweight symbolizes good nutritional status, and a greater chance of survival.

Low birth weight, defined as weighing less than 2500 g at birth, affects 8% of newborns in Brazil (UNICEF, 2007). Thirty percent of infants 6–9 months old are breastfed with complementary food, and only 17% remain breastfed at 20–23 months.

Six percent of Brazilian children under 5 years suffer from being moderately to severely underweight (UNICEF, 2007). Being severely underweight affects 1% of Brazil's children. Moderate to severe wasting was found in 2% and stunting in 11% of this particular population. The vast majority of households in Brazil (88%) consume adequately iodized salt.

Ninety percent of Brazil's total population uses improved drinking-water sources (UNICEF, 2007). Specifically, 96% percent of the urban population as compared with 57% of the rural population has access to improved drinking-water sources.

 COMMUNICATION AND COUNSELING TIPS

First and foremost, it is important to consider the client's primary language and, if necessary, offer the assistance of a professional interpreter to avoid misunderstandings. (Details regarding specific foods or beliefs can be missed if there is a significant language barrier.) Another important aspect to consider is the client's region of origin, as this can help identify typical food resources and culture. It is essential to address food security prior to discussing possible alterations or restrictions to the client's current diet. Moreover, the availability of foods will depend on rural or urban geography. For people who live in urban areas, affordability and access to high-fat and processed foods increase. These clients are at risk for becoming overweight and contracting chronic disease associated with high fat consumption. On the other hand, asking a client to eliminate foods, or to add foods that are beyond his or her financial means, would be inappropriate and likely unachievable. Encouraging a balance between modern conveniences and traditional foods is essential. Modifications in portion sizes and/or encouraging certain healthier cooking techniques may be another reasonable approach.

During interviews, always ask whether the person takes herbal medicines and what it is that he or she is treating. Also inquire about where he or she typically receives health and nutrition recommendations. This may help to identify whether he or she is avoiding or including certain foods in his or her diet based on the humoral theories.

FOOD NAMES WITH ENGLISH AND PHONETIC TRANSLATION

Food names with English and phonetic translation are as follows:

Brazilian Names	English
Abacate (ah-bah-KAH-tee)	Avocado
Arroz (ah-ROHS)	Rice
Bolo (bo-lo)	Cake
Cachaça (kah-SHAH-sah)	Brazilian alcohol made from sugarcane
Empanada (ehm-pah-nah-dah)	Turnover made from wheat
Feijoada (fay-ZHWAH-duh)	Brazil's national dish of meat, black beans, and vegetables
Mate (mah-tay)	Hot tea drink
Vatapa (va-ta-pa)	Dish of fish, coconut milk, and dende oil

Pão de Queijo

⅓ cup vegetable oil

½ cup water

⅓ cup milk

1 tsp. salt

2 cups cassava flour (tapioca flour)

¾ cup *queijo minas* (parmesan cheese)

2 beaten eggs

1. Preheat oven to 375°F.
2. Pour oil, water, milk, and salt into a large saucepan, and bring to a boil.
3. Remove from heat immediately upon boiling.
4. Stir in tapioca flour until smooth. Stir the cheese and egg until well combined. Allow the dough to set for 15–30 minutes.
5. Make small rounded balls (about 2–3 tbsp. dough) and place them onto an ungreased baking sheet.
6. Bake balls until puffy and the tops are lightly browned (about 15–20 minutes). Serve warm.

More recipes are available at http://nutrition.jbpub.com/foodculture/

REFERENCES

Bogumil, C. (2002). *Humoral theory in cultural food beliefs*. Retrieved August 29, 2008, from http://food.oregonstate.edu/ref/culture/humoral.html/

Box, B. (2005). *South American handbook*. UK: Footprint.

Foster, G.M. (1994). *Hippocrates' Latin American legacy: Humoral medicine in the New World*. Newark, NJ: Gordon and Breach.

Herbst, S., & Herbst, R. (2007). *The new food lover's companion*. New York: Barron's Educational Series.

Kiple, K., & Ornelas, K. (2000). *The Cambridge world history of food: South America* (pp. 1254–1260). New York: Cambridge University Press.

Lovera, J. (2005). *Food culture in South America*. Westport, CT: Greenwood Press.

Ortiz, E. (1979). *The book of Latin American cooking*. New York: Random House.

Pan American Health Organization. (2007). *Health in the Americas* (Vol. 1). Washington, DC: Author.

Tucker, K., & Buranapin, S. (2001). Nutrition and aging in developing countries. *Journal of Nutrition, 131,* 2417S–2423S.

Uauy, R., Albala, C., & Kain, J. (2001). Obesity trends in Latin America: Transitioning from under- to overweight. *Journal of Nutrition, 131,* 893S–899S.

UNICEF. (2007). *The state of the world's children 2007: Women and children, the double dividend of gender equality.* Retrieved April 14, 2009, from http://www.unicef.org/sowc07/statistics/tables.php

Victoria, C., Munoz, N., Horta, B., & Ramos, E. (1990). Patterns of mate drinking in a Brazilian city. *Cancer Research, 50,* 7112–7115.

CHAPTER 42

Argentina

Beth Klos, BS

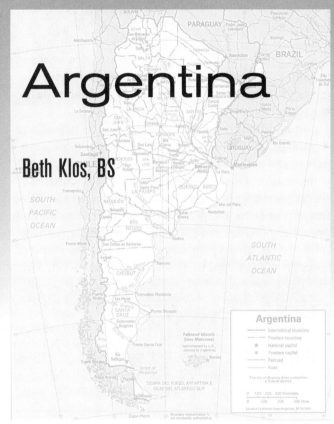

 ## CULTURE AND WORLD REGION

Argentine culture is a lively mix, strongly influenced by early Spanish immigrants, as well as more recent waves of immigrants, especially from Spain and Italy. Immigrants from other countries of Europe and the rest of the world have also impacted the culture. With 97% of the population descended from Europeans, it is easy to see how this is the case (U.S. State Department, 2008). Mestizos, indigenous peoples, and people of color make up a small part of the population (about 3%). While some areas retain the influence of these cultures, they have had a smaller impact on the common culture of Argentina. The religious makeup of the country is consistent with its ancestry, with 70% practicing Roman Catholicism, 9% Protestantism, 1.5% Muslim, about 1% Judaism, and 2.5% other religions. Two of Argentina's distinctions are a relatively large Jewish community, the largest in Latin America according to some sources, and an active Arabic commu-

nity with members of distinction, including a former president. Perhaps owing to the global marketplace, the influence of modern English, American, and other cultures cannot be ignored in Argentina, especially the interest in technology and other services and goods produced abroad.

Owing to the legacy of a forward-thinking former president, education is free or very low cost. Schooling is compulsory to age 18 years and 97% of the country is literate. Their life expectancy, not surprisingly in a literate country, is a little over 75 years. About a third of the workforce is employed in industry and commerce, a tenth in agriculture, and about half in service industries.

When Argentine culture is mentioned outside of Argentina, the tango and gauchos are often the first association. Beyond the stereotype that every Argentine must tango, this dance is an important part of Argentine culture. This graceful, passionate dance, thought to have been created in the brothels of unsavory parts of Buenos Aires, is enjoying a revival of popularity in Argentina. One of the most prominent Argentines in the 20th century, Carlos Gardel, was a tango musician in the 1930s who popularized this beloved music outside of Argentina, especially in Europe. Only then did tango become acceptable to the upper echelon of Argentine society, which had rejected it for its scandalous origins. As for gauchos, their image went from savages to icons in Argentina. The numbers of the adventurous cowboys of the Pampas are in decline, but their idealized image persists.

In addition to Carlos Gardel, there are two other Argentine cultural icons of the 20th century who are part of the national consciousness and often topics of conversation. One such icon is Diego Maradona, the soccer player who rivals Pelé from Brazil for the distinction of being the greatest player in history. Maradona has been retired for many years but remains a celebrity. His fame is not surprising in a country where soccer is the national pastime, perhaps only rivaled in popularity by polo. A visitor may notice impromptu soccer games cropping up in parks or any spare swatch of grass large enough to hold a game.

Arguably the most important figure of the 20th century is Eva Maria de Duarte Perón, known as "Santa Evita" (Saint Eva) or simply "Evita," which translates as "Evie" or "Little Eva." Wife of former president Juan Domingo Perón, she is both lionized as a populist hero and forward-thinking woman, and demonized for her sordid past and political tactics.

Argentina is in eastern South America, with neighboring Bolivia, Paraguay, Brazil, and Uruguay running west to east on its northern border. It shares a long, mountainous western border with Chile, and its eastern border is the Atlantic coast. Interestingly, this extensive coast does not figure strongly in the cultural identity of the country. Argentina's location makes it part of a region of South America called the Southern Cone, which is also comprised of Chile, Paraguay, and Uruguay. As the name Southern Cone implies, it is the southern part of the continent, which resembles a hooked arrow pointing at Antarctica.

The area of the land mass of the country has been compared to the United States east of the Mississippi River, although it stretches a more impressive distance north to south, comparable to the distance from the Hudson Bay in Canada to northern Mexico (Brown, 2003; U.S. State Department 2008). In this large mass of land lie four traditional climatic zones: the Pampas east of the Andes, with both humid and dry sections; the Andes mountains; the Gran Chaco, a semiarid region north of the plains; and the Rio de la Plata to the east and northeast, comprised of several large rivers, their basins, and estuaries. In this region lies the capi-

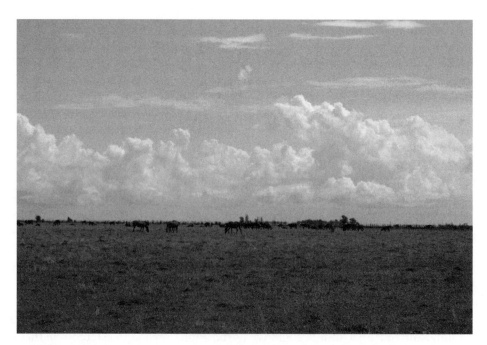

Horses and cattle graze on the "la pampa húmeda" (humid pampas) west of Mar del Plata.

Courtesy of the author

tal, Buenos Aires, sometimes called the Paris of South America for its French-inspired architecture. Buenos Aires is the third largest city of Latin America, which accounts for some of its influence on Latin culture. About a third of the country's population of about 40,301,927 live in the capital and surrounding region.

Patagonia stretches from the Rio Colorado in the north to the Strait of Magellan, flirting with Antarctica, and from the Andes in the west to its long Atlantic coastline in the east. It includes southeast Chile. It is a region of immigrants and large flocks of horses and sheep. In the central–western portion of Patagonia, the mountains and lakes, reminiscent of the Alps, drew many people of German descent who settled in Bariloche.

LANGUAGE

Spanish is the official language. In Argentina, however, Spanish is more commonly referred to as *Castellano* (Castilian), which indicates the regional Spanish roots of the language. Mixed with hints of the languages of the immigrants, especially Italian, and a tinge of the indigenous languages, it is a dialect that is representative of the people and history of Argentina.

There are communities that speak or still understand other European languages: Italian, British English, German, and French. In addition, Welsh is still spoken in the style of the immigrants who came in the late 19th and early 20th centuries, although it is disappearing. According to one source (World Investment News, 2001), 17 indigenous languages are still spoken, the more prominent of which are Quechua, Mapuche, Guaraní, Tobas, and Matacos.

CULTURE HISTORY

As in much of the Americas, the pre-Columbian colonization of Argentina is believed to have been accomplished gradually, by the descendents of Asians who crossed the Bering land bridge to North America. The result of this colonization was that numerous indigenous groups populated the country, none with a central government or part of an empire except those in the northwest corner. This region, separated from the rest of the country by the Cordoba Mountains, was briefly part of the Incan Empire before the arrival of Spanish conquistadors. The relative lack of wealth in the rest of the country left the Incas uninterested in its conquest. The Diaguita people, as well as other less dominant

groups, lived in this region and shared Andean culture. It is likely that they were hostile peoples, often in conflict, until the Incan rulers enforced peace. In the rest of the north, there were more organized groups, such as the Guaraní, with a tradition of the women acting as hunter-gatherers or agriculturalists, and the men as warriors and hunters. Warfare between neighboring groups was common, so when the first Spaniards arrived in 1536, Amerindians were prepared to resist. The south of Argentina was the least organized region, with groups of nomadic hunters not organized into tribes. This area was the most difficult for the Europeans to subdue. The 1879 Expedition into the Desert finally eliminated indigenous resistance to resettling the Pampas for the cattle industry.

Unlike the Aztec and Incan Empires, which gave the Spanish conquistadors a clear target for both political and religious conquest, these indigenous peoples of Argentina consisted of many language groups with dozens of ethic and cultural distinctions. Their loyalties were to small groups, a village, or a clan that controlled an area. Their conflicts with each other were brutal and intense in some areas, including retribution warfare and use of the skulls of the enemy as drinking vessels. Some groups continued successful resistance against colonization for about 400 years. Religious practices of these groups were largely polytheistic, with rites and folk medicine administered by shamans.

The capital city, Buenos Aires, was famously founded twice for a variety of factors, including indigenous resistance and the Spanish crown's lack of support for the region as an important trade area. After the first attempt to settle the area failed in 1536, it was not until 1580 that a second successful effort was made. Since the Spanish crown outlawed trade through Buenos Aires, it became a successful port city for contraband. Meanwhile, the cattle and horses left behind from the first failed Spanish settlement began multiplying and formed the basis for the cattle and horse industry of today.

After early disasters trying to conquer indigenous warriors, Spaniards instead began to gradually settle the country. It was a slow conquest, taking hundreds of years. Most arriving Spaniards were men who took indigenous wives or concubines, creating the first generation of Argentines who called themselves *Criollos* (Creoles). Denied the governmental and commercial power reserved for Europeans under colonial rule, they were the dominant class in society after independence from Spain and the flight of the Spaniards. The first phase of this independence came on May 10, 1810, in

Buenos Aires, with the establishment of the *Primera Junta* (First Ruling Junta). Independence was formally declared on July 9, 1816, in San Miguel de Tucumán. In 1853, a constitutional government was established that has been challenged by military rule many times.

Sephardic and Mediterranean Jews were present since the time of Spanish conquest and were soon followed by immigrants from France. In the late 19th and early 20th centuries, a wave of European immigration, especially from Italy, began. German and eastern European Jews were part of the same migration as Italians and other Europeans. World War I and the turbulence of the Spanish Civil War in the 1930s produced another influx of immigrants from Spain, hundreds of years after the first arrivals.

In the late 19th century, the sizable population that had descended from African slaves virtually disappeared. Speculation abounds as to the reason for this disappearance, with difficulty confirming whether it was disease, war, migration, or marriage with other ethnicities that was the cause. Genetic testing suggests that the latter is the most likely theory, although definitive proof is not possible.

Rising to power in the 1940s and holding the presidency until 1955, Juan Domingo Perón made a mark on Argentine politics that still resonates in the existence of the Peronist party. Considered a populist, because he drew support from ethnically and geographically diverse poor, disenfranchised *descamisados* (people without shirts), Perón, with the help of his wife Eva, formed a constituency of first-generation immigrants and indigenous and mestizo peoples from the provinces. A few years after Eva's death in 1952, Perón was forced into exile until 1973, when he was reelected to the presidency. After his death in 1974, as during his exile, military dictatorships sometimes won out over democracy due to instability.

Militarism and authoritarianism are strong themes in Argentine history. The infamous "Dirty War" started after the fall from power of Perón's third wife, Isabel, who was unseated by a military coup d'etat in the late 1970s. It was a time of brutal counterinsurgency, including large-scale kidnapping and torture. Support for the military government started to collapse in 1982, after defeat in the war against Great Britain in the Falkland Islands (Las Malvinas). Presidential elections and return to constitutional government occurred in 1983. The 1983 constitutional reforms made Argentina a more attractive investment opportunity, although economic instability has continued despite the current democratic government. The economy collapsed and unemployment soared in 2001, although it has since largely rebounded. Today, the legacy of class structure, some tension between the classes and races, and the history of tolerating violence are thought by some people to be the Achilles heel that prevents this vibrant culture from achieving more economic and political stability (Brown, 2003).

FOOD HISTORY WITHIN THE CULTURE

As the culture is a pastiche of indigenous and European traditions, so is the cuisine. Argentina has four traditional regions, each of which has its own cuisine: the northwest, northeast, central area, and Patagonian plateau. In all parts there is some mixture of indigenous ingredients and techniques with recipes and products brought by the Spaniards and subsequent immigrants. Most waves of immigration were from Europe and the Middle East, including Jewish and Arabic populations. Because Italians were the most populous immigrants, Italian food dominates the cuisine in Argentina, and especially in Buenos Aires. Pastas, sauce (*fileto*), coffee, and Italian pastries abound. In the past few decades, however, immigrants from Bolivia, Paraguay, Uruguay, Chile, Korea, and Indochina have become a presence. All groups have contributed elements of their own cuisine.

The inhabitants of the Andean settlements in the northwest, arguably the most advanced civilization in Argentina before the arrival of the Spaniards, raised alpaca and llamas for meat as well as other purposes. The Diaguita people, who share cultural ties with Peru, were the dominant group and lived in the area that is now the provinces of Salta and Jujuy. The Diaguita coexisted with numerous other cultural groups including the Atacameño, Humahuaca, Chica, and Lule. They lived under "imperial hegemony," the enforced peace of the Incas. They farmed corn, the staple grain of the Americas, and algarrobo pods, unique legumes that grow in a tree. The local fermented brew, somewhat similar to beer, was and still is made from algarrobo pods and corn. Today in the northwest, the cuisine is most strongly influenced by two groups: Spanish conquistadors and the original inhabitants. Subsequent immigration has not had a strong influence on the cuisine (except the wine).

In northeastern Argentina, the Guaraní people dominated in the pre-Columbian era. They probably descended from immigrants from the Brazilian

Amazon Basin. The women were cultivators of maize, beans, sweet potatoes, peanuts, squash, and cassava. Women also made *chicha*, a fermented beverage. The men contributed by fishing in rivers. In the northeast, the influence of the indigenous Guaraní is still evident, especially in the local produce. Jungles and rivers still also provide important parts of the diet.

Nomadic hunter-gatherers who lived off the land inhabited the central and southern parts of the country. For meat, they hunted partridges, nandùes, and vizcachas. Farther to the south, in the Andean foothills of Patagonia, roamed the guanaco, a reddish-brown ruminant mammal resembling the llama but related to the camel. In the woodlands, deer provided meat and gathering seeds provided additional nutrition. Along the coast, like in many other areas of the world, indigenous people hunted from canoes. The local fare included seal and fish. The current cuisine in Patagonia and the Pampas bears the influence of the Spanish and other more recent European immigrants, including English, Welsh, Germans, and Italians, in its empanadas, jams, and pastries.

Lively social life around eating has a long history in Argentina and merits mention. From the early days of Spanish men coming to Buenos Aires, largely alone, taverns took root in the culture. Cafés have existed at least since the 1700s and are still lively meeting places, much like the cafés of Europe.

MAJOR FOODS

Protein Sources

Beef Products

When the first unsuccessful Spanish settlers of Buenos Aires abandoned the settlement for what is now the city of Asunción, they left behind cattle, horses, and sheep that multiplied and created today's flocks and herds. Since the 16th century, meat products have been dominant in Argentine cuisine. The large Pampas, with its many *estancias* (ranches) provides ample pasture for grazing, so Argentines proclaim that all of their beef is free-range and take great pride in its quality. Beef is nothing short of a national obsession, available in a seemingly endless variety of dishes. Enough cannot be said about the love of the Argentines for meat, especially an *asado* or *parrilla* (both similar to a barbeque). For both preparations, the heat source, much like at a barbeque, can be of charcoal briquettes or a fire of wood or coal. For meat to be *asado* (roasted), it is cooked on a spit perpendicular to the heat source, often stuck into the ground. Among the types of spits used, a common tool is *la cruz* (the cross), which can support a whole animal carcass and is often used to cook a sheep, lamb, short cow, or piece of a cow. It is cross-shaped

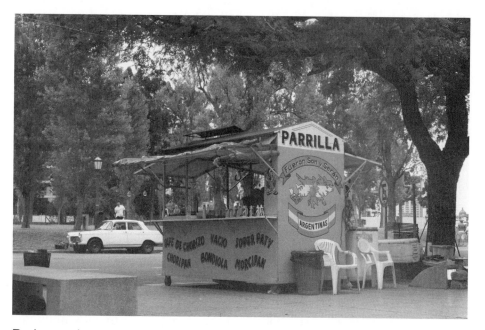

Barbequed meat is served everywhere from elegant restaurants to roadside stands such as this one in Puerta Madera, Buenos Aires.

Courtesy of the author

and secured to the floor leaning slightly forward in front of a large bed of embers or a gentle fire. Meat can be cooked *asado con cuero* (roasted with its hide) to preserve its juice. As the name implies, for a *parrillada* (grilled meat) a grill is used, which may or may not be adjustable over the heat source. A complete *parrillada* or *asado* includes cuts of beef, sausages, organ meats, blood sausages, and possibly side dishes of mutton or lamb, chicken, or a suckling pig. Salad, bread, and *chimichurri* or other sauces, as well as good red wine, round out the menu. Empanadas of meat or other fillings may be served as appetizers. The average guest at an *asado* eats about 1 lb. of meat. Restaurants that sell this kind of food abound, ranging from fine sit-down establishments to roadside vendors. Care and attention are given to slowly cook the meat to perfection.

Showing their affinity for beef, Argentines prepare meat in many other ways, including *charqui* (meat dried in the sun), a technique inherited from the Guaraní. Stew made with this jerky is called *charquicán* or *charquicillo*. It typically may also contain potatoes, carrots, the pith of other vegetables, beans, garlic, and other assorted seasonings. Another popular way to eat beef, as well as other meats and fish, is as thin filets, prepared *a la Milanesa* (breaded and lightly fried).

Pork

Although it is second to beef in preference, pork and pork offal are also popular dishes. Pork is often cooked *asado*, used to fill empanadas, and in numerous other dishes. One of the traditional dishes of Argentina, a stew called *locro*, commonly contains pork products. A novel type of pork for which Argentina is well known is the pork from the wild boars of Patagonia, which draw hunting expeditions.

Cheese

With an abundance of cattle, it is no wonder that cheese is another favorite protein. In the 19th century, production of cheese began in earnest, and the later influx of European immigrants added to its variety. There are scores of local variations of European favorites and original creations: Camembert, cheddar, fontina, provolone, gruyére, reggiano, and quesillo (goat cheese). Chubut, Huemel, and *mar del plata* cheeses show Dutch influence. A local version of mozzarella (called *muzzerella*) is popular on pizza, and the local version of provolone is often served with an *asado* and also on pizza.

Sheep

Lamb is the favored meat in Patagonia, where sheep ranches abound. It is often cooked *asado*, like beef in other areas. A stew with a base of sheep offal, evidence of Guaraní influence, is a favorite. One interesting cooking technique is that sheep is sometimes cooked with raisins for sweetness.

Indigenous Animals

Wild animals still serve as foodstuffs and available types differ by region. In Patagonia, deer and boar are hunted, both by locals and tourists. Boar meat is often stewed or roasted. In the central part of Argentina, partridges (flightless birds, smaller relatives of the ostrich), and vizcachas (a small rodent resembling a rabbit), are also protein sources.

In the northwest, the guanaco (a reddish-brown ruminant mammal from which llamas descended) still roam wild in their homeland in the Andean foothills. Some guanaco are herded as they were by the Araucano people, a tribe of the Mapuches. In the Central Andes, the vicuña, an endangered species, is still eaten. It is a small, llama-like animal with beautiful silky fleece once prized by Incan royalty. Vizcacha is used in stew or empanadas. Armadillo is also eaten, often roasted.

Chicken

Chicken is used in empanadas and other dishes, although it is generally considered to be vastly inferior to beef and other meats.

Freshwater Fish

Argentina's numerous rivers and lakes provide many varieties of fish, which contributes diversity to the cuisine. The rivers of Patagonia provide trout and salmon. Patagonia's lakes, originally stocked with salmon from the United States in 1904, also provide this delicacy, which is popular cooked in white wine. Southern Argentina sustains three varieties of trout: rainbow, brown, and salmon-like trout. Trout cooked in black butter is a favorite. Additionally, two varieties of trout, brown and black, live in the rivers near the Andes.

In the north of the country, fish from the Paraná and Uruguay rivers also are staple dishes. *El Dorado* ("the golden one"), known as dolphin fish in English, a large river fish with luminous gold, green, and blue–purple skin, is a seasonal delight in the summer. Called the "Tiger of the Paraná" for its feisty spirit when caught, its meat is white and exquisite, although the flesh is bony. In the province of Corrientes, *El Dorado* is often stuffed with onions, tomatoes, parsley, oregano, and breadcrumbs, coated with oil, more breadcrumbs, and bay leaves, and then grilled. Grilling is the favored cooking method to reduce the fat content, although it may be baked, boiled, or added to stew. Another popular river fish, *palometa*, has rosy, greasy meat, but with few bones. The fish called pejerrey is another river fish that lives in the northern rivers, seas, and lagoons. Its white meat lends itself to many cooking methods, including boiling, baking, or poaching. The Surubí, yet another river-dwelling fish, has soft, tasty, yellowish meat and is popular grilled and served with tomato sauce.

Ocean-Dwelling Fish and Shellfish

Along the Atlantic coast, a wide variety of fish and shellfish have a place in the local diet, although they may still be considered inferior to beef. Some of the varieties of fish and shellfish include cod, *brótola*, sole, hake scallops, mussels, clams, squid, southern king crab, and shrimp. On the coast of Patagonia, *curantos* are held, which are similar to clambakes. Fish and shellfish are roasted in a hole under stones. It deserves mention that golf sauce, a mixture of mayonnaise and tomato ketchup invented by Argentine Nobel Prize winner Dr. Luis Federico Leloir, is very often served with seafood in Argentina.

Nuts

Both indigenous and imported nuts are eaten in Argentina. Mapache Indians of the southern Andes harvest the pinecone of the araucaria tree (also called the *pehuén* tree in their language). This pinecone may be filled with around 300 pine nuts (called *nguillú* in the indigenous language). The taste is similar to chestnuts; however, the texture is much harder, so the nuts have to be boiled before they can be eaten. Additionally, this tree produces a crystalline resin in the lower branches that is eaten as candy. In the northwest, in the province of Mendoza, walnuts are cultivated. Although there are competing claims, Argentines assert that the peanut plant originated in northern Argentina and was used for food by the first inhabitants. Today, it is often seen cooked in the streets as *garrapiñada* or caramelized, although it is available plain, along with other imported nuts and seeds, in health food stores and groceries.

 Starch Sources

Breads, pastas, and indigenous starches abound in Argentina, perhaps second only to meat in importance at a meal. Bakeries and grocery stores sell an abundance of refined breads and rolls (including many varieties showing European influence), biscuits, and crackers. In Buenos Aires more options, such as whole grains and Japanese noodles and rice, are readily available.

Pasta and Pizza

One rarely sees foreign chain restaurants selling Italian food in Buenos Aires, as local varieties are strongly preferred. Pastas, often variations of well-known Italian dishes, are sold in a seemingly endless number of types. Noquis (small potato dumplings similar to Italian gnocchi), polenta, and raviolis are among the available varieties.

In the northwest, algarrobos pods (the fruit of a local shrub of the *Leguminosae* family) grow in both black and white varieties, serving as food as they did in pre-Columbian times. The indigenous people made flour and bread from the algorrobo. Potatoes also serve as grains, as they have since pre-Columbian times.

The fare in the northeast, where Guaraní influence is still strong, mostly resembles pre-Columbian cuisine. There the manioc, known elsewhere as yucca and cassava, is utilized by either being made into flour or roasted. It grows in the forests of the northwest as well. This trusty root, the starch of which is made into tapioca, is widely used in Latin America. It sometimes replaces corn flour as a staple.

For thousands of years, corn has served the Amerindians as a staple grain, much like wheat in other cultures. Although sometimes rivaled, corn is still commonly used in both the provinces of the northeast and northwest. It is used to make a long list of dishes, including *locro* and other stews and soups, *tamales*, *humitas*, *carbonada*, and *mazamorra*. It is also served on the cob, in a cup, or mixed in salads.

In mountainous areas where the elevation is too high for corn cultivation, potatoes become the starch of choice. The Incans widely cultivated potatoes, and it is tentatively believed that the potato plant originated in Peru. They are still eaten in indigenous areas and other parts of the country in numerous dishes and forms, including in stews and as mashed potatoes.

Sweet potatoes are another ancient food still cultivated in the provinces of Santiago del Estero, and

Cordoba, as well as along the Paraná River. The sweet potato made its way into the Spanish stew *puchero* when colonists needed to cook this dish with local ingredients. This stew is still an Argentine favorite. A food unique to Argentina is a preserve made from sweet potatoes, demonstrating the flexibility of this humble tuber.

Although rice is popular in Latin cuisine in other countries, it is not so in Argentina. It is popular as a side dish with the river fish pejerrey and in risotto, which arrived with Italian immigrants.

 Fat Sources

Both solid fats and oils are used in Argentine cuisine. Solid fats include butter, a modern variety of margarines purporting healthy benefits, lard, suet, *chicharrones*, and other animal fats. Various oils are available, with sunflower oil being especially popular.

 Prominent Vegetables

With beef the principal of Argentine cuisine, vegetables are decidedly a minor character. Greens in empanadas, salads as a side dish, and peppers cultivated in the northwest are notable dishes with vegetables. Pumpkin in the northwest, (from the Guaraní heritage) and central area is part of stuffed pumpkin and pumpkin stew. Vegetables are also complements to starch and meat in other stews, such as *puchero*, which contains onion, carrot, cabbage, turnips, tomatoes, scallions, leeks, celery, pumpkin, and peppers, in addition to meat and potatoes.

 Prominent Fruits

Fruits do not play a pronounced role in Argentine cuisine, although many types produced domestically and abroad are available, including apples, pears, oranges, pineapples, watermelon, peaches, and grapes. There are several regional specialties. In the subtropical northeast, papaya is a favorite that shows Guaraní influence. In the Andean foothills, residents of San Carlos de Bariloche, which draws Argentine and international tourists, cultivate native strawberries and *calafates*. Apples, originally cultivated by Jesuits who came shortly after the Spanish conquistadors, still grow in the province of Río Negro. Interestingly, although fruits do not play a large role in typical Argentine cuisine, denizens of the north prepare a sweet stew with dried peaches or apricots.

 Spices and Seasonings

Argentine food dispels the myth that all Latin American food is spicy. Argentines prefer mild spices. *Ají*, paprika, cumin, garlic, parsley, and oregano are typical seasonings. In the mountains of Cordoba, aromatic herbs, such as mint, *yerbabuena*, *carqueja*, and rosemary, are cultivated for the production of bitters for alcoholic drinks.

 Beverages

Mate

Often compared in flavor to green tea, mate is an integral part of Argentine life. This tea is made from the plant yerba mate, an evergreen of the *Aquifoliaceae* (holly) family. The most preferred way to drink mate is from a small mug-like utensil called a gourd that is filled to the brim with loose leaves and stalks. Aficionados drink mate through a metal straw called a *bombilla* that has slits at the bottom, which allow the tea to pass through while preventing loose particles from going up the straw. Warm, not hot water, is poured over the tea. When the gourd is empty, water is poured over the mate repeatedly, until it loses its flavor. Mate is often drunk away from home, so mate drinkers carry a thermos of warm water to refill the gourd. The gourd is often passed among friends to be enjoyed as a communal experience. Mate is also sold in tea bags, but the preferred way to drink it is from a gourd. It is claimed to have a mild stimulant effect, similar to caffeine, as well as health benefits for digestion, the nervous system, circulation, and memory.

Wine

Wine has a long and proud history, with the first vines arriving in 1566, cultivated in the province of Mendoza. After Argentine independence in 1810, Argentine wine become more popular, perhaps out of necessity. Later, the arrival of immigrants from Europe in the late 19th and early 20th centuries, people who were knowledgeable about winemaking, brought more skill to local winemaking. A wide variety and volume of red and white wines are now cultivated in Argentina, bringing the country to fourth in the world in volume of wine produced. Vineyards are located in the semiarid fringe at the foot of the Precordillera of the Andes, from the provinces of Salta in the north to Río Negro and Chubut in the south; however, about 75% of wine production still takes place in Mendoza. Cab-

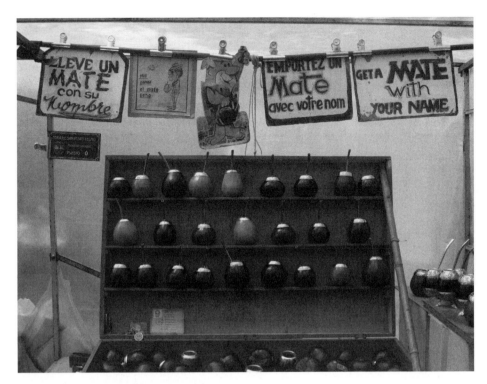

Mate gourds with bombillas for sale.
Courtesy of the author

ernet Sauvignon, Syrah, and the aromatic white wine Torrentés transplanted from Spain to La Rioja and Salta, are some of the many varieties produced. Cabernet Sauvignon used to be the national favorite but has been supplanted by Malbec, a varietal from Bordeaux that has flourished in the soil of Mendoza.

Other Alcoholic Beverages

There are many local alcoholic beverages produced in Argentina, including *chicha*, made of fermented cornmeal; liquor of *caraguata*, made from the fruit of that name, also considered a potent cough medicine; *aloja*, an Indian beer drunk at Christmas and carnival; *ullpada*, a corn-flour spirit; *caña* and *chavü*, sugarcane spirits; and *pilquillín*, a drink made from fermented pine nuts. Beer, whiskey, vodka, rum, and vermouth are also produced in Argentina, although they originated elsewhere.

Hot Beverages

With the influx of Europeans, especially the Italian immigrants, came coffee, now a favorite. There are many variations in coffee: regular coffee; coffee with a little milk, known as *café cortado* ("cut coffee"); *café doble* ("double coffee"), a large portion; and coffee with a lot

of milk (*café con leche*), a popular breakfast drink. Hot chocolate is also popular, particularly a type called *submarino*, which is made by putting a solid bar of chocolate at the bottom of a cup and filling the cup with milk. In another nod to Europe, Welsh tea is served in the teahouses of Patagonia.

Other Beverages

Sodas, particularly those *suavemente gaseosa* ("lightly carbonated"), and in distinctly Latin American flavors, such as grapefruit, are popular. As Argentines become more weight conscious, diet sodas have become available. There are also many other low-calorie or calorie-free options. Many types of juice are also available.

 Desserts

In artfully crafted Argentine pastries, the European influence shines brightly. Small pastries, or *facturas*, as the locals call them, dominate bakeries. Although Argentines use the word for bread bakery (*panadería*) to describe their bakeries, where one often finds a plethora of pastries and sweets and only a few rolls, sandwiches, and loaves of bread. The most famous and omnipresent of the *facturas* is the *medialuna* ("half-moon"). Although it is roughly the shape of a croissant, it is more

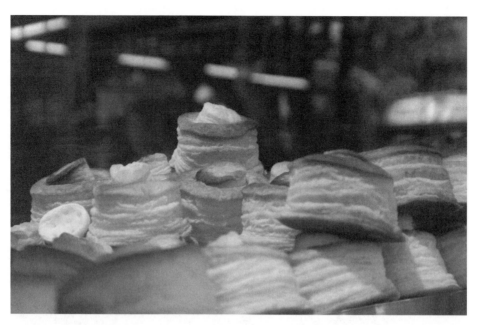

Fresh *criollitos* (Argentine biscuits) for sale at a bakery.
Courtesy of the author

bread-like in texture. Despite its French appearance, historical sources attribute it to Germanic influence. There are myriad other *facturas* with colorful names, including *caras sucias* ("dirty faces"), which are coated in brown sugar, *miguelitos* ("little Michaels"), and *palitos* ("little stakes"), which are long stick-like pastries.

Dulce de Leche

It is impossible to conceive of Argentine pastry without the very sweet, ever-present spread, *dulce de leche*, which is made by caramelizing milk and sugar. The name translates as "milk's candy" or "the sweet of the milk." Although eaten in many Latin countries, Argentines consider it their own creation. The debated Argentine legend of its creation takes various forms; one is that on July 17, 1829, in the province of Buenos Aires, a servant of Juan Manuel de Rosas was making sugar dissolved in milk for mate over a fire of embers, when she was interrupted and ran to get her master. When she returned, the milk had thickened, turned brown, and tasted wonderful.

Another ever-present Argentine dessert found in almost every bakery and grocery store is the *alfajor*. It basically resembles an Oreo cookie, with two layers and a filling (often *dulce de leche*). Fresh versions, bought in bakeries, are more popular than mass-produced types. The cookies may have a coating of chocolate or sugar.

There are many other desserts popular in Argentina, many of European origin. In the area around San Carlos de Bariloche, Argentines of German, Austrian, and Swiss descent make excellent chocolate. They also produce jams and pastries from native strawberries and blue–black *calafate* berries, as well as quince, apples, currants, cherries, and sour cherries. The Welsh community makes famous black cakes. Fruit salad or quince and cheese also serve as desserts.

Ice Cream

Ice cream is a national obsession that came with more recent immigrants. In the early evening in the summer, long lines form outside the popular ice cream shops. Although there are many brands, softer types sold by Freddo and Munchies are favorites in Buenos Aires.

Indigenous Desserts

From the northeast come a variety of sweets with eggs, including *flans* and *quimbos* (baked beaten egg yolks in syrup). Adding more variety is *ambrosía*, a fruit-flavored egg custard not related to the dessert by the same name in English. Another dessert from the northeast, *mazamorra*, features corn, not eggs. It is hominy enhanced with milk and sugar. Plain it accompanies meat, is indigenous in origin, and is now one of the most popular pastries nationwide. From the peanut, *garrapiñada de maní* is made by combining sugar with water, adding peanuts, and stirring as the mixture caramelizes and adheres to the nuts. Street vendors often

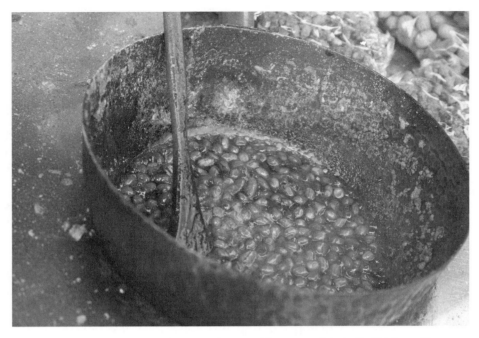

Garrapiñada de maní cooking at the weekly street fair in Sal Telmo, Buenos Aires.
Courtesy of the author

sell this in Buenos Aires, aided by the sweet, rich smell to draw customers. Other nuts, such as almonds, can also be cooked *garrapiñada*.

 ## FOODS WITH CULTURAL SIGNIFICANCE

In the early afternoon in Argentina, long lines form at empanada shops. Empanadas came to Argentina with the first Spanish immigrants and are now a cultural phenomenon. Every household has its own recipes, variations on a basic theme. True to its name, which means "rolled in bread," the outside of an empanada is made of dough, either regular bread dough or with embellishments, such as containing fat instead of water. The fillings vary from hearty types that make a meal, such as ground or finely cut beef, pork, chicken, lamb, vizcacha, fish, shellfish, cheese, greens, onions, potatoes, or humita, to sweet varieties made with jam. There are endless variations. In La Rioja, olives make an appearance as a filling, whereas in Catamarca empanadas are spicier. The inhabitants of San Juan prefer to add lots of condiments. In the northeast, the dough for the outer layer may be made of a blend of wheat and manioc flour.

To distinguish different contents, the cook makes empanadas in different shapes or with different edging, each using his or her own system. *Chimichurri,* a red sauce of mild spices and garlic, is often served with empanadas. Empanadas have the ease that makes finger food a delight—a delicious treat that does not require a fork or any formality. This flexible dish can be baked or fried, and served hot or cold. It is believed that the empanada's first aficionados needed it for the convenience of eating without utensils. Today, this down-to-earth history, combined with extreme care in providing high-quality ingredients, provides an interesting reflection of Argentine culture, which is undeniably proud of its sophisticated European roots.

Dishes made of beef, as already discussed, and especially the *asado*, are rituals of Argentine cuisine. Mate, *facturas*, pizza, pasta, and pasta sauces are also very important, even almost revered. Any locally produced foods, and foods eaten by their immigrant forbearers, inspire fierce loyalty in Argentina.

 ## TYPICAL DAY'S MENU

Breakfast typically consists of coffee and *facturas* or bread. Lunch often consists of empanadas. Afternoon snacks might be sweets or ice cream. Dinner consists of *asado* or barbequed meats and offal, perhaps with side dishes of bread and salad. Beverages are mate, tea, light or regular grapefruit soda, beer, or wine.

HOLIDAY MENUS

Celebrations descend from immigrants and Amerindian peoples of Argentina; thus, holidays and menus are not harmonized nationally. A few examples of indigenous celebrations include the winter festival of Pachamama, the goddess Mother Earth, celebrated August 1 in the provinces of Catamarca, Salta, and Jujuy in the northwest. A hole is made in the earth, and coca, wine, and desserts are put in as an offering. The celebrants eat *chicharrones*, *locro*, and empanadas, washed down with *chicha*, wine, and *api* (hot *mazamorra* made with sugar, lemon, and cinnamon, and thickened with corn flour). On this same date, other indigenous festivals are celebrated in the northeast province of Chaco, and in the northwest province of Santiago del Estero.

At holidays such as Christmas, Easter, and Good Friday, descendents of immigrants prepare the dishes of their forbearers, although they may be out of season in the southern hemisphere. People of German descent make *stollen*; Welsh, cakes with dried fruits; Spanish, *turrón*; and Italians, *panettone*, which resembles Neapolitan sweet bread. On Good Friday, empanadas made with vegetables, fish, and shellfish are popular. Easter Sunday brings ring-shaped cakes with hard-boiled eggs, chocolate hens, rabbits, and eggs, as in many other parts of the world. On Jewish holidays, traditional dishes are still eaten, although sometimes with modern variations.

HEALTH BELIEFS AND CONCERNS

Little research exists on Argentine health beliefs. When providing care to the members of such a diverse society, discuss beliefs and observe the practices and preferences of individuals, rather than assume homogeny. Health practices seem to follow trends in other developed countries, such as for patient-centered diabetes self-management. Alternative health measures are available, such as massage and homeopathy, as well as mainstream Western medicine. Although little data are available on the practices of Amerindians, it stands to reason that indigenous populations that live as a

community and speak their native language still value and use indigenous herbs and treatments.

GENERAL HEALTH AND NUTRITIONAL INDICATORS SUMMARY

Low birth weight, defined as weighing less than 2500 g at birth, affects 8% of newborns in Argentina (UNICEF, 2007). Four percent of the nation's children below 5 years suffers from being moderately to severely underweight. Moderate to severe wasting was found in 1% and stunting in 4% of this particular population.

The great majority (90%) of households in Argentina consume adequately iodized salt (UNICEF, 2007). Ninety-six percent of the total population uses improved drinking-water sources. Specifically, 98% of the population in the nation's urban areas, and 80% of the rural population, has access to improved drinking-water sources.

COMMUNICATION AND COUNSELING TIPS

Argentines are generally down-to-earth and like to converse with strangers. Even in Buenos Aires, one does not find the brusque manners that are common in many large capitals. If speaking in Spanish, many Argentines use the informal versions of you (*tu* or *vos*), even with strangers. There is always the possibility of meeting someone with more formal manners, so the general rule of using *usted* until the other party uses *tu* or *vos* will prevent possible offense.

To speak to most Argentines of giving up red meat would seem nothing short of lunacy. For people with high cholesterol or weight gain, limiting portions, gradually reducing frequency of consumption, and choosing leaner cuts are more reasonable goals. Including vegetables at meals and developing a taste for more variety in the protein group are also likely to be more reasonable goals.

PRIMARY LANGUAGE OF FOOD NAMES WITH ENGLISH AND PHONETIC TRANSLATION

Food names are like the language itself, a unique amalgam mostly of Spanish, with smatterings that can be traced to the languages of indigenous peoples and immigrants.

Argentinian Names	English
Alfajores (al-fa-hor-es)	Filled Argentine cookies
Asado (ah-sah-do)	Noun means a barbeque or barbequed meat; past participle means roasted or grilled
Bife de lomo (beef-ay day lo-moe)	Steak fillet
Choclo (chock-lo)	Sweet corn
Chorizo (chore-ee-zo)	Spicy sausage
Dulce de leche (dool-say day leh-che)	Caramelized milk and sugar
Empanada (em-pa-nah-da)	Pastry or sandwich-like food similar to a turnover

Argentinian Names	English
Facturas (fack-too-rah)	Assorted small pastries
Humita (oo-me-ta)	Dish similar to polenta, made with *choclo* boiled in its own husk
Locro (lo-crow)	Traditional stew
Mate (ma-tay)	Tea made from a holly plant
Medialuna (may-dee-a loo-na)	Pastry similar in shape to a croissant
Parrilla (parr-ee-ya)	A grill or restaurant serving grilled food
Salchicha (sal-chee-cha)	Sausage

FEATURED RECIPE

Empanada Dough and Filling

Dough for Empanadas

2¼ lbs. flour

14 oz. warm, melted lard

1–1½ cups lukewarm water

1 tsp. salt

1 tbsp. of paprika

Variation: use regular bread dough

Empanada Filling

1 lb. sirloin tips (finely ground)

1 lb. scallions (quantity to taste), finely chopped

1 red sweet pepper, finely chopped

2 tomatoes without the seeds, peeled, chopped

1 tbsp. paprika

1 tsp. cumin

1 tbsp. oregano

Salt to taste

1 olive per empanada

1 tbsp. raisins (optional)

2 hard-boiled eggs, thoroughly chilled (optional)

1. On a counter or cutting board, place the flour in the shape of a wreath, and put the paprika and lukewarm lard in the middle.
2. In a separate bowl, combine the salt and lukewarm water, then mix everything together, kneading well for 15 minutes until it is very smooth.
3. Leave dough covered with a dishcloth for 20 minutes.
4. Roll out dough with a rolling pin until it is about ½ inch thick.
5. Cut dough into medallions, sufficient to hold a few ounces of filling.

(continues)

**Empanada Dough
and Filling (Continued)**

6. Put a splash of oil in a saucepan and add the scallions, sweet red pepper, and tomatoes. Cook on low heat until they are tender.
7. Add the meat and stir until it is browned.
8. Remove mixture from the heat and add the raisins. Let the resulting mixture cool completely.
9. Add hard-boiled eggs.
10. Place this mixture on one side of a dough medallion and add one olive. Fold over and roll the edges together. Bake in a hot oven (350°F) for 10–12 minutes or until golden brown. (If both the mixture and the hard-boiled eggs are not thoroughly cooled when combined, the egg will not hold its shape. Note that empanadas can also be deep-fried.)

Yields 24 empanadas

More recipes are available at http://nutrition.jbpub.com/foodculture/

REFERENCES

Brown, J.C. (2003). *A brief history of Argentina*. New York: Facts on File.

Cabrera, F. (2004). *Manual pràctico del asador*. Buenos Aires, Argentina: Negocios Editoriales.

Central Intelligence Agency (CIA). (2008). *World factbook: Argentina*. Retrieved March 10, 2008, from https://www.cia.gov/library/publications/the-world-factbook/geos/ar.html/

Foster, D., & Tripp, R. (2006). *Food and drink in Argentina*. El Paso, TX: Aromas & Sabores.

Foster, D.W., Lockhart, M.F., & Lockhart, D.B. (1998). *Culture and customs of Argentina*. Westport, CT: Greenwood Press.

Hoss de le Comte, M.G. (2000). *Argentine cookery*. Buenos Aires, Argentina: Maizal.

Medina, I. (2005). *Cocina pais por pais: Argentina*. Buenos Aires, Argentina: Aguilar, Altea, Taurus, Alfaguara, S.A. de Ediciones.

Mundoandino.com. (2006). *The Andean world. Cuisine of Argentina*. Retrieved March 20, 2008, from http://www.mundoandino.com/Argentina/Cuisine-of-Argentina/

UNICEF. (2007). *The state of the world's children 2007: Women and children, the double dividend of gender equality*. Retrieved April 14, 2009, from http://www.unicef.org/sowc07/statistics/tables.php

U.S. State Department. (2008). *Background note: Argentina*. Retrieved March 15, 2008, from http://www.state.gov/r/pa/ei/bgn/26516.htm/

Vino! The World of Wine. (2000–2007). *Wine production in Argentina*. Retrieved May 10, 2008, from http://www.vino.com/country/argentina/wine/production.asp/

World Investment News. (2001). *Population, culture and sport*. Retrieved March 15, 2008, from http://www.winne.com/argentina/bf04.html/

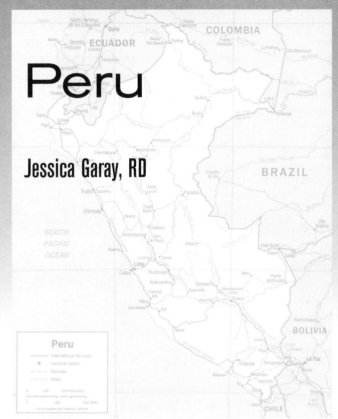

CHAPTER 43

Peru

Jessica Garay, RD

 CULTURE AND WORLD REGION

Peru is the third largest country in South America, bordered by Ecuador and Colombia to the north, Brazil and Bolivia to the east, Chile to the south, and the Pacific Ocean to the west. The 2005 census estimated that 27 million people reside in the country, which is divided into 25 regions. Approximately one third of the population lives in the urban area of the capital city, Lima. Other major cities include Arequipa, Chiclayo, Cusco, Huancayo, Iquitos, and Trujillo. The country is distinguished by three different climates: moderately tropical weather on the coast with little rainfall; Andes mountain region, which experiences variations of dry and wet weather, depending on altitude; and warm, rainy weather in the Amazon rainforest area. Such diversity creates distinct cuisines based on what types of food can be grown and the protein sources present in each region.

Peru also exhibits demographic diversity. The Inca people lived on the land that became Peru until the 16th century when the Spaniards conquered South America and destroyed the Inca Empire. Peru developed under Spanish control until it became independent in 1821. As a result, in modern Peru, the two dominant ethnic groups are the indigenous class (people of Andean descent who are direct ancestors of the Incas) and the "mestizo" group, which represents people who are a mixture of indigenous and Latin descent. Other ethnic groups present in Peru include growing African, Chinese, and Indian populations.

Because of the influence of the Spanish, Christian religions, in particular Roman Catholicism, are prevalent throughout Peru. A smaller number of Peruvians identify themselves as Protestants. In addition, many ancient Incan practices continue to be followed and celebrated, particularly in the Cusco region of Peru. Such ceremonies often involve music, singing, dancing, and food. Music and art both contribute to the cultural practices throughout Peru, with many musical instruments made from ingredients native to Peru, such as the *zampoña*, a wind instrument used in the Andean region. Many types of dances are used in ceremonies, such as the ritual hunting, war, and harvest dances. The most popular type of dance is reserved for courting purposes, the *marinera norteña*. Decorative pottery, earth-inspired sculptures, and Spanish baroque-style paintings represent the art produced in Peru.

LANGUAGE

Spanish is the language most widely spoken in Peru (80% of the population) followed by Quechua, the native language of the Inca people (16%). Both languages are official languages of the country. Another official language, spoken by a small number of indigenous Peruvians in the Andes region as well as in Bolivia and Argentina, is Aymara. In addition, throughout the Amazon jungle there are as many as 43 different dialects spoken.

CULTURE HISTORY

Peru is an independent democratic republic led by a president, according to the nation's 1993 constitution. In addition, the government is led by 120 members of Congress, and the Supreme Court of Peru. Each of the 25 regions in the country has its own government, and within each region there are multiple provinces that can contain local districts.

Evidence of civilization on the land now called Peru dates back to 6000 BC along the coast and in the highlands around the Andes. These early inhabitants survived by planting corn and learning to domesticate alpaca, llama, and guinea pigs. Growing and using cotton was also crucial to survival, along with basket weaving and pottery making. Such cultures include the Paracas, Moche, and Nazca people. Eventually, the inland populations began to grow in power to form city–states and then empires prior to the Incas. The 15th century brought about the first evidence of the Inca Empire, which eventually stretched across much of the west coast of South America. The total Inca population is believed to have been approximately 12 million people. The capital of the Inca Empire was Cusco, and the official language was Quechua. As the empire spread, conquered peoples were allowed to continue

their own religious practices, but they had to also worship the Inca sun god, Inti. The Incas built impressive fortresses and cities using large pieces of stone that in some cases were not native to the immediate area. It is unknown exactly how these structures were built by the Inca people.

Spanish explorers, led by Francisco Pizarro during the 1530s, were the first to name the land "Peru." The Inca Empire was successfully defeated by Spain in 1532 during a civil war among two Incan princes. Eventually, the city of Cusco was recreated into a Spanish settlement, which involved the construction of Spanish architecture over Inca-style buildings. Many ruins now contain both types of building materials and designs. The city of Lima was developed in 1535, and in 1542, Spain declared Peru a viceroyalty, which would last until the 19th century. At that time the counted population of Incas was slightly more than 1 million, a significant decrease related to war and contagious diseases (introduced by the Spanish invaders).

Peru's population began fighting for independence in the early 1800s, and by 1821, independence was declared; however, Spain did not formally recognize Peru until 1879, after fighting between the two countries took place in Peru in the 1860s. Regional disputes followed against Bolivia and Chile until the early 1900s. The political instability continued, because the country had 18 presidents until 1963, many of whom took on military or dictator-like leadership roles. Social conflict raged between the relatively conservative upper class and liberals who desired change. A democratic government was established with General Francisco Bermudez in 1980. Economic troubles plagued Peru during the 1980s, and a new president, Peruvian–Japanese Alberto Fujimori, was elected in 1990. He is credited with reducing crime and improving the economy during his 10-year presidency, but recently he was put on trial for human rights abuses.

FOOD HISTORY WITHIN THE CULTURE

Peru's unique blend of geography, demographics, and history result in traditional cuisine unlike that of any other country. During the Inca Empire, breakfast and dinner were the main meals of the day. Meals were centered on the abundant crops, namely corn (maize) and potatoes. Beverages were often consumed at the end of the meal, not during. A seasoning used by Incas that is widely used in modern Peruvian recipes is *ají*, which is a hot pepper used to make sauces for meat or vegetables. In many parts of the Inca Empire and modern Peru, guinea pig (*cuy*) has been traditionally consumed. The Spanish influence presents itself in the form of the hundreds of soup and stew recipes, particularly in the coastal region. In addition, wheat, sugarcane, and chicken were introduced by Spaniards. New "fusions" have emerged as the immigrant population increases from Europe, Africa, and Asia. *Chifa* is the term widely used to refer to Asian–Peruvian food combinations. *A la criolla* refers to foods with a blend of traditional Peruvian and European flavors.

 MAJOR FOODS

 Protein Sources

Because of Peru's location between the Amazon River and the Pacific Ocean, there are thousands of fish species present. The signature dish of Peru is ceviche, which is made with lemon juice-marinated raw fish or shrimp. In addition, many types of fish are cooked and served whole (skin, eyes, tail, all included). Near Lima and towns along the Pacific Ocean, sea bass or other white fish, scallops, and mussels are common.

Also along the coastal areas some traditional recipes include goat or lamb. Within the Amazon River region freshwater fish, such as trout, is consumed in addition to piranha and paiche, which is believed to be the largest freshwater fish in the world. An additional protein source in this region is wild boar, which is typically roasted. Chicken, and therefore eggs, are utilized as protein sources in almost all regions of the country. In the Andes region of Peru, trout and other freshwater fish is consumed, but more common protein sources include beef, pork, and guinea pig. Throughout Peru all of these protein sources can be located fresh at local markets, in some cases still alive. Methods of preparation for the various protein sources include broiling, frying, baking, and grilling fish, and stewing, roasting (including spit-roasting), and frying chicken, beef, pork, goat, or lamb.

 Starch Sources

Potatoes and sweet potatoes are grown in large quantities, with thousands of varieties produced of each type. The International Potato Center is headquartered in Lima, due to the fact that potatoes were originally discovered in Peru and transported to Europe. The varieties grown within the country even include a purple potato as well as a frost-resistant potato. A crop similar

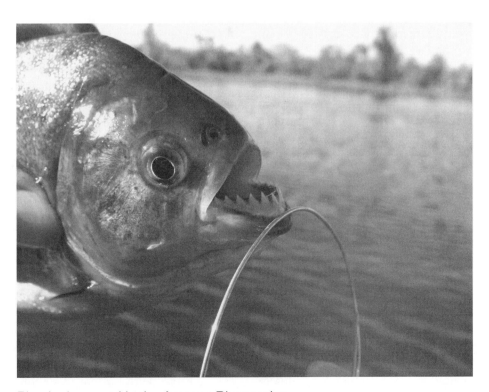

Piranha is served in the Amazon River region.

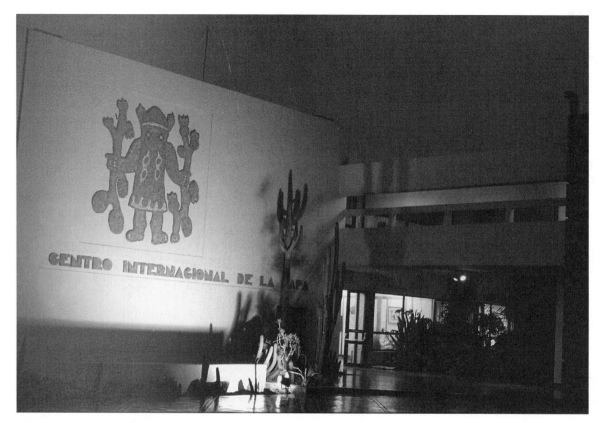

The International Potato Center is headquartered in Lima, due to the fact that potatoes were originally discovered in Peru and transported to Europe.

to potatoes that is prevalent in parts of Peru is called yucca, which is a starchy root vegetable that can be prepared like a potato (boiled, mashed, fried). A second very common native food grown in Peru is corn. There are more than 30 different kinds of corn grown and consumed in the country. While potatoes are served in some fashion in almost all Peruvian entree dishes, corn is used in other ways, such as to make beverages or as a side dish. A popular way to consume corn is called *choclo*, which is a large kernel type of corn served right off the cob by street vendors.

Grains native to Peru include quinoa and kiwicha, both of which are nutritional powerhouses. Quinoa is a small golden-brown grain that can be grown in a variety of altitudes and climates. It contains all the amino acids needed by the human body, making it a rare plant-based complete protein. In addition, it is gluten free, a good source of fiber, and rich in minerals such as iron. When prepared, it resembles couscous and has a nut-like flavor. Quinoa can be served as a stew, breakfast grain, or in place of rice. Kiwicha, which has a purple flowered appearance, is similar to quinoa in

the ease with which it can be grown and the high levels of protein, fiber, and iron. Kiwicha is often also referred to as amaranth. Interestingly, these grains are believed to have been outlawed by the Vatican when the Spanish conquered Peru but have since reappeared on the menus of Peruvian restaurants.

 Fat Sources

Because Peru was a meat-based society, much of their fat consumption came from animal fat. Beef and pork fat was present in heart stews, as well as sausage. Other foods were fried in leftover pork fat, adding to a high saturated fat intake.

 Prominent Vegetables

Peruvians have enjoyed squash, yams, beans, and yucca, a starchy vegetable that is often served boiled or fried as a side dish. A vegetable unique to Peru is called *maca* (a turnip-like root vegetable), which can be boiled and mashed to produce a thick liquid that can be mixed with milk or made into a flour. A bean native to Peru is the Lima butter bean (*pallares*), which is typically served in a mixed salad that resembles salsa. Lastly, Peru has several varieties of vegetable/fruit, meaning peppers and tomatoes, which serve as ingredients in many stews and stuffed appetizers.

 ## Prominent Fruits

Since the time of the Incas, fruits such as bananas, pineapple, avocado, plums, and papayas have been consumed. Spanish invaders brought citrus fruits, apples, and cherries to South America. Fruits unique to Peru include an estimated 650 types, such as *cherimoya* (custard apple), a creamy-tasting fruit that resembles an avocado; *lúcuma*, which is a nut-like fruit that tastes like maple syrup; *tuna*, a fruit (despite its name) that represents the edible portion of a cactus plant grown in Peru; *maracuyá*, similar to a passion fruit, which is often consumed in juice form; and *camu camu*, a reddish fruit similar to a cherry that contains a very high amount of vitamin C and can be found in the Amazon region.

 ## Spices and Seasonings

Peruvian cuisine is often made spicy by means of *ají* pepper, as are other types of chili peppers. Some Peruvian chili peppers are not spicy but serve to give taste and color to dishes. Peruvian cuisine has been influenced by such an array of cultures, that one may find a multitude of spices here.

 ## Beverages

Peruvian taste buds tend toward the sweet, and the drink options throughout the country are no exception. Fruit juices are consumed typically at the breakfast meal and can include papaya juice, among others. The most popular soft drink is a bubble gum-tasting, bright-yellow soda named "Inka Kola." (It is believed that this beverage was purchased by Coca-Cola because it was outselling Coca-Cola in Peru!) The most popular alcoholic drink in Peru is the pisco sour, which is made with pisco, a brandy, although beer is common also. Corn can be fermented to create a beer-like drink native to the Andes region called *chicha*. Another popular drink is *chicha morada*, which is made using purple corn. This beverage is commonly served at lunch as part of the daily menu. A unique drink is *mate de coca*, which is tea made from the leaves of the coca plant. This tea is recommended to visitors traveling to the Andes and Macchu Picchu regions to help prevent altitude sickness. (Street vendors sell these leaves as a type of chewing gum, but actually they are from the same plant used to produce cocaine!)

 ## Desserts

The most prevalent sweet treat throughout Peru is called *manjar blanco*, which is a candy similar to caramel, made from condensed milk and sugar, that is often used as a filling for pastries and cakes. A common bakery item filled with this is the *churro*, which can often be found at a street-vendor cart. A popular dessert for lunch is called *mazamorra morada*, which is made with purple corn and has a consistency like that of pudding. Other desserts include rice pudding (*arroz con leche*) and ice cream flavors based on popular indigenous fruits such as *lúcuma*. Yucca, the root vegetable, can even be turned into a dessert by creating dough balls that are deep fried and covered in sugar.

 ## FOODS WITH CULTURAL SIGNIFICANCE

The types of crops grown in Peru dictate the foods used in recipes and celebrations from the Inca period to modern times. Each geographic region of the country has a distinct offering of foods and preparation methods. Along the coast, seafood predominates most dishes and the use of *ají* is popular in making sauces. In the mountain region, alpaca is the meat of choice, and the method of cooking is called *pachamancha*, which involves cooking over hot stones under the ground to create moist, flavorful meat. In the Amazon Jungle, fish is typically the main dish. This area also contains a variety of exotic fruit. Throughout Peru a common appetizer or side dish is stuffed avocado (*palta rellena*) or pepper (*rocoto rellena*), which can contain grains and other vegetables. Overall, the cuisine of Peru from coast to jungle is based on various preparations of its staple crops: potato, corn, and hot peppers.

 ## TYPICAL DAY'S MENU

In many restaurants throughout Peru a *menú* is offered, which consists of a two- or three-course meal at a fixed price. Typically, each course has at least two options, but in some cases the traditional drink *chicha*

morada (made with purple maize) is served as one of the courses.

 ## HEALTH BELIEFS AND CONCERNS

Throughout Peru, many people obtain food at local open-air markets, which means that there are many potential concerns regarding food safety. Cheese may be left at room temperature for hours before being sold, and live chickens may be butchered on a cutting board used for other food items. In addition, Peru's drinking water contains bacteria in amounts that afflict tourists and newborns alike with diarrhea, nausea, and vomiting. Among native Peruvians, this process is normal for newborns and signifies their development; however, it

---

FEATURED RECIPE

Locro de la Nata

1 lb. white beans	3 onions, chopped
1 lb. hominy maize, coarsely chopped	1 sweet red pepper, diced
27 cups water	3 white and/or red chorizos (Spanish style)
1½ lbs. beef brisket	1 small cabbage, chopped
½ lb. pork bones	5 cups vegetable broth
6 oz. bacon cubed	Salt and pepper
3 medium sweet potatoes	Ground chili and red pepper
½ pumpkin or winter squash	

1. Soak the white beans in water overnight.
2. Wash the hominy and soak them in the 27 cups of water 1 day prior.
3. The following day, drain the white beans and boil them for 30 minutes or until cooked. Drain them and keep them in a bowl.
4. Boil the hominy in the same water you soak them in, for 1½ hours or until half cooked.
5. Add white beans to the hominy pot.
6. Cut the beef in cubes and add it to the pot of hominy and white beans.
7. Wash the pork bones and add them to the pot.
8. Cut the bacon in cubes and add them to the pot.
9. Let the pot boil at medium heat for 40 minutes, stirring occasionally with a spoon. (The mix should get thick due to all the starches.)
10. Take the skin off the sweet potatoes and pumpkin. Cut them into cubes and add them to the pot.
11. Add the onions and peppers to the pot.
12. Cut the chorizos in half and chop the cabbage, then add them to the pot.
13. Cook for 1 hour at moderate heat and, if needed, add broth.
14. Add salt and pepper to taste.

For the sauce:

1. Chop the onions and sweet red pepper, sauté them lightly, and add 1 tbsp. of ground red pepper (or to taste), and season with salt and pepper.
2. Serve the sauce in the middle of the soup dish.

(Courtesy of Luciana Ambrosi)

More recipes are available at http://nutrition.jbpub.com/foodculture/

often leads to nutrient deficiencies, and therefore agencies similar to the WIC program in the United States are available throughout the country to provide necessary medical services to these children.

A very common method of treating various illnesses is through use of an egg, which Peruvians believe has healing powers. The egg is not eaten but rather rubbed on the outside of the body by a healer (typically a woman trained by relatives in folk medicine). Afterward, the egg is placed in a glass of water to reveal what has been released from the body. In some cases the egg is broken before being placed in the water, allowing the healer to identify whether the egg whites appear translucent or hardened (the latter would be an indication of the illness having left the body). Other types of folk medicine include using plants, such as aloe and eucalyptus, in either a topical treatment or burning them to release a healing smoke.

 ## GENERAL HEALTH AND NUTRITIONAL INDICATORS SUMMARY

Low birth weight, defined as weighing less than 2500 g at birth, affects 11% of newborns in Peru (UNICEF, 2007). Sixty-four percent of children are exclusively breastfed during the first 6 months of life. Eighty-one percent of infants 6–9 months are breastfed with complementary food and 41% remain breastfed at 20–23 months.

Eight percent of children below 5 years suffer from being moderately to severely underweight (UNICEF, 2007). Moderate to severe wasting was found in 1% and stunting in 24% of this particular population. The great majority (91%) of households in Peru consume adequately iodized salt.

Eighty-three percent of Peru's total population uses improved drinking-water sources (UNICEF, 2007). Specifically, 89% of the population in the nation's urban areas and 65% of the rural population has access to improved drinking-water sources.

REFERENCES

Barrett, P. (Ed.). (2002). *Insight guide: Peru* (3rd ed.). Singapore: APA Publications.

Ferreira, C., & Dargent-Chamot, E. (2003). *Culture and customs of Peru*. Westport, CT: Greenwood Press.

Pearson, D.L., & Beletsky, L. (2005). *Travellers' wildlife guides: Peru*. Northampton, MA: Interlink Publishing Group.

UNICEF. (2007). *The state of the world's children 2007: Women and children, the double dividend of gender equality.* Retrieved April 14, 2009, from http://www.unicef.org/sowc07/statistics/tables.php

Oceania

Food, Cuisine, and Cultural Competency for Culinary, Hospitality, and Nutrition Professionals discusses three prominent regions in Oceania:

AUSTRALIA

Australia is a continent located in Oceania between the Indian Ocean and the South Pacific Ocean. Australia has an enviable, strong economy with a per capita gross domestic product on par with the four dominant western European economies. Emphasis on reforms, low inflation, a housing-market boom, and growing ties with China have been key factors over the course of the economy's 17 solid years of expansion. Robust business, consumer confidence, and high export prices for raw materials and agricultural products have fueled the economy in recent years, particularly in the country's mining states.

INDONESIA

Indonesia is located in southeastern Asia, between the Indian Ocean and the Pacific Ocean. Indonesia struggles with poverty and unemployment. Economic difficulties in early 2008 centered on high global food and oil prices, the impact of which was extremely detrimental to Indonesia.

PHILIPPINES

The Philippines are located in southeastern Asia, between the Philippine Sea and the South China Sea, east of Vietnam. Although the general macroeconomic outlook of the Philippines has improved significantly in recent years, the economy still faces several long-term challenges. The Philippines must maintain the reform momentum in order to catch up with regional competitors, improve employment opportunities, and alleviate poverty. The Philippines will need still higher, sustained growth to make progress in alleviating poverty, given its high population growth rate and unequal distribution of income.

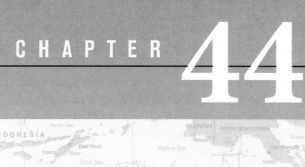

CHAPTER 44

Australia

Rebecca J. Scritchfield, MA, RD

 ## CULTURE AND WORLD REGION

Australia is a stable, democratic society with a skilled workforce and a strong, competitive economy. Australia's multicultural society includes its indigenous peoples and migrants from some 200 countries, including Vietnam, China, Greece, and the United Kingdom (UK). Cultural diversity has become a touchstone of Australia's national identity. Just one example of this diversity is the recent growth of Islam in Australia. Australia respects the right of all Australians to express and share their individual cultural heritage within an overriding commitment to Australia's democratic foundations (Australian Government Department of Foreign Affairs and Trade, 2008).

Today's Australians ("Aussies") are proud of their heritage and progress. Their ancestors, a nation of working-class citizens, built a modern egalitarian society on rugged and unforgivable terrain. Australians are often characterized as informal and "laid back," with the typical greeting among "mates" and "sheilas" used often: G'day (Good day). Their humor is often characterized as sarcastic, ironic, and self-deprecating. With this type of cultural personality, it is no wonder that Australians generally dislike the pompous and ostentatious (Encyclopedia Britannica, 2008).

Drinking and gambling have long been important aspects of Australian popular culture. Beer has traditionally been the drink of choice, but Australian wine production has exploded due to influences from Italy, Germany, and France. Australians of all ages socialize at pubs, and many young people are likely to seek out the disco or trendy bar or restaurant (Encyclopedia Britannica, 2008).

Australia hosts many festivals, which often attract a wide international audience. Particularly noteworthy arts events are the Sydney Festival (January), which features concerts and theater and is accompanied by fireworks displays; the biennial Adelaide Festival of Arts (March); and the Melbourne Festival (October).

Aboriginal arts festivals include the Barunga and Cultural Sports Festival (June) and Stompin Ground (October), held in Broome. Sydney's vibrant Gay and Lesbian Mardi Gras, held annually in February, attracts hundreds of thousands of revelers from around the world and is considered the world's largest celebration of its kind (Encyclopedia Britannica, 2008).

Australia is located in the Southern Hemisphere. It is part of the Oceania region, which includes Australia, New Zealand, Papua New Guinea, and the Pacific Islands. Australia, which is the smallest continent, is the sixth largest country in the world. Australia divides the Indian and South Pacific oceans. The total land area is 7,617,930 km^2 (nearly 3 million square miles), which is slightly smaller than that of the continental United States. The country is divided into six states and two territories: Australian Capital Territory, New South Wales, Northern Territory, Queensland, South Australia, Tasmania, Victoria, and Western Australia. Most of the 21,299,941 people who call Australia home are concentrated along the eastern and southeastern coasts (World Factbook, 2008). Based on the 2006 Australia Census, the largest cities are Sydney (4,119,190), Melbourne (3,592,591), Brisbane (1,763,131), Perth (1,445,078), and Adelaide (1,105,839).

LANGUAGE

Australians speak several different languages, although English is the official language. Based on the 2006 census, English is spoken by 78.5% of the population. Small proportions of the population speak other languages. The most common languages other than English are Italian (1.6%), Greek (1.3%), Cantonese (1.2%), Arabic (1.2%), and Mandarin (1.1%) (Australian Bureau of Statistics, 2007).

CULTURE HISTORY

The Latin word "Aborigine" means "original inhabitants." Aborigines consist of the native Australians, who migrated from places in Asia about 40,000 years before the first Europeans began exploration in the 17th century. The Aboriginal culture was primitive and one of the best-known ancient cultures of the world. Most tribes were nomadic hunters and gatherers, living off the land. With culturally diverse clans, the Aborigines shared many different "beliefs, customs, dialects, languages, rituals, art forms, painting styles, food and

hunting habits" (Maps of the World, 2008a). The Aborigines collectively spoke 200–250 different languages and over 700 dialects, making primitive Australia linguistically the most diverse society on earth.

No formal territorial claims were made on Australia until 1770, when Captain James Cook took possession in the name of Great Britain. Six colonies were created in the late 18th and early 19th centuries. They became the Commonwealth of Australia in 1901. The new country took advantage of its natural resources to rapidly develop agricultural and manufacturing industries, and to make a major contribution to the British effort in the World War I and II (World Factbook, 2008).

FOOD HISTORY WITHIN THE CULTURE

Aboriginal people survived off the native plants and animals of the Australian environment for thousands of years. Mammals and birds, such as kangaroo, wallaby, and emu, were regularly hunted and killed. Although animals were sometimes thrown straight onto the fire for cooking, there were a variety of preparation and cooking techniques. Other foods that seem less palatable to modern urban Australians, such as witchetty grubs, lizards, snakes, and moths, were greatly valued. "Bush foods," such as berries, roots, and nectars, were a vital part of the Aboriginal diet in many areas. In certain coastal areas, shellfish were plentiful and easily harvested. Aboriginals also caught fish in the oceans and rivers using hooks, spears, and fish traps. Aboriginal groups would often travel from season to season, moving to where they knew various food sources would be available (Australian Government Culture and Recreation Portal, 2008).

Early European settlers produced European crops and raised herd animals for food. The available meat was usually beef, pork, or mutton. Because there was no refrigeration, meat was usually salted or dried to preserve it. The settlers introduced European game animals, such as deer and rabbits, for hunting. Flour was a staple item of the early settler's diet. It was usually made into bread or damper dense, thick bread made without yeast. Tea was the staple drink and considered a necessity, even when other items were scarce. Rum brought over from Europe was eventually produced (Australian Government Culture and Recreation Portal, 2008).

Today's Australian cuisine is a product of international trends and the contributions of its Aboriginal and immigrant communities, most notably German,

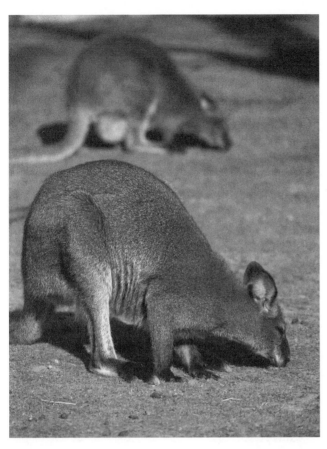

Kangaroo is sometimes cooked and eaten in parts of Australia.

Italian, Greek, Asian, and South African. It has been heavily influenced by the country's Anglo-Celtic heritage, with the traditional British supper still common. East and West "fusion" cuisine is popular countrywide. Australians are fond of both vegetarian and nonvegetarian foods consisting of pies, roasted cuts of meat, grilled steak and chops, and other forms of meat generally accompanied by vegetables. Barbecues ("the barbie") are a hallmark of Australian culture (Encyclopedia Britannica, 2008). Like their ancestors, Australians continue to use local fruits and plants. They have created unique culinary dishes such as calamari seasoned with lemon myrtle, lemon myrtle linguine tossed with scallops and prawns, and native spinach fettuccine with smoked salmon with creamy bush tomato and macadamia sauce.

Even though Australia has rough terrain and arid temperatures, it remains productive in agricultural crops: wheat, coarse grains (barley, oats, sorghum, maize, and triticale), rice, oilseeds (canola, sunflowers, soybeans, and peanuts), grain legumes (lupins and chickpeas), sugarcane, cotton, fruits, grapes, tobacco, and vegetables (Encyclopedia Britannica, 2008). The main livestock production of contemporary Australia is in sheep (wool and lamb), beef, pork, poultry, and dairy products. Many of these crops, including wool, cotton, wheat, barley, rice, fruit, and dairy products, are exported.

 ## MAJOR FOODS

 ### Protein Sources

Meat is a staple food in Australia. Beef, lamb, pork, chicken, and sometimes kangaroo dominate the meat sources of protein. Because the majority of Australians live on the coast, fish, oysters, prawns, crab, lobster, and mussels are abundant in the Australian diet. Eggs, dairy products, legumes, and tofu are also consumed. Nuts, including macadamia nuts (native to Australia), almonds, pistachios, and wattle seed (from Acacia trees), are sources of protein and fat in the Australian diet.

 ### Starch Sources

Starches in the Australian diet include cereals, bread, rice, pasta, potatoes, beans, peas, and lentils.

 ### Fat Sources

Fast food, avocado, nuts, and oils, including macadamia nut oil, are sources of fat.

 ### Prominent Vegetables

Popular vegetables include capsicum, broccoli, cauliflower, cabbage, lettuce, tomato, bush tomato ("desert raisin"), carrot, eggplant, cucumber, onion, pumpkin, potato, and spinach (native).

 ### Prominent Fruits

Available fruits include pineapples, passion fruit, mangoes, bananas, pawpaw, grapes, oranges, lemons, apples, pears, and peaches.

 ### Spices and Seasonings

The following native Australian bush foods are used as spices in Australian cooking (Gourmet Sleuth, 2007): lemon myrtle, mountain pepper, forest anise, forest peppermint, forestberry herb, pepperberry, rainforest rub, Red Desert seasoning, wildfire spice, and wild thyme.

Beverages

Australia has a booming wine industry and alcohol is very much part of the hospitality experience, whether it be at a fine-dining restaurant or at a barbecue in a friend's backyard. There are a wide range of food events and a great number of wine or brewery events throughout the year. Many areas of Australia base their tourism promotions on the local wine-producing industry and the associated gourmet food outlets.

Espresso coffee and tea are popular hot beverages that are frequently ordered in restaurants and cafes.

Desserts

There are a small number of desserts and sweet dishes that are popularly thought of as being unique to Australia:

- Anzac biscuits, traditional biscuits baked by anxious wives and mothers during World War I, packed in food parcels, and sent to the Australian soldiers in the trenches. They are made with rolled oats, desiccated coconut, flour, sugar, and butter.
- Frozie cup, a simple Australian dessert often sold for school fundraisers. It is a frozen cordial in a paper, plastic, or styrofoam cup similar to a popsicle.
- Lamingtons, a cube-shaped cake coated in a layer of chocolate icing and then desiccated coconut. They are sometimes served as two halves with a layer of cream or strawberry jam in between.
- Pavlova, a meringue dessert made with egg whites and topped with cream and fruit.

FOODS WITH CULTURAL SIGNIFICANCE

Vegemite is probably the most notable cultural food in Australia today. Similar to a British product, marmite, it became popular when marmite imports were disrupted after World War I. It is a dark-brown savory food paste made from yeast extract (brewer's yeast by-product of beer making), and various vegetable and spice additives. With a texture like peanut butter, the spread is used on sandwiches, toast, and cracker biscuits, as well as a filling of pastries. It has a salty, slightly bitter, and malty taste.

Several desserts are unique to Australia. Pavlova is a sweet confection made from sugar and egg-white

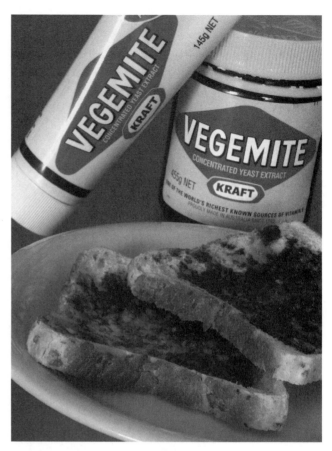

Vegemite is an Australian staple.

meringue, and then covered with whipped cream and seasonal fruits. Anzac biscuits are hard, crispy cookies made with rolled oats, coconut, and molasses. Soldier's cake is a boiled fruitcake that has a very long shelf life (Maps of the World, 2008b). Lamingtons are sponge-cake cubes coated in a layer of chocolate icing and coconut. They are sometimes served with a layer of cream or strawberry jam in between two halves.

Australians enjoy a special hand-sized meat pie made with meat and gravy and wrapped in a light pastry shell. Every establishment that sells food, including carry-outs and gas stations, has hot meat pies for sale. Traditional fillings include steak and kidney, mincemeat and onion, meat and mashed potatoes, meat and mashed peas, and meat and mushroom. From time to time, meatless pies are served as well, such as cheese and broccoli or cheese and egg (Australian Life Tips, 2008).

Other iconic national foods include the chiko roll, a deep-fried spring roll; violet crumble, a honeycomb chocolate bar; jaffas, an orange-flavored, candy-coated chocolate; tim tams, a chocolate biscuit; and the breakfast cereal Weet-Bix.

TYPICAL DAY'S MENU

There is no such thing as a "typical menu" in Australia because every household sits down to something different. Some eat fast food or restaurant meals, some prepare processed foods at home, and others make food from scratch. The cuisine varies by region too, with more seafood typically consumed in coastal areas and very traditional "meat-and-vegetable" meals based on fresh foods in outback towns.

Breakfast is normally an early meal before the heat of the day arrives. There are a variety of foods served based on local weather, local food tradition, and the amount of physical labor involved in one's day. Typical traditional foods include cereals such as Weet-Bix and Vita Brits (whole-wheat biscuits) with milk and honey; European muesli and fresh fruit; for winter, oatmeal with milk and a dab of butter; or toast and marmalade jam and other fruit jams, local honeys, and Vegemite. Heartier appetites feast on Aussie sausages, steak and eggs, bacon, baked beans, tomatoes, mushrooms, as well as bubble and squeak (fried leftovers of cabbage, potato, and pumpkin). A cup of tea is standard with an Aussie breakfast, but coffee, milk, and juices could also be included (Australian Life Tips, 2008).

The Australian lunch can be made up of a wide range of traditional Australian foods. An Aussie meat pie or sausage roll and a bottle of chocolate milk make a staple lunch. Sandwiches made with most any ingredient are common, including Vegemite, salads, baked beans, sweet corn, mushrooms and buttered sauce, fish paste, banana and sugar, and cold spaghetti. Hamburgers in Australia likely come with a fried egg, pickled beet root, and pineapple. Lunch is usually small because Australians break for morning and afternoon tea (Australian Life Tips, 2008).

The evening meal is the main meal of the day for most Australians and is often eaten with members of the immediate family or household. The dishes served vary widely according to the tastes and/or background of the family. Common choices include roast meat and vegetables, pasta, pizza, casseroles, barbecue meat, vegetables and salads, soup, and stir-fries. A typical Australian cafe or restaurant might offer sandwiches and foccacia; pasta, risotto, or curry dishes; steak, chicken, or other meat-based dishes; cakes or other desserts; and juices, soft drinks, beer, and coffee.

HOLIDAY MENUS

Good Friday and Christmas Day are celebrated with a traditional menu. Fish and seafood are served on Good Friday. Turkey, ham, roast vegetables, seafood, plum

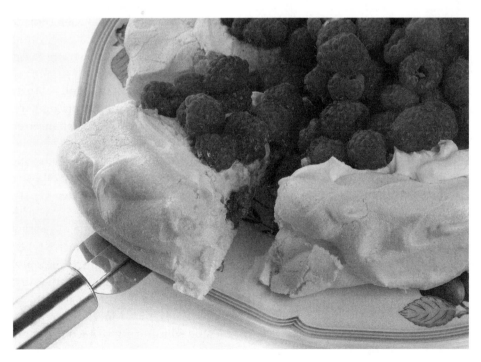
Pavlova

pudding, and trifle or pavlova make up the typical Christmas menu. Because Christmas falls at the height of summer, it can seem very odd to non-Australians to see a group of people eating a hot, roast meal on a hot day. Due to the heat over the Christmas holiday, many people will have cold ham and salads instead, or turkey terrine. Other holidays (New Years, Queen's Birthday, and Australia Day) are largely marked with barbecues.

 ## HEALTH PROVISION

Healthcare provision is managed by the states and territories, although broad national policies are framed by the federal government through the Department of Health and Aging. The national government also influences health service standards through its financial arrangements with the states and territories, through grants and benefits to individuals and organizations, and by regulating health insurance. Health care is also delivered by local governments and private enterprises. Public and private hospitals provide good-quality care and support medical research that has established an excellent international reputation. Private health insurance covers about one third of Australians (Encyclopedia Britannica, 2008).

 ## GENERAL HEALTH AND NUTRITIONAL INDICATORS SUMMARY

Because Australia is a developed country with a bountiful food supply, nutritional deficiencies are rare. In fact, Australia's nutrition-related health problems mirror the United States with obesity, heart disease, and diabetes being major public health concerns. Overweight or obesity affects 67% of Australian men, 52% of women, and 20–25% of children. Nearly 4 million Australians have heart disease, which is the primary cause of death of women in the country. Diabetes affects nearly 1 million Australians. At the current growth rate, about 300 Australians are diagnosed with diabetes each day (Australian Institute of Health and Welfare, 2009). Some contributing factors for the prevalence of these diseases include lack of exercise, frequent unhealthy meals outside the home, and large portion sizes of foods that are high in calories, sugar, and fat.

The most common deficiency in the world is iron deficiency. In Australia, low iron stores have been reported in up to one third of children ages 1–3 years. Risk factors for the development of iron deficiency in children include prematurity, low birth weight, gastrointestinal disease (malabsorption or blood loss), exclusive breastfeeding beyond 6 months, introduction of cow's milk as the main drink before 12 months, and high intake of cow's milk, delayed introduction of solids, low (or no) meat intake, and general poor diet in the second year. Recommendations for dietary approaches to support iron levels include daily consumption of between 65 and 100 g of meat, or between 80 and 120 g of fish, or a half to full serving of meat alternatives. Meat alternatives include half a cup of cooked dried beans, lentils, chickpeas or canned beans, 2 small eggs, and one third of a cup of nuts. In addition, including a food rich in vitamin C, such as tomato, capsicum, berries, orange, or mandarin, with nonmeat sources of iron will help improve the absorption of iron. (Department of Human Services Victorian Government, 2009).

Low birth weight, defined as weighing less than 2500 g at birth, affects 7% of newborns in Australia (UNICEF, 2007). One-hundred percent of the population in both urban and rural areas uses improved drinking-water sources.

 ## COMMUNICATION AND COUNSELING TIPS

Traditionally, Australians have viewed themselves as an egalitarian society, with a distrust of the rich and powerful. This belief continues today in the form of the "tall poppy syndrome"—when someone of higher economic, social, or political position attracts criticism. Australians have a very strong "underdog" attitude, which means that they will support those who appear to be at a disadvantage (unless Australia is in direct competition with another nation). This is most often seen in sports, where Australians are likely to root for the underdog in competitions.

"Mateship" is an Australian cultural idiom that embodies the working-class ethos: equality, loyalty, and friendship. There are two types of mateship, the inclusive and the exclusive; the inclusive is in relation to a shared situation (e.g., employment, sports, or hardship), whereas the exclusive type is toward a third party (e.g., a person who you have just met).

Counseling strategies for the Australian client are similar to the techniques used to provide nutrition counseling for an American client. In Australia, most dietetic educators have been using motivational interviewing, cognitive behavioral therapy, and coaching for the past decade.

FEATURED RECIPE

Balsamic Bean Salad with Grilled Fish Fillets

1 tbsp. olive oil

1 tsp. ginger (fresh or ground)

2 cloves garlic, chopped

½ tsp. cumin, ground

½ tsp. chili powder, ground

5 small fish fillets

Canned beans (chickpeas, black beans, or black-eyed peas)

½ medium English cucumber, seeded, diced

1 large tomato, chopped coarsely

½ onion, chopped

2 tsp. balsamic vinegar

2 tsp. olive oil

1 tbsp. each of mint and parsley, chopped

Pepper

1. In a flat dish combine oil, ginger, garlic, chili powder, and cumin.
2. Add fish and refrigerate.
3. In a bowl, mix together beans, cucumber, tomato, and onion.
4. Add vinegar, olive oil, herbs, and pepper. Toss to coat well.
5. Chill salad while grilling fish fillets.
6. Preheat char-grill pan, and grill or barbecue until hot.
7. Remove fish from dish and cook each fillet for 4 minutes each side or until cooked through. (When cooked, the fish flakes when tested with a fork.) Serve immediately.

Yields 5 servings

More recipes are available at http://nutrition.jbpub.com/foodculture/

REFERENCES

Australian Bureau of Statistics. (2007). *2006 census quickstats.* Retrieved April 20, 2008, from http://www.censusdata.abs.gov.au/ABSNavigation/prenav/ViewData?&action=401&tabname=Summary&areacode=0&issue=2006&producttype=QuickStats&textversion=true&navmapdisplayed=true&&breadcrumb=PLD&/

Australian Government Culture and Recreation Portal. (2008). *Australian food and drink.* Retrieved May 9, 2008, from http://www.cultureandrecreation.gov.au/articles/foodanddrink/

Australian Government Department of Foreign Affairs and Trade. (2008). *Australia today.* Retrieved April 20, 2008, from http://www.dfat.gov.au/facts/aust_today.html/

Australian Institute of Health and Welfare. (2009). *Chronic disease in Australia.* Retrieved April 13, 2009, from http://www.aihw.gov.au/subjectareas.cfm/

Australian Life Tips. (2008). *Australian food tips.* Retrieved May 15, 2008, from http://australian.lifetips.com/cat/59206/australian-food/

Department of Human Services Victorian Government. (2009). *Iron deficiency.* Retrieved April 12, 2009, from http://www.health.vic.gov.au/nutrition/child_nutrition/iron.htm/

Encyclopedia Britannica. (2008). *Australia.* Retrieved June 10, 2008, from http://library.eb.com/eb/article-228705/

Gourmet Sleuth. (2007). *Australian foods.* Retrieved May 30, 2008, from http://www.gourmetsleuth.com/australianfood.htm/

Maps of the World. (2008a). *Aboriginal Australian culture.* Retrieved April 26, 2008, from http://www.mapsofworld.com/australia/australiaculture/aboriginal-australian-culture.html/

Maps of the World. (2008b). *Australian culture food.* Retrieved May 16, 2008, from http://www.mapsofworld.com/australia/australia-culture/australian-culture-food.html/

UNICEF. (2007). *The state of the world's children 2007: Women and children, the double dividend of gender equality.* Retrieved April 14, 2009, from http://www.unicef.org/sowc07/statistics/tables.php

World Factbook (2008). *Australia.* Retrieved January 6, 2010, from http://www.cia.gov/library/publications/the-world-factbook/geos/xx.html

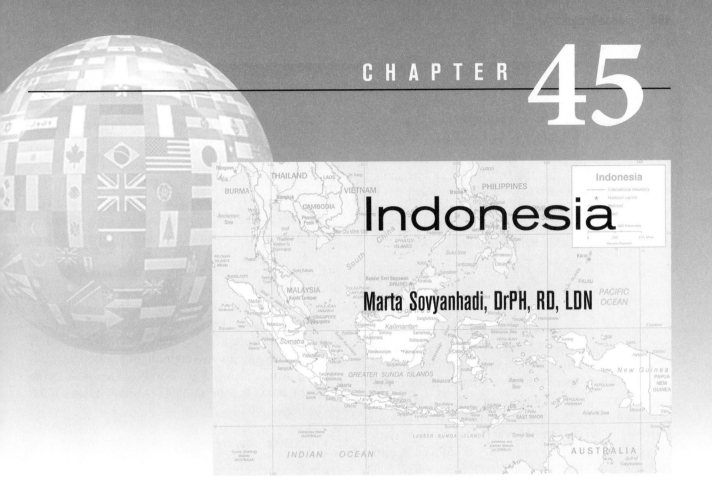

CHAPTER 45

Indonesia

Marta Sovyanhadi, DrPH, RD, LDN

 CULTURE AND WORLD REGION

Multiple foreign influences and decades of original indigenous customs have shaped Indonesian culture. Its potpourri of cuisine was largely influenced by Asian cultures, including Chinese and Indian, as well as by Western cultures. In the 15th century, Portuguese and Arabian traders arrived on the Indonesian shores trading both their spices and ethnic cultures. These immigrants from many different countries brought with them the culture and cuisine that is known to Indonesia today (Miller, 1996; Ricklefs, 2001; Taylor, 2003).

Indonesia is composed of a series of islands located at the southeastern Asia archipelago, between the Indian Ocean and the Pacific Ocean. Its people share a rich cultural heritage and enjoy a unique diet (Marks, 1989). The Republic of Indonesia consists of five large islands and thousands of smaller islands (about 6000 of which are inhabited), with a total area of 1,919,440 km² (741,100 square miles). Indonesia has a striving

agriculture industry with sugar as the largest commercial crop. Improved agricultural techniques during the 1980s and 1990s have also made it possible for the country to grow enough rice to meet its local demands. The country is also considered the world's third largest producer of coffee (after Brazil and Colombia), and the second largest producer of palm oil (after Malaysia) (Ricklefs, 1991, 2001; Dijk, 2001; Taylor, 2003).

 LANGUAGE

The Malay language was standardized and officially defined during Indonesia's independence in 1945. Aside from the national language, regional languages or local dialects, such as Minangkabau, Sundanese, and Javanese, are commonly spoken at home and within the local communities (Sneddon, 2004).

Indonesia has been influenced to varying degrees by trade and contact with the civilizations of India, China, and the Middle East, as well as Europe through Portuguese and Dutch colonialists. During the early 17th century, the Dutch East India Company (VOC) sought to control lucrative Indonesian trade through military and political domination. In 1800, VOC interest in Indonesia was nationalized into the Dutch East Indies; however, it was not until 1914 that the Dutch rule and hegemony extended across all parts of what is now modern-day Indonesia. The Indonesian islanders comprise a diversity of cultures, ethnicities, and languages (Ricklefs, 1991, 2001; Miller, 1996; Oostindie & Paasman, 1998).

 ## CULTURE HISTORY

Indonesia's strong cultural influences of Asia and the Western cultures were a result of ancient trading routes between the Far East and Middle East. These trading routes also influenced the cuisine of Indonesia, including the serving of food and use of spices. This complex cultural mixture has varied from its original version as seen by the many cultural practices and the varieties of religions, including Hinduism, Buddhism, Confucianism, and Islam (Witton, 2002; Brissendon, 2003; Anderson, 1995).

 ## MAJOR FOODS

The people of Indonesia are very health conscious. Their five-basic-food-groups message is "4 sehat, 5 sempurna" (which means "4 is healthy, 5 is excellent"). This message, which is recognized throughout the country, has been proven to be scientifically sound and is arranged in the following categories: carbohydrates, vegetables, dairy, fruits, and meat (Sihotang, 2002).

 ## Protein Sources

Dietary protein is provided from both plants and animals. The plant sources are provided from soybeans and soybean products such as tofu and tempeh, lentils, pinto beans, black beans, and peanuts. The animal protein sources are from eggs, beef, lamb, chicken, duck, and fish. In addition, most islanders also eat tiny fish, called *dilis*, which are about 0.5 in. long. They are swallowed whole. The bones are very soft and a good source of calcium. Milk is frequently not included in the menu because many Indonesians are lactose intolerant (Ethnic Cuisine, 2007; Biro Pusat Statistik, 2004; Government of Indonesia, 2000; Drajat & Ariani, 2004; McMillan, 2006).

 ## Starch Sources

Dietary carbohydrates include rice, corn, cassava, and potatoes; however, rice is by far the most common source. In fact, many Indonesians do not feel satiated or satisfied with a meal if it does not contain rice. The Indonesian word for rice is *nasi*, and it is eaten three times a day. For special occasions, such as birthdays, weddings, or New Years, a special rice dish called *nasi tumpeng* is prepared. (Ethnic Cuisine, 2007; Govern-

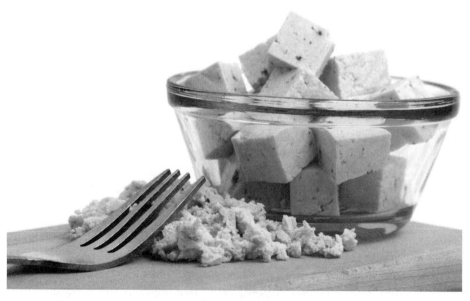
Tofu is a popular source of dietary protein.

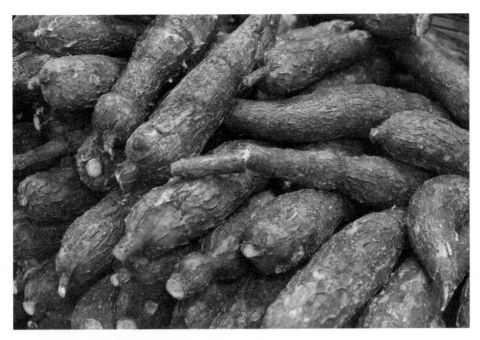

Common vegetables are the leaves of the papaya, spinach, cassava (pictured), pumpkin, and stems of bean sprouts.

ment of Indonesia, 2000; Department of Health Indonesia, 1993, 1994).

 Fat Sources

The edible fat products, from both vegetable and animal sources, are coconut oil, palm oil, kernel oil, sunflower oil, fish oil, pork oil/fat, cow fat, and bird fat.

 Prominent Vegetables

Common dietary vegetables are the leaves of the papaya, spinach, cassava, pumpkin, and stems of bean sprouts. They are eaten raw, steamed, or included in soups (Government of Indonesia, 2000; Department of Health Indonesia, 1993, 1994).

 Prominent Fruits

Mango, mangosteen, star fruit, papaya, banana, guava, rambutan, jackfruit, lychee, salak, sirzak, pomelo, and chiku are the fruits most often enjoyed in Indonesia. Oranges and pineapples are available year round. They are eaten fresh or mixed into a fruit gravy called *rujak*.

 Spices and Seasonings

Indonesia is a spice-rich country. *Kemiri* (candlenut), *cengkeh* (cloves), *ketumber* (coriander seeds), *pala* (nutmeg), *merica* (pepper), *tabiabun* (long pepper), *lenge* (sesame seeds), *lengkuas* (galangal), *jae* (ginger), *kencur* (resurrection lily), *kunyit* (turmeric), *bongkot* (torch ginger), *sereh* (lemon grass), *jeruk purut* (kaffir lime), *asam* (tamarind), *garam* (salt), *cabe* (chili), *bawang putih* (garlic), *bawang merah* (red shallot), *kemangi* (hoary basil), *daun pandan harum* (pandan leaf), and *daun salam* (salam leaf) are widely used to season daily dishes (Balinese Foods, 2007).

 Beverages

Indonesians enjoy their unique delicious beverages, both nonalcoholic and alcoholic.

The nonalcoholic beverages are as follows:

1. Cendol. It has gelatin-like consistency, green pieces of tapioca, is mixed with water and coconut milk (*santan*), and is sweetened by a liquefied brown sugar (*gula jawa*).
2. Es campus (mixed ice drink). It is somewhat similar to cendol but contains a variety of other things. In addition to different kinds of tapioca products, Indonesians add different kinds of fruits such as avocado, jackfruit, and so on.
3. Young coconut juice. It is fresh from the shell of the young coconut.
4. Various kinds of fruit juices from papaya, passion fruit (*markisah*), durian (*sirsak*), and so on.

5. Piña colada. A drink served inside a freshly hollowed-out pineapple.

6. Coffee (*kopi*) is served black, sweet, thick, and rich with the grounds floating on top. Indonesian *kopi* is sometimes laced with chicory or chocolate.

The alcoholic beverages are as follows:

1. *Tuak*. It is a sweet palm wine made from the juice of the coconut palm flower, which is stored for about 1 month for fermentation. It contains about 5% alcohol.

2. *Brem* (rice wine). It is made from black glutinous rice and coconut milk. The alcohol content is about 7–9% after 3 days of fermentation.

3. *Arak* (hard liquor). It is colorless, sugarless, and spirit distilled from either *brem* or *tuak* with 20–50% alcohol content (Global Gourmet, 2007; Jason, 2004, Balinese Foods, 2007).

 Desserts

Indonesians' healthy popular desserts are *juice alpokat* (an avocado drink), *rujak manis* (mixed fruits), *lemper* (sweet, stuffed sticky-rice roll), banana citrus cake with orange syrup, durian cookies, multicolor layer cake, *kue mangkup* (cupcake), *bolu kukus* (steamed spongy cake), *martabak manis* (sweet crepes), *kue lumpang* (cakes with a hole), and *bubur ketan hitam* (black glutinous rice porridge) (Indolists, 2007).

 FOOD WITH CULTURAL SIGNIFICANCE

Indonesian cuisine does not employ complex cooking tools. The essential cooking methods entail blanching, boiling, steaming, frying, and deep-frying. Two of the most basic tools are the wooden chopping block and heavy cleaver. These items provide everything that is needed, from cutting chicken to chopping down lemongrass to breaking open cardamom pods.

The first important task in cooking Indonesian cuisine is to break up and compress the important seasonings that are the foundation of Indonesian meals. *Sambel* (a sauce) originated in Indonesia. For preparing *sambel*, a saucer-shaped granite crushing stone with a granite pestle is needed. The basic ingredients of *sambel*, onion, garlic, turmeric, chili peppers, and coriander, are sliced into small quantities to grind. The pestle is then applied with a kneading motion until the contents are combined together into a smooth paste.

Sambel is commonly used as a dipping sauce or a seasoning sauce for meat, vegetables, or seafood. In addition, coconut milk is the main secret that enriches the flavor of the traditional Indonesian meal. Banana leaves are used to wrap the meat, vegetable, and fish dishes that are spiced with *sambel* and then cooked on top of burning charcoal.

Another important tool used in an Indonesian kitchen is the bamboo steamer. This kind of steamer is favored over the metal steamers because it soaks up more moisture instead of letting it drop back into the food and can fit inside a wok with steaming water. A wok is preferred over a deep-fryer because it needs less oil.

The traditional Indonesian meal does not involve courses that are served individually; instead, each dish is handed out collectively. Different portions of food are given depending on the region of Indonesia. These portions include foods such as *nasi goreng* (fried rice), *satay* (skewered meat), or *bakmi goreng* (fried noodles). Various parts of Indonesia have particular recipes and dishes that are made only in those regions. For instance, in Padang, which is located in the Minangkabau region, spicy dishes are made and usually cooked in front of the individual outside of the restaurant. This allows the customers to see the fresh ingredients that are used in each dish. It is also traditional to eat each dish with one's hands.

North Sulawesi is not a Muslim region; therefore, pork is widely used in dishes. On the other hand, in the Javanese regions many of the dishes include vegetables, soybeans, beef, and chicken, all of which are dipped in the *sambel*.

 TYPICAL DAY'S MENU

Indonesian cuisine is considered one of the world's most unique cuisines due to its combination of geographic and cultural diversity. Although meals are generally simple, the plentiful use of various roots, spices, and leaves adds zest to most dishes. Coriander is widely used in cooking; however, common use of the chili pepper may mislead some people to believe that all Indonesian dishes are spicy, whereas other spices, such as cumin and ginger, which are relatively mild spices, are often used in many Indonesian dishes. A popular meal throughout the country is plain rice served with a spicy sweet or hot sauce. This dish, with its contrasting flavors, is common in Indonesian cuisine.

In Maluku and Irian Jaya (Indonesian New Guinea) sago palm flour, sweet potatoes, and cassava reign supreme; however, rice is the main staple in all other parts of Indonesia. Meat, fish, and vegetables are condiments designed to flavor the staple, whereas sauces, such as fiery *sambel*, lend additional character.

With the base of most Indonesian meals being rice, the typical Indonesian menu is high in fiber, complex carbohydrates, and monounsaturated fatty acids. A heavy breakfast (*makan pagi*) normally containing a bowl of rice, noodles, or *soto* (meat and vegetable soup), accompanied by *Java kopi* (world-famous coffee) or tea, starts the day. Lunchtime (*makan siang*) often provides the main meal of the day. This meal is prepared all morning long and is served all at once. Most of the Indonesian families have helpers to cook the meals. Dinner (*makan malam*) is often eaten after the workday has ended. Lunch and dinner normally contain staples, meat or fish, vegetables, and condiments. (Bookrags, 2007; McMillan, 2006).

HOLIDAY MENUS

The five religious holidays celebrated and officially recognized in Indonesia are Islamic, Catholic, Protestant, Buddhist, and Hindu holidays. Ramadan (*Puasa*), a month-long observance of fasting and celebration, is the most important time of the year for Muslims. The fasting begins at dawn and is broken at sunset when groups come together for a large feast. Families that participate in this celebration rise as early as 3:00 AM to consume as much food as possible before dawn. Lebaran, also called Hari Raya or Idul Fitri (Muslim New Year), marks the end of *Puasa* as well as the return of regular eating habits. Muslims often prepare *ketupat* blocks, a rice recipe cooked in coconut or palm leaves. Cakes and cookies are served with a seemingly bottomless pot of tea.

The celebration of a new family, home, or business is a significant event practiced by most families where prayers are offered to a god. This uniquely Indonesian tradition, called *selamatan* (wedding party or housewarming party), is followed by a kickoff party. *Nasi tumpeng*, a cone-shaped mountain of steamed yellow rice, is sliced at the top and served.

Bali is home to the greatest Indonesian Hindu population, and the most elaborated celebration is Hari Raya Nyepi, the Hindu New Year. On New Year's Eve, food is prepared for the following day (homemade pastries and sweetmeats). Hindus refrain from all activities during the New Year celebration, including food preparation. Streets are deserted and tourists are often not allowed to leave their hotel.

Indonesia's Independence day, Hari Proklamasi Kemerdekaan, is celebrated on August 17. Everyone prepares for the festivities several weeks in advance. Money is raised for contests, such as the *krupuk udang* (shrimp crackers) eating contest and the women's baking contest, which is usually an attempt to make the largest *nasi tumpeng*.

The holiday to honor the first Indonesian female emancipationist, Raden Kartini's day, is celebrated on April 21. On that day women take a day off from household responsibilities such as taking care of the children, cooking, and cleaning. The menu is normally *nasi tumpeng*, *gado gado* (mixed vegetables), *teh halia* (hot ginger tea), and *pisang goreng* (fried banana cake as dessert).

For almost all kinds of special occasions, such as birthdays, anniversaries, or New Year, *nasi tumpeng* is prepared. Other rice dishes, such as *ketupat* (rice steamed in woven packets of coconut fronds), *lontong* (rice steamed in banana leaves), *intip* (rice crackers), desserts, noodles, *brem* (rice wine), and *nasi goreng* (fried rice), are included in the holiday/special-occasion meals (Koll, 2007, 2008; Freeman, 2007; Eu Hooi, 2007; Taylor, 2003; Witton, 2002; Dalton, 1995; Bigalke, 1981; Rodgers, 1981; Ramseyer, 1977; Nooy-Palm, 1979; Sitompul, 1974; Hooykaas, 1973; Belo, 1953).

HEALTH BELIEFS AND CONCERNS

The health beliefs of Indonesians are strongly associated with their main religion, Islam. Approximately 88% of the population, which is just over 200 million people, identify themselves as Muslims, thereby making Indonesia the most populous Muslim nation in the world. The Qur'an (the Muslim holy book) gives guidelines for the overall health of one's body, mind, and soul.

Muslims are mandated to observe Ramadan (Islamic New Year). To prepare for it, they fast for 30 days for both spiritual and social purposes. In addition, they fast from dawn to sunset and observe a strict way of eating. For instance, foods that are slow digesting are consumed during this period. Whereas fast-digesting foods last for only 3–4 hours, slow-digesting foods sustain fasting individuals for as much as 8 hours; thus, this regimen prevents them from becoming hungry often.

Foods that are considered slow digesting are complex carbohydrates, such as foods that contain grains and seeds like barley, wheat, oats, millet, semolina, beans, lentils, whole-wheat flour, and unpolished rice, whereas fast-burning foods are considered to be those that contain sugar and white flour (refined carbohydrates). A well-balanced diet is followed strategically during this time in order to maintain energy and electrolyte levels. Foods from each food group; that is, fruits, vegetables, meat/chicken/fish, bread/cereal, and dairy products, are eaten. Fiber-containing foods, such as bran, whole wheat, grains and seeds, vegetables (beans, peas, marrow, mealies, spinach) and other herbs (e.g., methie, the iron-rich leaves of beetroot), fruits with skin, dried fruit (especially dried apricots), and figs, are also consumed.

A dietary plan may consist of the following:

1. Bread/cereal/rice, pasta, biscuits, and crackers: 6–11 servings/day.
2. Meat/beans/nuts: 2–3 servings/day.
3. Milk and other dairy products: 2–3 servings/day.
4. Vegetables: 3–5 servings/day.
5. Fruits: 2–4 servings/day.
6. Added sugar (table sugar, sucrose): sparingly.
7. Added fat, polyunsaturated oil: 4–7 tbsp/day.

During Ramadan, breakfast (*iftar*) might consist of dates, three juice servings (4 oz. each), and vegetable soup with pasta or graham crackers (1 cup). Such a menu hydrates the body, maintains mineral balance, and provides an immediate energy source. A food highly utilized by Muslims is dates. They are excellent for people who are fasting as well as for pregnant and lactating women (who are excused from the Ramadan fast) because of its high sugar levels. Pregnant women are given foods that contain fruit sugar on the day they give birth, to help with energizing and revitalizing the mother's weakened body, and at the same time, to stimulate the milk hormones and increase the levels of breast milk, which is essential to the newborn baby.

The predawn meal (*sahur*) is a light meal that consists of foods from all food groups. Olive oil, or any other monounsaturated or polyunsaturated fats, may be added to a salad or cereal. Indonesian Muslims believe in the health benefits of consuming olives in their diet, including the leaf and oil. Olive oil, referred to as *zaytuha* in the Qur'an, is cited as one of the most highly recommended types of oil.

Muslims are advised to refrain from drinking tea during this time of the year, because it can cause frequent urination, which can take with it valuable minerals that the body needs during the day.

Pork is believed to be a harmful substance, and it is prohibited by the Qur'an for human consumption. One reason that it is considered not fit for humans is the potential presence of the trichina worm in the meat. Currently, it is possible to identify a pig that carries trichina, but in the past it was almost impossible to detect. Nevertheless, the Qur'an stood firmly against pig consumption, as mandated by Allah (Shakir, 1997; Berberoglu, 2007).

GENERAL HEALTH AND NUTRITIONAL INDICATORS SUMMARY

Malnutrition in Indonesia is so prevalent because of lack of access to sufficient food, and not choosing a variety of foods for a nutritious diet. Rice is overvalued and other nutritious foods are overlooked in many Indonesian communities. Due to the multiple micronutrient deficiencies, many women experience complications during childbirth. Around 20,000 mothers die every year, with maternal mortality remaining high at 307 deaths per 100,000 live births.

One local organization, Yayasan Ayo Indonesia, decided to help decrease the prevalence of malnutrition and micronutrient deficiencies by teaching the locals how to grow their own vegetables. They also shared the importance of eating three meals per day with foods from each of the three main food groups (energy, growth, and helper foods). Energy foods consist of rice, taro, sweet potatoes, corn, and cassava; growth foods are tempeh, tofu, fish, eggs, and beans; and helper foods include a variety of fruits and vegetables. The group also advised women and children to take vitamin A, iron, and iodine supplements to decrease their chances of developing a deficiency.

According to the Indonesian Bureau of Statistics (2006), 70% of women and children are anemic, and 44% of children 24–59 months have stunted growth. Iron deficiency has been known to affect children's brain and physical development, and to increase their chances of contracting immunity disorders. Prevention for this deficiency is to eat iron-rich foods such as meat, fish, tofu, green vegetables, and peanuts. Iron deficiency has also struck the pregnant population of Indonesia, with an estimated 6.4% of pregnant women having an iron deficiency (UNICEF, 2007).

Iodine is another micronutrient deficiency that plagues Indonesians. This deficiency can cause many things, but one particular symptom is the enlargement of the thyroid gland in the throat, commonly called the goiter. Lack of iodine is the main cause of endemic goiter, where the loss of iodine from the soil due to glaciating, erosion, high rainfall, snow, and flooding leads to a low iodine content of all food grown in it. Dietitians are advised to partner with agriculturalists and husbandry groups in these areas. In addition, iodine supplements, such as iodine salt, can be introduced to prevent this deficiency.

COMMUNICATION AND COUNSELING TIPS

In order to communicate with, and counsel, the Indonesian community, a person needs certain tools. First, a good rapport is necessary. In order to have a positive influence on an Indonesian family, the husband and mother-in-law need to be consulted on each topic because they are considered to be the heads of the family. This dynamic should be established at the outset. Sensitivity to Indonesian culture is also important.

Second, the counselor has to build a relationship of trust with the client. The client needs to feel assured of the counselor's presence, dependability, honesty, and earnest aspiration to give assistance when requested. This trust cannot be assumed; it must be earned.

The third necessity is to show respect, which, among other things, means understanding the client's circumstances as well as his or her general food and health practices. In addition, the counselor should attempt to establish empathy by looking beyond outward behaviors and perceiving the client's inward experiences.

Fourth, it is important to be sincere. Clients will be able to tell whether a counselor is not being genuine with them (Snetselaar, 2007; Holli, Calabrese, & O'Sullivan Maillet, 2003; Favin & Griffiths, 1999).

PRIMARY LANGUAGE OF FOOD NAMES WITH ENGLISH AND PHONETIC TRANSLATION

Table 45-1 gives the primary language of food names with English and phonetic translation.

TABLE 45-1   Primary Language of Food Names with English and Phonetic Translation

Indonesian	English	Phonetic Translation	Indonesian	English	Phonetic Translation
Nasi	Rice	Na'–see	Anggur	Wine	Ang–gur
Jagung	Corn	Ja–gūng	Gula	Sugar	Gū–la
Ubi kayu	Cassava	Ûbee–kayū	Daging	Meat	Da–ging
Kentang	Potato	Ken–tang	Susu	Millet	Sū–sū
Daun	Leaf	Da–ūn	Bawang	Onion	Ba–wang
Papaya	Papaya	Pe–pa–ya	Biji biji	Cereal	Bee–jee Bee–jee
Bayam	Spinach	Ba–yem	Kacang kedelai	Soybean	Ka–chang Ke–de–lae
Touge	Bean sprout	Tŏ–ge'	Kacang tanah	Peanut	Ka–chang Ta–na
Mangga	Mango	Mang–ga	Tomat	Tomato	Tŏ–mat
Pisang	Banana	Pee–sang	Ubi jalar	Sweet potato	Ûbee–Ja–lar
Jambu	Guava	Jam–bū	Kemiri	Pecan	Ke–mee–ree
Jeruk	Orange	Je–rook	Cengkeh	Cloves	Chang–ke'
Nenas	Pineapple	Ne–nas	Pala	Nutmeg	Pa–la
Kelapa	Coconut	Ke–la–pa	Merica	Pepper	Me–ree–cha
Kopi	Coffee	Kŏ–pee			

FEATURED RECIPE

Nasi Tumpeng

1 cup coconut milk

3 cups water

4 cups enriched rice, long grain

¼ cup turmeric powder

1 small bunch lemongrass

6 bay leaves

Salt to taste

1. Boil all ingredients together until the liquid is evaporated.
2. Transfer to steamer and cook until rice is done.
3. Mold it into a cone shape.
4. Garnish with sliced cucumber and tomato, scrambled eggs, *sambel* tempeh, and perkerdel dipped in *sambel*.

Yields 8–12 servings

More recipes are available at http://nutrition.jbpub.com/foodculture/

REFERENCES

Anderson, S. (1995). *Indonesian flavors.* Berkeley, CA: Frog Ltd.

Balinese Foods. (2007). *Drinks, spices and fruits.* Retrieved November 15, 2007, from http://www.murnis.com/culture/articlebalinesefoodsdrinksspicesandfruit.htm/

Belo, J. (1953). *Bali: Temple festival New York.* Seattle: University of Washington Press.

Berberoglu, H. (2007). *Health guidelines for Ramadan.* Retrieved March 25, 2008, from http://asiarecipe.com/indohealth.html/

Bigalke, T.W. (1981). *A social history of Tana Toraja 1975–1965.* PhD Thesis. Madison, WI: University of Wisconsin.

Biro Pusat Statistik. (2004). *Konsumsi kalori and protei penduduk Indonesia and propinsi.* Jakarta, Indonesia: CV Arief Brothers.

Bjom. (2005). *History of Indonesia #10.* Retrieved November 2, 2007, from http://www.indonesiaphoto.com/content/view102/4/

Bookrags. (2007). *Cuisine of Indonesia.* Retrieved November 15, 2007, from http:// http://www.bookrags.com/Cuisine_of_Indonesia

Brissendon, R. (2003). *South East Asian food.* Melbourne, Australia: Hardie Grand Books.

Bureau of Statistics. (2006). *Indonesia.* Retrieved November 12, 2007, from http://hivinsite.ucsf.edu/global?page=cr08-id-00

Dalton, B. (1995). *Indonesian handbook* (4th ed.). Chico, CA: Avalon Travel Publishing.

Department of Health Indonesia. (1993). *Menu seimbang dari berbagai makanan pokok seri 1.* Jakarta, Indonesia: Author.

Department of Health Indonesia. (1994). *Pesan dasar gizi seimbang.* Jakarta, Indonesia: Author.

Dijk, K.V. (2001). A country in despair: Indonesia between 1997 and 2000. Leiden, Netherlands: KITLV Press.

Drajat, M., & Ariani, M. (2004). *Perkembangan konsumsi pangan rumah tangga di Indonesia.* Paper presented at Widyakarya National Pangan and Gizi.

Ethnic Cuisine. (2007). *Indonesia.* Accessed November 15, 2007, from http://www.sallys-place.com/food/cuisines/indonesia.htm/

Eu Hooi, K. (2007). *Tourism Indonesia.* Retrieved March 25, 2008, from http://www.tourismindonesia.com/

Favin, M., & Griffiths, M. (1999). *Communication for behavior change in nutrition projects: A guide for World Bank task managers.* Washington, DC: World Bank, Human Development Network.

Freeman, N. (2007). *Ethnic Cuisine: Indonesia.* Retrieved March 25, 2008, from http://www.sallys-place.com/food/cuisines/indonesia.htm/

Global Gourmet. (2007). *Indonesian beverages.* Retrieved November 15, 2007, from http://www.globalgourmet.com/destinations/indonesia/indobevs.html/

Government of Indonesia. (2000). *National plan of action for food and nutrition, 2001–2005.* Jakarta, Indonesia: Department of Health Indonesia.

Holli, B.B., Calabrese R.J., & O'Sullivan Maillet, J. (2003). *Communication and education skills for dietetics professionals.* Philadelphia: Lippincott Williams & Wilkins.

Hooykaas, C. (1973). Religion in Bali iconography of religions series XIII, 10. Leiden, Netherlands: Institute of Religious Iconography, State University, Gronigen.

Indolists. (2007). *Indonesian kitchen at Indolists food.* Retrieved November 2007, from http://www.indolists.com/recipe/category/desserts/60 pdate/asc/

Jason, M. (2004). *The joy of Arak Madu.* Retrieved November 15, 2007, from http://www.arakmadu.com/

Koll, J. (2007). *Living in Indonesia.* Retrieved March 25, 2008, from http://expat.or.id/

Koll, J. (2008). *Selamat ceremony.* Retrieved March 25, 2008, from http://www.hebatindo.com/infopages/selamatan_eng.htm/

Marks, C. (1989). *The exotic kitchens of Indonesia: Recipes from the outer islands.* New York: Evans and Company.

McMillan, M. (2006). *Indonesian cuisine. Encyclopedia of modern Asia. Milk for schools.* Retrieved November 12, 2007, from http://81.21.76.62/milkforschools.org.uk/index.html

Miller, G. (1996). *To the spice islands and beyond: Travels in eastern Indonesia.* New York: Oxford University Press.

Nooy-Palm, H. (1979). *The Sa'dan-Toraja: A study of their social life and religion. Organization, symbols and beliefs* (Vol. 1).

The Hague, Netherlands: Verhandelingen Van Het Koninklijk Insituut Voor Taal-land en Volkenkunde.

Oostindie, G., & Paasman, B. (1998). Dutch attitudes towards colonial empires, indigenous cultures, and slaves. *Eighteenth Century Studies, 31*(3), 349–355.

Peterson, J. (1997). *Eat smart in Indonesia.* Madison, WI: Gingko Press.

Ramseyer, U. (1977). *The art and culture of Bali.* Oxford: Oxford University Press.

Ricklefs, M.C. (1991). *A history of modern Indonesia since c. 1300* (2nd ed.). Palo Alto, CA: Stanford University Press.

Ricklefs, M.C. (2001). *A history of modern Indonesia since c. 1200* (3rd ed.). Palo Alto, CA: Stanford University Press.

Rodgers, S. (1981). Adat, Islam, and Christianity in a Batak homeland. Athens: Ohio University Center for International Studies.

Sahanaya, W. (2006). *Study Indonesian dictionary.* South Melbourne, Victoria, Australia: Oxford University Press.

Shakir, M.H. (1997). *The holy Qur'an by prophet Muhammad* (M.H. Shakir, Trans.). Houston, TX: Institute for Islamic Knowledge.

Sihotang, S. (2002). *Empat sehat lima sempurna telah disempurnakan.* Jakarta, Indonesia: Kompas Cyber Media.

Sitompul, P.P. (1974). *Susila budhi Dharma: International mystic movement of Indonesia.* Claremont, CA: Claremont Graduate School Dissertation.

Sneddon, J. (2004). *The Indonesian language: Its history and role in modern society.* Sydney, Australia: UNSW Press.

Snetselaar, L.G. (2007). *Nutritional counseling for lifestyle change.* Boca Raton, FL: CRC/Taylor & Francis.

Taylor, J.G. (2003). *Indonesia: Peoples and histories.* New Haven, CT: Yale University Press.

UNICEF. (2007). *The state of the world's children 2007: Women and children, the double dividend of gender equality.* Retrieved April 14, 2009, from http://www.unicef.org/sowc07/statistics/tables.php

von Holzen, H., & Arsana, L. (1996). *Food of Indonesia.* Singapore: Periplus Editions Ltd.

Witton, P. (2002). *World food: Indonesia.* Melbourne, Australia: Lonely Planet.

CHAPTER 46

Philippines

Marcy J. Leeds, PhD, RD

Gemma L. and Jessie K. Padchonga

 CULTURE AND WORLD REGION

The Filipino culture is a mixture of diverse indigenous civilizations with characteristics introduced via foreign influences, including Spain, Mexico, the United States, and China. The people of the Philippines have taken the customs of all of these nations and blended them into their own unique way of life.

The Philippines is a Catholic nation (approximately 85%). The remainder of the country is primarily Protestant and Muslim, with a small percentage being Buddhist. As in most Catholic nations, families are typically large and divorce is illegal. Although native Filipinos still practice many beliefs that are considered primitive, such as ritualistically sacrificing chickens and pigs and "contacting" ancient ancestors, they attend church regularly and consider the church to be a center for their spiritual beliefs.

In the southern Philippines there is an island named Mindanao where most of the people are Muslims. The Muslim customs and traditions practiced there are unique compared with the rest of the Philippines.

Certain characteristics are common among all Filipinos wherever they reside. They tend to have close family ties, which are apt to grow stronger with distance. This includes a feeling of obligation to monetarily help support each other. Typically, if one family member is financially successful, he or she will share the wealth with all of the other family members. Sometimes more prosperous relatives will financially support parents, grandparents, siblings, nieces, and nephews. This sense of responsibility may go beyond the nuclear family to in-laws and other extended family members.

Filipinos believe in respecting elders. The elders in a community are turned to for advice and deferred to in important matters. Grandparents and parents are always respected and treated as figures of authority. Among siblings, the eldest has the highest ranking. Along with this ranking comes the responsibility of helping out all of the younger siblings with things such as college tuition and building a house.

Filipinos believe in repaying their debts, not just financial obligations but favors given to them or any family member. For example, when having a wedding celebration many people volunteer their time in food preparation, serving food to guests, and cleaning up after the wedding. This indebtedness is expected to be repaid in-kind in the future. When someone dies in the community, everybody helps with entertaining visitors and feeding the people who come to the wake. Again, in times of need these favors are returned. Many Filipinos who live in remote areas work together. For instance, if there are 10 people who own 10 rice fields, all 10 people go to work on one person's property on the first day. The next day they go to the next person's rice field, and so on. In this way, it is an enjoyable working environment; they can talk with each other while they get the work done. No money is exchanged.

Filipinos have a strong sense of personal and family pride, especially in acting appropriately in social situations. For example, when teachers discipline their students for inappropriate behavior, they may have the student squat for the entire period because they misbehaved. Students do not have the option of going home and complaining to their parents, because teachers have the right to discipline their students. Another example would be showing respect for older people when they give you advice, even if you do not agree with their suggestions. A third example is related to eating. When you are at a party or picnic, the children always eat first. Once the children are full, whatever is left is what the adults eat.

Filipinos are very hospitable to their guests; they give appropriate respect to anyone regardless of race, culture, or belief. If you are their guest, you are treated with nothing but kindness. A major part of being a guest is sharing food with your host. If someone offers you something to eat or drink, it is considered rude and disrespectful to not accept the offer. In fact, when entering someone's home it is expected that he or she will offer you the most delicious foods available. You need to be sure to enter with an appetite or you will most certainly insult your host.

Death is one of the most important occasions in the Filipino family. It is traditional, as with other aspects of the Philippine culture, to be hospitable to the guests; this is done by offering food and refreshments to those mourning with the family. The first-year death anniversary, as well as all of the following anniversaries of the deceased, is significant. In certain parts of the Philippines, a plate of food is offered for the deceased in hopes that he or she will spiritually visit and partake of the offering.

In terms of the arts, weaving is popular in the northern mountains of the Philippines. Wood carvings and bamboo crafts are found throughout the Philippines. Dancing and music are also at the heart of Filipino culture. Filipinos have unique folk dances. The most well-known dance is the *Tinikling*, in which two long bamboo sticks are knocked together while dancers jump in and out of them. In the northern part of the Philippines, known as the Mountain Province, a dance called the *Banga* is popular. In this dance the women wear hand-woven *tapis* (skirts) and balance clay pots on their heads; the men wear hand-woven G-strings (long, wide pieces that completely cover their groins). While dancing, musicians play gongs (metal hand drums) that create the rhythm for the dancers. In the southern part of the Philippines, there is another dance called the *Singkil*, which is mainly a dance that shows off extravagant Muslim royalty. The *Singkil* dance uses fancy silk clothing and umbrellas.

The Philippines is made up of 7107 islands. Located in Southeast Asia, it is bordered by the Philippine Sea on the east, the South China Sea on the west, the Luzon Strait on the north, and the Celebes Sea on the south. The total area of the Philippines is 299,404 km². From north to south the Philippines stretches for 1850 km and from east to west for 1100 km. The capital of the Philippines is Manila, which is located on the island of Luzon (Peters, 1994).

 LANGUAGE

The national language of the Philippines is called *Filipino*, which consists mainly of Tagalog. Tagalog is the language spoken in Manila, the capital; however, all schooling is in English, from preschool through university, other than the subject of *Filipino* itself. The other major languages spoken in the Philippines include Ilocano in the north, Kapampangan and Pangasinan in the central region, and Bicolano in the southern part of the main island. In the southern islands Cebuana, Visayan, and Illonggo are spoken. Also, in the remote areas each village has its own dialect, of which there are more than 100.

CULTURE HISTORY

Before the 1500s, indigenous Filipino culture was strongly influenced by Malaysia and Indonesia. Many customs and the way of life reflect these cultural influences. Chinese culture, along with Buddhism, had a strong impact on Filipino folklore.

The Spanish and Mexican cultures certainly played a major role in the Filipino culture. The Spanish colonized and governed the Philippines for more than 350 years (1521–1898). They brought Catholicism with them as well as many other customs and traditions. Filipino music, dance, art, and cooking all have a Spanish flavor to them. There are also many Spanish words intertwined into the many Filipino languages and dialects. Filipinos use Spanish numbers for telling time and counting. Their money is in pesos, similar to Mexico and other former Spanish territories.

The American culture had a strong impact on the Filipino lifestyle. The Philippines was an American territory for almost 50 years (1898–1946). The English language is widely used throughout the Philippines. In fact, more English is spoken there than in any other Asian country. The Philippines's educational system is modeled after the U.S. educational system, and as mentioned previously, English is the medium of instruction. Teachers speak English in their classrooms and students must read, write, and speak in English. One can also see American influences in Filipinos consuming fast foods and carbonated soft drinks, as well as in television programming, movies, and sports.

FOOD HISTORY WITHIN THE CULTURE

Filipino cuisine developed in stages. Before the arrival of the Spaniards, Filipino food habits were similar to those of most of Southeast Asia. Filipinos consumed a lot of rice and used soy sauce and fish sauce in food preparation. Filipino food was prepared by boiling, steaming, or roasting. The main protein foods at the time were pork, chicken, fish, shellfish, and water buffalo. There were a few remote locations where the diet also included lizards, locusts, and local birds.

Spanish colonialism brought many new Spanish and Mexican recipes that profoundly influenced Filipino cuisine. The Spaniards brought with them chili peppers, tomato sauces, corn, and the methods of sautéing with garlic and onions. They added vinegar and

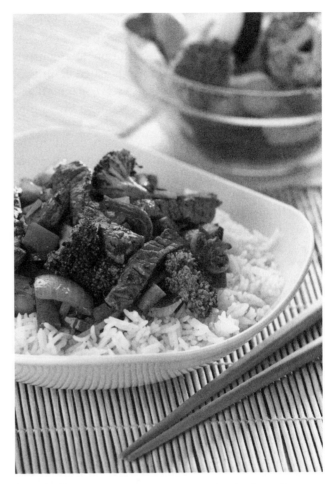

During the 1800s, Chinese food, including chop suey, became a staple of the noodle shops around the Philippines.

certain spices to foods to preserve them, due to lack of refrigeration. Local adaptations of Spanish dishes then became common, such as the transformation of *paella* into its Filipino version of *arroz valenciana* (rice prepared with sautéed vegetables and chicken, pork, and seafood), *chorizo* into its local version of *longanisa* (small Filipino sausage), and *escabeche* and *adobado* into pork or chicken adobo.

Filipino cuisine has also been influenced by China, India, Japan, the Middle East, and the United States. Surrounding Asian nations shared with Filipinos their methods of food preparation such as stir-frying and making delectable soups. The influence of the Chinese, who have been settling in the Philippines since precolonial times, is evident in the popularity of noodles. During the 1800s, Chinese food became a staple of the noodle shops around the Philippines. They served foods such as *sinangag* (fried rice) and chop suey (stir-fried mixed vegetables).

Relatively recent American influence on Filipino foods is seen with the availability today of many fast-food restaurants that serve the traditional hamburger, fried chicken, French fries, and carbonated beverages. Many of these fast-food chains also serve spaghetti and pizza. There are American donut shops in the Philippines as well.

Internationally, Filipinos are considered to be some of the best cooks (during the Bush administration a Filipina was the head cook at the White House), and Filipino foods are an integral part of Asian and international cuisines.

 MAJOR FOODS

 Protein Sources

The main protein sources include pork, chicken, beef, ox, caribou (water buffalo), goat, fish, dried fish, shellfish and other seafood, eggs, peanuts, navy beans, soybeans, and other legumes. Since the Philippines are a group of many islands, the majority of its residents have easy access to all forms of fish and seafood. In the rural areas most Filipinos raise their own pigs. In fact, it is difficult to partake of a Filipino meal without eating some pork. If pork is not one of the main dishes, it may be used to flavor a vegetable dish or little pieces may be added to the *pancit* (a rice or wheat noodle dish similar to lo mein).

 Starch Sources

The main sources of starch include rice, corn, *ube* (a purple-colored yam native to the Philippines), cassava (a root vegetable also known as yucca that is the base for tapioca), white potatoes, sweet potatoes, and *pancit*. In more recent years Filipinos have started to eat spaghetti and macaroni salad. Macaroni salad is often a special treat at holiday meals such as Christmas and New Year's Day.

Rice is the main staple in the Filipino diet. Most Filipinos eat a substantial amount of rice at every meal, three times a day. If rice is not served at a meal, many Filipinos will still feel hungry, even if they have consumed a large meal with bread or pasta as the starch. They simply do not feel satisfied without at least some rice. In fact, when they eat pancit, they typically serve it over their rice. Pancit is acceptable on its own as a snack but not without rice at a meal.

 Fat Sources

The Filipino diet can be very high in fat, much more so than most other Asian diets. It is also often high in saturated fats. Since lard and coconut milk are often easily accessible, they are common fats used in cooking. Margarine and vegetable oil are used in daily food preparation as well. Butter is expensive and therefore rarely used in home food preparation. Mayonnaise is used in preparing special foods, such as egg salad or macaroni salad, for a holiday treat.

Pork and chicken, and lesser amounts of beef, are the main animal sources of fat in the Philippines. In the Philippines, as opposed to the United States, pigs are raised to be high in fat, whether for personal use or for selling. Either way, Filipinos do not aim for lean cuts of pork. The fatter the pig, the more there is to eat or sell; hence, pork is one of the main sources of saturated fat in the Filipino diet. Most Filipinos prefer the fatty portions of the chicken, so chicken fat and chicken skin are certainly major sources of saturated fat. Typically, chicken adobo, one of the most popular Filipino dishes, is made with the drumsticks and thighs—the higher-fat dark meat—and not with the lower-fat white meat.

 Prominent Vegetables

There are many different vegetables consumed in the Philippines. The prominent vegetables include such leafy greens as *pechay* (bok choy), *lutud* (sweet potato leaves), cabbage, *kangkong* (swamp cabbage), and broccoli. Other popular cooked vegetables include green beans, Asian eggplant, carrots, chayote (a summer squash), snow peas, and various winter squash. Onion, garlic, green pepper, and tomato are added to flavor cooked dishes.

Filipinos typically eat their vegetables cooked. Chop suey is a popular stir-fried mixed vegetable dish. Sometimes they pickle vegetables to help preserve them without refrigeration. For example, they make pickled cabbage similar to sauerkraut. A few vegetables are occasionally consumed raw, such as cucumber, tomato, and onion; however in general, because few Filipinos own a refrigerator, they feel that food is "safer" when cooked.

 Prominent Fruits

Fruits are readily available to many Filipinos, especially in the rural areas. Tropical fruits are a main part of their diet, including mango, papaya, orange, grapefruit, calamansi (small limes), banana, guava,

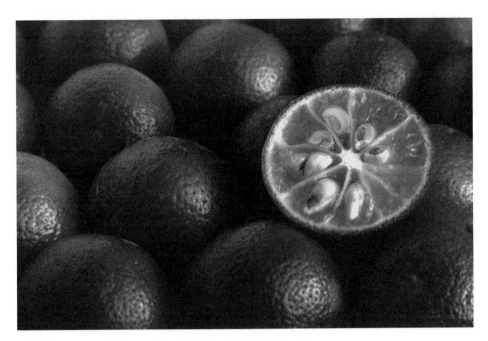

Calamansi are small limes grown in the Phillipines.

pineapple, watermelon, and jackfruit. In the northern areas they grow strawberries. Certain fruits are served more like vegetables before they ripen, including green mango, green papaya, and white jackfruit.

 Spices and Seasonings

Filipinos are known for their tasty foods; thus, spices are used generously in food preparation. Some of their main spices include ginger, chili peppers, soy sauce, patis (fish sauce), salt, black pepper (often freshly ground), tamarind powder, *bagoong* (a shrimp paste), white vinegar, light brown sugar, garlic, and onion. A touch of coconut milk is often added to dishes to give them that deliciously creamy taste.

 Beverages

Fluids regularly consumed by Filipinos include water, coffee with powdered milk and sugar, reconstituted powdered milk with added sugar, pineapple juice, tea (including native herbal teas such as ginger tea with sugar), juice drinks often sold in individual packets with straws attached, and sweetened carbonated beverages. Milon (a cantaloupe drink) is served on special occasions. Because few Filipinos have refrigerators in their homes, most beverages are drunk at room temperature except when dining at a restaurant. For this reason, Filipino Americans often still prefer their drinks at room temperature. Lack of refrigeration is also the reason why powdered milk is typically used.

Powdered milk is, however, often imported from Australia and relatively expensive; therefore, only the more affluent are able to provide milk for their children to drink at nutritionally recommended intakes.

 Desserts

Fancy desserts are reserved for holidays and other special celebrations, but fruit is readily available and is a more regularly consumed dessert. The most popular prepared desserts include sticky rice, *leche flan*, rice flour muffins, *puto* (steamed cake or muffins), mango-and-coconut ice cream, fried bananas, and *halo-halo* (crushed ice topped with fruits and other sweets). Some other special desserts include *biko* (sweet rice cakes), *buchi* (sweet rice balls), *cassava bibingka* (yucca cake), *ube* cake, carrot cake (sometimes with pineapple added to the recipe), and *budin* (bread pudding).

 FOODS WITH CULTURAL SIGNIFICANCE

Typically, when someone thinks of Filipino foods, the first thing that comes to mind is adobo. Adobo can be made with either chicken or pork and would thereby be referred to as chicken adobo or pork adobo, respectively. This is an everyday food as well as one served on special occasions. *Sinigang* is another popular dish. This is a type of fish soup often served at large gatherings.

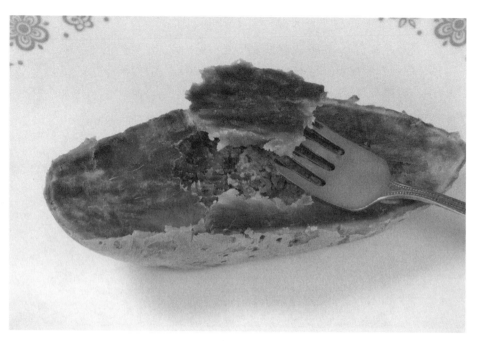

Ube is a purple-colored yam grown in the Philippines.

Tocino (sweet barbecued pork or chicken) is a fun food served as a snack or on special occasions. *Lumpia* (a Filipino egg roll) served with sweet-and-sour sauce is another culturally significant food.

Balut (a duck egg with a fertilized embryo) and *dinuguan* (blood stew made with pig liver, kidney, and/ or intestines) are two foods that certainly do not sound appetizing to the typical American but would certainly rouse excitement in a group of Filipinos. Another food unique to the Philippines is *ube*, a purple yam. *Ube* may be boiled and served as a cooked vegetable or used to make purple-colored cake or pudding.

The fact that rice is a dietary staple in the Philippines means that all of the aforementioned foods are served with it. Filipinos even eat their hot dogs with rice (not on a bun as Americans are used to seeing).

 TYPICAL DAY'S MENU

Filipinos traditionally eat three main meals and one snack every day: *almusál* (breakfast), *tanghalían* (lunch), an afternoon snack called *meriénda*, and *hapúnan* (dinner).

Breakfast may consist of dried fish cooked with tomato, fried rice, and coffee with powdered milk and sugar.

Lunch may consist of chicken adobo, steamed rice, *pechay* (bok choy), and fresh banana.

The afternoon snack may consist of *pancit sotanghon* (cellophane noodles with pork and vegetables) and coffee with powdered milk and sugar.

Dinner may consist of fried milkfish, steamed rice, *lutud* (sweet potato leaves), and fresh mango.

 HOLIDAY MENUS

Christmas Day

A sample menu for Christmas Day (*Araw ng Pasko*) is as follows:

> Appetizer: empanadas (meat turnovers)
>
> Main courses: chicken and pork adobo, *escabeche* (fish in a sweet-and-sour sauce)
>
> Side dishes: rice, *pancit sotanghon* (cellophane noodles), sticky rice, macaroni salad
>
> Vegetables: chop suey (a mixture of *pechay*, carrots, snow peas, and chayote)
>
> Desserts: fresh fruit, *leche flan*, *cassava bibingka* (special cassava cake), cookies
>
> Beverages: coffee, sweetened ginger tea, pineapple juice, sweetened carbonated beverages

New Year's Eve

A sample menu for New Year's Eve (*Bisperas ng Bagong Taon*) is as follows:

Observations from Gemma L. Padchonga (10 years old): Eating in the Philippines

When I go to visit my family in the Philippines, the foods I eat are very different than when I am in the United States. Every morning when I wake up, there is hot *pandesal* waiting for me. My mom and dad walk to the bakery and buy it fresh before I wake up. *Pandesal* is bread that is made from white flour and shaped like a roll. I eat *pandesal* with homemade peanut butter and fresh strawberry jelly. The peanut butter is made from peanuts that my grandmother grows. The jelly is made in Baguio from strawberries grown in Benguet, the strawberry capital of the Philippines. Some of my cousins in the Philippines think that *pandesal* is just a snack and not a meal. They eat rice and some type of meat for breakfast. But my grandmother and my cousin eat the same things that I do.

For lunch I eat rice that came from my grandmother's rice fields. I sometimes help my grandmother harvest the rice. I also eat vegetables. Some of the vegetables, like lutud, which are sweet potato leaves, come from my grandmother's garden. My grandmother also uses the lutud to feed the pigs. Other vegetables, such as *pechay*, come from the market. At the market there are many vegetable stands. The market also sells fruits. Another thing I eat for lunch is chicken. In the Philippines you go to the market and buy a live chicken and bring it home. Once it is home, you butcher it and cook it. The most typical ways that my family in the Philippines cooks the chicken are as chicken adobo or *pinikpikan*, a chicken soup cooked with salted pork and a green vegetable such as *pechay* or chayote.

For the afternoon snack my cousins and I often have crackers and milo (hot cocoa). The adults have crackers and coffee. Sometimes we have homemade banana pancakes instead of crackers. On special occasions we will all have doughnuts from Mr. Donut.

For dinner I eat the same thing that I eat for lunch. At dinner all of my cousins eat upstairs with me. My aunts, uncles, and grandparents join us for dinner. Sometimes there will be as many as 12 people upstairs. When we eat, the men eat with their hands and the women eat with silverware.

For celebrations like Christmas and New Year, my Auntie Rose will make macaroni salad. My aunt and older cousins will prepare the salad the day before the actual holiday. In the macaroni salad there is canned fruit, cheese, carrots, and raisins. Also, we have a barbeque on the rooftop on Christmas Eve and New Year's Eve. At the barbeque we have hotdogs, fish, and marshmallows. When the kids eat their hotdogs, they dip them in banana catsup with no buns. When the kids are finished eating their hotdogs, they eat roasted marshmallows. The adults eat fish with rice when they come back from midnight mass.

On the actual holiday we eat rice that my grandmother cooks. Also, we eat pork and chicken adobo that my uncles make. Then everybody, even our neighbors, will stop by to eat the macaroni salad. Lastly we eat *pancit*, which is rice noodles with cooked vegetables.

Do you think you would like eating the foods in the Philippines? I definitely do!

Appetizer: *lumpia* (Filipino egg rolls) with sweet-and-sour sauce

Main courses: *lechon* (whole pig roasted on a bamboo pole), chicken on a stick, barbecued milkfish (wrapped in banana leaves)

Side dishes: steamed rice, *pancit Canton* (wheat noodles garnished with shrimp and vegetables), egg salad

Vegetable dishes: *acharang gulay* (pickled vegetables), chop suey (made with cabbage, broccoli, carrots, and onions)

Desserts: fresh sliced mango, *ube* cake, fried bananas

Beverages: coffee, sweetened ginger tea, soft drinks

Good Friday

A sample menu for Good Friday, on which no meat is eaten (only fish), is as follows:

Appetizer: *ukoy* (shrimp-and-vegetable fritters)

Main course: *sinigang*

Side dishes: rice, *pancit bihon guisado* (rice noodles with sautéed vegetables)

Desserts: fruit salad, *biko* (sweet rice cake)

 HEALTH BELIEFS AND CONCERNS

Rural areas still have witch doctors and sacrifice animals (chickens, pigs, and caribou) to offer their ancient

ancestors in hopes of improving poor health. Spiritual healers and specific forms of voodoo are also common rituals used mainly in the more remote areas. *Mangkukulam* is the term used for people who cast spells. *Mambabarang* identifies the people who curse their enemies by putting insects inside their bodies. The healers of these curses are called *albularyo*.

The belief that "white is beautiful" is held by Filipino women and practiced by staying out of the sun to keep one from getting dark. From a young age girls are taught to practice this belief. Bias toward white skin came from influential occupations of the Spanish and Americans.

Fatness is often associated with wealth. Being too skinny is seen as a sign of poverty. If one wants to compliment your infant (and you) in the Philippines, they will tell you how fat he or she appears to be. Certainly in the United States many people would take offense to such a comment. The compliment implies that you are taking good care of your child by feeding him or her abundantly. In the urban areas of the Philippines this attitude toward body image has begun to change with access to American television. Filipino adolescents are now starting to aspire to be thin and stylish.

GENERAL HEALTH AND NUTRITIONAL INDICATORS SUMMARY

Low birth weight, defined as weighing less than 2500 g at birth, affects 20% of newborns in the Philippines (UNICEF, 2007). Thirty-four percent of children are exclusively breastfed during the first 6 months of life. Fifty-eight percent of infants 6–9 months are breastfed with complementary food and 32% remain breastfed at 20–23 months.

Twenty-eight percent of children below 5 years suffer from being moderately to severely underweight (UNICEF, 2007). Moderate to severe wasting was found in 6% and stunting in 30% of this particular population. The nation has an 85% vitamin A supplementation coverage rate for children 6–59 months. Fifty-six percent of households in the Philippines consume adequately iodized salt.

Eighty-five percent of the Philippines' total population uses improved drinking-water sources (UNICEF,

2007). Specifically, 87% of the population in urban areas and 82% of the rural population has access to improved drinking-water sources.

COMMUNICATION AND COUNSELING TIPS

Food is central to the Filipino culture. In the Philippines many people have limited resources; therefore, diets are restricted. When a Filipino immigrates to the United States and has access to a wider variety of foods, he or she often has difficulty in not overindulging. Changing such a person's food habits will probably only occur when that individual has great personal motivation. For example, if a family member has died of heart disease due to hypertension and/or atherosclerosis, when others realize that lifestyle changes might have saved that person's life, they might be motivated to start changing their own lifestyles.

Rice is an essential part of the Filipino diet and is consumed at least twice a day. Trying to remove rice from the diet, either partially or totally, will meet with much resistance. Filipino Americans typically buy rice in 50-lb. bags on a relatively regular basis.

There are times that for religious purposes pork or chicken must be consumed. These traditions have strong ceremonial ties and would be difficult to alter.

Like most Asians, Filipinos have a higher incidence of lactose intolerance; many avoid milk and cheese completely.

In the northern part of the Philippines, known as the Mountain Province, there are certain food restrictions after the death of a spouse or child. The spouse or parents will traditionally not eat certain foods for up to 1 year. Some of these food taboos include fish, beef, and vegetables when cooked in their own home. During this period of grieving, the main foods consumed are rice and beans.

PRIMARY LANGUAGE OF FOOD NAMES WITH ENGLISH TRANSLATIONS

The primary language of food names with English translations are as follows:

Philippino Name	English Translation
Adobo	Chicken or pork boiled in a soy sauce and vinegar mixture
Sinigang	Fish, shrimp, or pork soup with a sour, tamarind flavoring
Torta	Omelet
Lumpia	Meat or vegetable egg rolls
Pancit	A noodle dish
Pescado	Fried or grilled fish
Chorizo	Sausages
Longenisa	A sweet sausage
Hamonado	Pork sweetened in pineapple sauce
Lechon	A whole roasted pig
Pechay	Bok choy
Pandesal	Rolls
Mani	Peanuts
Mais	Corn
Lutud	Sweet potato leaves
Afritada	Chicken cooked in tomato sauce and vegetables

Philippino Name	English Translation
Kare-kare	Oxtail stew
Kaldereta	Goat stewed in tomato sauce
Pinakbet	Vegetable stew containing okra and eggplant
Utong	Long asian green beans
Balut	Boiled egg with a fertilized duckling inside
Tapa	Beef jerky
Chicharon	Deep-fried pork or chicken skin
Puto	Little white rice cakes sold at roadside stands as a snack
Halo-halo	Crushed ice with condensed milk, *leche flan*, and sliced tropical fruits
Bibingka	Rice cake with butter or margarine and salted eggs
Ensaymada	Sweet roll with grated cheese on top
Polvoron	Powdered candy
Tsokolate	Chocolate

FEATURED RECIPE

Pancit Canton, Madali (Chinese Egg Noodles, Quick and Easy)

2 tbsp. oil

1 lb. shrimp or 1 lb. chicken breast (boneless, skinless, boiled, and cubed)

1 medium onion, sliced

½ medium head cabbage, shredded

½ lb. carrots, peeled and thinly sliced in rounds

4–5 celery stalks, trimmed and thinly sliced

Premium oyster-flavored sauce (preferably Lee Kum Kee brand)

Water or broth

2 (8-oz.) pkgs. pancit Canton noodles (Chinese egg noodles)

1. Heat oil in a large skillet. Sauté the shrimp (or chicken) until heated through and then add the vegetables.
2. Stir-fry until vegetables are crisp–tender, adding a little water or broth if necessary.
3. Flavor with oyster sauce according to taste (start with 2 tbsp.).

(continues)

Pancit Canton, Madali
(Chinese Egg Noodles, Quick and Easy) (Continued)

4. Remove to a serving dish and keep warm.
5. In the same skillet, heat about ½ cup water or broth.
6. Add the noodles and stir-cook until soft, adding more water or broth as needed.
7. Flavor with oyster sauce (start with 2 tbsp.).
8. Combine with the shrimp and vegetables; mix lightly and cook until thoroughly heated. Serve hot.

(Reprinted with permission from Antoinette Angeles, from The Filipino American Association of Pittsburgh [2007] and Word Association Publishers.)

More recipes are available at http://nutrition.jbpub.com/foodculture/

ACKNOWLEDGMENTS

The authors express their appreciation to Antoinette Angeles, Robin M. Drogin, and Alice J. Leeds for reviewing the chapter.

REFERENCES

Filipino American Association of Pittsburgh. (2007). *Cooking with the Filipinos of Pittsburgh, PA* (4th ed.). Pittsburgh, PA: Filipino American Association of Pittsburgh.

Languages of the Philippines. (1994). National and official languages. Retrieved March 30, 2008, from www.kent.k12.wa.us/KSD/NO/E.S.L/Languages/phillipine.htm

Peters, J. (1994). *Philippines: A travel survival guide* (5th ed.).

UNICEF. (2007). *The state of the world's children 2007: Women and children, the double dividend of gender equality.* Retrieved April 14, 2009, from http://www.unicef.org/sowc07/statistics/tables.php

Middle East

Food, Cuisine, and Cultural Competency for Culinary, Hospitality, and Nutrition Professionals introduces the reader to six prominent regions in the Middle East:

The Middle East is a region that spans southwestern Asia, southeastern Europe, and northeastern Africa. The region has no clear boundaries and is often used as a synonym for Near East (as opposed to Far East). The term "Middle East" was popularized around 1900 in the United Kingdom. The Middle East comprises several regions and many countries, each characterized by both, similarities and differences. For example, Saudi Arabia and Iran both enjoy a rich economy partially provided by oil reserves. Turkey depends on agriculture, electronics, and clothing/textiles. Lebanon has a rich tourism industry. In the chapters on the Middle East, the reader can find interesting information on this very intriguing region.

ARABIAN PENINSULA

The Arabian Peninsula section contains information on the cultures of Bahrain, Kuwait, Oman, Qatar, Saudi Arabia, the United Arab Emirates, and Yemen. Saudi Arabia borders the Persian Gulf and the Red Sea, north of Yemen. Saudi Arabia, which has an oil-based economy and possesses more than 20% of the world's proven petroleum reserves, ranks as the largest exporter of petroleum. The petroleum sector accounts for roughly 80% of budget revenues, 45% of gross domestic product, and 90% of export earnings. High oil prices through mid-2008 have boosted growth, government revenues, and Saudi ownership of foreign assets.

ASSYRIAN REGION

The Assyrian region comprises Iran, Iraq, Turkey, and Syria.

TURKEY

Turkey is located in southeastern Europe and southwestern Asia (the portion of Turkey west of the Bosporus is geographically part of Europe), bordering the Black Sea, between Bulgaria and Georgia, and bordering the Aegean Sea and the Mediterranean Sea, between Greece and Syria. Turkey's dynamic economy is a complex mix of modern industry and commerce along with a traditional agriculture sector that still accounts for about 30% of employment. It has a strong and rapidly growing private sector, yet the government remains a major participant in basic industry, banking, transport, and communication. The largest industrial sector is textiles and clothing. Other sectors, notably the automotive and electronics industries, are rising in importance within Turkey's export mix. Real growth has exceeded 6% for many years, but this strong expansion has been interrupted by sharp declines in output in 1994, 1999, and 2001.

BILAD AL SHAM

Bilad Al Sham comprises Syria, Lebanon, Jordan, and Palestine.

LEBANON

Lebanon borders the Mediterranean Sea, between Israel and Syria. Lebanon has a free-market economy and a strong laissez-faire commercial tradition. The Lebanese economy is service oriented: the main growth sectors include banking and tourism.

PERSIA

Persia, also known as Iran, borders the Gulf of Oman, the Persian Gulf, and the Caspian Sea, between Iraq and Pakistan. Iran/Persia's economy relies on the oil sector. High oil prices in recent years have allowed Iran to greatly increase its export earnings and amass nearly $100 billion in foreign exchange reserves. Iran continues to suffer from double-digit unemployment and inflation, which climbed to a 28% annual rate in 2008. Underemployment among Iran's educated youth has convinced many of them to seek jobs abroad.

CHAPTER **47**

Arabian Peninsula

(Bahrain, Kuwait, Oman, Qatar, Saudi Arabia, the United Arab Emirates, and Yemen)

Dalal U.Z. Alkazemi, MSc, PhD Candidate

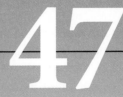

 CULTURE AND WORLD REGION

This chapter covers the rich cultural heritage of the Arabian Peninsula, which comprises Saudi Arabia, Yemen, Oman, the United Arab Emirates (UAE), Qatar, Bahrain, and Kuwait. In addition, Iraq is included because much of the region's historical, cultural, and food practices are influenced by, and shared with, Iraq. The region's heritage derives from its Arab founders and the Islamic religion. To the Arabs, ties of blood, clan, and tribal organizations are important. Values of mutual assistance, hospitality, loyalty, and generosity are highly prized. Life revolves around family and the preparation and serving of foods and drinks. Hospitality always involves invitations to meals, whether to share in a family lunch or a more formal occasion. Normal social life is interwoven with group activities and shared foods. Most Arabians are followers of Islam; however, both Christianity and Judaism are also practiced in the region. Most Arabian Muslims are tra-

ditionalist and practice their religion with respect and dignity. Islam sets guidelines for creating an integrated system of their lifestyle, family, and community.

The Arabian Peninsula lies in the southwest region of Asia. It is mainly a desert; however, there are long stretches of coastline along the Persian Gulf, the Arabian Sea (part of the Indian Ocean), and the Red Sea, with several major oases in the east. The Arabian Peninsula is mostly arid with inhospitable terrain and fertile regions nearly all around the periphery. Along the mountainous Arabian Sea coast to the south, rain-fed and irrigated highland areas support a rich agriculture. These mountains continue up to the Red Sea coast and are mostly arid. The southern area receives greater rainfall than the rest of the region. The climate is extremely dry; few places receive more than 178 mm (7 in.) of rain a year. Summer temperatures reach as high as 54.4°C (130°F) in some areas. The region owes its modern economic life to the vast reserves of petroleum and natural gas found largely in the area around the Persian Gulf. Major cities include Riyadh, Mecca, Aden, Jiddah, Sana'a (Sanaa), Abu Dhabi, and Kuwait. Generally, the countries of interest have small populations (except Saudi Arabia) with a high percentage of expatriates. In Kuwait, Qatar, and the UAE, the number of expatriates exceeds that of the national population. In the Gulf countries the percentage of expatriates ranges from 28% in Saudi Arabia to 64% in the UAE.

The rapid economic growth of those countries has led to a dramatic change in lifestyle, including health and nutrition status. Generally, two phases of development are distinguished: (1) pre-oil era (before 1940), and (2) oil discovery and boom period (1940 to the present). The rapid increase in income has led to a paradoxical situation in which affluence-derived nutritional problems, such as obesity and diabetes, coexists with anemia, growth retardation, and micronutrient deficiencies. The latter problems are due mainly to fast lifestyle change and lack of education.

LANGUAGE

The official language is Arabic; however, English is widely spoken and taught early in schools as a second language.

CULTURE HISTORY

The geographic location places a great deal of strategic importance on this region. On the world map, the Arabian Peninsula appears as a large land bridge suspended between the Mediterranean Sea and the Indian Ocean, and a crossroads between Africa, Asia, and Europe. Advanced civilizations flourished in the fertile parts of the peninsula. There were, at different times, *Tasm*, *Jadees*, *Saba'a*, and *Aad* in the south, and *Thamud* and *Madyan* in the north. The Arabs of the north were ethnically one people but were composed of two culturally opposite groups: nomadic (Bedu) and sedentary Arabs. Early sedentary settlers chose areas where they could farm, and herded flocks of sheep, goats, and camels. Domestication of the camel allowed pastoral nomads to inhabit even more arid parts of the peninsula. The camel caravan opened the Arabian Peninsula to regional and long-distance trade. The Arabs were skillful in transporting goods safely across the wide, barren stretches, guided by knowledge of astrology and intuition of nature. Towns developed along the trade routes, such as the inland towns of Mecca

and Medina. Mecca became a religious center that was a mixture of Bedouin polytheism, Judaism, and a little bit of Christianity, although most tribes remained polytheistic until the rise of Islam. Trade and migration brought luxury goods and wealth, and provided an environment for fostering knowledge and exchange of ideas in the growing communities.

Yearly pilgrimage in Mecca attracted scholars from around the world and encouraged the establishments of libraries and schools. The wealth and knowledge of the townspeople gave them a leading position. Nomadic herders, settled farmers, and townspeople shared an interdependent society. They depended upon one another for food, defense, and trade. A strong survival relationship developed between nomadic groups, farmers, and townspeople. Herders supplied meat, milk, and leather from their animals, farmers supplied grain for bread as well as dates, and traders supplied salt or spices in addition to long-distance trade goods such as silk, wool, and cotton cloth, spices, perfumes, jewels, gold, silver, and iron goods. Pastoral nomads became guides for townspeople, acting as a shipping service for merchant groups and providing skilled warriors and riders as security guards for the caravans.

FOOD HISTORY WITHIN THE CULTURE

Food Availability and Culinary Links

In the old days, the Arabic diet was very simple in ingredients and composition. It consisted of lamb, milk, and dates. Local sources of foods were meager. Fresh vegetables and fruits, such as squash, onions, radishes, okra, tomatoes, dates, oranges, and melons, were grown in oases and better irrigated lands in Basra and Bushire. Access to fresh vegetables and fruits was local and seasonal. Most herbs and aromatics, such as lemon, mint, chives, coriander, and dill, were eaten dried because it was the best method to preserve food in the hot climates. Imports from India, such as rice, cereals, spices, pulses, and tea, supplemented the diet, and Arabic coffee was supplied by Yemen. Rice became the region's stable food, and Indian recipes, such as spicy curries and biryani, became regular features in Arabic cuisine.

While some households had their own goats to provide milk and proteins, milk, butter, cooking fat, lamb and camel meat, and poultry were usually obtained from Bedu communities. Near costal regions, many families obtained their fish directly from fishermen or were themselves engaged in fishing. The warm waters of the region are home to abundant species of fish, from the Tigris and Euphrates rivers to the Persian Gulf and the Red Sea. Whole fried fish is the most preferred kind, served with whole stalks of spring onions. More elaborate recipes from Iraq and Iran are prepared from freshwater trout roasted on a stick over charcoal (*masgouf*). Spicy fish stews, such as *mahtf* and *mutabbug* (a rice-and-fish dish), are also eaten in the Gulf countries.

Social Status and Meal Patterns

In poor families meals are limited to bread, rice, and dates with some vegetables and an occasional serving of protein (fish in costal regions or lamb inland). Within this fairly restricted range of ingredients, menus tend to be repetitive. Breakfast is simple, consisting of bread and dates with coffee (for those who can afford it). The midday meal is the principal meal and is based on a communal dish of rice and meat or fish. The entire meal is cooked in one pot. Meat or fish together with onions and spices was first browned in the bottom of the pot, and water and rice are added to cover the meat. This would be allowed to simmer over a fire of palm leaves or a charcoal pit (*tanour*). Originally known as *tabeekh*, this method is still used with shrimp (*murabbian*) and legume (*mumawash* and *maaddis*) dishes, and is echoed in a number of others. The family would sit sharing it served in one pot.

In wealthy families, meals were elaborate especially when guests were entertained. Demonstration of wealth translated into using exquisite ingredients that show influences from sophisticated cuisines such as those from Persia, on the opposite side of the Gulf and Iraq to the north, and where Ottoman Turkish food traditions have penetrated. For example, rice *pilaus* of Persian cooking, flavored with saffron, shredded fried onions, and raisins, is served along with a side dish known as *maraq*, which is a meat stew with eggplant or okra in a tomato sauce. In addition, skewered minced meat (*kababs*) is served and *dolma*, which is a rice-stuffed vegetable dish that shows the influence of the Ottoman Empire. The meal is completed with dates and bowls of *leban*.

Mannerism and Respect

When it comes to social activities, men and women never socialize together. Food festivities that involve guests are served in *diwaneiyah*, where men gather to talk about life matters, politics, business, and so on,

whereas women always sit separately from men and share tea, food, family affairs, and gossip. Mealtime manners are simple and exacting. Shoes are removed and the meal is traditionally eaten sitting cross-legged on a cloth or mat (*soufrah*) spread on the floor. The meal begins with *bismillah* (in the name of God) and ends with *alhamdulillha* (praise to God). Most foods are eaten with the right hand. Fruits are eaten after the main course, then everyone washes their hands, and tea and coffee are served. The ritual of sprinkling the guest's hands with rose water and passing the incense burner containing *bokhur* (frankincense) are signs that the visit has come to an end.

Modern Arabia

In the 20th century, the region's significant stocks of crude oil gave it new strategic and economic importance. Mass production of oil began around 1945, with Saudi Arabia, Kuwait, Iraq, and the UAE having large quantities of oil. Along with money, cars, air conditioning, and other comforts has come a tidal wave of foreign foods flash-flooding the Gulf shores. The most immediately observable difference between the two periods (pre-oil and modern time) is in the range of foods now available. The selection of fresh and packaged foods now stocked on market stalls, in supermarkets, and in specialists' delicatessens is comprehensive. Green groceries are provided through improved local agriculture and imports, and include vegetables such as lettuce, cauliflower, and asparagus, and fruits such as avocados, pears, mangoes, and strawberries.

The staples of rice and bread are diverse. Popular types of rice include basmati, imports from Pakistan, and branded packages from America. Bread ranges from flat unleavened rounds and strips, which are either made daily in traditional bakeries attached to a supermarket or sold in plastic packages, and European-style block and plaited white and brown rolls. French, Italian, and Swiss natural and processed cheeses are available. Accompanying all these products is a rich selection of canned and packaged foods, preserves, and sauces. Fast-food chains and take-away restaurants spread rapidly across the region. Specialty sweet and confectionary stores opened on every corner offering a large selection of cakes and sweets such as the traditional Arabian *baklawa* (flaky layers of dough and nuts soaked in syrup), *ma'moul* (sweetened dough filled with nuts and dates), and European-style sponge- and fruitcakes, gateaux, biscuits, and assortments of roasted nuts and sugared almonds.

Elaborate and lavishly presented lunch parties continue to be a preferred way of entertaining guests. Much of the food tradition, dietary habits, and cooking methods remained in the region and were transferred from generation to generation. Home cooking with exquisite ingredients, and the acquired tastes of India and Persia, saturated the region along with the flood of expatriates to the Gulf countries. Menus stimulated by both the availability of a wide range of ingredients and the influence of the cooking habits of other nationalities were present in the region. The cuisines of other Arab countries has also been popular for some time, brought by Egyptians, Syrians, Palestinians, Jordanians, and Lebanese, or brought back by Saudi, Kuwaiti, and Bahraini students, businessmen, and vacationers. In addition, modern television advertisement, magazine articles, and cookbooks featuring Levantine and Egyptian Arabs inspired dishes, and collections of recipes from foreign cuisines transformed the regional cuisine into a mixture of both traditional home-cooked and convenience meals.

Dishes such as lasagna, macaroni, *sambosak* (Indian-style savory fried pastry stuffed with meat or vegetables), *molekheiyah* (mallow), and *kubbah* (wheat balls stuffed with mince meat) have been adopted into the regional cuisine. Influences on the average meal pattern emerge not only from the abundance of food but also from a notable change in lifestyle and the family unit. Most women are joining the work force, and foreign nannies and caregivers from East Asia are being employed to replace the mother in terms of household duties.

Indoor or outdoor buffet-style banquets are the preferred method for food-service industries, which also cater weddings and festivities. Hotel banquets and restaurants serve an international selection of foods that display a wide range of culinary influences of Persian, Indian, American, French, English, and Chinese cuisines. Menu items range from *foie gras truffe*, Beluga caviar, shrimp cocktail, smoked Scotch salmon, terrine of duck, tomatoes stuffed with Russian salad, and artichoke hearts filled with cheese, to Levantine appetizers such as *hummus*, *taboulah*, and *baba ghannouj* in the hors d'oeuvre section of the menu. The entree menu items include turkey meat loaf, shrimp lo mein, kebab halla, chicken curry, kufta, and sirloin beef with pepper sauce served along with rice, potatoes, and sautéed vegetables. Fancy desserts, such as crème brulée, chocolate eclair, cream bun, and many other European desserts, are also served.

 MAJOR FOODS

 Protein Sources

Protein sources are lamb, mutton, chicken, beef, camel, fish, shrimps, crabs, and eggs; dairy products: yogurt,

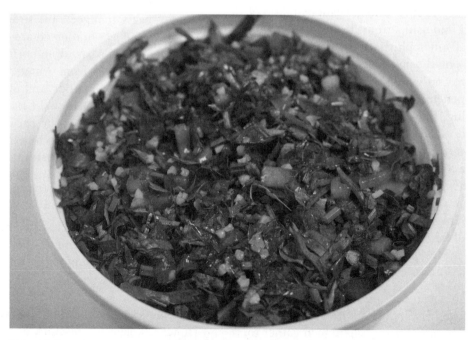

Taboulah salad is often served as an appetizer before the meal.

labnah, and white cheese; legumes: red lentils, fava beans, chickpeas, broad beans, split peas, and black-eyed peas.

 ### Starch Sources

Starch sources are rice (staple), wheat-derived products, such as cracked wheat used in meat porridges, bulgur, and semolina meal, and flour used in desserts and sweets, pasta, noodles, and *khoubz* bread.

 ### Fat Sources

Fat sources are corn oil (most used in the region), olive oil, butter, ghee (clarified butter imported from the Indian subcontinent; it is a butter that is cooked long enough to evaporate the water portion and caramelize the milk solids, which are then filtered out, resulting in a long shelf life without refrigeration), cream (could be *kishta*, made from cow milk, or *gaimar*, made from domestic buffalo milk), and adani (sheep fat primarily from the tail part, *cheffal*).

 ### Prominent Vegetables

Prominent vegetables include cucumbers, eggplant, okra, onions, and tomatoes. Leafy greens, such as parsley, dill, coriander leaves, and mint, are popular as seasonings in many dishes, and spinach is used in cooked dishes.

 ### Prominent Fruits

Prominent fruits include citrus fruits, apples, melons, grapes, and pomegranates, as well as bananas, dates, and figs.

 ### Spices and Seasonings

Common spices include turmeric, garlic, cumin, cardamom, cinnamon, black pepper, nutmeg, ginger, mint, coriander, thyme, *za'tar* (dried thyme mixed with sumac, salt, and sesame seeds, often sprinkled on *labnah* or mixed with olive oil to form a dipping paste with bread or as *fatayer's* filler), fenugreek, black lemon (sun-dried lemon *loumi aswad*, a very popular aromatic that originated from Oman, used in the entire region), and saffron.

 ### Beverages

Common beverages include coffee, tea, *karakade*, flower soak, *nagqe'el zebib*, raisin soak, *irq soos*, licorice drink, *tamr hindi*, tamarind drink, *quamar elddin*, dried apricot drink, *shineena* (or *leban*), and sour yogurt drink. Fruit juices and sherbet, made from especially

Observations from the Author (Dalal U.Z. Alkazemi)

As a nutritionist in Kuwait, I was always fascinated with what people ate and how they thought about food. My observation was that Kuwaitis and Arabs in general are attached to food and are emotional eaters. Food is comfort in sadness and in celebrations. In the hospital where I worked, clients' families would bring home-cooked foods to their own sick family member and bring along coffee service for drop-in guests. (They never follow hospital regulations and think of dietitians as food-service staff who handle complaints and food preferences.) Many of my outpatient clients read about nutrition in magazines and on the Internet, and they are quite educated and aware about their food habits and patterns. They can point exactly to what is making their waistline expand or their thighs jiggle, not to mention off-chart glucose and lipid values. They find it emotionally disturbing, however, when advised not to share the food normally prepared for the rest of the family in family gatherings and when socializing with friends and colleagues at work. They find it absolutely impolite to refuse the tempting beverages and chocolates they are offered when visiting the ill at the hospital, or new mothers, or a relative who just got back from a trip. Such frequent social habits are considered an obligation. Family gatherings occur twice a week or more, and during that time big banquets are offered. Why not cook a healthy meal for the whole family? Simply because this would cause a strike because it is an insult to serve rice without its sparkling oil sheen, topped with fried meat or fish with condiments such as *ma'abooche* (minced chili and garlic) and salads. One must also try a bit of the béchamel casserole and side dishes, in addition to the different types of desserts awaiting the end of the meal with tea (on a full stomach no doubt). Moreover, it is considered rude to refuse when your mother, mother-in-law, sister, cousin, neighbor, or auntie *umm Ali* offer you a serving of the items they prepared for this special occasion—during which they share the sweetest conversations on the latest diet trends and why they can never follow them.

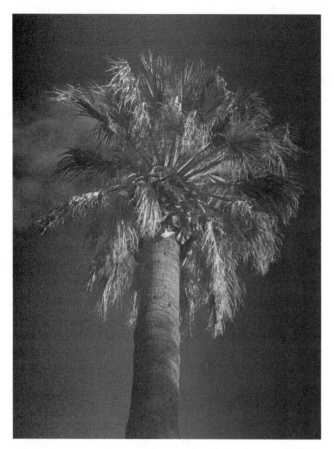

The palm tree is the only tree indigenous to the region.

pomegranate, watermelon, orange, and lemonade, are also popular.

 Desserts

Common desserts are *l'gaimat* (light and airy fried dough shaped in balls or a mesh-like pattern soaked in syrup), *sab elgafsha*, *zalabyah*, *halwa* (flour, sugar, and oil cooked until a caramelized paste is formed, flavored with saffron and cardamom), *rahash* (sesame paste and sugar syrup mixed with nuts, and some varieties are coated with chocolate), *zardah* (sweet rice pudding flavored with saffron and cinnamon, served with clarified butter), *mahalbiah* (rice or starch-based milk pudding flavored with cardamom and rose water), *girs ageiliy* (cake-textured bread flavored with saffron and cardamom, and topped with sesame seeds), *darabeel* (thin slice of unleavened bread dough folded and rolled into a cylindrical shape, topped with sugar icing, cinnamon, and dried cardamom), *ma'moul* (semolina-flour disks stuffed with nuts or dates and dusted with sugar icing), *kalei'chah* (in Iraq, wheat-flour biscuits

stuffed with dates; in the Gulf region, plain biscuits made from a mixture of chickpea flour, wheat flour, and sugar icing flavored with cardamom), *qataeif* (semolina-based pancakes stuffed with cheese or nuts, then fried and soaked with syrup), and *tamerea* (buttered dates with flour).

 FOODS WITH CULTURAL SIGNIFICANCE

Dates

Dates (*tamar*) are a delicacy cherished and demanded all year long. In fact, the palm tree is also highly prized and considered *barakah* (a blessing) in any proximity. It is the only tree indigenous to the region, the one that survived the desert heat. Dates are one of the many fruits repeatedly mentioned in the Qur'an. The habit of eating and storing dates has continued from generation to generation. Treasuring its nutritious value allowed Arabs to survive the scorching heat and scarce resources. In the early days, date paste was given to newborns to strengthen their immunity. The small, traditional oval kind of date is usually preferred over the large, imported *majool* dates. The seven most sought-after varieties of date come from Saudi Arabia, Iraq, and Iran, including *berhi*, *khalas*, *safari*, *zahdi*, *sukari*, *bisha*, and *qintar*.

Meat

Lah'ham (meat from lamb and/or mutton), the most widely consumed meat, is a delicacy in the peninsula. All parts of the meat are edible including the head, tongue, bones, fat, and organs. Usually the liver, kidneys, heart, and testicles are grilled on charcoal, whereas the head, tongue, and bones are cooked in the soup dish *bachah or pacha*. Arabs serve whole animals stuffed with rice and barbecued *qouzi* or *mendi* as a sign of hospitality and to show their guests that the animal is served to honor their presence. It is a ritual to slaughter a sheep as a sign of festivity and celebration at weddings, with the arrival of newborns, and at religious holidays (especially Eid al-Adha). It is the biggest religious festival celebrated by Muslims as a commemoration of Ibrahim's (the father of all prophets, also known as Abraham) willingness to sacrifice his son as commanded by God. People who can afford to do so sacrifice their best domestic animals as a symbol of Ibrahim's sacrifice. A large portion of the meat has to be given to poor and hungry people so that they can all join in the feast, which is held on Eid al-Adha. The remainder of the meat is cooked for the family celebration meal in which relatives and friends are invited to share.

Coffee

The ritual of coffee making is a sign that a guest is welcome and honored by his or her host. Whether in a modern Arab home or in the dessert, the traditional preparation and serving of Arabic coffee is carried out with immense care and is as intricate as a tea ceremony. Traditionally in the desert, an open fire was used, whereas today coffee is prepared using a low, rectangular brass brazier filled with hot coals. Coal is the preferred fuel because it adds a special flavor to the coffee that a gas stovetop does not provide. The coffee is always freshly ground and roasted before each preparation. In the Gulf region it is usually flavored with cardamom or ginger. In many first-class hotels in the Gulf, a traditional coffee corner fills the air with a fragrant aroma that invites guests to sample the coffee of Arabia.

Tea

Regarding tea (*chai*), mostly Ceylon is the preferred variety, a custom established with the early trading with the Far East. The tea-drinking ritual is observed after each meal. Some countries adopted the habit of afternoon tea, such as in Iraq; in Kuwait, it is mid-morning tea known as *chai eltha'ha*. Traditionally, water for tea is heated in a *samawer* over charcoal and tea is let to simmer on the gentle heat until it steeps. Modern electric kettles are used today and tea is made in advance and stored in vacuum flasks in case guests arrive. The tea is typically served in "wasp-waisted glasses" known as *istikans*. It is customary to put a thick layer of sugar in the bottom of the glass, which is placed on a small saucer. Into the saucer the tea is intentionally spilled over as a sign of generosity of the server. Tea is usually drunk plain, but some flavor it with cardamom or saffron, or with fresh mint. *Ligg'aah* water (essence derived from the flowers of the date palm trees) is sometimes sprinkled in the *istikans* for its admirable flavor and medicinal qualities. Herb teas of many varieties are enjoyed and also drunk for medicinal purposes. Blue tea from anchusa flowers is used for fever, violets to clear measles, thyme to fight colds, sage and marjoram for stomach flu, and cinnamon for menstrual cramps. Milk fresh or from powder flavored with any combination of cardamom, cinnamon, and saffron is served with tea (a combination known as *chai machbouse*, and in the Western world, *chai latte*) in the mornings and in the winter months.

Desert Truffles

Desert truffles (*fagga, faghea,* or *fagh*) are the jewels of the desert. After the rainy season, men usually go hunt for them in the desert. Both white and brown varieties are highly sought. They are usually served boiled over rice or sautéed in ghee with onions and eaten with bread. They are considered a sign of God's blessings and gifts with regard to the previous year. Arabian truffles are much milder in flavor than the European variety.

Honey

Honey (*assal*) is mentioned in the Qur'an as a healing agent. Most Arabs hail honey for its natural antibiotic properties for colds, flu, and infections. Even diabetics agree that honey has healing properties. The most popular honey is the *Yemini assal baladi* variety, which has a distinctive floral flavor.

Sour Yogurt Drink

Sour yogurt drink (*leban* or *shenina*) is the most popular drink in the region. It is believed to have originated from efforts to preserve milk as *leban* to be kept longer where no refrigeration was common. All varieties of milk, including goat and camel milk, are fermented into *leban*. Cow-milk *leban* is the most popular commercial type. The taste of *leban* resembles, to a great extent, that of *kefir* more than it does that of buttermilk.

 TYPICAL DAY'S MENU

Breakfast is often a quick meal that consists of bread and dairy products with tea and sometimes honey or jam. The most common dairy products are *labneh* and cream. *Labneh* is served with olives, dried mint, and dried thyme (*zata'ar*), and is drizzled with olive oil and eaten with flat bread. Pastries, such as *fatayer,* are often consumed stuffed with cheese or *zata'ar* paste. Breakfast sometimes includes heavier items such as boiled broad beans (*bajella*), chickpeas (*nakki*), or *foul medamas*, which consists of fava beans cooked with chickpeas, garlic, lemon, and olive oil. Falafel, grilled *haloumi* cheese, and fried eggplant-and-potato sandwiches are common breakfast items for people who work in offices. Breakfast cereal and milk are preferred items among the young.

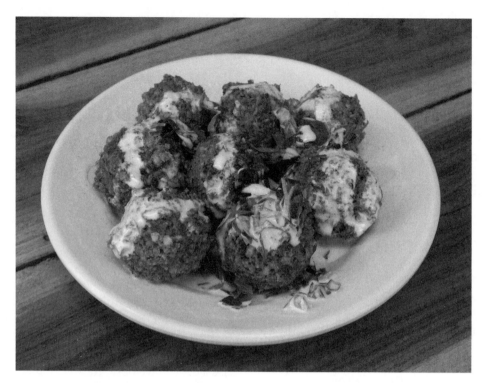

Falafel is a common breakfast item for the working class.

Lunch is considered the main meal of the day, traditionally eaten after the noon prayer. Meals comprise one main course, and salads and *maza* are served as side dishes. The meal consists mainly of protein, be it meat, poultry, or fish, accompanied by a large portion of rice known as *machbouse* or *kabsa*. Side dishes include cooked lentils and a portion of cooked vegetables in addition to the fresh ones, such as salad. Usually the vegetables and meat are cooked together in stews (*maraq*), which are usually tomato or tamarind based. Most households consume bread in addition to the rice. Drinks are not served with the food; however, *leban* and fruit juices are offered after the meal. Since the 1950s, Pepsi and similar soft drinks have been popular.

Dinner is often the lightest meal, although in modern times, and due to changing lifestyles, dinner has become more important. Dinner can be any combination, from fruit (e.g., watermelon and grapes) with bread and feta cheese or other dips with bread and olive oil, to a full meal similar to that of lunch. Pastries (*fatayer*) are also eaten for dinner stuffed with minced meat, sausage, or chicken. Other items most often consumed for dinner include scrambled eggs and charcoal-grilled food (*mashawi*) such as *kabab, farouj*, and *shawarma*. Fast food, such as pizza, burgers, and fried chicken, are mostly consumed among youth.

 HOLIDAY MENUS

Special attention is always given to the month of Ramadan when it comes to food preparation and menu festivities. Ramadan is the ninth month of the Islamic lunar calendar. It is when Muslims all over the world practice fasting simultaneously; thus, there is no eating in the daytime hours, but there is nightly feasting that begins at sunset and ends at dawn just before the morning prayer.

Religious custom (*sunna*) recommends that the daily fast be broken by eating dates and drinking water, and then soup is consumed just before the sunset prayer. The most popular soup is lentil soup, but a wide variety of soups are consumed, such as chicken, root vegetables, potato, and others. This is believed to gently accustom the stomach to food before the nightly feasting.

Fatour is the fast-breaking meal eaten at dusk. A typical *fatour* meal consists of the aforementioned ritual of dates, water, and soup, which is followed by a meat porridge (*jeereesh* or *hareesa*) and/or a rice-and-meat dish, such as *machbouse* or *maraq*, and/or *tashriba*, a lamb stew in which bread has been soaked. Cold drinks from dried fruits and flower petals are also served, such as *karakade* (petals soak), *nagqe'el zebib* (raisin soak), *irq soos* (licorice), *quamar elddin* (dried-apricot soak), and *tamr hindi* (tamarind).

During Ramadan sweets are consumed much more than usual. Sweets and fresh fruits are served between meals. Although most sweets are made all year long, such as *knafah*, *baklawa*, and *basboosa*, some are made especially for Ramadan, such as *qataeif* and *l'gaimat*. A smooth-textured Turkish rice pudding, *muhallabiah*, is also prepared flavored with rose water, cardamom, and chopped nuts such as pistachios and almonds.

Ghab'gah is a small meal eaten between *fatour* and *sahour* after the lengthy prayer of *Taraweeh*, a special prayer recited during the month of Ramadan. *Ghab'gah* is common only in the Gulf countries. It is of great importance because it is the time of the night when families and friends visit each other. Such social activity is especially encouraged during Ramadan. The meal usually consists of a selection of finger foods, such as *kubbah*, *sambosak*, and saltine pastries, stuffed with meat, vegetables, and cheese, or it consists of mini-sandwiches. Simple salads, such as *fatoush* and *taboulah*, are also served. Traditionalists serve cooked broad beans (*bajella*) and chickpeas (*nakki*). Ramadan sweets, fruit salads, and fruit juices are also served with tea to complement the meal.

Suhur is the meal eaten just before dawn when fasting must begin. It is usually a light meal that consists of items similar to those served for dinner, such as dips with bread, sandwiches and soups, and any *fatour* leftovers, especially *jeereesh* and *hareesa*.

Eid al-Fitr starts the day after Ramadan ends and is verified by the sighting of the new moon. Muslims give money to the poor and wear their best clothes. On the day of the celebration, families awake very early, do the first daily prayer, and are required to eat something to signify the end of Ramadan. They then attend special congregational prayers held in mosques. After the special prayers, festivities and merriment are commonly observed with visits to the homes of relatives and friends to thank God for all blessings.

 HEALTH BELIEFS AND CONCERNS

Fasting in Ramadan

The concept of "every individual is the judge of his or her own health" is applied when Muslims make decisions regarding whether to fast during Ramadan. Fasting is obligatory to every Muslim who is adult and healthy. Teenagers start fasting once they reach puberty and parents do encourage half-day fasting for young children (as young as 7 years) to teach them respect for

Ramadan as a shared religious activity. Healthy pregnant women usually practice fasting; however, women should prioritize their health and their baby's well-being if it is determined by health professionals that there are risks associated with fasting. Even individuals with type-2 diabetes fast during the month of Ramadan, but special attention should be given to spacing meals in the course of the day and any hypoglycemic agents and/or medications. If any health risk (e.g., high fever, epilepsy, heart disease, severe anemia) is determined regarding any other medical condition, then fasting is not obligatory.

Childbirth

Nifas is the 40-day period following childbirth. New mothers usually reside in their mother's or mother-in-law's house to receive care. Special attention is given to the new mother's diet. Water is usually restricted, as are fruit juices, because it is believed that this practice promotes healing. Lots of herbal tea, especially fenugreek, is given to encourage milk production and thereby breastfeeding. *Hesou* or *louhoom* (herbal remedies made from fenugreek), spices such as cinnamon, fennel seeds, and turmeric, almonds, and dates cooked in oil are recommended to be consumed several times a day. This is believed to cleanse the blood from the uterus and strengthen the bones. Women are usually confined to bed and discouraged from doing any physical activities. The best-known dish for new mothers in Gulf countries is *gabout*, which is made from stewed mutton, tomatoes, whole-wheat dumplings, and spices.

 GENERAL HEALTH AND NUTRITIONAL INDICATORS SUMMARY

Bahrain

Low birth weight, defined as weighing less than 2500 g at birth, affects 8% of newborns in Bahrain (UNICEF, 2007). Thirty-four percent of children are exclusively breastfed during the first 4 months of life. Sixty-five percent of infants 6–9 months are breastfed with complementary food and 41% remain breastfed at 20–23 months.

Nine percent of children below 5 years suffer from being moderately to severely underweight (UNICEF, 2007). Being severely underweight affects 2% of Bahrain's children. Moderate to severe wasting was found in 5% and stunting in 10% of this particular population.

One hundred percent of the nation's urban population uses improved drinking-water sources.

Kuwait

Low birth weight affects 7% of newborns in Kuwait (UNICEF, 2007). Twelve percent of children are exclusively breastfed during the first 4 months of life. Twenty-six percent of infants 6–9 months are breastfed with complementary food and 9% remain breastfed at 20–23 months.

Ten percent of children below 5 years suffer from being moderately to severely underweight (UNICEF, 2007). Being severely underweight affects 3% of Kuwait's children. Moderate to severe wasting was found in 11% and stunting in 24% of this particular population.

Oman

Low birth weight affects 8% of newborns in Oman (UNICEF, 2007). Ninety-two percent of infants 6–9 months are breastfed with complementary food and 73% remain breastfed at 20–23 months.

Eighteen percent of children below 5 years suffer from being moderately to severely underweight (UNICEF, 2007). Being severely underweight affects 1% of Oman's children. Moderate to severe wasting was found in 7% and stunting in 10% of this particular population. The nation has a 95% vitamin A supplementation coverage rate for children 6–59 months. The majority (61%) of households in Oman consume adequately iodized salt.

Qatar

Low birth weight affects 10% of newborns in Qatar (UNICEF, 2007). Twelve percent of children are exclusively breastfed during the first 4 months of life. Forty-eight percent of infants 6–9 months are breastfed with complementary food and 21% remain breastfed at 20–23 months.

Six percent of children below 5 years suffer from being moderately to severely underweight (UNICEF, 2007). Moderate to severe wasting was found in 2% and stunting in 8% of this particular population. One-hundred percent of the total population, both in urban and rural areas, uses improved drinking-water sources.

Saudi Arabia

Low birth weight affects 11% of newborns in Saudi Arabia (UNICEF, 2007). Thirty-one percent of children

are exclusively breastfed during the first 4 months of life. Sixty percent of infants 6–9 months are breastfed with complementary food and 30% remain breastfed at 20–23 months.

Fourteen percent of children below 5 years suffer from being moderately to severely underweight (UNICEF, 2007). Being severely underweight affects 3% of Saudi Arabia's children. Moderate to severe wasting was found in 11% and stunting in 20% of this particular population. Ninety-seven percent of Saudi Arabia's urban population uses improved drinking-water sources.

United Arab Emirates

Low birth weight affects 15% of newborns in the UAE (UNICEF, 2007). Thirty-four percent of children are exclusively breastfed during the first 4 months of life. Fifty-two percent of infants 6–9 months are breastfed with complementary food and 29% remain breastfed at 20–23 months.

Fourteen percent of children below 5 years suffer from being moderately to severely underweight (UNICEF, 2007). Being severely underweight affects 3% of children in the UAE. Moderate to severe wasting was found in 15% and stunting in 17% of this particular population. One-hundred percent of the total population in both urban and rural areas uses improved drinking-water sources.

Yemen

Low birth weight affects 32% of newborns in Yemen (UNICEF, 2007). Twelve percent of children are exclusively breastfed during the first 6 months of life and 76% of infants 6–9 months are breastfed with complementary food.

Forty-six percent of children below 5 years suffer from being moderately to severely underweight (UNICEF, 2007). Being severely underweight affects 15% of Yemen's children. Moderate to severe wasting was found in 12% and stunting in 53% of this particular population. The nation has a 20% vitamin A supplementation coverage rate for children 6–59 months. Thirty percent of households in Yemen consume adequately iodized salt.

Sixty-seven percent of Yemen's total population uses improved drinking-water sources (UNICEF, 2007). Specifically, 71% of the population in the nation's urban areas and 65% of the rural population has access to improved drinking-water sources.

Iraq

Low birth weight affects 15% of newborns in Iraq (UNICEF, 2007). Twelve percent of children are exclusively breastfed during the first 6 months of life. Fifty-one percent of infants 6–9 months are breastfed with complementary food and 27% remain breastfed at 20–23 months.

Twelve percent of children below 5 years suffer from being moderately to severely underweight (UNICEF, 2007). Being severely underweight affects 3% of Iraq's children. Moderate to severe wasting was found in 8% and stunting in 23% of this particular population. Forty percent of households in Iraq consume adequately iodized salt.

Eighty-one percent of Iraq's total population uses improved drinking-water sources (UNICEF, 2007). Specifically, 97% of the population in the nation's urban areas and 50% of the rural population has access to improved drinking-water sources.

COMMUNICATION AND COUNSELING TIPS

Communication and counseling should be based on the following factors:

- Islamic laws influence the kinds of food chosen and/or how the foods are combined.
- Muslims do not eat any form of pork, or any meat that has been slaughtered without invoking God's name (known as *halal* meat or *thabiha*), although some consider any nonpork meats to be *halal* and substitute *thabiha* for kosher.
- Muslims do not drink alcoholic beverages or foods flavored or cooked with alcohol.
- Different rules apply to fish. For instance, fish with scales are always *halal*, whereas it is debated whether shellfish and fish without scales, such as catfish, are *halal*, *haraam* (not allowed), or *makruh* (prohibitively disliked). The majority of Muslims consider all shellfish (including crabs, lobsters, shrimp, crayfish, and all nonpoisonous mollusks) to be *halal*.
- Arabians prefer fermented forms of dairy products and have a high incidence of lactose intolerance.
- Body contact, such as touching and hand shaking, is allowed only between people of the same gender.
- Body language, such as nodding and eye contact, remains an important tool in effective communication during counseling.
- Cooking styles differ from one household to another (e.g., one cook may use more hot peppers, another more fat, or some families may prefer fish over meat), but the basic cooking techniques, spices, and ingredients, however manipulated, are particularly Arabian.
- Because of the complexity of the Arabian dishes, whereby they require multiple ingredients and both proteins and carbohydrates are cooked together, such as in *maraqs* and *kabsa*, it is difficult to analyze their diet based on reported intakes.
- A form of written food diary or a food log should be encouraged, with emphasis on including cooking methods and food-preparation techniques.
- For assessment of the adequacy of nutrient intake, food-composition reference books and databases exist and represent generally reliable sources for the nutritive value of dishes served in the region.
- Semiquantitative food-frequency questionnaires have been developed for research purposes in the Gulf region.
- Nutrient data on raw foods, which are mostly imported to the region, are also available.

PRIMARY LANGUAGE OF FOOD NAMES WITH ENGLISH AND PHONETIC TRANSLATION

The primary language of food names with English and phonetic translation is given in Table 47-1.

TABLE 47-1   Primary Language of Food Names with English and Phonetic Translation

Arabic	English	Phonetic Translation	Arabic	English	Phonetic Translation
الألبان منتجات	Dairy products	Muntajat elalban	ليمون	Lemon	Laiymoon
حليب	Milk	Haleeb	عيش)أرز(	Rice	Aish (Arouz)
جبن	Cheese	Jibn	بقوليات	Legumes	Bo'qouleiyat
روب	Yogurt	Roobe	مكسرات	Nuts	Mo'kasarat
لبن	Yogurt drink	Leban	حلويات	Sweets	Halaweiyat
لحم	Meats	La'haam	أسماك	Fish	Assmak
زبده	Butter	Zibdah	اته)كاكاو(شيكولت	Chocolate	Kakao (chicolatah)
زيت	Oil	Zaiet	سلطه	Salads	Salatah
خضار	Vegetables	Khodar	خبز	Bread	Koubz
تفاح	Apple	Touffah	معكرونه	Pasta	Ma'karounah
موزه	Banana	Mouzah	بهارات	Spices	Bu'harat

FEATURED RECIPE

Machbouse La'haam (Kabsa) (Meat with Rice)

1 lb. lamb or mutton (typically containing bones and fat)

2 medium onions, finely chopped

4 cups basmati rice, washed and soaked for an hour

2–3 tbsp. oil

1 cup split peas, washed, cooked, and strained

¼ cup golden raisins washed and strained

¼ cup rose-water mix with a pinch of saffron (about 1 g)

3 tsp. mixed spices (equal amounts of grounded cardamom, saffron, clove buds, black pepper, turmeric, and cinnamon)

1 medium cinnamon stick

4 whole buds of cardamom

3 whole buds of cloves

Salt and pepper to taste

1. Place the meat in a pot and cover with about 1 inch of water.
2. Add the cinnamon stick, clove, cardamom buds, pepper, and salt.
3. Cook until meat is tender.
4. Remove the meat from the broth.
5. Strain the rice from the soak water and place the rice in the meat-broth pot.
6. Make sure that you use no more than 6 cups of meat broth and cook on medium heat until the rice is cooked and the broth is absorbed.

(continues)

**Machbouse La'haam
(Kabsa) (Meat with Rice) (Continued)**

7. Heat the oil in a frying pan.
8. Brown the onions and then add the meat and cook for a few minutes.
9. Add the cooked split peas and raisins; mix well and heat well.
10. Add the mixed spices and remove from the heat.
11. Arrange the fried mixture on top of the rice.
12. Add the rose water and saffron mixture.
13. Cover the pot and cook for 45 minutes over low heat until steam starts venting from the pot.

More recipes are available at http://nutrition.jbpub.com/foodculture/

REFERENCES

Al-Nesf, N., Al-Sultan, Y., & Helmi, M. (1980). *Nutritive values of Kuwaiti foods.* Kuwait: AlQabas Press (in Arabic).

Food and Agriculture Organization of the United Nations (FAO). (1982). *Food composition tables for the Near East.* (Report no. 26). Rome: FAO.

Heine, P. (2004). *Food culture in the Near East, Middle East, and North Africa.* Westport, CT: Greenwood Press.

Hussaini, M.M., & Sakr, A.H. (1983). *Islamic dietary laws and practices.* Chicago: Islamic Food and Nutrition Council of America.

Kittler, P.G., & Sucher, K.P. (2004). *Food and culture.* Belmont, CA: Thomson/Wadsworth.

Musaiger, A., & Al-Dallal, Z. (1985). *Food composition tables for use in Bahrain* (1st ed.). Bahrain: Bahrain Ministry of Health.

Musaiger, A.O. (1987). The state of food and nutrition in the Arabian Gulf countries. In G.H. Bourne (Ed.), *Nutrition in the Gulf countries. Malnutrition and minerals.* Basel, Switzerland: Karger.

Pellett, P., & Shadarevian, S. (1970). *Food composition tables for use in the Middle East.* Beirut, Lebanon: American University of Beirut.

Rodinson, M., Arberry, A.J., & Perry, C. (2001). *Arab cookery/essays and translations.* Devon, England: Prospect Books.

Rowland, J. (1950). *Good food from the Near East: 500 favorite recipes from twelve countries.* New York: Barrows.

Sawaya, W.N., & Al-Awadi, F.A. (1995). *National food composition table: Phase II.* (Report No. 4616). Kuwait: Kuwait Institute for Scientific Research.

Shabbuh, I. (2004). *The cuisine of the Muslims.* London: Al-Furqan Islamic Heritage Foundation.

UNICEF. (2007). *The state of the world's children 2007: Women and children, the double dividend of gender equality.* Retrieved April 14, 2009, from http://www.unicef.org/sowc07/statistics/tables.php

van Gelder, G.J.H. (2000). *Of dishes and discourse: Classical Arabic literary representations of food.* London: Curzon.

Zubaida, S., & Tapper, R. (2000). *Culinary cultures of the Middle East.* New York: St. Martin's Press.

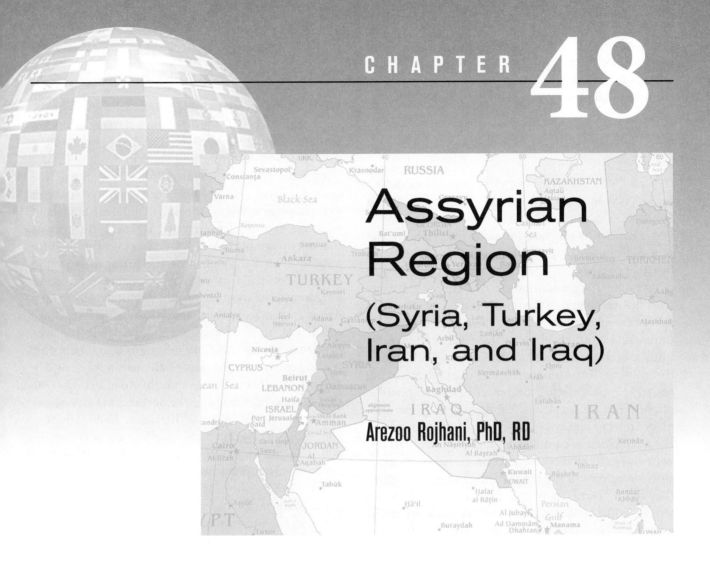

CHAPTER **48**

Assyrian Region
(Syria, Turkey, Iran, and Iraq)

Arezoo Rojhani, PhD, RD

 CULTURE AND WORLD REGION

It is estimated that there are between 2,500,000 and 3,000,000 Assyrians worldwide (Aprim, 2007b), which includes those living in Syria, Turkey, Iran, and Iraq. Today, nearly one third of Assyrians live in diaspora, split into rival churches and political factions (Parpola, 2004).

Religion

Assyrians were the first people to accept Christianity at the time of the Apostles themselves (Aprim, 2007a). While modern Assyrians belong to various Christian denominations, including Assyrian Church of the East, Roman Catholic (Caldean Assyrians), the Ancient Church of the East, Syriac Orthodox, Syriac Catholic, and almost every Protestant and Evangelist denomination (BetBasoo, 2006; Aprim, 2007b), originally all Assyrians belonged mainly to the Assyrian Church of

the East and, to a lesser degree, to the Catholic Church (Baumer, 2006).

The Assyrian Church of the East was formed in what in ancient times was Parthia (modern-day Iraq and Iran) and gradually spread to the east. The church was formed by splitting from the early Christian Church as a result of the Nestorian schism in 431 AD. In fact, in the West, the Assyrian Church of the East is often referred to as the Nestorian Church (Baumer, 2006).

Family Roles and Organization

Little is known about the early family system and kinship structure of Assyrians. Based on limited available evidence, the Assyrian family structure has traditionally been and remains patriarchal, with the final authority in the hands of the senior male member of the family (Ishaya, 1985; Benjamin, n.d.). The men have the responsibility of providing for the family's economic needs, while women, even those with formal education, are expected to give priority to managing the house and caring for the children.

Attitudes, Beliefs, and Practices

Assyrians remain strongly committed to monogamy (Ishaya, 1985). Marriage is viewed very seriously, because it is seen as a union of both the couple and their families (Benjamin, n.d.). In fact, until recently divorce was considered a disgrace and occurred rarely (Benjamin, n.d.); however, when it happens, it can be initiated by either partner.

Among Assyrians, family ties are very strong, with the well-being of the family taking priority over that of the individual (Ishaya, 1985). It is normal for unmarried adult children to live with their parents until marriage, although with increased affluence, the tendency for unmarried sons to continue living with their parents has decreased. Despite possible physical distance, a strong feeling of loyalty and allegiance toward family persists among family members. For example, it is common for elderly parents to live with their eldest son (married or unmarried), or in close proximity to the home of their children, where they can be regularly visited. Furthermore, there is a strong sentiment against committing one's parents to a nursing home, because it is perceived as dishonorable (Ishaya, 1985).

Regardless of what Christian denomination they belong to, Assyrians celebrate several distinct life events (Assyrian International News Agency, n.d.). These events include baptism, engagement, and weddings. Mourning the dead is very passionately expressed and is followed by a prolonged period of grieving. As a sign of their sorrow, female relatives often wear black or dark-color clothing for several months. Funerals are followed by several days of visitation to the residence of the deceased or their immediate family (Assyrian International News Agency, n.d.).

LANGUAGE

Modern Assyrian language (adapted around 750 BC) has its roots in ancient Aramaic and Akkadian (Assyrian International News Agency, n.d.; BetBasoo, 2006). Until the 3rd century BC, the Assyrian alphabet was based on cuneiform script. Subsequently, the Aramaic alphabet was adapted (see Table 48-1).

CULTURE HISTORY

The ancient Assyrians were people who lived in the northern reaches of Mesopotamia starting from before 3000 BC (Hooker, 1996). The first religion of the Assyrians was Ashurism and the word "Assyria" is derived from the words *mât Aššur*, which mean "the country of god" (Kuhrt, 1995). In fact, Assyrians refer to themselves as *Ashuri* (or *Aturi*) and their homeland as *Ashur* or *Atur*. The first official royal inscriptions that document the rule of Assyrian kings appear from around 2000 BC (Saggs, 1984). During this period Assyria consisted of various city–states and small kingdoms. The most important city–state was named *Ashur* (taken from the name of the Assyrian God), which was also the main trading center in the area (Kuhrt, 1995). At this time Assyrians also established trading colonies in the Anatolian plateau (present-day Turkey) (Bertman, 2005). Shamshi-Adad I (1813–1791 BC) conquered *Ashur* and the neighboring city–states in northern Mesopotamia (Bertman, 2005). His son, Ishme-dagan, inherited the kingdom but was eventually overthrown by Hammurabi, king of Babylon (southern Mesopotamia). Eventually, Ashur-uballit I (1365–1330 BC), through his conquests, was able to make Assyria an independent state again (Kuhrt, 1995). In the subsequent centuries, Assyria was vastly expanded; however, following a prolonged civil war, the empire ultimately fell in 612 BC (Parpola, 1999). In the subsequent centuries Assyrians continued the traditions of their fathers by pursuing scholarly activities in literature, mathematics, physics, and architecture, and contributing to the well-being of the societies where they were now subservient to their former subjects (Talia, 1980).

In 1915 and during World War I, the Ottoman (present-day Turkey) government forced the Assyrians to flee to the city of Urmia in Azerbaijan province (northwest of present-day Iran) (Aprim, n.d.a, 2007a; Stafford, 1935). In addition, approximately 20,000 Assyrians followed the Russians back to Russia (Aprim, n.d.a). Many of those who were left behind were forced to evacuate Azerbaijan and flee to the south to seek the protection of the British army stationed in Hamadan, Persia. The Assyrians were later put in a refugee camp in Baquba (Iraq) to await the negotiation of peace between Britain, Iraq, and Turkey (Aprim, n.d.a, 2007a; Stafford, 1935). It is reported that two thirds of the Assyrian total population was killed during World War I (1914–1918) (Aprim, n.d.a).

TABLE 48-1   Aramaic Alphabet

Character	Sound	Greek/Latin/English Equivalent	Character	Sound	Greek/Latin/English Equivalent
ܐ	Alap	Alpha/A	ܡ	Meem	Mew/M
ܒ	Beet	Beta/B	ܢ	Noon[a]	Nu/N
ܓ	Gamal	Gama/G	ܣ	Simkat	Sigma/S
ܕ	Dalat	Delta/D	ܝ	Yodh	Y
ܗ	Heh	H	ܦ	Peh	Pi/P
ܚ	Khet	KH	ܩ	Qop	Q
ܛ	Teth	Teta/T	ܪ	Resh	Rho/R
ܘ	Vav	V	ܨ	Sadeh	S
ܙ	Zain	Zeta/Z	ܫ	Sheen	Sh
ܥ	Aih	E	ܬ	Taw	Tau/T
ܟ	Kap[a]	Kappa/K	ܠܐ	Tawalap	TA
ܠ	Lamad	Lambda/L			

[a]The three displayed characters are different representations of the same letter. The first character is the normal form of the letter. The second character is a representation of the letter when it is the last letter in a word ("final connected"). The third letter is a representation of the letter when it is the last letter in a word but not connected to the rest of the letters in that word ("final nonconnected").

After the defeat of the Ottoman Empire in 1918, the army of the newly formed country of Turkey exiled hundreds of thousands of Assyrians into present-day Syria (Aprim, n.d.a, 2007a). As a result, the population of Assyrians in southern Turkey dwindled to only a couple of thousand (Aprim, n.d.a). Other ethnic clusters of Assyrians were created in Lebanon and Palestine in 1933 following the independence of Iraq (Aprim, 2003).

During World War II, and for many years after, political upheaval in the Middle East created new waves of Assyrian refugees (Ishaya, 2003). Later, with the help of Assyrian political organizations, such as the Assyrian Universal Alliance and World Council of Churches, many Assyrians were admitted into the United States (Ishaya, 2003); thus, a combination of the aforementioned events led to an exodus of increasingly more Assyrians from their ancestral homelands to the United States and other Western nations.

Based on available estimates, the United States is home to the third largest Assyrian population in the world. It is estimated that approximately 120,000 Chaldeans (Catholic Assyrians) reside in Detroit, Flint, and surrounding areas in Michigan. There are 90,000 Assyrians in Chicago, Illinois, 10,000 in Phoenix, Arizona; in California there are 15,000 in San Francisco and San Jose, 25,000 in Modesto/Turlock, 25,000 in San Diego, and 5000 in Los Angeles. There are also roughly 5000 Assyrians on the East Coast in Hartford/New Britain, Connecticut, and several thousand more in eastern Massachusetts, New York, and New Jersey.

FOOD HISTORY WITHIN THE CULTURE

Although in ancient times scarcity of food threatened man's survival, in Mesopotamia bountiful supply of food was produced in the fertile soil between the Euphrates and Tigris rivers. Several domestic varieties of sheep (Nickles, 1973), as well as cattle, oxen, buffalo, and even bison, were bred in Mesopotamia (Aprim, n.d.b). The great winged bulls, the tutelary genii that guarded the gates of the Assyrian capital city Khorsabad (Dur-Sharrukin), represented a memory of the bison, which was by far the most dangerous animal in Mesopotamia. Artwork from that era suggests that the hump-backed ox was also bred in Mesopotamia by 3000 BC. In fact, evidence from the time of the Assyrian King Sargon II suggests that the economy in Mesopotamia was based at least partially on animal husbandry and agriculture (Aprim, n.d.b).

Fish was popular in ancient Assyria and the rivers flowing through the region provided an ample supply (Saggs, 1965). The Assyrian's knowledge of the breeding habits of fish was considerable and fertilized eggs were collected and placed in special lakes for propagation. Building dams was another means by which Assyrians maintained an adequate supply of fish. The canals were also useful as a source of edible fish; in fact, fishing appears to have been pursued as an occupation (Aprim, n.d.). Fishing was done mainly on a line, but various kinds of net were also employed (Saggs, 1965). Both fresh and dried fish were important elements in the Assyrian diet. The larger fish were dried, gutted, filleted, and hung on a line, as is still done in Norway (Aprim, n.d.b) and by the Inuit. Smaller fish were left in the sun and then compressed into a solid block from which the required quantity could be cut off (Aprim, n.d.b).

Much of the information regarding use of milk and milk products comes from literary, ceramic, and art evidence. Probably cow and goat milk were the most used by early Assyrian communities. The use of butter, sour milk, and cheese must have quickly followed the use of milk, based on drawings available from this period (Aprim, n.d.b). In one milking scene, the method used by the shepherds is shown as a man seated and rocking a large narrow-necked jar lying on its side, while to his left two other men are straining the resulting liquid in order to extract the butter. Assyrians referred to all fat as simply "fat." Some evidence suggests that a product similar to butter or curd was used. Another form

of fat employed in cooking and baking was sesame oil (Aprim, n.d.b).

The current state of knowledge regarding early domestication of birds in Assyria is scant. The appearance of fowls on Assyrian seals as early as the 8th century BC, however, attest to their existence. The wild birds of that period included the ibis, crane, and heron (of which seven varieties have been counted), which frequented the marshes, and the pelican, which was trained for fishing, while the fields were home to thrushes, blackbirds, sparrows, and larks. Quails were rare, but partridges and francolins bred in the country, and we can see the latter being hunted with a bow on a bas-relief in artwork from the time of King Sargon II, on display in the Louvre Museum (Aprim, n.d.b). All of this signifies the importance of protein-containing foods since the emergence of humans.

Barley and wheat are the cereal grains that occur most frequently at Mesopotamian archaeological sites (Nickles, 1973; Aprim, n.d.b). Because barley was naturally abundant in the region, it was the primary grain used for bread making (Saggs, 1965). The starchy grain known as spelt was indigenous to Mesopotamia as well but was never as common or as important as barley (Aprim, n.d.b). Based on available evidence, four varieties of "bread" were consumed by Assyrians of that period, of which the commonest was an unleavened bread in the form of thin crisp disks made from whole-meal barley flour (Saggs, 1965). This bread was likely baked in a hot brick oven (about 500°F) creating in just a few seconds a balloon-like empty chamber inside the flat loaf (Abdalla, 1996). The other varieties of bread consumed were similar to modern-day pastries, because they contained ingredients such as sesame oil and something called "honey." The confusion about the latter term is that the same *Akkadian* (language spoken by Assyrians and Babylonians) word sometimes means honey from bees and sometimes date syrup (Saggs, 1965). Textual evidence from the time of Assyrian King Sargon II attests to the importance of dates to Assyrians and the widespread consumption of date syrup as compared with that of honey (Aprim, n.d.b).

Among vegetables in common use at that time were cucumbers, peas, beans, lentils, pumpkins, and plants such as cress, garlic, onion, and leek (Saggs, 1965). The onion was regarded as a peasant food. They were usually eaten raw with bread and were sold in strings. Gardens in fertile Mesopotamia flourished, and onion, leeks, and garlic were among the most frequently cultivated plants. A good meal consisted of vegetables, such as lentils, which, like beans, have always been grown in the area, boiled millet, barley prepared as rice is prepared today, and possibly maize. There was also a kind of truffle that was considered a great delicacy, and there is mention of baskets of them being sent to the king (Aprim, n.d.b). By far the most commonly consumed fruit was the date, but grapes, figs (Saggs, 1965), apples, pears, plums, and apricots are also mentioned (Aprim, n.d.b). Banana may also have been consumed by Assyrians based on bas-relief sculptures that show finger-like objects attached at the base among fruits on the table. Banana may have been brought from present-day Syria, which was part of the Assyrian Empire at the time (Aprim, n.d.b).

It is not clear when Assyrians learned of and drank beer and wine, but a large number of tablets that record wine trade have been discovered. Furthermore, a clear distinction between fermented and unfermented liquor was made, and wines that aged without fermenting were highly prized. It appears that the beer was produced locally from a barley base, and palm-tree wine was obtained by tapping the top of the trunk of the palm tree and collecting the sap (Aprim, n.d.b). Once fermented for 2–3 days, this wine became extremely intoxicating. Wine was also imported from the kingdoms to the north and northeast (Saggs, 1965).

Although Assyrian food habits have evolved over the years, some elements of their earlier dietary habits, such as their love for fruits and vegetables, have been retained. After the fall of the Assyrian Empire, for nearly two centuries the Assyrians formed ethnic clusters primarily in the mountainous *Hakkiari* district of southern Turkey, the plains and mountains of northern Iraq, and villages scattered throughout the region west of Lake Urmia in northwestern Iran (Ishaya, 2002). Because they were isolated from the mainstream cultures in these primarily Muslim regions, they had to be self-sufficient to provide for their families and build a community of their own. Raising livestock for their meat, cultivating vegetable gardens, and planting fruit orchards were means of achieving autonomy and self-reliance. Many of them continued to pursue agricultural and pastoral subsistence; however, political instability in the Middle East during the past 100 years has resulted in the scattering of Assyrians throughout many parts of the world (Aprim, 2007a; Stafford, 1935). Due to the fact that Assyrians are minorities in all places they inhabit, their local cuisine may vary and

also contain elements of the popular cuisine in their locale. For example, many aspects of Iraqi cuisine, including a variety of spices, are incorporated into Iraqi Assyrian cuisine, and the same is the case for Assyrians of Iran, Syria, and Turkey.

MAJOR FOODS

Protein Sources

Meat remains an important element of the Assyrian diet, with beef and lamb consumed most often. Unlike Muslim and Jewish neighbors of the countries they originated from, Assyrians consume pork, although not frequently. This may be due partly to the influence of their Muslim neighbors and also the unavailability of pork at local butcher shops, where many Assyrians in the Middle East continue to purchase their meat.

Meat is often incorporated into stews and is braised with vegetables and spices. Many of the stews are tomato based. A popular stew with relatively few ingredients is *shurwa*, which contains lamb shoulder or beef cubes, potatoes, tomato paste, onions, green pepper, and paprika. Iraqi and Syrian Assyrians serve *shurwa* over a bed of rice, whereas Iranian Assyrians eat their *shurwa* along with wheat bread and sometimes pickled vegetables. *Kurush* is another popular stew, made of a mixture of beef and assorted vegetables seasoned with paprika. The assortment of vegetables used in many of these main dishes not only enhances the taste of the food but also contributes to the nutritional value of these traditional meals.

Kipte, which in its simplest form consists of balls of minced lamb or beef mixed with egg, onion, and spices, and is cooked in a tomato-based sauce, is a hearty, versatile dish that is sure to warm you on a cold day. The meat is often mixed with other ingredients such as rice or bulgur and aromatic herbs and vegetables. Some Assyrians place a hard-boiled egg inside their *kipte*.

Among species of bird, chicken is consumed most. All types of meat, whether beef, lamb, or chicken, are marinated, charcoal-broiled, and served over rice. Assyrians, similar to other Middle Eastern cultures, are fond of charcoal-broiled organ meats (Nickles, 1973), such as liver and heart, which, although rich in many B vitamins and iron, harbor a lot of cholesterol (Whitney & Rolfes, 2008). Ducks and geese are also raised and consumed in the countryside. Wild birds,

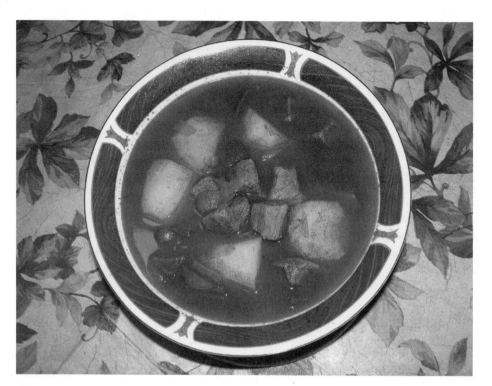

Shurwa
Courtesy of the author

such as quail and pheasant, are commonly hunted from open grasslands of mountainous valleys in northwestern Iran. The rivers running through this part of Iran and northern Iraq (the region known today as Kurdistan) also provide a bountiful supply of fish.

Eggs are for the most part considered a breakfast food and are prepared in many different ways, including scrambled, sunny-side up, or hard-boiled. Iraqi Assyrians also add parsley and dried beef sausage (*bastirma*) to their scrambled eggs for special occasions such as Christmas or Easter. The Assyrian omelet, popular with Iranian Assyrians, consists of sautéed green pepper, onion, tomatoes, and eggs seasoned with salt and pepper. The omelet is generally eaten as the main meal for lunch or dinner.

Being devout Christians and observing Lent necessitated abstinence from meat and dairy products (Abdalla, 1996). Observance of Lent and the high cost of meat products in their original homelands has led Assyrians to create a plethora of tasty meatless meals made from legumes, mainly beans and lentils. The protein-rich beans and lentils, which are also an excellent source of minerals, such as calcium, iron, zinc, and selenium, along with B-vitamin folate and fiber, are prepared many different ways in Assyrian cook-

ing. A common method of preparing kidney beans and pinto beans involves soaking the beans overnight followed by discarding the soaking water and boiling the beans in cold fresh water until tender, with a bit of fresh garlic and green pepper added. Assyrians knew that the soaking step rid the beans of gas-causing agents long before scientific evidence proved that the oligosaccharides (sugars) present in beans were the cause of flatulence (Price, Lewis, Wyatt, & Fenwick, 1988; Sat & Keles, 2002). The human body does not produce the enzymes that break down the oligosaccharides, and soaking followed by boiling the beans in cold fresh water reduces the concentration of these gas-causing sugars (Vidal-Valverde, Frias, & Valverde, 1993). *Mashee*, a sauce that consists of sautéed onions, a bit of paprika, and tomato paste, is another recipe for adding flavor to the boiled beans. *Mashee* can also be prepared with the addition of beef. Chickpeas (*garbanzo* beans), a legume less familiar to the American palate until relatively recently, are not only added to soups, and toasted and salted, they are consumed as snacks. These tasty puffed beans also make excellent cocktail nibbles and are crunchier than peanuts.

Due to unavailability of refrigeration in earlier times and high rates of lactose intolerance, Assyrians frequently turned milk into yogurt, cheese, and butter. This custom has continued throughout the generations. They are masters at making homemade yogurt (*mesta*), fermented by a culture or starter saved from the previous batch. Yogurt is not only frequently consumed as a side dish to the meal; it also constitutes an important ingredient in one of the oldest Assyrian dishes, a creamy soup called *Boushala*, which can be served hot or cold. Yogurt and grains are mixed in an enticing manner in this traditional Assyrian soup, a peppery pottage of green leafy vegetables and bulgur wheat. The result is a wholesome, nutritious soup that is not only a good source of complete protein but also provides an assortment of vitamins, minerals, and antioxidant nutrients (Whitney & Rolfes, 2008).

Traditionally, Assyrians have made butter from yogurt by mixing it with water and churning the mixture while the fat separates. What remains is a milky liquid rich in protein, calcium, and notably the B vitamin riboflavin (McWilliams, 2005). To maximize use of available food sources, water is drained from this milky liquid until a solid dry consistency is formed. Mixed with a small amount of butter, onion, and aromatic vegetables, such as dill and coriander, it is used as a cheese spread called *jajik*. In making *daweh* (a yogurt drink), yogurt is mixed with water and the mixture is lightly salted. *Daweh* is an excellent thirst quencher that is commonly served as a complementary drink with meals.

The long-held Assyrian belief regarding the supremacy of yogurt as a health food is consistent with our current understanding of the health benefits of the probiotics naturally found in these fermented dairy products. Probiotics are live microorganisms that, when present in the diet in adequate amounts, confer a health benefit on the host. A growing body of research regarding these "beneficial microorganisms" suggests that they can be used to treat a wide range of medical conditions that have been linked to pathogens; for example, gastrointestinal problems, such as irritable bowel syndrome and inflammatory bowel disease (i.e., Crohn's disease, ulcerative colitis, respectively), various infections, such as vaginal and skin infections, and diseases of the oral cavity such as tooth decay and periodontal disease (Huffnagle & Wernick, 2007). Some studies suggest that probiotics are effective in preventing and possibly even treating food allergies (Huffnagle & Wernick, 2007; Majamaa & Isolauri, 1997).

Another milk by-product consumed by Assyrians as a breakfast item is *kaymak*, a creamy product similar

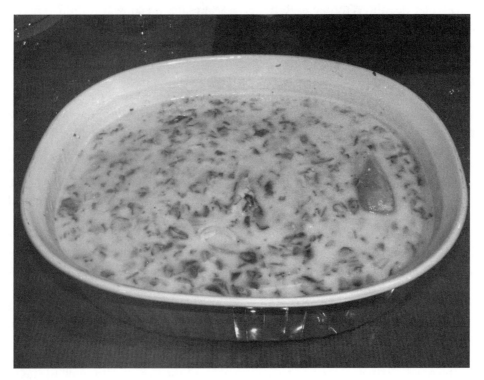

Boushala
Courtesy of the author

to sour cream but with a subtle, sweet taste. The traditional method of making *kaymak* consists of boiling the milk slowly followed by simmering it for 2 hours over a very low heat. After the heat source is shut off, the cream is skimmed and left to chill (and mildly ferment) for several hours or days. The end product has a thick, creamy consistency and a rich taste. It has a high percentage of milk fat (typically about 60%), much of it in the form of saturated fat. Traditionally, *kaymak* was made from the milk of water buffalos, although it can be prepared from cow's milk as well.

A variety of seeds and nuts that are considered meat substitutes rich in protein and high in beneficial polyunsaturated fats (Whitney & Rolfes, 2008) are consumed as snack foods or as ingredients in dishes. The most common varieties of nuts eaten are walnuts, hazelnuts, and almonds. The majority of nuts and seeds, with the exception of walnuts, are eaten roasted and salted. Walnuts are of special significance in the Assyrian diet, because they were traditionally used as an important protein source during the Lenten period. Walnuts are served in different ways: along with raisins as a snack, added to desserts, and even as part of a main dish. Nutritionally, walnuts are known for their high content of omega-3 polyunsaturated fats, which are believed to have many health benefits including that of cardiovascular health (Whitney & Rolfes, 2008). Tahini, a paste of ground sesame seeds mixed with date syrup, is often eaten as an accompaniment to breakfast by Iraqi and Syrian Assyrians.

Regardless of where they live, the custom of eating sunflower, pumpkin, and melon seeds is practiced almost universally by Assyrians. They are, without a doubt, masters at the task of cracking the seeds open with the teeth and getting the flesh out with the tongue, without using the hands. The skill and rapidity with which they strip off the hard shell to obtain the tiny kernel must be seen to be appreciated. Although the amount of seeds consumed by a typical family has not been quantified, based on the author's personal experience and available reports (Abdalla, 1996), it is substantial. It has been reported that when sunflower seeds packed in small plastic bags began to appear in Swedish shops in the 1970s, Assyrian emigrants would buy the entire stock. Until that time, bird breeders had been the principal buyers of seeds. When Assyrians later discovered that the seeds they purchased also contained sand, they continued to buy the product and sifted the sand at home (Abdalla, 1996). Nutritionally, seeds are not only a good source of protein; they are rich in vitamin E, an antioxidant nutrient. Antioxidant nutrients prevent cellular damage, a common pathway for aging and chronic diseases such as cancer and cardiovascular disease (Whitney & Rolfes, 2008).

 Starch Sources

Assyrians prefer the taste of bread made with wheat flour to that of other grains. Ample archeological evidence suggests that wheat, the oldest cultivated crop, was first domesticated about 9000 years ago in a mountainous grassy region of the Middle East (Nickles, 1973). This area covers large parts of eastern Turkey, northern Iraq, and northwestern Iran. Both northern Iraq and northwestern Iran are home to large communities of Assyrians who are indigenous to these regions; therefore, it is no surprise that wheat bread is an important staple in the Assyrian diet. If bread is not homemade, it is bought from local bakeries fresh and warm, sometimes twice a day. Many varieties of wheat bread are consumed; a favorite is the *lavash*, a thinly rolled-out dough that is traditionally baked on *tanura* (a clay-coated pit where fire is kindled) walls. *Samoon*, a fluffy bun, is popular with Assyrians who live in the United States, especially those residing in Chicago and its suburbs.

Besides bread, wheat flour is used to make stuffed dumplings of unleavened dough that often contain minced beef or lamb meat, potatoes, onions, cheese, or any combination of these ingredients. These semicircular dumplings, called *piroshke*, are pan-fried and served hot (similar to *pierogi*, which is strongly linked to Slavic culture). *Piroshke* was likely added to Assyrian cuisine upon migration of Assyrians to Russia. It is estimated that approximately 25,000 Assyrians reside in Russia.

Wheat is also used to make bulgur. This is done by parboiling the wheat, a unique technology rooted in ancient Assyria and still used by modern Assyrians (Abdalla, 1992, 1996). After parboiling the wheat until soft, it is allowed to dry in the sun. The outer covering of the wheat kernel is then removed by pounding it in a special mortar called *khasholta*. Using a simple milling instrument called *jarusta*, the wheat is ground. Finally, the by-product is sieved into different fractions. Presently, bulgur is considered a universal and versatile grain product that is consumed in many parts of the world. Although all stages of bulgur production have been automated (at least in the West), the original technology has its roots in ancient Assyria (Abdalla, 1992). *Kibbi, kibbeh, kobba,* or *kubba* (name used in Iraq) is a family of dishes made from a shell or crust of bulgur and minced meat, onions, and spices, stuffed with the same meat mixture, and is popular in many parts of the Middle East (Nickles, 1973). Some variations of *kubba* are very specific to the Assyrian community; one is *kubbah hamouth*, where the dough used to make the shell is made with crushed rice. The dough is then filled with the meat mixture and cooked in a tomato-based soup, much like *kipte*. The other *kubba* often eaten during the long Lent is *kubba d-khoumsa*, the vegan version of *kubba*, made with a chickpea filling.

Another way wheat is used in Assyrian cooking is in the form of wheat berries. When preparing whole-wheat berries, they use light-colored peeled ones, which cook more rapidly than the non-hulled kind. An age-old specialty that is uniquely Assyrian is *harissa*, a rich porridge made from cooked, deboned, and shredded chicken or turkey and cooked, de-hulled wheat berries. It is flavored with roasted, finely ground coriander seeds as well as butter. Variations of the Assyrian *harissa* are prepared by the Arabs and Iranians, the main difference being elimination of the ground coriander and sprinkling of sugar and cinnamon on the surface of the porridge before serving.

Although this has not historically been the case, rice is considered a staple grain in the Assyrian diet. Even though all recipes, without exception, call for the use of long-grain rice similar to the basmati variety, there are some regional variations in the method of preparation of rice. Iranian Assyrians prepare their rice by soaking it in salt water overnight. The next day, the soaking water is drained and the rice is parboiled in fresh water until a firm thread remains in the middle. Then it is rinsed with lukewarm water to get rid of excess saltiness and starch. Finally, the rice is transferred back to the pot, steamed on the stovetop, and garnished with saffron. Although of lower nutritional value, due to loss of many water-soluble vitamins after soaking and boiling in a large amount of water and rinsing, this method results in exceptionally fluffy rice with the grains not sticking together. It also creates a golden rice crust at the bottom of the pot. (For variety, bread or potatoes can be fried at the bottom of the pot for a different type of bottom crust.) Another variation of the basic rice recipe, the so-called Assyrian rice or *reza rikta*, calls for adding homemade noodles made from wheat flour to the rice prior to steaming or baking it. Some Assyrians, rather than steaming the rice on the stovetop, bake it in the oven.

 ## Fat Sources

For centuries the only sources of fat available to Assyrians were butter and animal shortening. Then in the 1970s technology for production of vegetable shortening became available. At the same time many consumers were cautioned by health professionals about the detrimental effects of regular consumption of butter and animal shortening high in saturated fat on cardiovascular health; hence, many Assyrians slowly switched to using vegetable shortening. Currently, the main sources of fat used by the younger generations are liquid vegetable oils; however, many older Assyrians accustomed to their old dietary habits and the rich taste of butter have difficulty giving it up completely. It is therefore not uncommon to encounter an elderly Assyrian who insists on frying his or her morning egg in butter or prefers butter as an accompaniment to meals.

 ## Prominent Vegetables

By far one of the most nutritious aspects of the Assyrian diet is consumption of large amounts of vegetables. Modern Assyrians use many of the same vegetables used by their ancestors, such as onions, garlic, leek, cucumber, peas, beans, and lentils (Aprim, n.d.b; Saggs, 1965). This author has come across few main dishes that do not include either onions, garlic, or both, and tomatoes in some form are used in many recipes. Not only do addition of onion and garlic add pungency to the food, it may be a healthful practice as well. It is believed that the organosulfur compounds found in garlic may lower blood cholesterol (Whitney & Rolfes, 2008). Tomato not only enhances flavor; its high lycopene content appears to inhibit growth of cancer cells and may protect against cardiovascular disease (David, 2004; Whitney & Rolfes, 2008).

Other commonly consumed vegetables include potatoes, cabbage, a variety of peppers, celery, zucchini, squash, okra, and eggplant. Potatoes were introduced to Assyrians by Europeans about 160 years ago (Abdalla, 1996). Today, potatoes constitute an important ingredient in more than 20 different Assyrian dishes, including many stews (Abdalla, 1996). Potato chap patties, which consist of ground beef, onion, parsley, and a mixture of spices, deep-fried or pan-fried, are popular with many Assyrians. Tomato, peppers, and zucchini are considered New World vegetables and were most likely introduced to Assyrians by Europeans. Eggplant, although not indigenous to the Middle East, has been used there for many centuries (Nickles, 1973).

This Middle Eastern favorite is the main ingredient in an appetizer called *baba ghannooj*, which is made of pureed, charbroiled eggplant, tahini, garlic, salt, and lemon juice.

Assyrians combine vegetables with meat in an ingenious way in the form of a class of dishes called *dolma*. Although *dolma* is a part of Turkish cuisine and the cuisine of several other countries that were once part of the Ottoman Empire (Nickles, 1973), none compares with the way Assyrians make theirs. There are three main types of *dolma*, which include *dolma darpe* (stuffed grape-leaf *dolma*), *dolma kalama* (stuffed cabbage-leaf *dolma*), and *dolma makhlot* (stuffed mixed-vegetable *dolma*). The latter *dolma* is composed of a variety of hollowed-out and stuffed vegetables and fruits such as eggplant, zucchini, tomato, green pepper, quince, and green apple. The ingredients used as filling are fairly similar for the different *dolmas*. They include beef or lamb mixed with a variety of herbs and spices. One big difference in the way Assyrians make their *dolmas* is in using cooked, shredded beef rather than ground beef or lamb, and including stuffed fruits.

The Assyrian cook has at his or her command a variety of aromatic green leafy vegetables, such as parsley, dill, cilantro, mint, tarragon, basil, and *marzeh* (not consumed in the West), that may be used fresh or sun-dried for winter months. These vegetables are not only often added to recipes to enhance flavor and aroma, they are frequently trimmed, washed, and eaten raw, much like a salad. Many vegetables receive little processing prior to consumption (Abdalla, 1996). For example, cucumbers are often consumed without peeling, and no one discards radish leaves. *Tabbouleh*, a salad of chopped tomatoes, green and white onions, parsley, mint, and bulgur, popular in many Arab countries, is eaten by Syrian and Iraqi Assyrians; however, bulgur, similar to *baba ghannooj*, is not considered an authentic Assyrian food and was most likely adopted as a result of cultural assimilation.

The love Assyrians have for raw vegetables is reflected in the common practice of pickling, which is employed to preserve Jerusalem artichokes, carrots, cabbage, celery, peppers, beets, cauliflower, garlic, grapevine leaves, semiripe tomatoes, and cucumbers. Pickling is an economical means of preserving vegetables. It enabled Assyrians to have access to vegetables during long winters in times when modern food-transportation systems were not available. This custom of pickling vegetables in early fall and using them during the winter has been passed down from

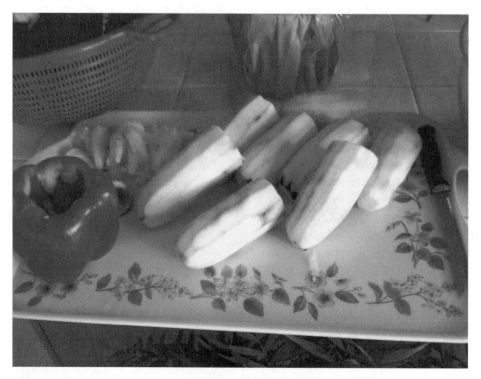

Dolma Makhlot
Courtesy of the author

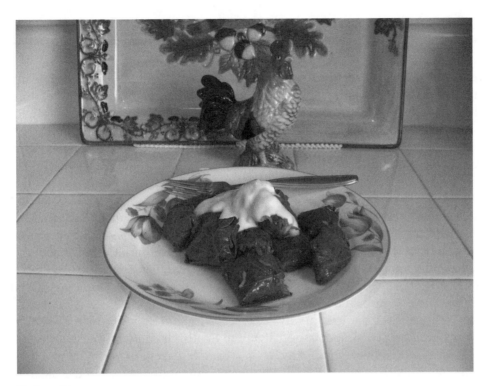

Dolma Darpe
Courtesy of the author

generation to generation. Today, many Assyrians living in the East and West continue to enjoy the taste of pickled vegetables at dinner. Sun-drying, which is another preservation method, was not used only for aromatic vegetables, such as parsley and cilantro, but also for other vegetables, such as tomatoes, that were hard to obtain during winter and were therefore preserved in the same manner.

Another important element of the Assyrian diet are vegetables that grow wild, such as mallow, endive, chicory, purslane, sorrel, stroksbill, wart cress, thistle, hawsbeard, hawweed, shepherd's needle, wood sorrel, and many others (Abdalla, 1996). Although transfer of knowledge from older generations to the young regarding the nutritional and medicinal properties of these vegetables and herbs has lessened over the years, some of them, including those belonging to the mallow species, are still consumed. Some of these wild vegetables are more popular because they are juicier, have less hairy leaves, and when cooked, they give off a pleasant aroma and a slightly sour taste. For example, depending on the occasion, a mallow dish is made without any animal products, with some oil (Lenten period) or with butter, eggs, and *qaliyyo* (potato-size pieces of beef and mutton preserved by

salting and melting with tallow in a large pot over a fire) (Abdalla, 2004).

 Prominent Fruits

Although Assyrians consume many varieties of fruits, grapes have always held a special place for them. Grapes are not only consumed fresh (*verjuice*); the sour juice of unripe grapes was used as a flavoring agent in cooking (Abdalla, 1996), long before Assyrians were introduced to lemons. Distilled liquor is also made from grapes and raisins. In this century-old process, the sugar in the grapes or raisins is fermented by the yeast, resulting in production of alcohol. The alcohol content is then separated from the fermenting fruit mixture (mash) by distillation. The end result is a neutral spirit with little color, aroma, or flavor. Assyrians refer to this liquor as *arak*. The distiller sometimes blends this neutral spirit with other alcohol or flavorings and may or may not leave it to age until the desired flavor and aroma is achieved before bottling. Iranian Assyrians ferment cherries in sugar and add the resultant mixture to distilled liquors for a fruity flavor.

Grapes are also turned into grape syrup, for which there are regional differences in the method used to make it. Iranian Assyrians add ash obtained from the nearby mountains to fresh, unfermented grape juice and let the mixture sit overnight. Next the mixture is decanted, strained to remove all sediment, and reduced by boiling. The resulting syrup is highly concentrated and has a fairly long shelf life. Until the 1950s the only sweetener available to Assyrians was grape syrup, and to a lesser extent, date syrup (Abdalla, 1996). Grape syrup is used to make other products as well. After thickening, flour is added, and the mixture is put into a shallow pan to cool. It is then dried in various shapes of varying thickness, texture, and size (Abdalla, 1996); often, these are flavored with nuts. To entertain children, wheat and syrup pulp are also used to produce edible animal shapes for the New Year's celebrations (Abdalla, 1996). Assyrians's high consumption of grapes, grape juice, and wine is consistent with good health, primarily due to naturally occurring phytochemicals in grapes. Grapes, especially red grapes and red wine, contain high levels of a class of phytochemicals known as flavonoids (Vita, 2005; Whitney & Rolfes, 2008).

The method used by Assyrians to produce raisins is very interesting. Grapes are dipped into a boiling solution containing dissolved ash of burnt maize stems or rock salt. The solution contains ions of metals, the most important being that of calcium (Abdalla, 1996). These ions react with the pectins naturally present in the fruit, making the latter stronger. As a result of this treatment, the fruit does not give off juice during heating and drains easily during drying, producing the desired glossy appearance (Abdalla, 1996).

 ### Spices and Seasonings

Spices and herbs add much to Assyrian cooking. For centuries this region was the gateway through which caravans transported incense, oils, and spices to the rest of the Middle East and Europe (Nickles, 1973). Today, many of the spices commonly employed in cooking in the West, such as black pepper, curry powder, bay leaf, and cloves, are used in Assyrian cooking. There are also some unusual spices, such as *sumak*, which lends a tart taste to meats and is frequently sprinkled on charbroiled meats and chicken prior to serving. Ground coriander imparts a pleasant, subtle aroma and flavor to meat and grain mixtures such as *harissa*. The aromatic spice turmeric, which lends not only a pleasant smell but also an interesting yellowish color to food, either alone or in combination with other spices, is added to many stews and main dishes. Curcumin, the major

pigment in turmeric, has been shown to possess both anti-inflammatory and antioxidant properties as well as a chemopreventive effect.

Animal studies have demonstrated inhibition of colon cancer from dietary administration of curcumin (Kawamori et al., 1999). Colorectal cancer is the third leading cause of cancer deaths in both men and women in the United States (Jemal, Siegel, Ward, Murray, & Jiaquan Xu, 2006). It is noteworthy that ethnic populations, such as east Indians, who use spice mixtures containing turmeric have lower incidence of colon cancer (Mohandas & Desai, 1999). Saffron, with its yellowish–orange color, contributes to the color and taste of rice dishes. Cumin is added to a special feta-type cheese that is shredded and placed in glazed clay pots to prevent moisture loss. The lid is then sealed tightly and the cheese is refrigerated. This cheese is called *gupta domorta* in Assyrian, which translates to English literally as "buried cheese." The reason for this odd cheese name is the practice of burying clay pots containing cheese in the cellar ground to keep it from spoiling. This was done long ago due to lack of refrigeration.

Although in the West lemons or lemon juice are often used to add tartness to recipes, Assyrians have traditionally mixed *verijuice* (sour liquid derived from unripe grapes) or dried whole limes with other ingredient to create a subtle tartness and awaken the taste buds. Iraqi Assyrians make use of a mixture of spices called *baharat* in making their exotic *biryani*, a dish of rice, assorted meats, vegetables, hard-boiled eggs, spices, and roasted slivered almonds.

 ### Beverages

Although there is some evidence to suggest that beer was invented in Mesopotamia (Saggs, 1965), after the fall of the Assyrian Empire, wine was the basic drink of these ancient people. It was not until 100 years or so ago that beer was once again introduced to Assyrians. The amount of wine consumed varies depending on the geographic region. For example, some Assyrians, such as those who reside in northwest Iran, may drink wine daily. For people who prefer a stronger drink, liquor distilled from grapes or dates, called *arak*, is available. These distilled liquors are fairly potent, which explains the reason for the practice of serving the drink along with appetizers. In the Shapour region, in northwest Iran, a common custom is to remember the deceased over dinner by toasting their memory with a glass of wine or a shot of liquor. After the deceased is buried, a

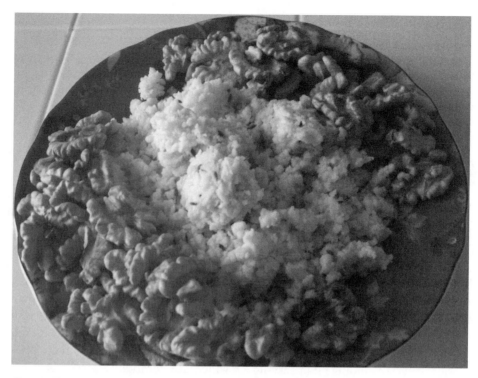

Gupta Domorta
Courtesy of the author

bottle of *arak* is spread over the grave site as a symbol of the person's last drink.

Although coffee is fairly regularly consumed, it takes second place to black tea brewed from loose tea leaves. The beverage of choice for breakfast for most Assyrians is tea, which is drunk hot and sweet. Tea is prepared in an elaborate vessel called a *samovar* (a Russian word that means "self-brewer"), which was introduced to the Assyrians by the Russians. The vessel is used to heat and boil the water and has a section on top that holds and heats a teapot filled with tea. Other than the morning tea, which may be sweetened by directly mixing sugar with it, at other times during the day when tea is drunk (which can be numerous times), pieces of hard sugar cube are placed in the mouth to impart a sweet taste as one sips the tea.

Even though tea is considered to be the most widely consumed beverage in the world, it has been only in the past two decades that scientists have discovered its numerous health benefits (Stangl, Lorenz, & Stangl, 2006). A growing body of scientific evidence suggests that flavonoids, the phytochemicals naturally present in tea in relatively high concentrations, may be effective in preventing cardiovascular disease, in particular atherosclerosis and coronary heart disease (Kris-Etherton & Keen, 2002; Riemersma, Rice-Evans, Tyrrell, & Clifford, 2001;

Stangl et al., 2006). Contrary to the habit of adding milk to tea, as is prevalent in the West, Assyrians, like many other Middle Eastern cultures, drink their tea black. This in itself appears to be of value healthwise, because some studies have suggested that lactose, the primary naturally occurring sugar in milk, may have an atherogenic effect, counteracting the protective effects of tea flavonoids (Segall, 1997).

Assyrians are fond of coffee as well. Using a small narrow-neck, long-handle pot called a *jezve*, coffee is made by boiling finely powdered roasted coffee beans with sugar and cream and serving it into small cups where the dregs settle. The end product is a thick, strong coffee similar to Italian espresso but sweeter. Coffee is generally served at social gatherings; for example, when women get together to socialize after they are finished with domestic tasks. A ritual practiced at social gatherings is to serve coffee followed by fortune-telling, known as tasseography in the West. This involves interpreting patterns in the coffee grounds that have sedimented to the bottom of the cup after the cup has been inverted over the saucer. (This author has rarely attended a social gathering with Assyrian women where coffee and fortune-telling were not included.) Generally, all predictions by the fortune-teller are of a positive nature, bearing an assortment of good news for one to anticipate. Coffee is also traditionally served at funerals.

Nothing works as well as a tall glass of fruit-syrup drink mixed with water and ice to quench one's thirst, and Assyrians are certainly very skilled in preparing these flavorful drinks. Before the advent of carbonated beverages, fruit-syrup drinks made from quince, sour cherry, and rhubarb were quite popular and in demand during the summer.

 Desserts

The usual Assyrian dessert is fruit. By far one of the most universally cherished desserts by Assyrians young and old is the sweet bread *kadeh*, which is a yeast-leavened bread made from flour, sugar, eggs, baking powder, salt, and a large amount of butter. Butter is not used only to make the dough, it is also incorporated in its filling. *Kadeh* is commonly eaten as a breakfast bread. Due to its high saturated fat content, most health-conscious Assyrians indulge in a serving of this delectable sweet only occasionally. *Nazoochi*, a triangular-shaped pastry similar to *kadeh* but sweeter, is often served with afternoon tea at social gatherings. *Kulaicheh* are small cakes stuffed with coarsely ground walnuts, or shredded coconut, mixed with sugar.

There are also several varieties of halva, a sweet made with different types of flours, sweeteners, butter, and nuts. Halva with a tahini (sesame paste) base is popular with many Assyrians as an accompaniment to breakfast. It is often eaten with butter and *lavash* bread. Another type of halva more familiar to Iranian Assyrians is made with grape syrup. Once allowed to harden, it can be cut into pieces. At times, the latter halva is mixed with a larger amount of water and made into a pudding called *hassida*, which is often prepared and offered to women soon after giving birth. A simpler form of halva is one made of semolina, oil, and plain sugar.

Baklava, which is usually associated with Greek cuisine, is also a popular dessert with Assyrians. It is made much the same way Greeks make theirs, with honey as the sweetener and the addition of walnuts. Cakes, such as walnut cake made with ground walnuts, flour, milk, and sugar, as well as sugar cookies, are also favored.

Assyrians are fond of fruit preserves and jams, which are commonly served at breakfast along with bread and butter. Whole-fruit preserves are also sometimes served as an accompaniment to mid-morning or afternoon tea. A fruit made into a fine preserve, but for the most part is not familiar to Westerners, is quince. In addition to quince, sweet-and-sour cherries are fre-

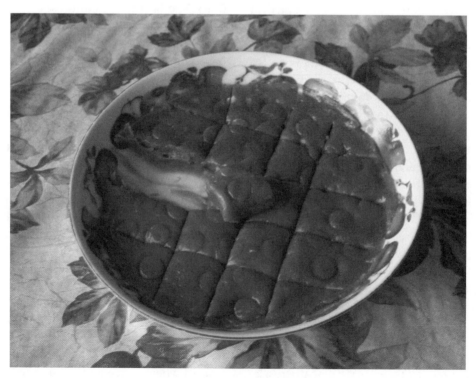

Halva
Courtesy of the author

quently turned into preserves, whereas apples and figs are used to make jam.

FOODS WITH CULTURAL SIGNIFICANCE

The majority of Assyrian celebrations involve food and are closely tied to religion in some way. Next to religion and language, foods and special ways of preparing them that have been passed down the generations have been an important thread in unifying Assyrians and allowing them to maintain their identity despite living in diaspora.

The two most important holidays for Assyrians of all Christian denominations are Christmas and Easter; however, generally Easter is considered the more important of the two. As a result, it is called *eida gura* (big holiday) (Assyrian International News Agency, n.d.). On both occasions great feasts are held and special foods are prepared. For Assyrians, Easter is a grand community celebration. Each family, to the best of its ability, prepares meals, drinks, and desserts for visitors. In many cities, the city is divided into geographic and neighborhood areas and a day is assigned for visitation of the inhabitants of each area. Visitors can range from family and friends to total strangers who may drop by to bless the host's Easter and partake in a drink (traditionally wine, *arak*, which is distilled liquor, fruit juice, and tea), appetizers (*maza*), and desserts such as walnut cake. Many of the appetizers are foods that can be served cold and handled easily. Some of the most common appetizers include sliced roast beef flavored with spices, potato chap patties, roasted chicken, and boiled garlic-flavored lamb and beef tongues. The table on which food is set is adorned with cut flowers and eggs colored red by boiling them in vinegar and onion skin.

The younger generations congregate in church courtyards to play and dance. Very young children also participate in an egg-cracking game in which two participants take turns and gently tap the head and tail of their eggs together. The person who cracks the other person's egg is the winner and gets to keep both eggs.

Traditionally, Christmas has been more immediate-family oriented, a time when children in particular receive the presents for which they had wished. Typical foods prepared for the big Christmas celebration include *harissa* (made of cooked, deboned, shredded chicken and de-hulled wheat berries), grapevine *dolma*, *reeshaw aqle* (tripe), a soup made of the innards of lamb or beef (some Assyrians serve this soup at Easter), and *patcha*, a soup made much the same way as *reeshaw aqle* but with lamb or calf feet. Based on this author's personal experience, *harissa* holds a special place in Assyrian cuisine because it is prepared and served at all major celebrations. Among desserts, it is customary to bake *kadeh* and *kulaicheh* for Christmas (Benjamin, 1996).

Feasts are also held in memory of various patron saints. The celebrations can range from small family gatherings to large community picnics (Assyrian International News Agency, n.d.). Everyone who is present partakes in a dish of boiled lamb stew and bread. Then they all join in traditional Assyrian group dances. The most commonly commemorated saints include Mart Maryum (St. Mary), Mar Gewargis (St. George), Mar Zaia, Mar Odisho, Mar Bishu, Mar Sliwa, Solten Madu, and Mar Pithyu. Some of these traditions have been practiced by Assyrians for well over 1500 years.

TYPICAL DAY'S MENU

A typical breakfast consists of *lawash* bread, *jajik*, feta cheese or Assyrian cheese, honey or jam, *kaymak*, butter, and sweetened hot tea. Lunch consists of *lawash* bread, *kipte*, mixed green leafy vegetable and herb salad, mixed roasted and salted nuts and seeds, and tea. The afternoon snack consists of grapes and peaches, feta cheese or Assyrian cheese, and bread, as well as tea and Assyrian coffee. Dinner consists of steamed white rice, charbroiled lamb and chicken kebabs, charbroiled tomatoes, green peppers, onions, *somak* to sprinkle on

Observations from the Author (Arezoo Rojhani)

My first exposure to Assyrian *dolma* was right after my husband and I got engaged and my in-laws invited us over for dinner. My mother-in-law had prepared stuffed mixed-vegetable *dolma*. Since my mother came from Turkish descent, I had frequently eaten *dolma* while growing up, but my mother-in-law's *dolma* was in a class by itself. It had a special blend of spices that gave it a pleasant and mildly spicy flavor. Also, I had never seen stuffed quince and apples thrown into the mix!

kebabs, mixed green leafy vegetable and herb salad, mixed pickled vegetables, watermelon and cantaloupe, wine or a shot of *arak*, and tea.

HOLIDAY MENUS

For breakfast on Christmas Day, the menu might consist of *harissa* topped with ground coriander seeds and butter, *kadeh* with honey or grape syrup, sweetened hot tea, and a shot of *arak*. For lunch on Easter Day, a typical menu would be *lawash* bread, *reeshaw aqle* (tripe), mixed green leafy vegetable and herb salad, wine or *arak*, assorted seasonal fruits, and tea. The afternoon snack might be walnut cake, *nazoochi* or *kulaicheh*, *lawash* bread with feta cheese, assorted seasonal fruits, and mixed roasted and salted nuts and seeds, as well as tea and Assyrian coffee. Easter dinner might consist of mixed vegetable *dolma*, yogurt, mixed green leafy vegetable and herb salad, assorted seasonal fruits, wine or *arak*, and tea.

HEALTH BELIEFS AND CONCERNS

Given that the Assyrian civilization dates back many centuries, they possess a fairly comprehensive folk-medicine system that has been tried and tested. There are specific practices that are thought to be important for good health and prevention of illness.

Assyrians firmly believe that keeping oneself and one's surroundings clean prevents illnesses and guarantees good health. For example, a newborn baby is given daily baths to ensure proper growth. Although this may seem ordinary in Western countries, where most people have access to running hot water, Assyrians practiced this principle in the days when indoor plumbing was not readily available. Keeping dry and warm and eliminating undue exposure to drafts is also considered to be consistent with good health, especially as it relates to preventing colds and coughs.

A good diet is considered essential for physical and psychological health. Eating three square meals a day and possibly an afternoon snack is believed to provide the body with the energy it needs to stay healthy. The older generations of Assyrians frown upon intentional food deprivation in the form of dieting or skipping meals for the purpose of losing weight. It is felt that such practices weaken the body and make it prone to illness. The majority of Assyrians believe that cooking the Assyrian way is overall healthier due to the large amount of fruits and vegetables incorporated into Assyrian rec-

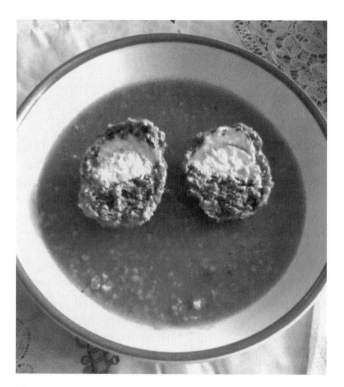

Kipte
Courtesy of the author

ipes. Due to their cohesiveness, stemming from their involvement with the church and civic organizations, even second- and some third-generation Assyrians have retained their traditional culinary practices. On a recent visit to the home of her husband's uncle, this author was pleasantly surprised by the assortment of Assyrian dishes prepared by the uncle's wife, who was born and raised in the United States. Some Assyrians also believe that consuming alcoholic beverages (especially wine) in moderation promotes good digestion and contributes to an overall sense of well-being.

Table 48-2 lists many of the popular folk-medicine practices in the form of dietary prescriptions. Because many Assyrians are devout Christians, their strong religious beliefs appear to play an important role in assisting them through the difficult moments in life, including recovery from illnesses.

GENERAL HEALTH AND NUTRITIONAL INDICATORS SUMMARY

Syria

Low birth weight, defined as weighing less than 2500 g at birth, affects 6% of newborns in Syria (UNICEF, 2007). Eighty-one percent of children are exclusively

TABLE 48-2   Assyrian Folk Remedies

Illness	Folk Remedy
Anemia	Red wine, charbroiled liver, spinach
Diarrhea	Caramelized sugar or rice and yogurt
Stomach ache	*Vishnoka* (distilled liquor) mixed with sour cherry stems or mint essence
Toothache	Crushed cloves placed around aching tooth
Tapeworm	Massive consumption of pumpkin seeds
Kidney stone	Dried and crushed corn husk mixed with water or beer
Gallbladder stone	Chicken gizzard
Antiseptic	Crushed alfalfa
Cough	Starch mixed with milk
Small bleeding cuts	Sprinkling powdered sugar on affected area
Jaundice	Eating raw fish
Sore throat	Crushed quince seeds or ginger powder mixed with sweet tea
Swollen tonsil	Gurgling *arak* (distilled liquor)
Eye irritation	Cold brewed tea used as eye wash
Constipation	Prunes, olive oil, or flaxseed oil
Baby colic	Crushed incense and crystalline sugar mixed with water
Prickly heat	Rubbing skin with the inside of watermelon rind

breastfed during the first 4 months of life. Fifty percent of infants 6–9 months are breastfed with complementary food and 6% remain breastfed at 20–23 months.

Seven percent of children under 5 years suffer from being moderately to severely underweight (UNICEF, 2007). Being severely underweight affects 1% of Syria's children. Moderate to severe wasting was found in 4% and stunting in 18% of this particular population. The majority (79%) of households in Syria consume adequately iodized salt.

Ninety-three percent of Syria's total population uses improved drinking-water sources (UNICEF, 2007). Specifically, 98% of the population in the nation's urban areas and 87% of the rural population has access to improved drinking-water sources.

Turkey

Turkey's population is about 72 million people (2008). Life expectancy at birth is 71.5 years. Turkey is the 17th

largest economy in the world. The nutritional status in Turkey has aspects that represent the problems of both developing and developed countries. There are considerable differences in nutritional status with respect to the regions, seasons, socioeconomic levels, and urban–rural residence. One of the main reasons is unequal income distribution. This situation has an effect on the degree of nutrition problems and frequency of occurrence. According to 2005 data, 0.87% of the Turkish population cannot afford a diet of 2100 calories/day. On the other hand, as they migrate from rural areas to urban areas, Turkish people are starting to change their eating habits. More processed, fast-food-type meals are commonly consumed, especially among young people. As a result, obesity, diabetes, and heart disease rates are increasing in Turkey.

Turkey's infant mortality rate is 22.6 per 1000 live births, and the under-5-years mortality rate is 25.1 per 1000 births (2006). In addition, 16% of infants are born with low birth weight (UNICEF, 2007). Lastly, 3.9% of children under 5 years are underweight (2003). Much of the infant and child mortality related to growth disorders is attributable to insufficient nutrition. Such preventable diseases are the result of insufficient protein, carbohydrate, vitamin, and mineral consumption.

The Turkish Ministry of Health offers free immunization programs (about 80% of the population receives this service). In recent years, with the encouragement of the Ministry of Health, all the salt sold in stores is iodized. Also, in some cities, Turkish bakers have started adding vitamins to their breads.

Table 48-3 lists the demographic and health indicators for Turkey.

Iran

According to UNICEF (2007), from 1998 to 2005, 7% of Iran's infants had low birth weight. This was similar to the United States, which had an 8% rate during the same period. In Iran, 44% of infants are exclusively breastfed for the first 6 months of life. The life expectancy of an Iranian is 71 years as of 2007. Ninety-four percent of the population consumes iodized salt. Moderate to severe underweight for children under 5 years is 11% (UNICEF, 2007).

Iraq

According to UNICEF (2007), 15% of Iraq's infants had low birth weight. In Iraq, 25% of infants are exclusively

TABLE 48-3   Demographic and Health Indicators for Turkey

Total population	71,517,100 (2008)
Life expectancy at birth (years)	71.5 (2006)
Birth rate/1000 population	18.7 (2006)
Crude death rate/1000 population	6.3 (2006)
Infant mortality rate/1000 live births	22.6 (2006)
Under-5-years mortality rate/1000 live births	25.1 (2006)
Maternal mortality ratio/100,000 live births	44 (2005)
Adult literacy rate > 15 years	88.1 (2006)
Human development index	0.798 (2006)

Data are from the Turkish Statistical Institute.

breastfed for the first 6 months of life. The life expectancy of an Iraqian is 67 years as of 2007. Seventy-seven percent of the population has improved drinking water. Moderate to severe underweight for children under 5 years is 8% (UNICEF, 2007).

COMMUNICATION AND COUNSELING TIPS

Assyrians have historically assimilated well into American society (Ishaya, 2003). One of their most remarkable characteristics is their sense of hospitality, in which they take pride. They are naturally warm and sociable toward both friends and strangers (Benjamin, 1996). Visiting back and forth between relatives and friends is frequent. No appointment is necessary for casual visits and the guest is always welcome in the home. Assyrians receive visitors with hugs and kisses of greeting. In their manners, the Assyrian people are frank and open; in their discourse, they are modest and reserved. Contrary to what has been reported with other Middle Easterners (Kittler & Sucher, 2001), they do not gesture with their hands or talk loudly (Benjamin, 1996).

Evidence suggests that effective nonverbal communication skills, such as using the right body language, can have an impact on the patient's satisfaction with the quality of care delivered (DiMatteo, Taranta, Friedman, & Prince, 1980). Facial expressions, such as smiling while talking and using a calm tone of voice, were considered by Syrian Muslim women to be expressions of a caring attitude (Wehbe-Alamah, 2006). It is logical to assume that these factors may positively affect a client's receptiveness to verbal information and help to establish trust with the client. Common courtesy, such as acknowledging one's arrival by greeting him or her at the door, and respecting people who are older, is closely observed among many cultures (Kittler & Sucher, 2001; Brannon, 2004), including Assyrian culture; hence, undue informality, such as calling an older client by his or her first name during the initial visit, may be considered rude. Bodily contact with members of the same gender, such as shaking hands or patting someone on the shoulder, are also quite common and may imply a sense of satisfaction and closeness. Men hug and kiss each other, as do women. Although awareness of the verbal and nonverbal cues, such as those described previously, are important for more effective communication, healthcare practitioners must avoid stereotyping clients by assuming that all Assyrians think or behave alike; hence, allowance needs to be made for individual differences such as variance in age, gender, education level, socioeconomic status, and time lapsed since migration to the United States (Harris-Davis & Haughton, 2000).

Acknowledging their origin and cultural heritage is very important to Assyrians, given that as religious and linguistic minorities in the Muslim countries they once inhabited, they were denied their Assyrian identity. For instance, in Iran, they were often grouped together with Armenians and collectively referred to as "Iranian Christians." In fact, even though this author was born and raised in Iran, and graduated from high school in Tehran, she had never heard of Assyrians as a distinct ethnic minority in Iran. There was no mention of them in history books, even though, based on ample evidence, they were indigenous to the northwestern part of the country (Ishaya, 1985, 2002). The situation of Iraqi and Syrian Assyrians, as well as those who migrated to the United States from other Arab countries, is similar, because they were often referred to as "Arab Christians," the term of choice by Arab nationalists (Lewis, 2003).

Given that family relations are extremely important to Assyrians, healthcare providers will do well in getting to know their clients and becoming familiar with their families. It is also advisable to begin counseling sessions by first seeking information about the well-being of the client as well as showing interest in their children, parents, and so on. It is not uncommon to encounter immediate family members, such as the husband or wife and adult children, or even extended family, accompanying the client to counseling sessions and getting involved in decision making regarding health care (Kittler & Sucher, 2001; Brannon, 2004). This phenomenon has been reported in other cultural groups as well. Showing empathy toward one's troubles and demonstrating a caring attitude is inherent to Assyrian culture. When appropriate, healthcare providers should attempt to imitate these behaviors. These counseling tips may be especially important when working with older Assyrian clients who have stronger ties to their heritage.

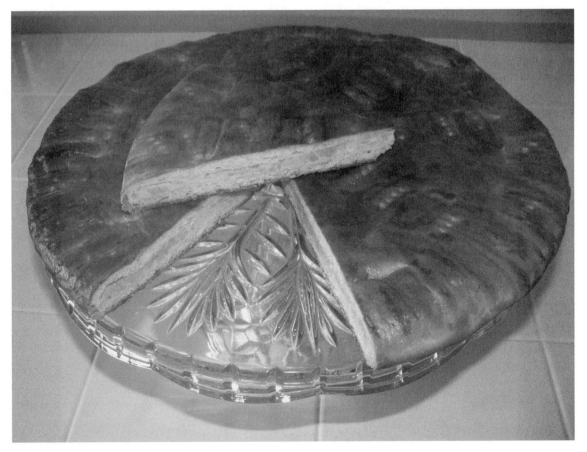

Kadeh
Courtesy of the author

FEATURED RECIPE

Kadeh (Butter Bread)

Dough:

1 lb. (4 sticks) butter, cut into small chunks

2 cups milk

7 cups flour

½ cup sugar

5 eggs

1 tbsp. baking powder

3 oz. baking yeast

Filling:

1 tbsp. salt

1½ lbs. butter (6 sticks)

7 cups flour

To prepare the dough:

1. In large bowl mix flour, salt, baking powder, and butter chunks. (This mixture will be referred to as the dry mixture.)
2. In a small bowl mix sugar and yeast, and let stand until yeast is activated.
3. Boil the milk and then cool it until lukewarm.
4. In a third bowl beat eggs thoroughly and then add the lukewarm milk to it.
5. Add the yeast–sugar mixture to the milk-and-egg mixture and blend thoroughly.
6. Pour the resulting liquid mix on the dry mixture and blend well.
7. Cover and let the dough mixture rise in a warm place for about 2 hours.
8. Knead the dough and let it rise again for an additional hour.
9. Divide the dough into five round balls. Let the dough balls rise for an additional 20 minutes.
10. To prepare the filling, slowly melt the butter and add flour while mixing constantly until the mixture starts to soften. (This should take about 40 minutes. The constant mixing ensures that the mixture does not burn.)
11. Sprinkle flour on a clean table or large cutting board and roll each ball into a strip about 20 inches long and 5 inches wide.
12. Spread 1 cup of filling on half of strip and fold the other half over to cover the filling. Firmly pinch edges together.
13. Roll out the resulting stuffed dough until it is in the shape of a thin cylinder (about ½ in. thick).
14. Brush beaten egg yolk on top. Use a fork or other utensil to prick the top of the kadeh. (This is done for esthetic reasons as well as to ensure that water vapor can safely escape from inner layers.)
15. Place on a cookie sheet and let rise for another 15 minutes.
16. Preheat oven to 400°F and bake for about 15 minutes on lowest rack and for an additional 15 minutes on highest rack (ensures that the top is browned).
17. Let it cool. Refrigerate for longer shelf life.

More recipes are available at http://nutrition.jbpub.com/foodculture/

ACKNOWLEDGMENTS

The author thanks Bateshva Eivaz, Dr. Edwin Ghahramani, and Bella Kamber for clarifications to this chapter.

REFERENCES

Abdalla, M. (1992). Bulgur: A key to contemporary Assyrian cuisine. *Journal of Assyrian Academic Society, 6*(1), 3–17.

Abdalla, M. (1996). The evolution of Assyrian traditional culinary practices. *Journal of the Assyrian Academic Society, 10*(1), 19–26.

Abdalla, M. (2004). Wild growing plants in the cuisine of modern Assyrians in the eastern Syrian–Turkish borderland. *Journal of the Assyrian Academic Society, 18*(2), 50–58.

Aprim, F.A. (2003). *Indigenous people in distress.* Retrieved February 14, 2008, from http://www.nineveh.com/Indigenous PeopleinDistress.html/

Aprim, F.A. (2007a). *Assyrians: From Bedr Khan to Saddam Hussein.* Verdugo City, CA: Pearlida.

Aprim, F.A. (2007b). *Who are Assyrians?* Retrieved February 10, 2008, from http://www.fredaprim.com/who_assyrians. php/

Aprim, F.A. (n.d.a). *The Assyrians of San Joaquin valley: From early settlements to the present.* Retrieved February 14, 2008, from http://www.nineveh.com/The%20Assyrians%20of% 20the%20San%20Joaquin%20Valley,%20California.html/

Aprim, F.A. (n.d.b). *Food and diet in Assyria.* Retrieved February 20, 2008, from http://www.nineveh.com/Food%20 and%20Diet%20in%20Assyria.html/

Assyrian International News Agency. (n.d.). *Assyrians of Chicago.* Retrieved February 9, 2008, from www.aina.org/

Baumer, C. (2006). *The church of the east: An illustrated history of Assyrian Christianity.* London: I.B. Tauris.

Benjamin, Y. (1996). Assyrians in Middle America: A historical and demographic study of the Chicago Assyrian community. *Journal of Assyrian Academic Society, 10*(2), 18–46.

Benjamin, Y. (n.d.). *Assyrian rituals of life-cycle events.* Retrieved February 14, 2008, from http://www.aina.org/articles/yoab. htm/

Bertman, S. (2005). *Handbook to life in Mesopotamia.* New York: Oxford University Press.

BetBasoo, P. (2006). *Brief history of Assyrians.* Retrieved February 10, 2008, from http://www.aina.org/aol/peter/brief. htm/

Brannon, C. (2004). Cultural competency: Values, traditions, and effective practice. *Today's Dietitian, 6*(11), 14–20.

David, H. (2004). Vegetables, fruits and phytoestrogens in the prevention of diseases. *Journal of Postgraduate Medicine, 50*(2), 145–149.

DiMatteo, M.R., Taranta, A., Friedman, H.S., & Prince, L.M. (1980). Predicting patient satisfaction from physicians' non-verbal communication skills. *Medical Care, 18*(4), 376–387.

Harris-Davis, E., & Haughton, B. (2000). Model for multicultural nutrition counseling competencies. *Journal of the American Dietetic Association, 100*(10), 1178–1185.

Hooker, R. (1996). *Mesopotamia: The Assyrians.* Retrieved February 10, 2008, from http://www.wsu.edu/~dee/meso/ assyria.htm/

Huffnagle, G.B., & Wernick, S. (2007). *The probiotics revolution: The definitive guide to safe, natural health solutions using probiotic and prebiotic foods and supplements.* New York: Bantam.

Ishaya, A. (1985). Family and household composition among the Assyrians of Iran: The past and the present. In A. Fathi (Ed.), *Women and the family in Iran* (pp. 212–225). Leiden, Netherlands: E.J. Brill.

Ishaya, A. (2002). From contributions to diaspora: Assyrians in the history of Urmia, Iran. *Journal of the Assyrian Academic Society, 16*(1), 25–41.

Ishaya, A. (2003). *Assyrian Americans: A study in ethnic restructuring and dissolution in diaspora.* Retrieved February 21, 2008, from http://www.nineveh.com/ASSYRIAN-AMERICANS.html/

Jemal, A., Siegel, R., Ward, E., Murray, T., & Jiaquan Xu, C. (2006). Cancer statistics, 2006. *Cancer Journal for Clinicians, 56,* 106–130.

Kawamori, T., Lubet, R., Steele, V.E., Kelloff, G.J., Kaskey, R.B., & Rao, C.V. (1999). Chemopreventive effect of curcumin, a naturally occuring anti-inflammatory agent, during the promotion/progression stages of colon cancer. *Cancer Research, 59,* 597–601.

Kittler, P.G., & Sucher, K.P. (2001). *Food and culture.* Belmont, CA: Wadsworth/Thomson Learning.

Kris-Etherton, P.M., & Keen, C.L. (2002). Evidence that the antioxidant flavonoids in tea and cocoa are beneficial for cardiovascular health. *Current Opinions in Lipidiology, 13,* 41–49.

Kuhrt, A. (1995). *The Ancient Near East: C. 3000–330 B.C.* London: Taylor and Francis.

Lewis, E.L. (2003). Iraqi Assyrians: Barometer of pluralism. *Middle East Quarterly, 10*(3), 1–4.

Majamaa, H., & Isolauri, E. (1997). Probiotics: A novel approach in the management of food allergy. *Journal of Allergy and Clinical Immunology, 99,* 179–185.

McWilliams, M. (2005). *Foods: Experimental perpective* (5th ed.). Upper Saddle River, NJ: Prentice-Hall.

Mohandas, K.M., & Desai, D.C. (1999). Epidemiology of digestive tract cancers in India: Large and small bowel. *Indian Journal of Gasteroenterology, 18*(3), 118–121.

Nickles, H.G. (1973). *Middle Eastern cooking.* New York: Time Life Books.

Parpola, S. (1999). *Assyrians after Assyria.* Retrieved February 12, 2008, from http://www.nineveh.com/Assyrians%20 after%20Assyria.html/

Parpola, S. (2004). National and ethnic identity in the neo-Assyrian empire and Assyrian identity in post-empire times. *Journal of Assyrian Academic Society, 18*(2), 5–22.

Price, K.R., Lewis, J., Wyatt, G.M., & Fenwick, G.R. (1988). Flatulence: Causes, relation to diet, and remedies. *Nahrung/ Food, 32*(6), 609–626.

Riemersma, R.A., Rice-Evans, C.A., Tyrrell, R.M., & Clifford, M.N. (2001). Tea flavonoids and cardiovascular health. *Quarterly Journal of Medicine, 94,* 277–282.

Saggs, H.W.F. (1965). *Everyday life in Babylonia and Assyria.* Retrieved February 5, 2008, from http://www.aina.org/books/eliba/eliba.htm/

Saggs, H.W.F. (1984). *The might that was Assyria.* London: Sidgwick & Jackson Ltd.

Sat, I.G., & Keles, F. (2002). The effect of soaking and cooking on the oligosaccharide content of sekera dry bean variety (*P. vulgaris, L*) grown in Turkey. *Pakistan Journal of Nutrition, 1*(5), 206–208.

Segall, J.J. (1997). Epidemiological evidence for the link between dietary lactose and atherosclerosis. In C.A.L.S. Colaco (Ed.), *The glycation hypothesis of atherosclerosis* (pp. 185–209). Austin, TX: Landes Bioscience.

Stafford, R.S. (1935). *The tragedy of the Assyrians.* Retrieved February 8, 2008, from http://www.aina.org/books/tota.htm/

Stangl V., Lorenz M., & Stangl K. (2006). The role of tea and tea flavonoids in cardiovascular health. *Molecular Nutrition & Food Research, 50*(2), 218–228.

Talia, P. (1980). *Our yesterday, today and tomorrow: History, dilemma, and destiny of the Assyrian people.* Chicago: Covenant Publications.

Turkish Statistical Institute. (2008). *Statistics.* Retrieved February 16, 2010, from http://www.turkstat.gov.tv

UNICEF. (2007). *The state of the world's children 2007: Women and children, the double dividend of gender equality.* Retrieved April 14, 2009, from http://www.unicef.org/sowc07/statistics/tables.php

Vidal-Valverde, C., Frias, J., & Valverde, S. (1993). Changes in the carbohydrate composition of legumes after soaking and cooking. *Journal of the American Dietetic Association, 93*(5), 547–550.

Vita, J.A. (2005). Polyphenols and cardiovascular disease: Effects on endothelial and platelet function. *American Journal of Clinical Nutrition, 81*(Suppl), 292S–297S.

Wehbe-Alamah, H. (2006). Generic and professional health care beliefs, expressions and practices of Syrian Muslims living in the United States. *Dissertation Abstracts International, 66*(11), 5908 (UMI No. 3197399).

Whitney, E., & Rolfes, S.R. (2008). *Understanding nutrition* (11th ed.). Belmont, CA: Wadsworth/Thomson Learning.

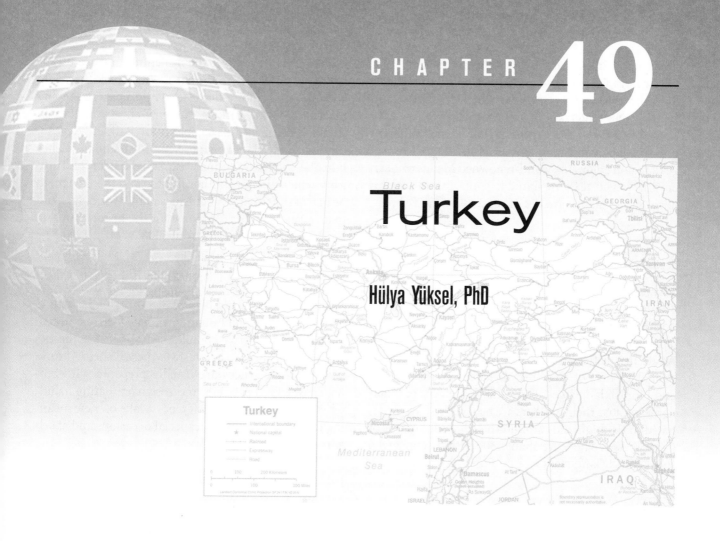

CHAPTER 49

Turkey

Hülya Yüksel, PhD

 CULTURE AND WORLD REGION

Turkish culture is diverse and fascinating. The majority of the population is Muslim, with small numbers of Christian Armenians and Jews. There are many other ethnic groups, such as the Laz, Cerkez, Bosnak, Arnavut, and Kurds, that are interrelated because they have been cohabitating the region for centuries. As a result, their folk dances, music, and food customs are similar.

Turkey bridges two continents of the East and West (Asia and Europe, respectively) at the crossroads of three continents (Europe, Asia, and Africa). The European part of the country is called Trakya (Thrace) and the Asian part is known as Anatolia or Asia Minor. Turkey is bordered to the northwest by Greece and Bulgaria, to the east by the relatively new republics of Georgia, Armenia, and Azerbaijan (part of the former Soviet Union), as well as Iran, and to the south by Iraq and Syria.

Because of its geographical location, the mainland of Anatolia has been the birthplace of many great civilizations. Turkey is a land of myth, a cradle of various civilizations, a cornucopia of nature's bounties, and a confluence of varied streams of culture. Owing to its strategic position, it has long been prominent as a center of commerce due to its land connections to three continents and the sea surrounding it on three sides.

Turkey is divided into seven regions based on climate and geographical characteristics. Although there are unifying underlying themes, each region has its own food culture, folk dances, and costumes. For instance, the central, eastern, and southeastern parts of Turkey are famous for oily and spicy meat dishes, kebabs, and dishes made with grains and legumes (beans, lentils, and chickpeas). The Black Sea region is known for dishes made with anchovies and corn. In the Marmara, Aegean, and Mediterranean regions, more greens, vegetable dishes, dishes made with grains, legumes, beans, fish, olive oil, lemon juice, yogurt, and feta cheese are used. There are, however, many foods common to all regional kitchens. Central Anatolia, with 455 different foods and drinks, is at the top of the list. Eastern Anatolia comes in second with 425 varieties of food, followed by southeastern Anatolia, with 397 different food types. The Mediterranean and Marmara regions have 184 types. Finally, the Aegean region has 162 different types of foods and beverages (Meral, 2008). The Aegean region enjoys the world-renowned Mediterranean cuisine, which uses an abundance of olive oil, lemon juice, garlic, many varieties of vegetables, and fish.

LANGUAGE

Turkish is the official language of the country, but there are also about 40 other languages spoken by ethnic minorities. The Turkish language is not an Indo-European language; it belongs to the Altaic branch of the Ural-Altaic linguistic family. Its grammatical structure is related to that of the Korean, Japanese, Mongolian, and Finnish languages. The Altaic languages get their name because their speakers are believed to have originated in the highlands around the Altai Mountains of Central Asia. There are about 150 million people who speak Turkic languages around the world.

CULTURE HISTORY

Turkish culture is a rich amalgam of elements fused through its long history. The original homeland of the Turks is Central Asia, bordering China. They migrated westward more than a thousand years ago. Along the way to Asia Minor, the Turks have interacted with Chinese, Indian, Middle Eastern, European, and earlier Anatolian civilizations. Today's Turkish culture interweaves motifs from each of these diverse cultures.

For centuries, Anatolia has hosted a succession of civilizations, from the Hittites, Phrygians, Greeks, and Romans, to the Byzantine, Seljuk, and Ottoman empires, and today's Turkish Republic. Catal Huyuk in Anatolia was one of the first towns ever built. There is evidence of agricultural settlement in Asia Minor dating back to 5700 BC.

FOOD HISTORY WITHIN THE CULTURE

The splendid diversity of Turkish cuisine is attributable to several factors. The variety of natural products offered by the land and sea, interchanges among numerous cultures over the millennia, and the inventive styles developed in the palace kitchens of the Seljuk and Ottoman empires have all played a part in shaping the character of Turkish culinary culture. Ottoman palace cuisine blends elements of Balkan, Aegean, Caucasian, Syrian–Lebanese, and Anatolian dishes into one pot. Many culinary experts consider the Turkish kitchen, along with the Chinese and the French, to be one of the three great cuisines of the world. It is said that travelers in Turkey "come for the history but stay for the food" (Turkey For You, 2008).

Turkish cuisine comprises dishes prepared with cereals, various vegetables and some meat, soups, cold dishes cooked with olive oil, pastry dishes, and dishes made from wild plants. Healthful foods, such as *pekmez*, yogurt, and bulgur, originated there. Turkish cuisine does not have complex sauces because there is no need for sauces to add taste to these dishes (Akturk, 2005). Simple sauces are usually prepared with butter, crushed red peppers, and rosemary. Eating habits, which reflect regional preferences, take on new meaning (and even sanctity) on special occasions and at celebrations and ceremonies.

The variety and savor of Turkish cuisine offer a paradigm for healthy and balanced diets with a profusion of vegetarian dishes. Maria Yordanidu, a Greek writer from Istanbul, claims that Easterners (including the Chinese) value food greatly. She gives the following example: "Confucius divorced his wife because she was not able to cook the rice well and cut the meat thinly. When he married again he married to a good cook. He had said our destiny is not in the hand of gods but in the hands of women who cook our food." (Savkay, 2000).

In Turkish culture, eating is far more than merely filling the stomach. It has profound social significance. Turkish people socialize around big family dinners, wedding feasts, and special meals during the religious holidays such as Ramadan (the month of fasting in Islamic tradition). Food has been a way of creating and fostering relationships. Especially in rural areas, among traditional families, the head of the household (the father) sits at an honored place at the dinner table (usually on the floor, around a big round tray) and all the family members eat from the same dish. The best part of the food (meat) is offered to the head of the household. In big cities, the entire family gets together around the dinner table in the evenings. The Prophet Mohammed enjoined the faithful to "Eat the family meals together with the whole family, because they bring prosperity to the whole family." (Republic of Turkey Ministry of Culture and Tourism, 2008).

Wedding feasts have special importance in Turkish culture; to a lesser extent, so do circumcision celebrations. The food offered at wedding feasts is meant to show the social status and prestige of the host. (Less affluent people can only afford humble wedding meals.) Dishes made with meat would be the most valued food on the table. Also, there would be some typical regional specialties. The month of Ramadan, the holiest period for the Islamic faith, is very important in Turkish cuisine and is known as the sultan of the year.

The Ottoman Imperial Kitchen has greatly influenced Turkish cuisine. The capital city of Istanbul was the center of this elaborate cuisine. The staples of Ottoman cuisine were wheat, flour, meat (lamb, mutton, beef, chicken), rice, butter, olive oil, and sugar, as well as fruits, vegetables, milk and milk products, and spices (Bilgin, 2004); however, with globalization and industrialization, food culture has been changing from more traditional dishes to more fast food, especially in large cities among young people.

The Ottoman Empire was very wealthy at the time of the discovery of the New World. As a result, the Ottomans were introduced to new crops such as green peppers, zucchini, corn, green beans, tomatoes, and potatoes before many European countries adopted them. (Previously, meat, yogurt, and grains were the staples of the Turkish diet) (Unsal, 2004). An important characteristic of eastern Mediterranean cooking is that meat is eaten sparingly or not at all. Varieties of vegetables, spices, and oil are brought together to cook delicious meatless dishes. Another important characteristic of this cuisine is a wood-fire stone oven that is used to cook meat, bread, and other pastries. Also, copper pans are commonly used, although these days they are being replaced with steel pans.

Islam, because it forbids consumption of pork and alcohol (also in cooking), has naturally had some influence on Turkish cuisine, which used milk, dairy products, and other meats. Traditionally, Turkish people ate more meat in Central Asia, but when they migrated to Anatolia fresh vegetables and legumes became more prominent in Turkish cuisine. Meat was expensive and used sparingly in vegetable stews. Turkish cuisine values vegetables and legumes. In the past, another important characteristic of Turkish cuisine was that everything was cooked in its season (Savkay, 2000); however, in today's food markets (bazaar), people can find summer vegetables all winter long.

Reform movements in the 19th century resulted in modernization in many areas of Ottoman culture and government. Turkish cuisine has also been influenced widely by Western culinary traditions, especially the French. In the 21st century, the impact of globalization, modernization, industrialization, urbanization, and women's participation in the business world have shortened the time spent in the kitchen. In luxurious

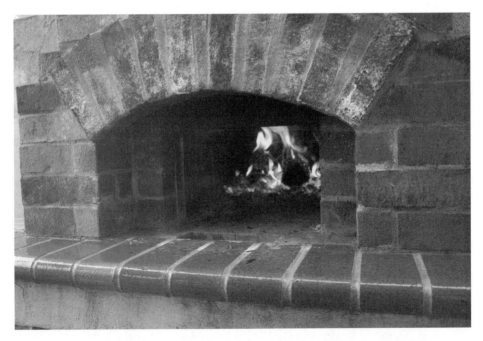

A wood-fired stone oven is often used to cook meat, bread, and other pastries.

restaurants in big cities, the influence of French, Italian, Chinese, Japanese, and Mexican cuisines has increased. Turkish people are starting to eat fast food more often, especially in big cities, where going to McDonald's or Burger King is fashionable among kids and young adults. Turkish *pide* (grilled flatbread with meat or cheese) is being replaced with pizza and hamburger shops; simultaneously however, the growing movement toward a healthier diet is driving urban restaurants to cook more traditional home-style dishes.

In summary, the hallmarks of Turkish cuisine include healthy ingredients, simple cooking techniques, and openness to innovation.

 MAJOR FOODS

 Protein Sources

Meat (mutton, lamb, beef) is fundamental to Turkish cuisine, because animal husbandry has always had economic value in the culture. Lamb and mutton are especially favored, with spit-roasted and grilled meat being characteristic of the cuisine. Eating liver, kidney, and brain is popular among many people. There is also *kokoreç*, a Turkish dish of Balkan origin, made of skewered lamb intestines. It is sold by street vendors and also served in some specialized restaurants.

All types of legumes are used at almost every meal, among them white beans, chickpeas, and lentils (orange, yellow, green). Grains, such as wheat, bulgur (cooked, then dried and crushed wheat), as well as dairy products, feta cheese, yogurt, and eggs, are also major protein sources in the Turkish diet. Yogurt, a Turkish invention, plays a central role in the Turkish kitchen.

 Starch Sources

According to the *Guinness Book of World Records* in 2007, Turkey is the highest consumer of bread in the world, with 200 kg of bread per person eaten annually. Also, rice pilaf, pastas, *eriste* (homemade pasta), couscous, and *börek* (filo dough stuffed with vegetables or meat) are often found on the everyday menu. *Simit*, a circular bread with sesame seeds, is so popular in Turkey that many people eat it for breakfast, lunch, and as a snack. In addition, varieties of pastries are esteemed.

 Fat Sources

With regard to fat sources, olive oil has, throughout the centuries, largely replaced the butter once used by the nomadic Turks. Olive oil is used mostly for salads everywhere in Turkey; however, it is the principal fat used for cooking in the Aegean, Marmara, and Medi-

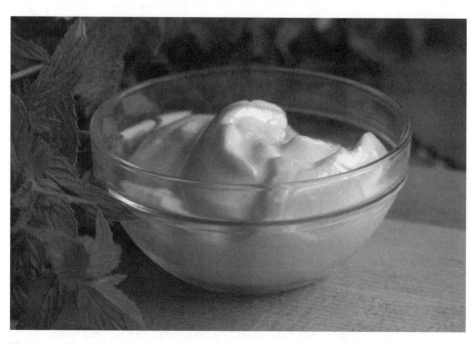

Yogurt, a Turkish invention, has a central role in the Turkish kitchen.

terranean regions. Vegetable oils (sunflower seed oil, corn oil), butter, and margarines are widely used. Also, the tail fat of sheep is used for kebabs and for some pastries.

 Prominent Vegetables

Fresh fruits and vegetables, grown in abundance, are consumed in great quantities (fresh in season and dried in winter). The following are the commonly used vegetables: onion, tomato, garlic, spinach, cauliflower, leek, lettuce, parsley, arugula, carrot, turnip (white, black, red), scallion, red cabbage, white cabbage, cucumber, green and red peppers, eggplant, zucchini, green bean, celery, okra, fava bean, artichoke, and broccoli.

Summer vegetables are preserved for winter use, pickled in salt and vinegar. Also, tomatoes, peppers, green beans, zucchinis, and eggplants are sun-dried. Tomatoes are consumed by the kilo during the summer in every household in Turkey. Families in rural areas prepare tomato paste in large amounts for the winter. People who live in cities usually buy commercial tomato paste.

 Prominent Fruits

Turkey grows almost all the fruits, except the tropical ones. Apples, oranges, cherries, sour cherries, tangerines, oranges, strawberries, blackberries, plums (red, green, yellow), pears, mulberries, pomegranates, persimmons, dates, figs, apricots, peaches, grapes (red, yellow), watermelon, honeydew, bananas, kiwi, and quince are popular.

During the summer these fruits are eaten fresh or as compotes. In winter they are canned, dried, and made into jams. Raisins, dried apricots, figs, and currants are also valued in Turkish cuisine.

 Spices and Seasoning

The most commonly used seasonings and condiments are cinnamon, cumin, coriander, dill, garlic, mint, thyme, saffron, mustard, onions, and parsley. Sumac (a sour spice), chili peppers, sesame seeds, cinnamon, clove, Damascus fennel flower, and yogurt are often served as side condiments.

 Beverages

In terms of beverages, Turkish people consume mainly fruit compotes (e.g., sour cherry, apple, apricot, quince), sherbet (infusions, unfermented grape juice, rose-leaf sherbet), and *ayran* (a yogurt drink) as beverages.

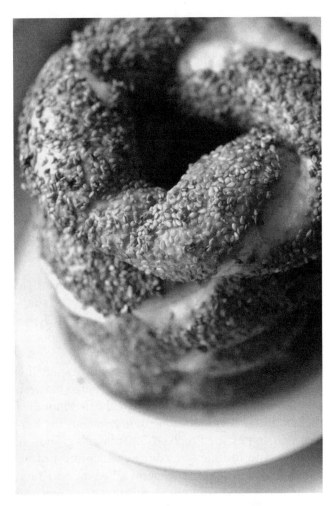

Simit, a circular bread with sesame seeds, is so popular in Turkey that many people eat this for breakfast, lunch, or snacks.

Turkish coffee and black tea (*çay*) are the most valued drinks in Turkish culture. They are always part of every ritual. During winter some people drink herbal teas made of linden, chamomile, mint, lemon, or sage. In some regions, turnip juice is widely consumed, especially with kebabs. *Salep* is another traditional drink for winter months. It is prepared from the root of an orchid with milk and sugar, topped with cinnamon. It is believed to help with coughs and sore throat during winter. In the past 20 years, carbonated drinks have entered the list of beverages.

 Desserts

The Turkish people are known for their love of desserts. There are even sayings such as "Let's eat dessert so we can talk sweetly." Dessert is always associated with positive things in Turkish culture: it brings people together and helps them mingle. When people think about dessert in Turkey, baklava is the first one that comes to mind. Although every region has this dessert, the southeastern city of Gaziantep is famous for its baklava.

Dinners typically end with a beautifully presented selection of seasonal fruits. Grape syrup and all kinds of nuts, especially almonds, hazelnuts, and pistachios, are considered essential when preparing desserts. Rose water is also added to some desserts with syrup. Traditional Turkish sweets, such as *lokum* (Turkish delight), baklava, *kadayif*, halva, or rice pudding, conclude the meal during holidays or special gatherings. Right after dessert, demitasse cups of strong Turkish coffee are offered.

Pekmez (made with all kinds of grapes without adding any sugar), which is similar to molasses, is consumed commonly especially during winter. It is believed to provide heat for cold winter days. *Pekmez* is also given to people who are anemic.

Asure is a dessert with religious significance. It is a ceremonial sweet that is generally prepared between the 10th and 20th days of Muharrem, the first month of the lunar year. This occasion commemorates the Kerbela uprising by the Prophet Mohammad's grandson, Hussein, and his followers, during which most of his family members and friends were killed by the Khalif of the time, Yazid. Tradition holds that *asure* was also the last meal prepared on Noah's Ark at the end of the flood. It contained 40 different ingredients, the final remnants of the supplies. During the month of *Asure*, every family makes its own *asure* and distributes it to neighbors, relatives, and friends.

The confection called *halva* also has religious and ceremonial significance. When someone dies, halva is distributed to relatives, acquaintances, and neighbors. Halva is also cooked as an offering to God.

FOODS WITH CULTURAL SIGNIFICANCE

The beginning of spring (Nevruz, March 21) and the beginning of summer (Hıdırellez, May 6) are celebrated in Turkey. During the Hıdırellez celebration, most people in Turkey go on picnics. In general, Turkish people love picnics by the rivers or any green area. They especially like to have barbecues (*mangal*) with lamb meat, meat balls, and sausage, but they would also be happy with tomatoes, green peppers, feta cheese, hard-boiled eggs, watermelon, and white bread (French bread). In some areas there is a tradition of eating eggs, pilaf, rice pudding, and yogurt.

According to Turkish tradition, everything starts with eating sweets. At birth, a baby is welcomed with halva (although this tradition is vanishing). When someone dies, halva is made again for the farewell. When a woman gives birth, very sweet fruit infusions (sherbet) are made, often with cinnamon sticks, cloves, and ginger added. Friends, relatives, and neighbors visit women who have given birth, and bring soup, milk, yogurt, and eggs. Guests are also served sherbet, biscuits, milk, and deserts. It is believed that a woman who has given birth must have milk, onion, sherbet, wheat, and lentils, and must not eat chickpeas, beans, or drink cold water if she wants to have sufficient milk to feed her child.

In addition, at other significant events, such as weddings, circumcisions, and engagement ceremonies, dessert is always offered. For the Muslim feast of Kandil, halva, *lokma* (dessert made with flour and fried in oil and soaked in syrup), and baklava are customary. In a house of mourning, food is not cooked for 3–7 days (depending on the region), and neighbors bring food to the grieving family. Serving food on the 3rd, 7th, 40th, and 52nd days after death still continues. *Lokma* is commonly made on the 7th day after someone dies, for remembrance. *Lokma* is considered to be the seal of the Prophet Mohammed.

At weddings and circumcision ceremonies, rice, vegetables, green beans, okra, and fruit compote (made as *ayran*) are served. In almost every region, *keskek* (pounded wheat with meat), rice, and meat are served at weddings. Desserts are usually halva, rice pudding, and baklava.

 ## TYPICAL DAY'S MENU

Soups, served as starters in Turkish cuisine, are among the most important foods. They are usually served hot, but in some regions there are also cold soups for the summer season. *Tarhana* is one of the distinctive Turkish soups. *Tarhana* is usually prepared during the summer from tomatoes, chickpeas, yogurt, and red peppers, and is sun-dried for the winter. It takes about a week to prepare this healthy soup, for which almost every region in Turkey has a variation.

In a typical day's menu, vegetable dishes are central, particularly green beans, *turlu* (a mix of six or seven different vegetables), eggplant, and okra. Rice or bulgur pilaf, couscous, or *eriste* (noodles) are usually served with vegetable dishes.

Side dishes and salads made with tomatoes, cucumbers, onions, green peppers, arugula, lettuce, and parsley are very common. *Ayran* and *cacik* (made with cucumber, yogurt, and garlic) are also very popular. During winter pickled vegetables are usually served. (People still make their own pickles, even in the big cities.) There are special stores that sell all sorts of vegetable juices and pickling supplies.

During winter a dish composed of white beans with olive oil or meat is highly esteemed in Turkey. It is usually eaten with bulgur or rice pilaf and pickled vegetables.

The breakfast menu is also very distinctive in Turkish cuisine. Especially during the summer, fresh tomatoes, cucumbers, and green peppers are part of the morning meal. Also, green and black olives as well as feta cheese are mandatory for a Turkish breakfast. Homemade jams (apricot, sour cherries), honey, *pekmez* (grape molasses), butter, eggs, and *sucuk* (Turkish sausage) are also part of the sumptuous Turkish breakfast menu.

 ## HOLIDAY MENUS

Month of Ramadan

The month of Ramadan is a holy month. All month long, relatives and friends get together after sundown around amply supplied dinner tables. Foods associated with breakfast are served as the first course (small samples of cheese, jams, olives, and dates). Then soup (e.g., wedding soup, yogurt soup, *tarhana*), a main dish (usually with some meat in it), vegetable dishes, salads, other side dishes, and of course baklava and other types of dessert are served. The second Ramadan meal is served before sunrise (when fasting begins). This meal is designed to be filling but not thirst-inducing, because no food or beverage may be consumed during the day.

An important Turkish dish is *dolma* (stuffed vegetables), especially *dolma* made with grape leaves, which is served for holidays. Vegetables are stuffed with bulgur, rice, meat, hazelnuts, pistachios, and spices. *Dolma* is a Turkish word, which indicates that these delicacies

became well-known from the Balkans to North Africa during Ottoman rule. *Dolma* is usually made for special occasions only, because it takes such a long time to prepare.

New Year's Eve is also celebrated in Turkey, but very religious people usually do not observe it. People who are more secular celebrate by eating big dinners with family or going out to restaurants or hotels.

 ## HEALTH BELIEFS AND CONCERNS

Turkish people classify diseases on the basis of a cold-and-hot dichotomy (Türkdoğan, 1991). When people get sick due to cold, flu, pneumonia, or bronchitis, warm food is consumed. Drinking cold water is discouraged. For people who suffer from respiratory complaints, rest, to sweat under thick blankets and covers, and to drink linden tea and hot soups would be recommended. On the other hand, when people have fever, they should drink *ayran*.

Turkish people also believe in the evil eye. People who have blue eyes are believed to have the power to bewitch those around them. The characteristic blue glass amulet in the shape of an eye is used for protection of goods, property, and animals against this malignant influence. Another measure taken against the evil eye includes the use of talismans such as the *muska* (a necklace that contains hidden prayers). To avert the evil eye, some Turks pour molten lead, toss salt, and burn incense.

In Turkish culture some foods are used for healing. People with high blood pressure should eat garlic. On the other hand, when someone suffers from low blood pressure, *ayran* (the salty yogurt drink) is recommended. Mint and lemon teas are recommended for colds. The 11th-century Turkish writer Yusuf Has Hacip had some health recommendations for food and drinks which have been translated below:

If you feel thirsty because you have eaten hot food, drink cold beverages. If cold is felt heavily then it should be balanced with heat. If you are

Observations from the Author (Hülya Yüksel)

When I started living in the United States, I was shocked by the amount of ice served in water glasses and soft drinks. Most Turkish people would believe that they would get a sore throat if they drank iced beverages. Also, I found that everything had high-fructose corn syrup, even the pickled vegetables. For Turkish people this would be unacceptable, because if something is expected to be salty and sour, then it should be that way, not sweet. Turkish people do not like to mix salty and sweet tastes together.

young, eat cold things because your blood will warm it up. But if you are over sixty, you are to stay away from cold food in winter. If you have eaten a lot of cold and dry food, eat hot and raw food to balance it. If your nature is hot then strengthen your body with cold. By the same token, if your body type is cold, balance it with hot food. If a person wants to be healthy s/he should eat in moderation and live that way.

GENERAL HEALTH AND NUTRITION INDICATORS SUMMARY

Sixteen percent of Turkish infants are born with low birth weight, with 21% of infants 6 months or younger exclusively breastfed. Four percent of children younger than 5 years suffer from moderate to severe underweight, and only 64% use iodized salt. Ninety-six percent of the population has improved drinking water. Life expectancy in Turkey is to age 70. Vitamin A and D deficiencies are noted (UNICEF, 2007).

COMMUNICATION AND COUNSELING TIPS

Turkish people are famous for their warm hospitality. When one travels in Turkey, one will always find friendly people trying to help. People love to offer Turkish coffee and tea. Refusing these refreshments can be offensive. There is a saying in Turkish (*Bir fincan kahvenin 40 yıl hatırı vardır*) that means that the memory of a cup of coffee lasts 40 years. This means that if you offer coffee to someone, you will be friends for 40 years.

If you are invited for a meal in a Turkish house, you can thank the host by saying *eline saglık* (literally translated as "health to your hands"). The lady would reply by saying *afiyet olsun!* This term is similar to the French *bon appétit*.

PRIMARY LANGUAGE OF FOOD NAMES WITH ENGLISH AND PHONETIC TRANSLATION

Turkish is a phonetic language and simple to pronounce, because it is pronounced as it is written. Table 49-1 lists the primary language of food names with English and phonetic translation.

TABLE 49-1 Primary Language of Food Names with English and Phonetic Translation

Turkish	English	Phonetic Translation
Çorba	Soup	Chor-ba
Pilav	Pilaf	Pilaf
Dolma	Dholma	Dholma
Sarma	Sarma	Sarma (a or a short, as in "ant")
Baklava	Baklava	Baklava
Taze Fasulye	Green beans	Taze fasulye

FEATURED RECIPE

Yayla Çorbası

6 cups chicken or beef broth

1 tbsp. flour

1½ tbsp. rice

2 cups yogurt

1 egg

1 tsp. crushed mint

Salt

1. Bring chicken broth to boil, then add the rice.
2. In another cup mix the egg, yogurt, and flour.
3. Add some of the boiling chicken broth to this mixture.
4. Slowly add the mixture to the boiling soup. Serve with the mint.

More recipes are available at http://nutrition.jbpub.com/foodculture/

REFERENCES

Akturk, A.I. (2005). *Osmanli mutfagi: Turabi efendi*. Istanbul, Turkey: Donence.

Ardakoc, B. (2003). *Seçme Türk yemekleri*. Istanbul, Turkey: Geçit Kitabevi.

Bilgin, A. (2004). *Osmanlı saray mutfağı*. Istanbul, Turkey: Kitabevi.

Glenday, C. (2010). *Guinness World Records*. New York: Guinness Media, Inc.

Meral, B. (2008). *Hangi ilin ne yemegi meshur*. Retrieved January 20, 2010, from http://www.e-hayat.net/hangi-ilin-ne-yemegi-meshur/

Republic of Turkey Ministry of Culture and Tourism. (2008). *The Ottoman cuisine*. Retrieved December 7, 2010, from www.turizm.gov.tr/EN/Genel/t.ashx?17A16AE30572D313 1055CFC3A8A961D4D157CB4DF4A46466

Savkay, T. (2000). *Osmanlı mutfagı*. Istanbul, Turkey: Sekerbank.

Toygar, K. (1994). *Turk mutfak kulturu uzerine arastirmalar: Geleneksel ekmekcilik hamurisi yemekler*. Ankara, Turkey: Ankara Universitesi Basimevi.

Türkdoğan, O. (1991). *Kultur ve saglik hastalik sistemi*. Ankara, Turkey: Milli Egitim Basimevi, Bilim ve Kultur Eserleri Dizisi 522, Arastirma-Inceleme Dizisi 17.

Turkey For You (2008). *Turkish food*. Retrieved December 7, 2010, from http://www.turkeyforyou.com/travel_turkey_turkish_food/

UNICEF (2007). Turkey Statistics. Retrieved December 7, 2010, from http://www.unicef.org/infobycountry/Turkey_statistics.html?q=printme#0

Unsal, A.T. (2004). Ayintab'tan gaziantep'e yeme icme. Istanbul, Turkey: Iletisim.

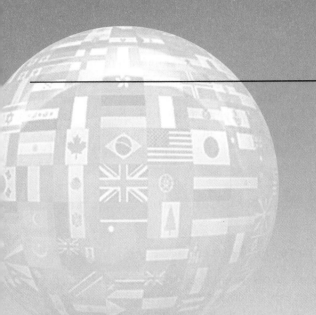

CHAPTER 50

Bilad Al Sham

(Syria, Lebanon, Jordan, and Palestine)

Roula Barake, MSc, PhD Candidate

CULTURE AND WORLD REGION

"Bilad Al Sham" was a term used by historians before the 20th century to describe "Greater Syria." Although the term "Levant" was also used to describe the same area, it is not a very precise synonym because it tends to describe a much larger area geographically. In this chapter we refer to Syria, Lebanon, Jordan, and Palestine as "Bilad Al Sham," because these countries share a common culture, cuisine, and economy, although actually the term is no longer used because each country/territory is now independent.

Bilad Al Sham is located on the eastern Mediterranean coast, covering a wide range of coastal cities, rugged mountains, fertile valleys, and deserts. The climate ranges from the pleasant Mediterranean mild climate, to snow-capped mountains, to sizzling-hot desert. Water resources come from a number of small rivers in Lebanon, Syria, Palestine, and the only river in Jordan, the Jordan River. Artificial lakes and dams were also constructed; rainfall is an additional minor source, which limits agricultural activities in desert areas.

LANGUAGE

Although Arabic is the official spoken language, English, French, and Armenian are widely spoken in this region. Classical Arabic is taught at schools along with the aforementioned languages, and is used in official written communications; however, spoken Arabic comes in different dialects among these countries, although it is still understood by all Arab countries. In Lebanon, people speak a patois of some of, or a combination of all, the four languages.

CULTURE HISTORY

This area has witnessed several successive civilizations and cultures over time. Lebanon, for example, has been known as home to the Phoenicians, after which came the Assyrians, Persians, Greeks, Romans, and Arabs. In more recent history, the Ottoman Empire ruled the area from the early 1500s through the early 1900s, after which the people were under either French (Syria and Lebanon) or British (Jordan and Palestine) mandates until they gained their independence. The region is also known to be the birthplace of Judaism and Christianity. Islam is the most practiced religion in Bilad Al Sham; the Muslim majority comprises Sunni, Shiite, Durzi, Alawi, Ismaili, and other sects. In addition, Arab Christians from Maronite, Catholic, and Protestant churches comprise an important part of the population. Jews were also part of the fabric of these countries; however, the majority have migrated to Israel.

FOOD HISTORY WITHIN THE CULTURE

The region has been a melting pot of several civilizations and cultures, which has enriched culinary traditions and influenced dietary practices. Strict rules apply to all practicing followers of religion. In accordance with the food laws, *halal* (food slaughtered in the name of God) and *kosher* foods are allowed, whereas pork consumption (*haram*, i.e., forbidden food) is prohibited for Muslims, as are alcoholic beverages. (Alcohol is permitted in Bilad Al Sham, however, because it is a more lenient society.)

Hospitality is an important feature of the region; people always welcome visitors, and food is always offered whether or not the visit was planned. What foods are offered may differ from one region to another depending on whether the region is urban, rural, or nomadic. The offering can range from fruits plucked from the host's own garden in rural areas, to slaughtering a camel or cattle in nomadic areas. Coffee is also often offered, but the time for serving it may vary by region. For example, in Lebanon, coffee is served as soon as a guest arrives, whereas in Palestine it is the last thing offered.

Arabs have had a tradition of documenting culinary practices since the Abbasid Period, when the first such documentation was recorded. Today, the Arab world, being part of the cyber world, has websites about

Arabic cuisine, websites for famous chefs, and satellite television and radio programs that broadcast recipes, cooking methods, and food-related topics on a daily basis. Food in this part of the world goes beyond just taste, with special attention given to producing dishes that are rich in color, aroma, and flavor.

MAJOR FOODS

Protein Sources

Protein sources include beef, mutton, veal, lamb, goat, organ meats (liver, kidney, sweetbread), chicken, pigeon, quail, turkey, fish, shrimp, crab, squid, lentils, chickpeas, fava beans, broad beans, black-eyed peas, milk, cheese, *laban*, *labneh*, *kishk*, *jameed*, and *shanklish*.

Meat

Meat is served primarily as a composite dish in most Middle Eastern countries, cooked mainly with different vegetable stews and rice. Meat is also a main ingredient of the most famous Lebanese dish, *kibbe*, a kind of meat dumpling that is served different ways, one of which is *kibbe nayie* (raw *kibbe*, similar to steak tartare) prepared from fresh meat with bulgur after grinding them manually (in a mortar, which is the traditional way) into a paste-like texture garnished with fresh mint, olive oil, and onions, and seasoned with pepper and salt. Fried *kibbe* is another format, in which the meat and bulgur paste is shaped into an American football-like shape stuffed with cooked ground meat, onions, and pine seeds, and is seasoned with sumac and then deep-fried to a crispy crust. *Kibbe bil sanieh* is a third method of preparing *kibbe*, in which two layers of the meat-and-bulgur paste sandwich the ground meat, onions, and pine seeds. The upper layer of the paste is beautifully shaped into geometrical designs and then baked in the oven. *Kibbe* grilled on charcoal is yet another method of preparation. Sumac may be used as a seasoning in all *kibbe* preparations, and a refreshing salad of yogurt and cucumber, with a hint of mint, may be served as a side dish.

When meat is consumed as a main dish, it is predominantly lamb or beef. Beef may be served as steak; however, lamb and beef are served as kebab, which is meat on skewers grilled on charcoal for a delicious smoky flavor. Lamb is usually ground with parsley and seasoned with a rich blend of spices such as allspice, cinnamon, nutmeg, and many others, and hand kneaded to finger-like form on the skewer. Beef is usually chopped into small pieces and marinated with zesty spices. Usually pieces of onions, capsicum, and cherry tomatoes are embedded between meat pieces to add a juicy flavor to the mixed grill.

Ground meat is also a major ingredient of stuffed vegetables, which are famous in the Lebanese and Syrian cuisines. Cooked ground meat with onions is added to rice and seasoned with spices, and used as a stuffing for vine leaves (*dolma* type), marrow, eggplant, tomato, capsicum, turnips, carrots, potatoes, and cucumbers. Each dish is prepared with different types of mouthwatering sauces, such as tomato, tamarind, tahini (sesame cream), or yogurt. Shawarma is also a very famous meat preparation (similar to doner kebab) and is served as a platter or, perhaps more often, in sandwich wraps seasoned with tahini, green peppers, pickled turnips, and parsley.

Mansaf is the national Jordanian dish. It is prepared with large chunks of lamb meat cooked with dried goat or sheep milk, known as *jameed*, along with rice.

Poultry

Chicken is also widely used as another source of protein. Chicken is served roasted, grilled, or as *shish tawook* charcoaled on skewers. It is also served as shawarma. Also, chicken may be stuffed with rice and ground meat, pine seeds, and other seasonings, and served at special occasions. The most famous traditional Palestinian dish is *musakhan*, which comprises mainly stone-oven-baked bread drenched with olive oil, onions, and sumac, served with chicken. Turkey, quail, and pigeon, although eaten in this part of the world, are less frequently consumed.

Fish and Seafood

Syria, Lebanon, and Palestine share a long coastal line on the Mediterranean Sea; hence, fish and seafood are commonly consumed. Local fish is fried and served with fried pita bread and a tahini-and-parsley sauce known as *tarator*. *Sayyadieh* is fried fish with rice seasoned with spices (cumin being the dominant spice). As for Jordan, fish is rarely eaten.

Pulses and Legumes

Lentils are widely used in cooking. *Mujaddarah* is a popular dish served year round in which lentils are cooked with rice and cumin and garnished with crispy golden caramelized onions. Lentil soup is also popular, served more commonly in winter and during Ramadan (the Muslim fasting month). Hummus, prepared from chickpeas, is another internationally renowned appetizer and is consumed almost daily in these countries. *Foul*, made from fava beans boiled and garnished with tomatoes, parsley, onions, and olive oil, is consumed either as an appetizer or as a main dish especially at breakfast. Falafel, prepared from chickpeas, fava beans, and greens, then deep-fried and eaten with tahini sauce and pickles, is another popular food. *Harra'a usba'o* is a famous Damascus (Syrian) dish made with lentils, greens, and pastry or fried bread, garnished with fried onions and lemon.

Dairy Products

Dairy products are an important part of the cuisine. Milk is consumed as a beverage or as a main ingredient in white sauce and béchamel preparations. Also, unsweetened yogurt is a refreshing side dish served with finely chopped cucumbers and a sprinkle of mint. *Laban*, a mixture of yogurt diluted with water, with a dash of salt and mint, is also a refreshing summer drink. *Labneh*, strained yogurt that has a creamy texture, is favored as a breakfast or dinner serving. It is prepared with olive oil, olives, and mint. *Shanklish* is another milk product, made from goat's milk in the form of solid balls rolled in dried thyme, wild thyme, or sumac; this is one method of preserving milk. *Shanklish* is usually served with chopped tomatoes, chopped onions, and a lot of olive oil. Dairy products are a main component of desserts.

 Starch Sources

Starch sources include wheat for bread (staple), pita bread, *tannour* bread, *markook* bread, *mashateeh*, *maftool*, *freekeh*, *maftool*, bulgur, rice, and potatoes.

Pita bread is the staple in this part of the world. It is consumed with every meal. Other types of bread, such as toast, buns, sesame bread (*ka'k*), thin format (*markouk*), and several other forms of bread, are also consumed. *Mana'eesh*, stone-oven-baked bread with either thyme or cheese, is consumed at breakfast. Rice and bulgur come next in line and are widely served with stews or as part of other food preparations, as mentioned previously. Potatoes are also consumed as part of stews, stuffed with ground meat, baked, boiled, or as French fries. All varieties of pasta are well liked in this region. *Maftool*, usually cooked with both meat and chicken, chickpeas, and onions, is the Bilad Al Sham version of Moroccan couscous.

 Fat Sources

Fat sources include olive oil, corn oil, sunflower oil, ghee (clarified butter), butter, cream (*qashta*), sheep tallow, and tahini. Olive oil is the predominantly used oil, whether consumed with thyme, hummus, or *foul*, as a garnish, or added at the final stages of cooking stews, or used to marinate fish or chicken. Corn oil and sunflower oil are also used in frying and cooking. Ghee, prepared from clarified butter, known as *samen hamawi*, is used in cooking and desserts in small quantities to add a special aromatic effect and enhance taste. Butter and fresh cream are also common ingredients in main meals and desserts. Tahini is also a main ingredient in Bilad Al Sham's cuisine.

 Prominent Vegetables

Prominent vegetables include squash, okra, eggplant, green beans, pumpkin, cucumber, tomatoes, carrots, lemon, peas, artichoke, spinach, mallow, chicory, vine leaves, Swiss chard, cabbage, colocasia, radish, grindelia, purslane, garlic, onion, and leek.

Vegetables are an essential component of all meals. The vast variety of salad preparations is unsurpassed. Mixed green salads or raw vegetables are enjoyed with meals or as snacks. *Fattouch*, also known as bread salad, is made of tomatoes, cucumbers, lettuce, onions and garlic with olive oil, sumac, and of course bread, which gives it its name. Bread is cut into small pieces and mixed with the salad, and may be fried or baked. *Tabbouli*, also known as parsley salad, is consumed all over the region and has gained international recognition. It is prepared from parsley, tomatoes, onions, freshly chopped mint leaves, and soaked bulgur in lemon juice. Cooked vegetable salads and green salads are also favored as part of the meal, as well as chicory salad cooked with onions, olive oil, and a hint of lemon juice. The eggplant is truly glorified in Bilad Al Sham cuisine. *Baba gannouj* is a famous dip prepared mainly from eggplant and tahini in addition to lemon juice; yogurt may be added in some recipes, garnished with pomegranate seeds and olive oil. *Raheb* is another eggplant-based salad. Eggplant is also eaten fried, grilled, and cooked with rice (*makloobeh*) or stuffed with ground beef, rice, and chickpeas (*mahshi batinjan*). Marrow is also eaten either as a stew, cooked as a cold salad, or stuffed with rice (*mahshi kusa*), similar to eggplant. Almost all vegetables are cooked in a stew

preparation and served with rice. Spinach is also served in stew, salad, and most commonly in a savory pastry form known as *fatayer sabanikh* (spinach turnovers). *Mulokhiyeh* is another leafy vegetable widely consumed in this part of the world, served in stews along with rice, vermicelli, and meat or chicken. Turnips, cauliflower, cucumber, tomatoes, and other vegetables are also pickled and served alongside many other foods.

 Prominent Fruits

Prominent fruits include apple, orange, grape, banana, guava, pomegranate, persimmons, cherry, loquat, peach, pear, prickly pear, quince, raspberry, and strawberry.

Fruit grows abundantly in Syria, Lebanon, and Palestine, but less so in Jordan because of limited water resources. A variety of citrus fruits, such as mandarins, oranges, and grapefruits, are consumed raw, in juices, as ingredients in desserts, and as compotes and jams. Dried fruits, such as figs, apricots, dates, and prunes, are also consumed. Berries, raspberries, strawberries, bananas, watermelons, apples, and an endless variety of other fruits are available. Persimmon, loquat, prickly pear, custard apple (also known as cherimoya), guava, and pomelo are also seasonally available and enjoyed by the majority of the population. A unique practice in this region is to preserve orange blossoms in syrup and use them in dessert preparations. Also, orange blossoms are distilled in a liquid (*ma'zaher*) that is used for desserts as well as for medicinal purposes.

 Spices, Condiments, and Nuts

Common spices, condiments, and nuts include sumac, turmeric, cumin, cardamom, cinnamon, caraway, anise seed, allspice, nutmeg, mastic (gum), mint, coriander, parsley, pistachio, walnut, pine seeds, lupine, watermelon seed, pumpkin seed, almond thyme, fenugreek, dill, sage, rosemary, cloves, ginger, basil, orange blossom, rose water, and orange-blossom water.

Perhaps what makes the food of Bilad Al Sham unique are the zesty aromas that accompany the different dishes and give a distinct flavor to each dish. Sumac is one of the main spices used to season both salads and main dishes, and it is an excellent source of antioxidants. Cumin is widely used as a powder or as roasted seeds. Cardamom is used extensively in beverages, cookies, stews, and sweets. Cinnamon accompanies various food preparations. Nutmeg, although used in moderation, adds a distinct flavor to many dishes. Turmeric and saffron are also used as food coloring for special rice dishes. Caraway is also used in main dishes and desserts.

Herbs, such as coriander, parsley, and thyme, are also used as seasonings or as a main ingredient in some food preparations. Herbs are a major component of the meal; women grow them on their balconies for both their culinary use as well as their aromatic properties.

 ## Beverages

Common beverages include Turkish coffee, tea, *z'hoorat* (herbal tea), *sahlab, inar* (cinnamon drink), *jallab, irq sous,* tamarine, *qamar eldinn, arak,* beer, wine, soft drinks, and fruit juices.

Turkish coffee with cardamom is the most-consumed drink. It is a rich, dense coffee similar to espresso, with a much stronger aroma. Herbal teas contain a mix of sage, chamomile, anise, lemongrass, rose petals, and others, each with a different medicinal use. Other drinks, such as *sahlab* (a milk-based drink) and *inar* (a cinnamon drink), are more winter beverages, whereas raspberry drink, rose drink, *jallab* (a drink prepared from dried raisins), and tamarind drink with crushed ice chips, are more summer drinks. *Matte* is another herbal drink consumed by mountaineers in Lebanon

and Syria, especially among the Druze. Local beers, wines, and the traditional Lebanese *arak* made from anise seed (similar to Greek *ouzo*) are the common alcoholic beverages. American coffee, tea, milk, and soft drinks are also consumed.

 ## Desserts

Popular desserts include *muhalabiya*, rice pudding, *halawet el jibn, halawet el riz, baklawa, burma, ma'moul, ghraybeh, knafeh,* cakes, pastries, *osmalliyyeh, ish-el-bulbul, jazariyeh, hareeset,* and *znood-el-sit*. Jams include apricot, apple, marmalade, eggplant, fig, and watermelon, and molasses is also consumed.

A vast variety of desserts are offered in Bilad Al Sham, with *knafeh*, a sweetened cheese dessert with semolina on top, bathed in syrup, being the most popular in Lebanon and Syria. The topping is made of orange-dyed vermicelli in Palestine and Jordan, and named *knafeh nabilsiyeh* due to its origin, Nablus (West Bank). *Ma'moul bil fustuq* (pistachio) and *jouwz* (walnut) are made from a semolina paste stuffed with sweetened crushed pistachio or walnuts, baked in the oven and served with sugar icing. *Awammat* (spoon doughnut) is another sweet made with special dough,

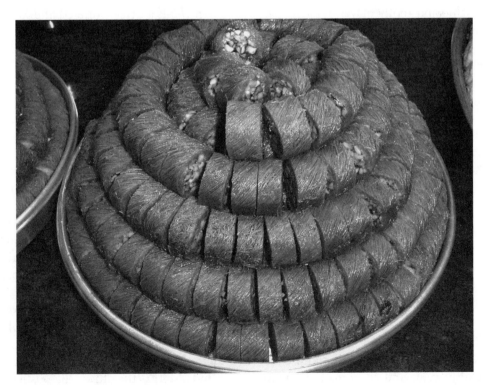

Burma
Courtesy of the author

Observations from the Author (Roula Barake)

Middle Eastern cuisine is described by Westerners as a burst of flavors, which results from an explosion of aromatic herbs and spices. Even though the cuisine is fancied and acquired by the Western palate in general, some people find the pungent flavor of sumac, the exquisite aroma of cardamom (*hal*) and the earthy flavor of coriander (*kusbarah*) a bit overwhelming and somewhat repulsive. Such enhancement of flavor is conditioned by the aromatic olive oil, which replaces butter and margarine in Bilad Al Sham's culinary practices. A typical custom of eating thyme and olive oil (*za'atar* and *zeit*) as a dip, or combining strained yogurt and olive oil (*labneh* and *zeit*), is difficult to conceive as breakfast habits in Western cultures. The extensive use of garlic in Middle Eastern cuisine is also not preferred by Western taste. The slightly smoky taste of eggplant that results when it is grilled is an appreciated culinary technique that has been adopted by non-Arabs. Middle Easterners do not consider meat to be a main component of their meals, but it strikes others as being fundamental to the cuisine. Meat and vegetables are "overcooked" by Western standards, and bread accompanies all Middle Eastern meals. The two main ingredients in dessert making, rose water (*ma'wared*) and orange-blossom water (*ma'zaher*), are used as flavoring agents in many traditional sweets and pastries. Westerners usually require repeated exposure to them to get conditioned to their distinctive floral—almost "perfumy"—taste. Nuts in general, and pine nuts in particular, are used in both savory foods and desserts, in addition to their use as snacks. Westerners enjoy the wide range of desserts offered in Middle Eastern cuisine, although they are often described as "too syrupy."

Middle Eastern cuisine requires a great deal of patience in preparation, because cooks take pride in the presentation and have to stuff a large variety of vegetables. They pay special attention to offer a *sofra* (a Turkish word that means coffee table, used in Bilad Al Sham to describe a food setting), which is appetizing for both the eye and the palate. The variety of herbal teas offered, coffee preparation, and the wide array of beverages served are also appreciated by Western consumers. The overall eating experience of people from the West is described as enjoyable, owing to the myriad flavors, varieties, colors, and aromas of Middle Eastern cuisine.

fried in small ball shapes and drowned in heavy syrup. *Burma* is a cylinder of vermicelli stuffed with pistachio or pine seeds, and *baklawa* is a phyllo pastry bottom topped with pistachio and another layer of phyllo pastry cut into diamond-shaped pieces. *Halawet el jibin* and *halawet al riz* are sheets of cheese or rice flour cooked with semolina, served with fresh cream and syrup, and garnished with crushed pistachio and sweetened orange blossom. A variety of cookies, such as *grayybeh* (sugar cookies) and *barazik* (sesame cookies), enrich the dessert selection in the area. The passion for preparing homemade preserved fruit compotes and jams has been passed from one generation to the next, but more recent food-preparation techniques are being practiced. Jams are considered an important component of desserts.

❤ FOODS WITH CULTURAL SIGNIFICANCE

Honey, grapes, figs, dates, yogurt, olives, and olive oil are all mentioned in the Qur'an (the holy book for Muslims); hence, they all have religious significance and Muslims tend to value and consume them regularly, and they believe that those food items all possess medicinal properties.

Basterma is a kind of dried meat introduced to the area by Armenian immigrants that has gained popularity.

Mughli is a dessert offered after a birth. It is made by combining and cooking rice powder, a variety of spices and condiments (such as cinnamon and caraway), and sugar, and is garnished with pistachios, almonds, and walnuts.

A feast is customarily offered at weddings, and special sweets are offered after an infant boy's circumcision. Food items may differ across different faiths as well as rural, urban, and nomadic cultures.

After burial of the dead, a three-day period of mourning takes place during which close friends, relatives, and neighbors offer a big lunch. Unsweetened coffee is offered in several rounds throughout mourning, and in some places sweets are offered on the last day.

Eid al-Adha is a religious festival celebrated by Muslims as a commemoration of Ibrahim's (Abraham's) willingness to sacrifice his son Ishmael for God. Lamb is the main dish offered on this occasion.

Qamar el din and *qatayef* are a drink and sweet, respectively, offered mainly during Ramadan, and *zalabiah* is offered on Prophet Mohammad's birthday.

Eid al-Fitr is the other religious festival celebrated by Muslims. Sweets such as *ka'k-el-eid*, which is made from semolina balls stuffed with pistachios, walnuts,

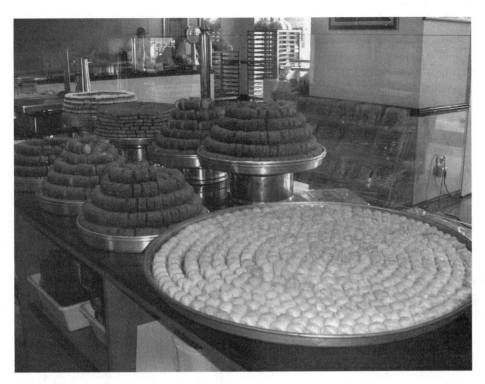

Lebanese Sweets
Courtesy of the author

or dates, are essential. Friends and family members gather and exchange visits during all three days of celebrations where these sweets are offered.

Practices differ during Lent between occidental (Catholic) and oriental (Orthodox) Christians. They refrain from eating meat and other animal products. Orthodox Christians refrain from eating fish as well; some refrain from eating until 12:00 noon every day, and others eliminate foods that they like; some omit meat products on Fridays, or both, Wednesdays and Fridays.

Burbara pudding is prepared from crushed, peeled, shelled wheat, with raisins, fennel, sugar, cinnamon, and some nuts offered exclusively on St. Barbara's Day.

Mezze is usually a variety of appetizers, both cold and hot, that may exceed 100 plates, and is served with *arak* in Lebanese and Syrian cuisine.

 TYPICAL DAY'S MENU

A typical breakfast menu consists of *mana'eesh* (pita-bread-like dough topped with dried thyme and olive oil, baked in a stone oven). Mint leaves may be added. A variety of cheese jams and eggs are common breakfast substitutes. *Labneh* and olives is another alternative. Tea or coffee is consumed. Lunch may consist of green salad (*salata khadra*), rice with vermicelli (*mloukiyeh*), or any vegetable stew, boiled chicken or stewed meat, chopped onions with vinegar, and *laban* drink. The afternoon snack may consist of tea or coffee and fruits or dessert. Dinner may consist of *labneh*, pickles, olives, olive oil, mint, *markouk* bread, apricot jam, and butter or cream. Dinner is very similar to breakfast. Turkish coffee with cardamom is a favorite drink and may be offered all day long.

 HOLIDAY MENUS

A typical holiday breakfast may consist of fried eggs, hummus, *foul*, mint, olives, chopped vegetables, and tea or coffee. Lunch might feature green salad and stuffed whole lamb (*kharouf mihshi*; a whole lamb is rubbed with seasoning inside and out, stuffed with rice and ground meat, almonds, pistachios, pine nuts, and a variety of spices, and then roasted in the oven) or a combination of stuffed eggplant/vine leaves and zucchini, *laban* drink with mint, and salad. The afternoon snack might be a dessert, such as date cookies (*ma'moul-bil-tamer*) and/or pistachio/walnut cookies (*ka'k bil-gawz/ fustuq*). Dinner may consist of cheese, *labneh*, jam, honey, butter or cream, and fruits.

HEALTH BELIEFS AND CONCERNS

Herbal medicine is highly regarded in this part of the world. The *Attar* is the person who sells the herbs. (It is a vocation usually passed from one generation to the next.) People tend to consult the *Attar* for treatments for different ailments, in conjunction with or as a substitution for Western medicine. The most common herbs used are cinnamon for menstrual problems, chamomile as a sedative, anise as a calmative, and sage for enhancing memory as well as relief of hot flushes and as a carminative. Ground rice pudding (*mughli*), the sweet offered after a birth, is thought of as milk secretagogue. Orange-blossom water (*ma'zahr*) is also used as a treatment for colic; it can either be added to water or consumed alone in moderation (because of its bitter taste). There seems to be a consensus on not mixing fish, yogurt, and tamarind, but no clear reason has been given.

GENERAL HEALTH AND NUTRITIONAL INDICATORS SUMMARY

Jordan

In Jordan, low birth weight, defined as weighing less than 2500 g at birth, affects 12% of newborns (UNICEF, 2007). Twenty-seven percent of children are exclusively breastfed during the first 6 months of life. Seventy percent of infants 6–9 months old are breastfed with complementary food and 12% remain breastfed at 20–23 months.

Four percent of children under 5 years suffer from being moderately to severely underweight (UNICEF, 2007). Being severely underweight affects 1% of Jordan's children. Moderate to severe wasting was found in 2% and stunting in 9% of this particular population. The majority (88%) of households in Jordan consume adequately iodized salt.

Ninety-seven percent of Jordan's total population uses improved drinking-water sources (UNICEF, 2007). Specifically, 99% of the population in the nation's urban areas and 91% of the rural population has access to improved drinking-water sources.

Palestine

Chronic malnutrition affects nearly 10% of children under age 5. The situation is most acute in Gaza, where 50,000 children are malnourished. About half of children under age 2 are anemic and 70% have vitamin A deficiency. To combat malnutrition, UNICEF and its partners raised awareness of the importance of breastfeeding and advocated for flour fortification and salt iodization. Additionally, approximately 10% of girls ages 15–18 are pregnant or already have a child (UNICEF, 2007).

Lebanon

UNICEF (2007) has provided a Better Parenting Initiative to promote parental and community education in health, nutrition, and psychosocial care practices. This includes promoting breastfeeding, proper complementary feeding practices, and implementing the International Code of Marketing of Breast Milk Substitutes, and support to national efforts to eliminate iodine deficiency disorders. All is being accomplished through monitoring support, and to control iron-deficiency anemia, through a comprehensive approach including fortification, supplementation, and health and dietary education.

COMMUNICATION AND COUNSELING TIPS

Generosity is one of the many good traits that define the people of Bilad Al Sham. For example, it is not customary for people to accept what is offered the first time; usually, they accept it after the third offer (which means that the host is obliged to offer it three times).

Religious practices are expressed strongly. Although most people shake hands when introduced, many Muslims may not respond to a handshake with the opposite sex; instead, they may place their hand on their chest with a slight bow as a form of reciprocating the greeting.

Residents of Bilad Al Sham are more westernized than people in other parts of the Arab world; hence, it is not likely that one will encounter conflicts in either verbal or nonverbal communication.

PRIMARY LANGUAGE OF FOOD NAMES WITH ENGLISH AND TRANSLATION

Table 50-1 gives the primary language of food names with English and phonetic translation.

TABLE 50-1   Primary Language of Food Names with English and Phonetic Translation

Arabic	English	Phonetic Translation	Arabic	English	Phonetic Translation
زبدة	Butter	Zibdeh	بطاطا	Potato	Batata
جبن	Cheese	Jibneh	ليمون	Lemon	Laymoun
حليب	Milk	Haleeb	ورق عنب	Grape leaves	Warak enab
مربى	Jam	Mrabba	تفاح	Apple	Tuffah
عسل	Honey	Asal	موز	Banana	Moz
زيتون	Olives	Zaytoon	برتقال	Orange	Burtuqal
زيت زيتون	Olive oil	Zeit zytoon	دراق	Peach	Durrak
مناقيش زعتر	Thyme bread	Mana'eesh	رمان	Pomegranate	Rumman
خبز	Pita bread	Khubz	صبير	Prickly pear	Subbair
عصير	Juice	Aseer	توت	Raspberry	Tout
رز	Rice	Riz	بطيخ	Watermelon	Battikh
عدس	Lentils	Adas	فروج / دجاج	Chicken	Farrouj/dajaj
خيار	Cucumber	Khiyar	بقلاوة	Baklava	Ba'lawah
بندورة	Tomato	Banadourah	كنافه	Cheese and semolina pastry	Knafeh
بقدونس	Parsley	Bakdunes	غريبة	Sugar cookies	Ghraybeh
بصل	Onion	Basal	معمول	Date/nut cookies	Ma'moul
ثوم	Garlic	Toom	قهوه	Coffee	Ahweh
خس	Lettuce	Khass			

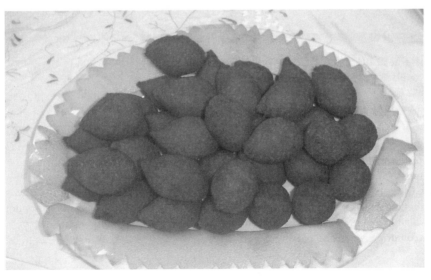

Kibbe
Courtesy of the author

FEATURED RECIPE

Lamb Kibbe (*Kibbeh*)

2 lbs. lean lamb, cubed

1 lb. fine bulgur

½ tsp. allspice

½ tsp. cinnamon

1 tsp. salt

1 large onion

½ cup olive oil or vegetable oil

Stuffing:

3 medium onions

1 lb. meat (beef or lamb), finely minced

1 cup vegetable oil

1 tsp. salt

½ tsp. allspice

Pinch of black pepper

1 cup pine seeds

1. Wash and soak bulgur for 30 minutes. Drain and squeeze dry.
2. Grind lamb and onions twice in a food processor.
3. Knead the ground lamb and onions with bulgur using hands. (You may wet hands with cold water repeatedly while kneading.)
4. Grind the mixture again in a food processor.
5. Add salt and spices to mixture, and knead once more to form a paste.
6. Peel onions and chop finely. Saute onions until golden.
7. Add minced meat, pine seeds, and all other seasonings and spices in a pan at medium heat until meat is cooked.
8. Grease the bottom of a round baking tray with oil and smooth approximately half the prepared kibbe paste in the baking tray.
9. Spread the cooked meat stuffing over the kibbe layer. Cover with the remaining slightly thicker layer of kibbe paste.
10. Cut into diamond shapes with a sharp knife.
11. Sprinkle with olive oil. (You can also make a hole in the middle with your thumb and fill it with olive oil.)
12. Bake at 350°F in a preheated oven for 30–45 minutes until it is well done with a brown and crisp top. Kibbe can be served hot or cold with yogurt and cucumber salad.

Yields 10 servings

More recipes are available at http://nutrition.jbpub.com/foodculture/

REFERENCES

Heine, P. (2004). *Food culture in the Near East, Middle East and North Africa*. Westport, CT: Greenwood Press.

Pellet, P.L., & Shadarevian, S. (1970). *Tables for use in the Middle East*. Beirut, Labanon: American University of Beirut.

Rowland, J. (1950). *Good food from the Near East: 500 favorite recipes from twelve countries*. New York: Barrows.

UNICEF. (2007). *The state of the world's children 2007: Women and children, the double dividend of gender equality*. Retrieved April 14, 2009, from http://www.unicef.org/sowc07/statistics/tables.php

Zubaida, S., & Tapper, R. (1994). *Culinary cultures of the Middle East*. London: University of London.

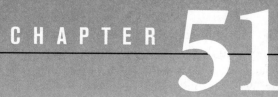

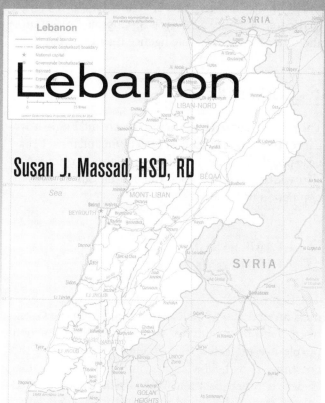

CHAPTER 51

Lebanon

Susan J. Massad, HSD, RD

CULTURE AND WORLD REGION

Lebanon, the home of the great Phoenician civilization, was settled more than 7000 years ago. It was known for the creation of the first alphabet and the colonization of the western Mediterranean. Phoenicians lived on the Mediterranean coast north of Palestine from approximately 1200 to 800 BC. Their cities were the southern Lebanon towns of Tyre and Sidon. Lebanon's rich, combined, East–West culture was shaped by Phoenician, Greek, Roman, Islamic, Ottoman Turkish, and French cultures, and by the Crusades. The religious and ethnic diversity of Lebanon is made up of Christians, Muslims, Arabs, Armenians, Kurds, and Assyrians.

Anglo-French forces captured Syria from the Ottoman Empire in 1918. Lebanon gained its independence from Syria in 1920. Lebanon became a French mandate in 1920 and was granted independence from France in 1943, with final withdrawal of French forces in 1946 (Mackey, 2006). Civil war from 1975 to 1990 devastated the country, but Lebanon has since made progress toward rebuilding its political institutions.

Lebanon's government is parliamentary, with a centralized, multireligious, and multiparty ruling based on "confessionalism." This requires a Maronite Christian president, a Sunni Muslim prime minister, and a Shi'a Muslim speaker of parliament. The country's population is 3,925,502 people (2007 estimate). The capital is Beirut, with an estimated population of 1,916,100 people (metropolitan area; 1,171,000 people in the city proper). Other large cities include Tripoli, with a population of 212,900 people, and Sidon, with a population of 149,000 people. The monetary unit is the Lebanese pound. The adult literacy rate is 87.4% (Central Intelligence Agency, 2008). Prior to the civil war (1975–1990), the literacy rate was closer to 95%. The world region where Lebanon is situated is the Middle East, bordering the Mediterranean Sea, between Israel and Syria. The ethnicity/racial makeup is Arab 95%, Armenian 4%, and other 1%. Religions include Islam 60% (Shi'a, Sunni, Druze, Isma'ilite, Alawite/Nusayri), Christian 39% (Maronite, Melkite, Syrian, Armenian, and Roman Catholic; Greek, Armenian, and Syrian Orthodox; Chaldean; Assyrian; Coptic; Protestant), and other 1% (Central Intelligence Agency, 2008).

LANGUAGE

The official language is Arabic. French and English are part of the standard school curriculum and most Lebanese people are fluent in both languages. Armenian is also widely spoken among the substantial Armenian population in Lebanon.

FOOD HISTORY WITHIN THE CULTURE

The first settlers arrived in what was known as Phoenicia around 3000 BC. Its name came from the Greek word "land of the purple" named after the color of a purple dye extracted from mollusks found along the coastline. The Phoenicians became the first navigator-traders between East and West. Their trade included spices, grains, dried and preserved foods, and wine. Lebanese cuisine evolved through its long history of successive invasions by outsiders, including the Egyptians,

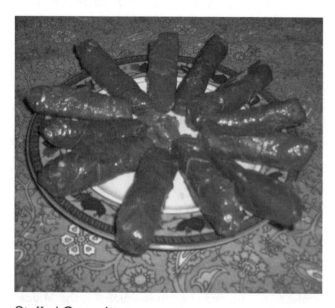

Stuffed Grape Leaves
Courtesy of the author

Assyrians, Babylonians, Persians, Greeks, and Romans. The Crusaders arrived in the 11th century and brought Western influence by making Lebanon part of the kingdom of Jerusalem (Helou, 1994). The Ottoman Turks dominated from 1516 to 1914. The Ottoman Empire broke up after World War I and Lebanon became a French Mandate from 1920 to 1946. This history of incursion has shaped the varied cuisine, as it is known today. Herbs and spices are used in many Lebanese dishes. Condiments are used in moderation. With the exception of a fish dish known as *samkeh harrah*, hot spicy dishes of Asia are seldom part of Lebanese cuisine. The typical spices and flavorings used are garlic, onion, salt and pepper, saffron, cumin, sumac, lemon, allspice, cinnamon, "seven-spice mixture" (sweet paprika, hot paprika, ground cumin, freshly ground black pepper, ground ginger, turmeric, and ground cinnamon), and *za'tar* (a mixture of thyme, sumac, sesame seeds, and salt), which is not used for flavoring other dishes, but rather on its own, with olive oil and bread.

The Arab association with spices goes back to before the birth of Christ at which time Arab merchants already dominated the spice trade. Acting as middlemen, they transported exotic herbs and spices to the Mediterranean region and beyond. The Arab dominance of commerce continued until the 16th century when the Portuguese captured the Arab-controlled ports and trade routes. The dominance was so strong that in the Middle Ages Arabic was considered to be the language of traders. When Columbus attempted to reach India by sailing westward, he took an Arabic-speaking interpreter with him (Salloum, 2000).

In the past few decades, the newly discovered oil wealth in the Arabic Gulf countries has lured millions of workers from around the world. The foods brought by these migrants from the Indian subcontinent, Iran, and the Far East have enriched the cuisine of this part of the Arabian peninsula with an array of mouth-watering meatless dishes (Salloum, 2000).

Vegetable appetizers, pickled turnips, salads, legumes, and yogurt dishes are either served as part of main courses or as side dishes. Vegetables such as cabbage, squash, peppers, and vine (grape) leaves, stuffed with rice and either meat or legumes, make tasty entrees. The herbs (parsley, mint) and flavorings (garlic, lemon) used in the stuffing blend with the vegetables and boost their taste. Canned vegetables and preservatives are rarely used. Everything from simple appetizers to elaborate main dishes are prepared with attention to detail and presented with pride to family and guests.

MAJOR FOODS

 Protein Sources

Protein sources include beef, chickpeas, fava beans, lamb, lentils, feta cheese, fish, kashkaval cheese (sheep's milk cheese), poultry, Syrian cheese, and yogurt.

 Starch Sources

Starch sources include bulgur (cracked wheat), legumes, *marqouq* ("mountain bread"; i.e., paper-thin, unleavened bread), potatoes, Syrian bread, and rice.

 Fat Sources

Fat sources include almonds, clarified butter, olives (harvested in abundance; olives and olive oil are stored in large quantities, often for an entire season), olive oil, pine nuts, and walnuts.

 Prominent Vegetables

Prominent vegetables include artichoke, arugula, asparagus, beet (pickled), cabbage, cauliflower, cucumber, eggplant, green beans, okra, onion, pepper, scallion, spinach, squash, tomato, and watercress.

 Prominent Fruits

Prominent fruits include apricot, apple, banana, date, fig, grape, orange, peach, pear, plum, and pomegranate.

 Spices and Seasonings

Common spices include allspice, anise, cinnamon, cardamom, clove, nutmeg, turmeric, *za'tar* (thyme mixture), and "seven-spice mixture" (sweet paprika, hot paprika, ground cumin, freshly ground black pepper, ground ginger, turmeric, and ground cinnamon).

 Beverages

Common beverages include *arak* (alcoholic beverage made from distilled grape juice and flavored with anise), fresh-squeezed juice, and Lebanese wine, as well as Turkish and Arabic coffee.

 Desserts

Popular desserts include baklava, cookies (shortbread type, with almonds), dates and date pastry, rice pudding, semolina cake (*nammourah*), semolina stuffed with walnuts or pistachios (*maamoul*), sesame seed-based cookies (*barazek*), sesame seed-based sweet (*simsimieh*), and walnut triangles.

 FOODS WITH CULTURAL SIGNIFICANCE

Listed below are many of the dishes that reflect the cultural history of Lebanon. The historical explanation of some of the foods used in these dishes can be found in the previous section, *Food History Within the Culture.*

- Ain-Zibdeh: Hareeseh (wheat and chicken)
- Baalbek: Safiha Baalbakieh (meat-stuffed puff pastry)
- Baino: Kebbe and Lahme bil-khal (meat mixed with crushed wheat and meat soaked in vinegar)
- Baskinta: Makhlouta (meat, rice, and nuts)
- Beirut: Samkeh Harra and Akhtabout (spicy fish and octopus), roasted nuts
- Beit Mery: Kebbe Lakteen (pumpkin-flavored meat)
- Beit Shabab: Riz bi-Djaj (chicken with rice)
- Beiteddine: Kafta Bithine (spiced meat with sesame concentrate)
- Broummana: Deleh Mehshi (stuffed rib cage of lamb)
- Bsharri: Koussa bil-Laban (meat and rice-stuffed zucchini cooked in yogurt)
- Deir al-Kamar: Fatet Batinjan (yogurt, fried bread, and aubergine)
- Dhour Choueir: Shish Barak (dough balls stuffed with ground beef and cooked in yogurt)
- Douma: Laban Immo (cooked yogurt and lamb with rice)
- Ehden: Kebbe Zghartweih (oven-cooked meat and crushed wheat blend)
- El-Koura: Abu Shoushe (topinambur and lentils stew)
- Firzel: Freikeh (cooked wheat with meat)
- Hammana: Fasoulya Hammanieh (kidney bean stew)
- Ihmej: Ghameh (stuffed cow intestines)
- Jbeil: Koussa and Wark Inab bil-Kastaletah (stuffed zucchini, grape vines, and steak)
- Kfar meshki: Kebbe bil-Kishk (meat mixed with wheat and yogurt)
- Ras al-Metn: Fatet (yogurt, fried bread, and nuts)
- Rashana: Mjadrat Fasoulya (lentils and kidney beans)

- Rashaya Al-Wadi: Kebbe Heeleh (meatballs)
- Saghbeen: Zankal bil-Laban (meat-filled pastry and yogurt)
- Sidon: Riz bil-Foul (rice and fava beans)
- Tripoli, Lebanon: Mjadrah and Fattoush (crushed lentils and salad)
- Tyre: Saiyadit al-Samak (rice and fish)
- Zahle: Kebbe Zahleweieh (meat and crushed wheat blend)

TYPICAL DAY'S MENU

A typical breakfast menu may consist of *laban* or *labneh*, Syrian bread or *manakeesh* (baked *za'tar* and olive oil baked on pizza-like dough), black olives, fava beans, coffee, and fruit. For lunch, lentil soup, kebabs (beef, lamb, or chicken) or stuffed vegetables, rice pilaf or lentil pilaf, salad (*tabouleh* or *fattoush*), and olives may be served. A typical dinner menu may consist of *mezze* (selection of hors d'oeuvres), stuffed grape leaves, *tabouleh*, *laban*, and Syrian bread. Dessert could feature dried fruit, Turkish or Arabic coffee, and rice pudding. For the evening snack, fruit and tea (typically served in small glass cups) would be served.

RELIGIOUS AND HOLIDAY MENUS AND CUSTOMS

Muslim and Christian religious practices each include some dietary laws and holiday food customs. Ramadan is the most important Muslim observance and is followed for a full month. It marks the month that the Qur'an (holy scripture) was given. Fasting (*sawm*) is done from sunrise to sunset. People typically break the fast by consuming a date. This symbolizes what Prophet Mohammed ate at the end of each day of fasting. This is followed by a main meal. Many people who observe Ramadan get up before dawn to eat the *suhoor* (predawn) meal and perform their prayers. They break their fast when the fourth prayer of the day, *maghrib* (sunset), is due. As the Ramadan fast is broken each day after sunset, prayers of appreciation are given for the food and all of life's gifts and blessings. The Feast of Breaking of the Fast, known as Eid al-Fitr, marks the end of Ramadan. Pregnant women, the elderly, and children under 12 years are all exempt from fasting (Culinary Kingdom, 2006).

Eid el-Kebir, or Eid ul-Adha, which means the "Festival of Sacrifice" or "Slaughter of the Lamb," is the second most important holy day, and is observed by Muslims and Druze. This occasion is observed in remembrance of the story of Abraham's willingness to sacrifice everything for God, including the life of his son Ishmael. Eid ul-Adha annually falls on the 10th day of the last month of the Islamic lunar calendar. The festivities last for 2–4 days. Eid ul-Adha occurs the day after the pilgrims conducting *hajj*, the annual pilgrimage to Mecca (in Saudi Arabia) by Muslims worldwide, descend from Mount Arafat. It happens to be approximately 70 days after the end of the month of Ramadan. In this tradition, an animal is slaughtered, usually a sheep or lamb, and its meat is given to family, friends,

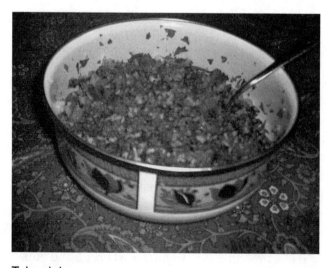

Tabouleh
Courtesy of the author

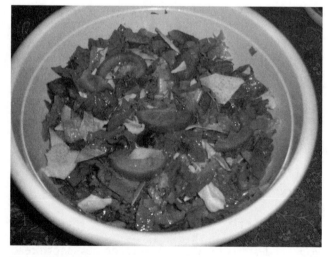

Fattoush
Courtesy of the author

Observations from the Author (Susan J. Massad)

When I visited Lebanon in 2005, one of the things I loved most was the *souks* (shopping bazaars) in Beirut and Tripoli where you can buy fresh bread, fruits, vegetables, olives, spices, handmade soap, and even some clothing and crafts. Fresh, tasty, nutritious foods abound in these marketplaces and in the restaurants. The Lebanese version of fast food is typically falafel (fried balls or patties made from spiced fava beans and/or chickpeas) or shawarma (a Middle Eastern-style sandwich made with shaved lamb, beef, or chicken).

One thing that stood out for me was the difference in the standard breakfast fare. Although the typical American breakfast items (eggs, toast, cereal, quick breads) are available, breakfast there usually consists of any variety of *labneh* (strained yogurt), olives, tomatoes, Syrian bread, *zar'tar* mixture, or fava beans. The Lebanese love coffee and consume lots of it; typically the stronger Turkish or Arabic coffee is served in a demitasse with sugar and no milk.

Even though the Lebanese have experienced war and economic hardship, especially during the civil war from 1975 to 1990, they have a nice rhythm of life, tend to be friendly, and have *joie de vivre*. Walk down any city street and you will see men playing *tawlie* (backgammon), and people laughing and talking, sipping coffee, or smoking from their water pipes, unrushed and enjoying the moment.

and also poor people (as a special act of charity). Lamb dishes are common during this season for that reason (Culinary Kingdom, 2006).

Most Muslims observe the practice of consuming *halal* meat. *Halal* means permitted or lawful in Arabic. Observant Muslims cannot consume certain foods and ingredients (called *haram*, or "forbidden" in Arabic). These items include pork and pork products, animals that were dead prior to slaughter, anything with animal blood, alcohol, carnivorous animals, birds of prey, and land animals without external ears. Animal foods must come from animals that were slaughtered humanely. (When an animal is slaughtered, the jugular vein is cut and the blood is allowed to drain from the animal.)

Christian holidays are celebrated in Lebanon and during Easter (or Eid il-Fasih). Traditional foods include *tabouleh*, ham or lamb meat, and *malamoul* (walnut-stuffed pastries). *Ka'ak* (slightly sweetened small, round bread) is often included. Easter eggs are traditionally dyed using onion skins to produce a deep orange/red color.

Practicing Orthodox Christians may fast during Lent—the 40 days prior to Easter, excluding Sundays, from sunrise to sunset—and break the fast in the evening with a light meal. The meals tend to be simple and primarily vegetarian. Typical Lenten meals include rice, beans (such as fava beans, chickpeas, or lentils), vegetables, *laban*, salad, olives, and bread. Meat is not eaten on Fridays. Eid il-Milad (Christmas) means "Festival of Birth." Typically, baklava, a sweet pastry made with filo dough, nuts, spices, and honey, is served. Baklava is eaten at most holidays in the Middle East.

Other Foods for Special Occasions

Meghli is a special Lebanese dessert traditionally prepared when a baby is born. The dessert is a cinnamon and ground rice custard and is usually prepared in large quantities and offered at home; the rest is sent to relatives and friends so that they can join the celebration.

Umuh is a special snack prepared in observance of a death. Made from cooked wheat berries, raisins, and candy-coated almonds, it symbolizes rebirth. When the wheat berries fall to the earth, they grow again, which is why *umuh* is given this symbolic meaning. It is served following a funeral.

 HEALTH BELIEFS AND CONCERNS

Good nutrition is highly valued, and a variety of vegetables and grains are more predominant than meat. Emphasis is on fresh foods. Weight management is a high priority. The obesity rate in Lebanon is significantly lower than that in North America.

A typical Lebanese meal features vegetables and rice as the main dish, with small amounts of meat as the side dish. Lunch is often the main meal. It is customary for Lebanese people, if their work schedule permits, to take a nap after lunch and a walk after dinner.

Family time is a top priority. Dinnertime tends to be a time of leisure, and families often sit for several hours in the evening and talk at length about family matters, politics, and social issues. This type of interchange is usually a way to sort out personal issues that

North Americans might instead settle through psycho-therapy and counseling.

GENERAL HEALTH AND NUTRITIONAL INDICATORS SUMMARY

Low birth weight, defined as weighing less than 2500 g at birth, affects 6% of newborns in Lebanon (UNICEF, 2007). Twenty-seven percent of children are exclusively breastfed during the first 4 months of life. Thirty-five percent of infants 6–9 months are breastfed with complementary food and 11% remain breastfed at 20–23 months.

Four percent of children under 5 years suffer from being moderately to severely underweight (UNICEF, 2007). Moderate to severe wasting was found in 5% and stunting in 11% of this particular population. The great majority (92%) of households in Lebanon consume adequately iodized salt. One-hundred percent of the total population, in both urban and rural areas, uses improved drinking-water sources.

COMMUNICATION AND COUNSELING TIPS

In a professional nutritionist/client setting, communication and counseling is similar to the way it would be in North America, with a few exceptions. Lebanese people are typically friendly, generous, and hospitable. For them it is considered impolite to walk into a room without greeting the people around you. If you show any interest in their cuisine, it would not be unusual for them to offer to bring you a specially prepared dish. There is one gesture that may be confusing to North Americans: Lebanese people nod upwards (just once), look up, and click their tongue once to say "no," instead of nodding their heads from side to side.

PRIMARY LANGUAGE OF FOOD NAMES WITH ENGLISH AND PHONETIC TRANSLATION

The primary language of food names with English and phonetic translation is as follows:

English	Lebanese	Phonetic Translation
Allspice	b'har helo	b'hăr hē'lo
Anise (seeds and powder)	yansoon	yăn soón
Apple	tuffaha	tŭffă'hă
Baked fish with tahini	sa'mak bil-tahi'neh	să'măk bĭl tăhē'nēh
Baked kibbeh	kibbeh bil-sani'yeh	kĭb'bee bĭl sănee'yĕh
Baklava	bakla'wa	băk'lēă'wă
Black and white pepper	b'harr swad wa abyab	b'hăr a'swăd' wă ŭ'byăb
Bread	al khobz	ál-khŭbz'
Bread dough	ajeenet al khobz	ăjē'enĕt ăl-khu'bz
Broad beans with fresh coriander and garlic	fool a'khdar bil-ki'zbra'h	fool a'khdăr bĭl-kĭ'zbră'h
Bulgur	burghul	būr'ghūl
Buttermilk	aray	ăy'răn
Cheese	jibneh	ji'bnēh
Chicken wings marinated in garlic	jawaneh d'jej bil toom	jă'wă'nĕh d'jĕj' bĭl-tūm'
Chickpea dip	hommus	hō'mmŭs
Cinnamon	e'rfeh	ērfĕh
Cinnamon and ground rice custard	meghli	mĕghli

(continues)

English	Lebanese	Phonetic Translation
Clarified butter	*sa'mneh*	sămněh
Coffee	*qa'hwah*	a'hwēh
Crescent and triangle pastries	*aje'ent al-fata'yer wa al-sam boo sak*	aje'ent al' fata'yer wa' al' sam bōō
Dairy products	*alban*	a'lbăn
Dried broad beans and chickpea rissoles	*falafel*	fălăa'fěl
Dried figs	*teen na'shef*	teen nă'shěf
Eggplant puree	*baba ghanooge*	bă'bă ghăn nūje'
Eggplant with chickpeas in tomato sauce	*moossaka'a*	mūsă'kă
Eggs	*be'yd*	bī'yd
Fava beans cooked in olive oil and lemon	*fool m'dammas*	fūl m'dămmăs'
Fish	*See'yadeeyeh*	see'yădăayěh
Fried cauliflower	*ar'nabit mi'li*	ăr'năbĭt mĭ'lē
Fried eggplant	*batinje'n mi'li*	bătĭnjě'n mĭ'lee
Fried fish with rice and caramelized onions	*sa'yadiyeh*	să'yădĭ'yěh
Fruit	*fawa'kihah*	făwă'kĭhăh
Garlic	*toom*	toom
Green beans in tomato sauce	*loo'byeh bil-zeyt*	lū'bēă bĭl zěyt'
Grilled eggplant salad	*batinje'n m'tabbal*	băt-ĭn'jě'n m'tăb-băl'
Herbal tea	*shay al-a'shăb*	sha̅'y' ăl-a'shăb'
Hors d'oeuvres	*mezze*	mě'ză
Kafteh and kebabs	*ka'ftah wa la'hem me'shwi*	kŭ'ftăh wă lă'hěm mě'shwee
Kibbeh balls	*rass kibbeh*	ărr ăss' kĭb'bee
Lamb or beef, ground, mixed with cracked wheat	*kibbe*	kĭb'bee
Lemon and garlic dressing	*zeyt bil-toom*	zīyt' bĭl-toom'
Lentil and onion soup	*shour'bet a'dass*	shoor'bět ă'dăss
Lentil and Swiss chard soup with lemon juice	*adass bil-hamod*	ă'dăss bĭl-hă'mŏd
Lentil, chickpea, and bean soup	*shour'bet makh'loota*	shoor'bět măgh'lootă
Lentils and rice	*m'ja'ddarah*	ūm jă'dăddăh
Milk	*halli'b*	hăll-eeb'
Minced lamb with bulgur and chopped onion	*kibbeh*	kĭb'be
Mixed herb and toasted bread salad	*fatto'osh*	fŭtt oosh'
Okra in tomato sauce	*ba'mya bil-zeyt*	ba'mya bil-zeyt

(continues)

English	Lebanese	Phonetic Translation
Olives	*zeyto'on*	zī toon'
Olive oil	*zeyt zeytoon*	zīte zī toon'
Orange-blossom water	*ma't el-zahr*	ma't ĕl-zăhr'
Parsley, tomato, and bulgur salad	*tabboo'leh*	tăboo'lee
Pastries	*hal waya't*	hăl wăyă't
Pickles	*kabe'es*	kăbē'ēs
Pine nuts	*s'noobar*	snŭ'bŭd
Pomegranate syrup	*rebb el-rumman*	rĕbb' ĕl-rŭmmăn
Raw kibbeh	*kibbeh nayeh*	kĭb'be nă'yĕh
Rice pudding	*meghli*	mĕ'glee
Roasted green wheat	*fre'ekah*	frē'kăh
Rose water	*ma'el-ward*	mă'ĕl-wărd'
Sandwich, rolled (lamb, chicken, or beef)	*shawarma*	shwear' mă
Sausage	*maqaneq wa suju*	mă'kăn-ĕk' wă sū'jū
Semolina	*smeet*	smēēt
Sesame seeds	*se'msum*	sĕm' sūn
Spinach triangles	*fatayer bil-s'banegh*	fătă yĕr' bĭl-s'bă'nĕgh
Steak tartare, Lebanese	*habrah nayeh*	hă'brăh nă'yĕh
Sumac	*sumak*	sū'măk
Sweetened bread	*ka'ak*	gaak
Syrian (pita) bread	*khobz arabi*	khŭbz ă'răbi
Tahini (sesame seed paste)	*tahineh*	tahē'nee
Tahini sauce	*tarator*	tă'dă tood
Thyme bread	*manae'esh bil za'tar*	mă'nă ē'sh bĭl-ză'tăr
Thyme mixture	*za'tar*	ză'tăr
Turmeric	*kurkum*	kūr'kŭm
Turnip	*lefet*	lĕ'fĕt
Vegetable and lamb soup with rice	*shour'bet mowzat ma khodrah*	shoor'bĕt mŏw'zăt mă khŏd'răh
Very thin flat bread that gets rolled up	*marqooq*	mărkŭk
Wild endive in olive oil	*hindbeh bil-zeyt*	hĭnd'bĕh bĭl-zĕyt'
Yogurt	*laban*	lă'băn
Yogurt (strained)	*labneh*	lă'bnee
Yogurt and cucumber salad	*kh'yaar b'lubban*	kh'yăr b'lūb'băn

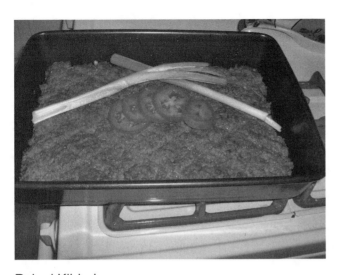

Baked Kibbeh
Courtesy of the author

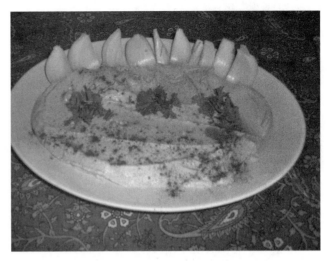

Hommus Bi Tahini
Courtesy of the author

FEATURED RECIPE

Hommus Bi Tahini

1 (16-oz.) can chickpeas

3 tbsp. tahini

1 clove fresh garlic, crushed

1 tsp. salt

Juice of 1 lemon

Paprika

3 sprigs parsley

1. Drain half of liquid from can of chickpeas.
2. Blend chickpeas and remainder of liquid in food processor or blender.
3. Add tahini, garlic, lemon juice, and salt.
4. Blend until smooth, pour into serving platter, and garnish with parsley and paprika.
5. Pour some olive oil on top (if desired). The mixture can be stored up to 1 week in a tightly covered container.

Yields 6–8 servings

More recipes are available at http://nutrition.jbpub.com/foodculture

REFERENCES

Central Intelligence Agency. (2008). *Lebanon*. Retrieved March 17, 2008, from http://www.cia.gov/library/publications/the-world-factbook/geos/le.html/

Culinary Kingdom. (2006). *Festival foods, religious influences, Middle East*. Retrieved March 30, 2008, from http://www.culinarykingdom.com/articles_festivalfoods_religious.htm/

Helou, A. (1994). *Lebanese cuisine: More than 250 authentic recipes from the most elegant Middle Eastern cuisine*. New York: St. Martin's Griffin.

Mackey, S. (2006). *Lebanon: A house divided*. New York: W.W. Norton.

Middle East Institute. (2005). *Lebanon*. Retrieved March 17, 2008, from http://www.mideasti.org/country/lebanon/

Salloum, H. (2000). *Classic vegetarian cooking from the Middle East and North Africa*. New York: Interlink Books.

UNICEF. (2007). *The state of the world's children 2007: Women and children, the double dividend of gender equality*. Retrieved April 14, 2009, from http://www.unicef.org/sowc07/statistics/tables.php

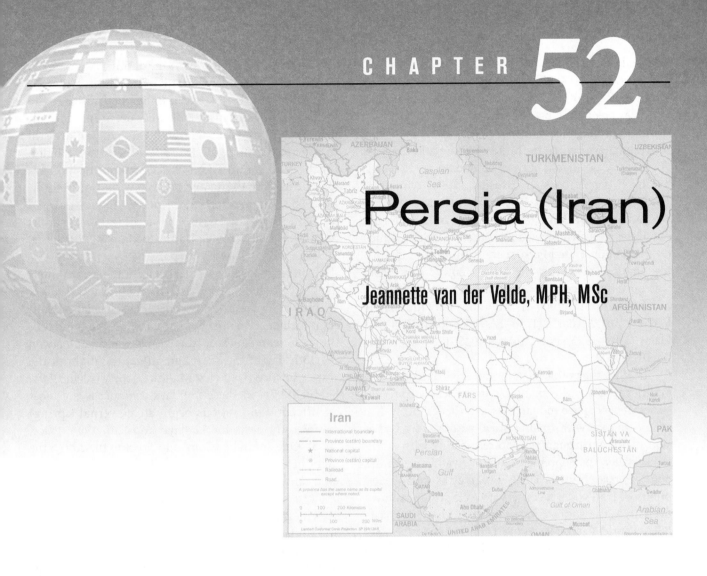

CHAPTER 52

Persia (Iran)

Jeannette van der Velde, MPH, MSc

CULTURE AND WORLD REGION

Iran, known as Persia until 1935, is situated in the Middle East and shares its borders with Afghanistan, Armenia, Azerbaijan, Iraq, Pakistan, Turkey, and Turkmenistan. Three bodies of water border Iran: the Gulf of Oman, the Persian Gulf to the south, and the Caspian Sea to the north (CIA World Factbook, 2008; Daniel & Mahdi, 2006; Price, 2005). Iran boasts a diverse geography from mountains, the Zagros and Alburz ranges, to desert and interior basins (Badripour, 2004). The Iranian plateau is a landlocked basin with a dry climate and a general lack of water, which greatly affects the area of cultivatable land (Badripour, 2004; Barthold, 1984; Daniel & Mahdi, 2006). In the mountainous regions, agriculture is dependent on irrigation, and most of the rivers (except the main rivers) have been diverted for that purpose (Barthold, 1984; Olmstead, 1948). A notable exception is the region nestled between the southern end of the Caspian Sea and the

Alburz mountain range, which is an area rich in agriculture attributable to the humid, tropical climate (Badripour, 2004; Daniel & Mahdi, 2006).

One of the longest-surviving cultures, the beginning of the Persian culture dates back to 550 BC, although archeological evidence indicates that nomadic tribes settled in the region as early as 3000 BC (Olmstead, 1948; Price, 2005). Cyrus the Great, the first king of the Achaemenids, is credited with founding the Persian Empire in 550 BC (Daniel & Mahdi, 2006; Olmstead, 1948). For the next 200 years, the Persians conquered regions stretching from Egypt to India and Greece, creating the first multiethnic and multireligious empire (Olmstead, 1948; Price, 2005). This laid the foundation for strong notions of monarchy, central governance, and religious and ethnic tolerance. According to Price (2005, p. 8), the "rulers called themselves the kings of 'many lands' or 'many peoples.'" Centuries of fighting with various empires (Greek, Roman, and Byzantine empires) left the Persian Empire weak, allowing for an Arab/Muslim invasion in 653 AD (Olmstead, 1948; Price, 2005).

The effects of the Arab invasion were long lasting, and Islam as a religion and way of life overshadowed Iranian culture (Shafii, 1997). After almost 200 years of Arab rule, a return to Iranian culture and dynastic governance occurred, only to be quelled in 1249 AD by the Mongol invasion (Moslehi, 1994; Olmstead, 1948; Price, 2005; Shafii, 1997). While the Mongols destroyed much of Persia, over time the conquerors adopted the Persian language and other traditions, which clearly demonstrated Persian constitution and character (Shafii, 1997). From the 16th to 20th century Iran was once again centrally governed by a succession of monarchs; in chronological order they were the Safavid (1502–1736), Afsharid (1736–1797), Zand (1750–1794), Qajar (1794–1925), and Pahlavi (1925–1979) dynasties (Shafii, 1997).

In 1979, the political landscape of Persia underwent another seismic shift, changing dramatically from centuries of successive monarchies to a theocratic system of governance with final political authority and decision making, through veto power, resting with a religious leader, the Supreme Leader or Ayatollah (Daniel, 2001). Persia (Iran) officially became the Islamic Republic of Iran when a conservative clerical movement overthrew the ruling monarchy, the Pahlavi Dynasty (CIA World Factbook, 2008; Daniel, 2001). Decades of progress and modernization, as well as ethnic and religious tolerance, abruptly halted and reversed, and large numbers of Iranians voluntarily and involuntarily emigrated to Europe and North America. Cleric conservatives quelled attempts at reform and retained power through the complex system of religious and democratic governance (CIA World Factbook, 2008). Although the Iranian populace elects a president, potential presidential candidates are vetted and screened by the Supreme Leader (Daniel, 2001). Additionally, the president remains a figurehead, with the ultimate power resting with the Guardian Council (CIA World Factbook, 2008).

The latest figures place Iran's population at more than 65 million people, with more than 75% of the population under 25 years of age (U.S. Census Bureau, n.d.). The demographic breakdown is as follows: 23.2% between 0 and 14 years, 71.4% between 15 and 64 years, and 5.4% over 65 years. For each age cohort the gender ratio is approximately equal; for the first two cohorts males slightly outnumber females; and in the over-65-years cohort females slightly outnumber males (U.S. Census Bureau, n.d.).

The oldest religion in Iran, dating back to 1200 BC, is Zoroastrianism (Daniel & Mahdi, 2006; Olmstead, 1948). While the number of Iranians who practice Zoroastrianism is steadily declining, the cultural traditions associated with this religion are still in practice (Daniel, 2001). Today, the major religion practiced in Iran is Islam (98%); 89% of Muslims follow the Shi'a tradition and 9% follow the Sunni tradition. The remaining 2% of the population are devoted to the Zoroastrian, Jewish, Christian, and Baha'i faiths (CIA World Book, 2008; Daniel & Mahdi, 2006; Price, 2005).

Although largely secularized, Iran's national holidays are rooted in Zoroastrian tradition (Daniel & Mahdi, 2006; Price, 2005). These four special celebrations include: *Chaharshanbesuri*, the last Wednesday of the solar year; *Nowruz*, New Year's Day; *Sizdah bedar*, the 13th day of the year; and *Yalda*, the night of the winter solstice (Daniel & Mahdi, 2006; Moslehi, 1994; Shafii, 1997). Of these holidays, *Nowruz* is the most significant. Celebrations begin at the vernal (spring) equinox and lasts for 12 days (Moslehi, 1994; Price, 2005). One special custom is to prepare the *sofreh* the night before the New Year, a table on which different foods and seven items (*haft sin*) starting with the Farsi letter "s" are placed (commonly used are apples, garlic, vinegar, sprouted seeds of grain, coins, hyacinth, and sumac) (Batmanglij, 2000; Moslehi, 1994). In addition, the *sofreh* includes a mirror, eggs, candles, a book of poems, rose water, goldfish, a bowl with an orange floating in water, and a variety of sweets (Batmanglij, 2000). All items on the *sofreh* are symbols that represent earth and its place in the universe, rebirth, and the good things one wishes for the coming year (Batmanglij, 2000; Daniel & Mahdi, 2006). According to Shafii (1997, p. 76) "growing greens is a symbol of the fertile season, when everything is revived and nature wakes up from the long winter sleep."

Family life is central to Iran's social fabric and family relationships take priority over any other social ties. Although the nuclear family is generally quite small, the extended family is intimate (Daniel, 2001). Mothers are highly regarded within the family structure and are extremely involved in their children's activities, especially education. Inquiries about wives and female relatives are considered inappropriate, and females are considered to need constant protection (Moslehi, 1988; Shafii, 1997). Generally, traditional gender roles are seen in the family structure, with responsibility for the home resting with the female (Moslehi, 1988).

LANGUAGE

Throughout its history and enjoying varying degrees of freedom, many distinct ethnic groups have called Iran home. Today, there are nine distinct ethnic groups, which consist of Persians 51%, Azeri Turks 24%, Gilakis and Mazandaranis 8%, Kurds 7%, Arabs 3%, Lurs 2%, Baluchis 2%, Turkmen 2%, and Bakhtiyaris 1% (CIA World Factbook, 2008; Price, 2005). The primary spoken and official language is Persian or Farsi, which comprises 58% of spoken language. Other languages, spoken by the ethnocultural minority groups, are 26% Turkic and Turkic dialects, 9% Kurdish, 2% Luri, and 1% each Baluchi, Arabic, and Turkish (CIA World Factbook, 2008; Price, 2005).

FOOD HISTORY WITHIN THE CULTURE

Admiration and appreciation for fine food and wine has been extensively chronicled in centuries of Persian art, prose, and poetry. The most famous compilation was written by Ferdowsi, entitled *Shahnameh* (The Book of Kings), an epic poem that traces the history of Iran from creation to the first Arab invasion in 653 AD.

Historically, the national diet was divided regionally: people who grew rice consumed rice almost exclusively and those who produced wheat consumed wheat almost exclusively. Today, every Iranian consumes both rice and wheat equally (Daniel & Mahdi, 2006). Traditionally, and even today in some rural areas, it is customary to eat sitting on the floor. A large cloth is spread on the floor on which platters and bowls of food are placed. The types of bread baked in Iran are a remnant of traditional eating habits: flat bread was used as a plate to hold food and as a utensil to ladle food (Daniel & Mahdi, 2006). Utensils are used today, with most meals being eaten using a spoon and fork. (Food is prepared in such a way that a knife is rarely needed.)

As with other cultures, food patterns and dietary habits change after exposure to different customs (e.g., use of nonnative ingredients, eating habits, fast-food restaurants) and as a result of modernity (i.e., more women working, less time to prepare foods, travel, changing gender roles, moving away from extended families). Western ingredients that were incorporated into Persian cuisine include most notably tomatoes and potatoes (Daniel & Mahdi, 2006). Recently, another change in eating patterns is occurring: a move away from high-protein diets and a rekindled interest in traditional basic foods (vegetable-based stews and breads). According to Shakoori (2001, p. 122), this shift is the result of political policy: "The scarcity of most food products at affordable prices and the heavy subsidization of wheat simultaneously caused a reduction in per capita consumption of protein products . . . and an increase in that of wheat and potatoes." Wheat and rice are consistently within the top five imports for Iran (Food and Agriculture Organization [FAO], 2008). Due to Iran's current political situation, its limited trading partners include the European Union, Japan, China, and South Africa (European Commission External Trade, 2008).

MAJOR FOODS

As with every country there are regional variations and differing dietary habits/customs between rural versus urban and rich versus poor populations. Iran is not an exception. Persian food is diverse and each region has unique methods of preparation. This chapter limits its discussion on the mainstream culinary tradition associated with the urban population.

Protein Sources

Sheep and goat are the preferred meat sources, although some beef is also consumed. In 2004, Iran's livestock numbers included "cattle 8,800,000; goats 26,500,000; and sheep 54,000,000" (Badripour, 2004). In 1952, Iran's poultry industry began through a mandate by the late Mohammad Reza Shah (Pahlavi Dynasty) to diversify the economy and increase jobs (Aresvik, 1976). Since then, consumption of poultry has grown exponentially to the point that Iran is now the number one exporter of poultry in the Middle East (Mirzaei, Yazdani, & Mostafavi, 2006). For Iranians living along the coastlines, fish is their main protein source; however, for the general population living inland, fish consumption is low, on average 6 kg per capita per year (FAO, 2008). Iran is a Muslim country, and according to Islamic precepts, seafood (e.g., shellfish, mollusks, lobster) and pork are considered unclean; thus, consumption of these foods is strictly forbidden. Even though they are illegal, these meats are available on the black market.

An important source of vegetable protein comes from beans (fava, broad, white, and red varieties), chickpeas, and lentils. These beans are consumed on

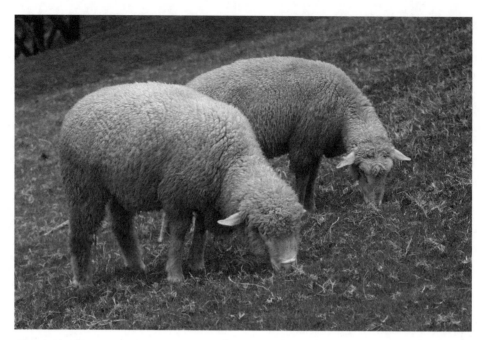

Sheep and goat are the preferred meat sources, although some beef is also consumed.

an almost daily basis as additions to stews, mixed with rice, and/or toasted and salted for snacks (Aresvik, 1976; Batmanglij, 2000). Nuts provide another source of protein; the most commonly consumed include pistachios, almonds, walnuts, and filberts (Aresvik, 1976; FAO, 2008). Iran is the world's leading exporter of pistachio nuts and exported nearly 140,000 metric tons in 2004 (FAO, 2008).

Starch Sources

Wheat, barley, rice, maize, and millet are the main sources of starch for Iranians (FAO, 2008; Shakoori, 2001). The latest data available indicate that Iran produced over 11 million metric tons of cereals (wheat, rice, and barley) in 2000, down from 13.5 million metric tons in 1990. Rice and wheat production cannot keep up with demand; Iran's population has increased significantly during the past two decades and the agricultural improvements have not substantially increased yield (FAO, 2008). For example, in 1999 over 8 million metric tons of cereal were imported (mostly rice) and only 4000 tons were exported (FAO, 2008).

Although Iran is an arid country, receiving on average 10 cm of rain annually, wheat and rice are grown in nearly all regions. Rice forms the staple of most meals and is usually prepared as *chelow* or *pollo* (Daniel & Mahdi, 2006; Shakoori, 2001). *Chelow* is rice that has

been soaked and parboiled (where water is drained and rice is steamed), producing nonsticky rice (Batmanglij, 2000). More significantly, this method leaves a golden crust on the bottom of the pan, called *tah-deeg*. Children and adults alike fight over this crust! *Pollo* is similar to *chelow* except that after draining the rice, other ingredients (frequently herbs such as parsley, dill, etc.) are added in layers and then steamed together (Batmanglij, 2000). Bread is another staple in the Iranian diet (Shakoori, 2001). There are over 40 different kinds of bread and it is present at every meal. The sweeter variations of breads, where the bread is made with milk instead of water, are usually served at breakfast or with tea (Batmanglij, 2000).

Prominent Vegetables

Vegetable consumption depends largely on the climate and what is produced locally, and varies from region to region. Iran boasts a climate ranging from subtropical to temperate that is conducive to growing a large diversity of vegetables year round (Aresvik, 1976; Benedictos, 1990). Iran's vegetable production has more than doubled during the past decades, due in part to better agricultural techniques. The most significant vegetable crops grown include potatoes, onions, tomatoes, cucumbers/gherkins, squash, eggplant, and some leafy vegetables (Benedictos, 1990). The potato and tomato are not native Persian vegetables; they were brought to Persia as a result of conquests by the Ottoman and Byzantine empires. Potatoes are consumed more as a side dish than a staple, except in areas where potatoes are grown (Batmanglij, 2000). For example, sliced potatoes will be added to the bottom of the rice pan to create an even thicker *tah-deeg* or crust.

Vegetables are rarely served on their own; instead, they are mixed with rice, stews, and meat dishes, especially vegetables such as eggplant, pumpkin, spinach, green beans, broad beans (lima beans), zucchini, squash, and carrots (Batmanglij, 2000). Tomatoes, cucumbers, and spring onions are served raw as accompaniments to the lunch and dinner meals (in much the same way as a salad). A sweet variety of cucumber is often served as a fruit.

 ## Prominent Fruits

As with other produce, fruit production depends largely on geography and varies from region to region. Iran's climate is conducive to growing a large diversity of fruits (Aresvik, 1976). Although great care is taken in the arrangement and presentation of fruits, fruits are more than simply a display on Persian tables. Fruits are usually consumed fresh as dessert or as snacks throughout the day (Batmanglij, 2000). Iran is one of the leading producers of dates and figs. For centuries, Iranians have been eating various fruits and vegetables whose health benefits are only now being appreciated by other countries (pomegranates are a good example). Also, fruits are combined in unique ways with meats in stews and as accompaniments to the main dish (e.g., rice with dates and chicken, or lamb stew with pomegranates). The list of fruits includes citrus fruits, apricots, grapes, dates, sweet and sour cherries, peaches, apples, plums, pears, pomegranates, quinces, figs, persimmons, strawberries, and mulberries, as well as a wide variety of melons (Aresvik, 1976; FAO, 2008). When fresh fruits are not in season Iranians consume dried fruits, most notably dates, figs, apricots, raisins, and sweet and sour cherries (Aresvik, 1976).

 ## Spices and Seasonings

Regional diversity is evident in the use of seasonings. What is common throughout Iran and what is unique to Persian cuisine is the restrained use of delicate flavorings in all preparations from soups to desserts. Although onions and garlic are used in cooking, these are added in small amounts. The most distinguishing flavorings include cinnamon, cloves, cardamom, nut-

meg, turmeric, and saffron (Batmanglij, 2000). The unique tartness in many Persian dishes is due to the addition of dried lemons, vinegar, lemon or lime juice, dried citrus peel, sumac, or tamarind (Batmanglij, 2000). Herbs that are commonly used include mint, dill, parsley, fenugreek, basil, coriander, and cilantro (Batmanglij, 2000). Except for traditional dishes from southern Iran, Iranian dishes are rarely spicy.

 ## Beverages

Tea (*chai*) is the most common drink and is served on every occasion, from breakfast to late evening (Batmanglij, 2000). It is estimated that during the 1970s, 1 kg of tea was consumed per person annually, and in 2003, 1.2 kg of tea was consumed per person per year (Aresvik, 1976; FAO, 2005b). Tea is usually sweetened with lumps of sugar. Most Iranians sip their tea through these lumps of sugar by placing the lump inside their cheek. A traditional drink that accompanies certain Iranian dishes is called *doogh*, which is a combination of yogurt, water, and dried mint (Batmanglij, 2000). *Doogh* is an excellent digestive aid and therefore is frequently served with heavier meals (e.g., kebabs). Many fruits are made into juice, specifically cantaloupes, watermelons, and pomegranates. During the summer, these juices are readily available at street kiosks. Some special-occasion drinks include *aab-e havij*, a carrot juice made into a sherbet garnished with cinnamon and nutmeg. Today, soda drinks are also readily available and consumed.

Since the time of Ferdowsi, Rumi, and other poets, wine has been a part of Persian culture. Prior to 1979, the major wine-producing regions in Iran included Qazvin, Orumiyeh, Shiraz, and Isfahan (Batmanglij, 2000). Since the Islamic Revolution of 1979, alcoholic beverages have been strictly banned (Daniel & Mahdi, 2006). Over the years, one exception to the strict governmental regulations is that non-Muslim minority groups (e.g., Zoroastrians and Christians) are entitled to produce wine for their own consumption. It remains illegal for them to sell to other Iranians or foreigners.

 ## Desserts

As mentioned previously, fresh fruits are often served as dessert; however, sweeter confections are also enjoyed and range from cakes and pastries to ice creams and sherbets. The sweets can be divided into moist and dry sweets (*shirini tar* and *shirini khoshk*, respectively). The moist sweets are inspired by European pastries and filled with whipped creams and custards topped with glazed fruits. Adding saffron, pistachios, and walnuts make these desserts uniquely Persian (Shafii, 1997). *Shirini khoskh* are the traditional cookies and cakes made from rice and chickpea flour, some with a walnut or fig filling and others with the addition of raisins or saffron (Batmanglij, 2000). Orange-flower water and rose water add fragrance and subtle flavor to many of the sweets. Unique Persian sweets include ice cream flavored with saffron or rose water, and heavy cream chunks and sorbets made from starch noodles and rose water. Another classic Persian dessert is halva, a saffron-flavored brownie that is usually served after a death and on certain dates of mourning (Batmanglij, 2000).

 TYPICAL DAY'S MENU

A typical day starts off with a light breakfast of flat breads, butter, cheese, and a variety of fruit spreads, followed by tea. A more elaborate breakfast, called *haleem*, is made with wheat, meat, lentils, and spices. This dish requires 7–8 hours of simmering; thus, preparation begins the night before. *Haleem* is high in calories and is usually reserved for the holy month of Ramadan. In southern Iran *haleem* is served year round.

Lunch and dinner are similar meals that consist of rice, stews, and seasonal vegetables, flat bread, and cheese. Fresh fruits follow as dessert. Throughout Iran, certain side dishes are always on the lunch and dinner table; these include fresh herbs (typically a combination of basil, coriander, cilantro, fenugreek, tarragon, and/or watercress), flat breads, feta-like cheese, cucumbers, tomatoes, onions, yogurt, and lemon juice. Depending on the region, pickles and gherkins may also be present (Batmanglij, 2000).

Between meals, Iranians snack on toasted nuts (pistachios, almonds, walnuts) and seeds (pumpkin, sunflower, and melon), fresh fruits, and tea. One customary mixture of nuts and seeds is one that has been simmered in lime juice, salted, and toasted (Batmanglij, 2000).

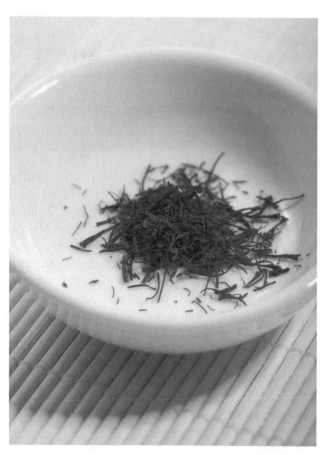

Shirini tar, moist desserts inspired by European pastries, are often topped with saffron (pictured).

 HOLIDAY MENUS

The *Nowruz* menu includes white fish served with green-herb rice (*sabzi pollo e mahi*), fresh-herb omelet (*koukou*), noodle soup made with green herbs (*ashe-resteh*), and sweets such as halva and baklava (Daniel & Mahdi, 2006; Moslehi, 1994; Shafii, 1997). The herbs used in all *Nowruz* dishes include parsley, coriander, chives, and fenugreek (Batmanglij, 2000; Daniel & Mahdi, 2006).

The traditional wedding menu may include sweet rice made with raisins, orange zest, and almonds (*shirin pollo*), stuffed whole lamb, pomegranate and fresh-herb stews, and potato omelet (Batmanglij, 2000).

 HEALTH BELIEFS AND CONCERNS

Many Iranians believe in "hot" and "cold" properties of food, and making a dish that combines foods with opposing properties is the cornerstone of a balanced diet (Batmanglij, 2000). "Hot" properties "thicken the blood and speeds the metabolism," whereas "cold" properties "dilutes the blood and slows the metabolism" (Batmanglij, 2000, p. 10). Similarly, disease is believed to be the result of an imbalance that can be treated by eating foods that contain the missing nutrient(s) (Fieldhouse, 2002). Many Iranians also believe that ill health can be the result of an "evil eye" or jealousy on the part of another person. Because many Iranians follow the Muslim faith, many have a strong belief in prayers, fasting, and charity as having healing qualities and contributing to general well-being (Khan, 2007). According to Fieldhouse (2002, p. 84), Iranian health beliefs are "a unique blend of Quranic and Hippocratic medical principles and practice emerged which later blended with modern scientific medicine to produce a spectrum of beliefs."

 ## GENERAL HEALTH AND NUTRITIONAL INDICATORS SUMMARY

Optimal health and well-being is influenced by nutrition, which can be monitored and evaluated through a variety of demographic and health indicators. The United Nations Development Programme (UNDP) established the human development index (HDI) to assist in evaluating where countries rank in terms of human progress and development. The HDI is a composite measure of three dimensions of human development: life expectancy, adult literacy, and standard of living in economic terms. The HDI for Iran is 0.777 (medium human development). Although the HDI does provide a general indication of the population's well-being, it is important to note that indicators for gender and income equality, human rights, and political freedoms are not included (UNDP, 2008).

Iranians live an average of 71 years. The country has a birth rate of 1348 per 1000 (UNICEF, 2007). The infant and under-5-years mortality rates are 31 and 36, per 1000 live births, respectively. The maternal mortality rate is 76 per 100,000 births (UNICEF, 2007). In Iran, 77% of adults are literate; however, a significant gender difference exists: 84% of men and 70% of women are literate (UNDP, 2008). Low-birth-weight babies (i.e., weighing less than 2500 g) have higher risk for serious health problems and lasting disabilities, in some cases even death. In Iran, 7% of children are born with low birth weight (UNICEF, 2007). Childhood nutritional indicators reveal that 15, 13, and 5% of children under 5 years are stunted (height for age), underweight (weight for age), and wasted (weight for height), respectively (UNICEF, 2007).

One consequence of inadequate nutrition, specifically iron deficiency, is anemia. Anemia occurs when there are insufficient red blood cells or when the red blood cells do not contain sufficient hemoglobin (World Health Organization [WHO], 2008). Although not the sole cause of anemia, iron deficiency is by far the most common. The prevalence of anemia in children under 5 years is 35% (nearly 2.2 million children). For nonpregnant women the prevalence is 30% (i.e., more than 6.2 million women with anemia). For expecting mothers, the prevalence of anemia increases to 40%, or over 500,000 women (WHO, 2008).

 ## COMMUNICATION AND COUNSELING TIPS

Iranians are extremely polite and well mannered. From a young age, children are taught to respect and go along with adults' opinions, even if the outcome may not be desirable (Moslehi, 1988). Iranians practice a form of civility that emphasizes humility; a host is obliged to offer a guest anything he or she may want, and a guest is equally obliged not to refuse it (Moslehi, 1988). Iranians show great respect for elders. This is supported by a study that examined the impact of nutritional education on the growth indices of Iranian children, and demonstrated that in order for these programs to be effective, it is imperative to approach influential individuals within the family and community first (Salehi, Kimiagar, Shahbazi, Mehrabi, & Kolahi, 2004). One gesture to caution against using is the "thumbs up" sign. The "thumbs up" sign means something completely different for Iranians; it is an obscene gesture. In Iran, the equivalent of the North American "thumbs up" is to hold up one hand and make a "V" sign with the fingers, similar to the North American "peace" sign (Persian Mirror, n.d.).

PRIMARY LANGUAGE OF FOOD NAMES WITH ENGLISH AND PHONETIC TRANSLATION

Table 52-1 gives the primary language of food names with English and phonetic translation.

TABLE 52-1 Primary Language of Food Names with English and Phonetic Translation

Persian	English	Phonetic Translation	Persian	English	Phonetic Translation
Talebi	Cantaloupe	TA-leh-bee	*Panir*	Cheese	Pan-ier
Hendevaneh	Watermelon	Hen-deh-voun-eh	*Shir*	Milk	Shier
Anaar	Pomegranate	An-ar	*Mast*	Yogurt	Mast
Sib	Apple	Sieb	*Bareh*	Lamb	BA-reh
Khorma	Date	Qor-ma	*Boz*	Goat	Boz
Anjir	Fig	An-ier	*Gooshte-gof*	Beef	Gousht-eh-gof
Beh	Quince	Beh	*Jujeh*	Chicken	Jou-jeh
Porteqal	Orange	Por-the-xal	*Nokodchi*	Chickpea	Nog-od-chi
Alu	Plum	Al-oo	*Adas*	Lentil	Adas
Albalu	Cherry	Al-BA-loo	*Khoresh*	Stew	Qor-esh
Angur	Grape	An-gour	*Aash*	Soup	A-sh
Gheisi	Apricot	Qei-shi	*Nan*	Bread	NAn
Tutfarangi	Strawberry	Tout-FAR-angi	*Chelow*	Rice (plain)	Chel-ow
Khiar	Cucumber	Qiar	*Pollo*	Rice (steamed with other ingredients)	Pol-low
Gojehfarangi	Tomato	Goj-eh-FAR-angi	*Pesteh*	Pistachios	Pesht-eh
Piaz	Onion	Pi-az	*Badam*	Almonds	BAD-am
Sir	Garlic	Sier	*Gerdu*	Walnuts	Ger-dou
Sib-samini	Potato	Sieb-SA-mini	*Cha'i*	Tea	CHAH-ie
Lubia	Bean	Loob-ia	*Doogh*	Yogurt drink	Doog
Esfenaj	Spinach	Es-fen-aji			
Havij	Carrot	HA-vij			

FEATURED RECIPE

Khoresht-Ghaimeh (Lentil Stew)

1 lb. lamb or beef, cubed

1 cup lentils, soaked in water overnight

2 medium-sized onions, thinly sliced

3 potatoes, peeled and cubed

3 tbsp. olive oil

2–3 tbsp. tomato paste

3–4 limes, crushed, dried (½ cup freshly squeezed lime juice can be used instead)

Salt and pepper to taste

1 tsp. turmeric

1 tsp. paprika

(continues)

**Khoresht-Ghaimeh
(Lentil Stew) (Continued)**

1. Fry onions in olive oil until golden brown.
2. Add meat and saute until browned.
3. Add 3 cups of water and bring to a boil.
4. Turn to simmer for 1–1½ hours until mostly cooked, adding more water if needed.
5. Add potatoes, lentils, salt, pepper, turmeric, paprika, and tomato paste. If using dried limes, add these as well. If using lime juice, add at end and cook for an additional 3–4 minutes.
6. Cook slowly until meat is very tender. (Add more water if needed.) Serve with plain rice.

More recipes are available at http://nutrition.jbpub.com/foodculture/

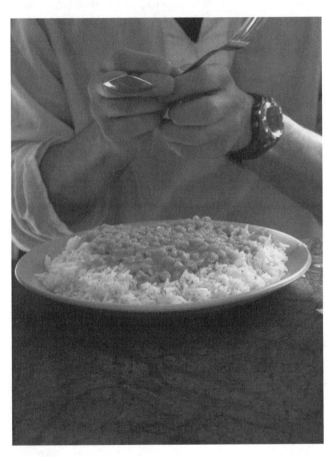

Lentil stew is a favorite Persian dish usually served with white rice.

REFERENCES

Aresvik, O. (1976). *The agricultural development of Iran.* New York: Praeger.

Badripour, H. (2004). *Country pasture/forage resource profile: Islamic Republic of Iran.* Retrieved March 4, 2008, from http://www.fao.org/ag/AGP/AGPC/doc/Counprof/Iran/Iran.htm/

Barthold, W. (1984). An historical geography of Iran. C.E. Bosworth (Ed.), and S. Soucek (Trans.). Princeton, NJ: Princeton University Press.

Batmanglij, N.K. (2000). *New food of life: Ancient Persian and modern Iranian cooking and ceremonies.* Washington, DC: Mage Publishers.

Benedictos, P. (1990). Agroclimatic conditions in relation to the timing of vegetable field production in Iran. *Acta Horticulture, 267,* 253–260.

CIA World Factbook. (2008). *Iran.* Retrieved February 29, 2008, from http://www.cia.gov/library/publications/the-world-factbook/geos/ir.html/

Daniel, E.L. (2001). *The history of Iran.* Westport, CT: Greenwood Press.

Daniel, E.L., & Mahdi, A.A. (2006). *Culture and customs of Iran.* Westport, CT: Greenwood Press.

European Commission External Trade. (2008). *Iran.* Retrieved March 5, 2008, from http://ec.europa.eu/trade/issues/bilateral/countries/iran/index_en.htm/

Fieldhouse, P. (2002). Food and health in the Baha'i faith. *Journal for the Study of Food and Society, 6*(1), 82–87.

Food and Agriculture Organization (FAO). (2005a). *Fishery country profile: Islamic Republic of Iran.* Retrieved March 4, 2008, from http://www.fao.org/fi/fcp/en/IRN/profile.htm/

Food and Agriculture Organization (FAO). (2005b). *Tea market studies: Egypt, Islamic Republic of Iran, Pakistan and Turkey. Intergovernmental Group on Tea.* Retrieved March 4, 2008, from http://www.fao.org/docrep/meeting/009/j5278e.htm/

Food and Agriculture Organization (FAO). (2008). *Asia Pacific food situation update.* Retrieved March 4, 2008, from http://www.fao.org/world/regional/rap/update_may_2008.pdf

Harbottle, L. (2000). *Food for health, food for wealth: The performance of ethnic and gender identities by Iranian settlers in Britain.* New York: Berghahn Books.

Khan, L. (2007). *Health beliefs of Muslim women living in the United States and implications for cultural competency in physical therapy evaluation and treatment*. Retrieved March 6, 2008, from http://papers.ssrn.com/sol3/papers.cfm?abstract_id=1005283/

Mirzaei, F., Yazdani, S., & Mostafavi, S.M. (2006). The dynamics of Iran's chicken meat export patterns in the Middle East region. *International Journal of Poultry Science, 5*(1), 93–95.

Moshki, M., Ghofranipour, F., Hajizadeh, E., & Azadfallah, P. (2007). *Validity and reliability of the multidimensional health locus of control scale for college students*. Retrieved March 4, 2008, from http://www.biomedcentral.com/1471-2458/7/295/

Moslehi, S. (1988). *Ask me, about me: A guide to understanding the Iranian culture*. Palo Alto, CA: Peninsula Printing.

Moslehi, S. (1994). *An introduction to Iranian culture*. Canoga Park, CA: Eqbal Printing and Publishing.

Olmstead, A.T. (1948). *History of the Persian Empire*. London: Universiy of Chicago Press.

Persian Mirror. (n.d.). *Persian culture*. Retrieved March 20, 2008, from http://www.persianmirror.com/culture/distinct/distinct.cfm#art/

Price, M. (2005). *Iran's diverse peoples: A reference sourcebook*. Santa Barbara, CA: ABC-CLIO.

Salehi, M., Kimiagar, S.M., Shahbazi, M., Mehrabi, Y., & Kolahi, A.A. (2004). Assessing the impact of nutrition education on growth indices of Iranian nomadic children: An application of modified beliefs, attitudes, subjective-norms and enabling-factors model. *British Journal of Nutrition, 91*, 779–787.

Shafii, R. (1997). *Scent of saffron: Three generations of an Iranian family*. London: Scarlet Press.

Shakoori, A. (2001). *The state and rural development in postrevolutionary Iran* (pp. 99–125). New York: Palgrave.

UNICEF. (2007). *The state of the world's children 2007: Women and children, the double dividend of gender equality*. Retrieved April 14, 2009, from http://www.unicef.org/sowc07/statistics/tables.php

United Nations Development Programme (UNDP). (2008). *Fighting climate change: Human solidarity in a divided world. Human Development Report 2007–2008*. Retrieved April 14, 2009, from http://hdr.undp.org/en/

United States Census Bureau. (n.d). *Country summary: Islamic Republic of Iran*. Retrieved March 10, 2008, from http://www.census.gov/ipc/www/idb/

World Health Organization (WHO). (2008). *Worldwide prevalence of anemia 1993–2005: WHO global database on anemia*. Retrieved April 14, 2009, from http://whqlibdoc.who.int/publications/2008/9789241596657_eng.pdf/

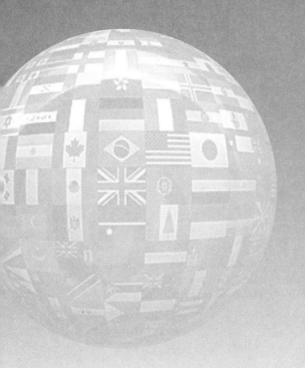

Index

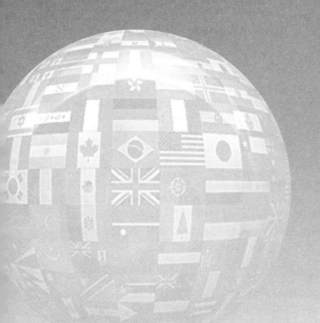

Photo Credits

globe with flags image © Kts/Dreamstime.com; **globe icon** © Bet Noire/ShutterStock, Inc.; **talk bubble icon** © Michael D. Brown/ShutterStock, Inc.; **scroll icon** © mart/ShutterStock, Inc.; **cauldron icon** © Sergey Yakovlev/Dreamstime.com; **cart icon** © N-a-s-h/ShutterStock, Inc.; **fish icon** © Hobart Design Group, LLC/ShutterStock, Inc.; **bread icon** © Miguel Angel Salinas Salinas/ShutterStock, Inc.; **carrot icon** © MisterElements/ShutterStock, Inc.; **apple icon** © twentyfourworks/ShutterStock, Inc.; **teacup icon** © losw/ShutterStock, Inc.; **pie icon** © marie kelley/ShutterStock, Inc.; **butter icon** © Miguel Angel Salinas Salinas/ShutterStock, Inc.; **salt shaker icon** © Miguel Angel Salinas Salinas/ShutterStock, Inc.; **place setting icon** © Ellen Beijers/ShutterStock, Inc.; **menu icon** © Vallentin Vassileff/Dreamstime.com; **bow icon** © U.P.images_vector/ShutterStock, Inc.; **pyramid icon** © OneO2/ShutterStock, Inc.; **caduceus icon** © James Steidl/ShutterStock, Inc.; **people icon** © Slobodan Djajic/ShutterStock, Inc.

Chapter 1

Opener © Monkey Business Images/ShutterStock, Inc.; **page 4** © Monkey Business Images/ShutterStock, Inc.; **page 5** © Bochkarev Photography/ShutterStock, Inc.; **page 6** © Steve Woods/Dreamstime.com

Chapter 2

Opener © Distinctive Images/Dreamstime.com; **page 8** © Distinctive Images/Dreamstime.com; **page 9** © Studiotouch/ShutterStock, Inc.; **page 10** © Elena Elisseeva/ShutterStock, Inc.; **page 11** © Lorraine Kourafas/ShutterStock, Inc.

Chapter 3

Opener © Etzbieta Sekowska/ShutterStock, Inc.; **page 26** © 5824998161/ShutterStock, Inc.; **page 27** © Harris Shiffman/ShutterStock, Inc.; **page 34** © Etzbieta Sekowska/ShutterStock, Inc.

Chapter 4

Opener © Elena Elisseeva/Dreamstime.com; **page 38** © Elena Elisseeva/Dreamstime.com; **page 40** © Riley MacLean/ShutterStock, Inc.; **page 42** © Andrea Skjold/ShutterStock, Inc.; **page 43** © Elena Elisseeva/ShutterStock, Inc.

Chapter 5

Opener Courtesy of the U.S. Central Intelligence Agency/University of Texas Libraries; **page 49** © Sunflowerhike/Dreamstime.com; **page 50** © Alexander Mychko/

ShutterStock, Inc.; **page 488** Courtesy of the International Potato Center

Chapter 44

Opener Courtesy of the U.S. Central Intelligence Agency/University of Texas Libraries; **page 497** © Alex Kuzovlev/ShutterStock, Inc.; **page 498** © Neale Cousland/ShutterStock, Inc.; **page 499** © Douglas Freer/ShutterStock, Inc.

Chapter 44

Opener Courtesy of the U.S. Central Intelligence Agency/University of Texas Libraries; **page 504** © Lana Langlois/Dreamstime.com; **page 505** © Jakub Pavlinec/Dreamstime.com

Chapter 45

Opener Courtesy of the U.S. Central Intelligence Agency/University of Texas Libraries

Chapter 46

Opener Courtesy of the U.S. Central Intelligence Agency/University of Texas Libraries; **page 515** © Dusan Zidar/ShutterStock, Inc.; **page 517** © Eduardo Wee/Dreamstime.com; **page 518** © Ken Brown/ShutterStock, Inc.

Chapter 47

Opener Courtesy of the U.S. Central Intelligence Agency/University of Texas Libraries; **page 528** © Paul Cowan/ShutterStock, Inc.; **page 530** © luchschen/ShutterStock, Inc.; **page 532** © f/stop/ShutterStock, Inc.

Chapter 48

Opener Courtesy of the U.S. Central Intelligence Agency/University of Texas Libraries

Chapter 49

Opener Courtesy of the U.S. Central Intelligence Agency/University of Texas Libraries; **page 563** © Kasiden/Dreamstime.com; **page 564** © Ewa Rejmer/Dreamstime.com; **page 565** © Friedel Grant/Dreamstime.com

Chapter 50

Opener Courtesy of the U.S. Central Intelligence Agency/University of Texas Libraries

Chapter 51

Opener Courtesy of the U.S. Central Intelligence Agency/University of Texas Libraries

Chapter 52

Opener Courtesy of the U.S. Central Intelligence Agency/University of Texas Libraries; **page 594** © Rickshu/ShutterStock, Inc.; **page 596** © Oliver Hoffmann/ShutterStock, Inc.; **page 599** © Marlies Plank/Dreamstime.com

Unless otherwise indicated, all photographs and illustrations are under copyright of Jones and Bartlett Publishers, LLC, or have been provided by the authors.